The Complete Guide to Aromatherapy

Second Edition

The Complete Guide to Aromatherapy

Salvatore Battaglia

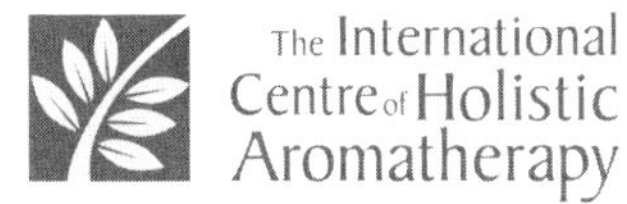

First published in 1995 by
Perfect Potion
90 Northlink Place
Virginia QLD 4014
Australia

ISBN 0 646 20670 2

Reprinted 1997, 1998, 1999, 2000, 2001, 2002

Second edition published in 2003 by
The International Centre of Holistic Aromatherapy
PO Box, 653, Albert Street,
Brisbane QLD 4002
Australia
www.icha.edu.au

Reprinted 2003, 2004, 2005, 2007, 2008, 2009

Note
Medical knowledge is constantly changing. As new information becomes available, changes in treatment, procedures, equipment and the use of drugs become necessary. The author and the publishers have, as far as it is possible, taken care to ensure that the information given in this text is accurate and up to date. However, readers are strongly advised to confirm that the information complies with the latest legislation and standards of practice.

National Library of Australia Cataloguing-in-Publication data:
Battaglia, Salvatore.
The complete guide to aromatherapy.

Bibliography.
Includes index.
ISBN 0 646 42896 9.

1. Aromatherapy. 2. Essences and essential oils --
Therapeutic use. 3. Oils, Volatile -- Therapeutic use.
4. Alternative medicine. I. International Centrel of
Holistic Aromatherapy. II. Title.

668.542

Cover design by Mandii Benson of Corporate Creations
Text design by Andrea Rinarelli of Australian Academic Press, Brisbane.

Typeset in Times by Australian Academic Press, Brisbane.
Printed in Australia by Watson Ferguson and Company, Salisbury QLD 4107

Contents in Brief

Contents in Detail

Acknowledgements

This book provides a complete aromatherapy training manual for people wishing to have a thorough understanding of aromatherapy. I am grateful for all the sources of information referenced throughout the book. The sources of information for this book include:

- text books which have outlined the principles of anatomy and physiology, aromatherapy, chemistry, pathophysiology, naturopathy, nutrition and other health related issues
- technical books and journals on aromatherapy, essential oils, holistic health and medicine
- personal accounts of others, and,
- my own experiences.

I am also indebted to the following people:

I gratefully acknowledge the professional associations who have endorsed *The Complete Guide to Aromatherapy* as a text book. I acknowledge the contributions that many of my colleagues, educators, researchers, therapists and clinicians have made to aromatherapy, to ensure its success.

All my teachers and people who have inspired me to pursue my career in natural therapies and aromatherapy. I am grateful to have had the opportunity to train with Madame Micheline Arcier, a person whose dedication and commitment to aromatherapy has taught me humility and respect. She has always been a major source of my inspiration.

All my past present and future students who are responsible for creating the inspiration I required to write this book.

John Kerr, a friend, colleague and the editor of *Aromatherapy Today*, who has always supported and promoted my book. John has played a very important role in the international success of the book.

Bob and Rhiannon Harris, from Essential Oil Resource Consultants for their technical expertise and advice on certain sections of the book.

In terms of the presentation of this book, Stephen May and the team at Australian Academic Press have done an outstanding job with the typesetting, design and layout of this book. I am indebted for the advice and professional support provided by Hilary Beaton from the Queensland Writers Centre and the fastidious John Sims of Sims Editing and Proofreading.

A very special thanks goes to the wonderful team at Perfect Potion and The International Centre of Holistic Aromatherapy, for ensuring the business ran smoothly while I was writing this book.

Simon Sparkes at Soyatech International for his expertise in the field of vegetable oils and for providing the typical fatty acid profiles of each of the cold pressed vegetable oils.

John Fergeus at Australian Botanical Products for providing the GC/MS traces of lavender and spike lavender on page 41.

Ruth Zorde, Melinda Smith and Shantal Walker for many of the illustrations.

The photograph on page 23 has been reproduced, with the kind permission of Inkata Press, the publisher of the book *Eucalyptus Leaf Oils: Use, Chemistry, Distillation and Marketing,* 1991, edited by D.J. Boland, J.J Brophy and A.P.N House, ACIAR/CSIRO, Canberra.

Last, but not least, I am indebted to my wife Carolyn Stubbin, for her constant support, patience and encouragement.

I almost forgot Chopper my pet beagle, who would patiently wait by my side for his daily walk, while I would say 'just a few more minutes, as soon as I finish this next sentence we will go for a walk.' A few minutes often became an hour later!

Salvatore Battaglia
2003

Preface to Second Edition

Eight years have passed since the publication of the first edition. During this period aromatherapy has blossomed into one of the most popular complementary health care modalities.

Through my own training, new research and feedback from other educators in aromatherapy, students, and aromatherapists, I have been able to expand on many of the existing chapters and add five new chapters.

The essential oil profiles have been extensively updated. I have included new categories on pharmacological and clinical studies, the energetics of the essential oils, the subtle effects of essential oils and the personality profile of essential oils.

There is now a considerable amount of research, which has scientifically validated much of what we know of the essential oils. For this, I am indebted to Bob Harris, who has provided us with the most comprehensive database on scientific research dedicated to aromatherapy.

I have included a section on the energetics of essential oils. As an acupuncturist, I have always utilised the essential oils using the principles of Traditional Chinese Medicine (TCM). I must acknowledge the work of Gabriel Mojay and Peter Holmes, who have made the principles of TCM accessible to aromatherapists.

I have included a category on the subtle effects of each essential oil — that is how the essential oils may influence our subtle bodies, chakras and spiritual wellbeing. For this, I am indebted to Patricia Davis and Valerie Ann Worwood, who have nurtured, promoted and created an awareness of this wonderful facet of aromatherapy.

In each essential oil monograph, I have included a section on method of administration. This provides the reader with clear advice on the most appropriate methods of use. In some cases, I have played the devil's advocate in suggesting internal ingestion. I do not teach internal ingestion, myself, and I certainly do not expect you to start recommending ingestion — especially without the appropriate medical and clinical training. I have cited *The German Commission E Monographs,* which recommends the ingestion of some essential oils. I believe that it is important for us to be aware that many phytotherapists have been successfully using essential oils by ingestion. This gives us an opportunity to broaden our knowledge and skill base. However, we should exercise some caution, and ensure that any move to promote ingestion of essential oils is backed up by comprehensive and authoritative training relevant to ingestion and that relevant government legislation regarding the prescribing of therapeutic substances is not breached.

While it is important to have excellent skills and knowledge to be a good aromatherapist, to be a successful aromatherapist it is also important to have sound business skills. I have therefore included information necessary to develop these business skills in the chapter, *Requirements for Professional Practice*.

The safe use of essential oils in aromatherapy has created some controversy in the last 5 years or so. While it is better to err on the safe side — especially when it comes to our client's safety, I believe that this has led to dogma within our industry. Therefore in some cases, I may sound ambiguous when I cite opposing views regarding safety and don't necessarily 'take sides'. This has been done intentionally — I hope that this encourages healthy debate and discussion, which will ultimately benefit aromatherapy.

I am also excited to have introduced five new exciting chapters. The main reason I became involved in complementary medicine in the first place was because of my fascination with the subtle anatomy — it is therefore with great pleasure that I have introduced a chapter on *Subtle Aromatherapy*. I can now confidently say that this book is 'complete'. While much research has been conducted into the chemistry and pharmacology of essential oils, I believe it is the subtle vibrational effects of essential oils that will make aromatherapy the holistic medicine of the 21st century.

Aromatherapy has become an integral part of mainstream health care in many hospitals and nursing homes. It is therefore appropriate that the important role that aromatherapy is now playing in mainstream health care be addressed in the chapter on *Aromatherapy for the Health Professional*.

A criticism of many books on aromatherapy has been the lack of information in developing skills to blend essential oils. This has been addressed in this edition with an entire chapter dedicated to blending of essential oils.

Many aromatherapists hunger for new and exciting essential oils to use in aromatherapy. I have introduced a new chapter on essential oils that may not necessarily be new or novel, but are not typically part of mainstream aromatherapy. Adventurous aromatherapists will find the chapter on *Exotic Essential Oils* very exciting.

The role of aromatherapy in skin care is as old as the origins of aromatherapy itself, however an exciting new phenomena in the last 8 years has been the rise of the day spa industry. Aromatherapy has played a critical role in the success of the spa industry. For individuals wishing to know more about the spa industry and how aromatherapy can complement it, the chapter on *Aromatherapy and Day Spas* is a must.

I hope that you find this new edition provides you with a very strong platform on which you can confidently practise aromatherapy.

Best Wishes,

Salvatore Battaglia
2003

Preface to First Edition

The booksellers' shelves are crammed with aromatherapy books. Much of the information is usually recycled from earlier English or French texts. While books such as *The Art of Aromatherapy* by Robert Tisserand and Tricia Davis's book *Aromatherapy: An A–Z* have become classics and are useful reference books, the majority of books on aromatherapy are not as useful as one would wish. They often provide an entertaining series of recipes an often misguided information, sometimes making unsubstantiated claims.

This makes it difficult for the modern holistic aromatherapist who needs to be a multidisciplined practitioner with training in remedial therapies, counselling, chemistry, botany, pharmacology, anatomy, physiology and pathophysiology.

The Complete Guide to Aromatherapy addresses all the topics listed above. This is the first time a book on aromatherapy has been aimed specifically at people with a serious interest in aromatherapy and the health professional working in the field of aromatherapy. While this book addresses in detail both the theoretical and practical aspects of aromatherapy, I have ensured that it remains true to the main principles of holistic healing which embraces three basic principles:

- a holistic approach to health which treat the patient as an individual
- the wisdom of the past and the validity of traditional empirical knowledge; and
- the analytical back-up provided by modern pharmacology and chemistry.

I believe that the future of aromatherapy as a powerful, safe and effective form of natural healing is embodied in the issues that I have raised in this book and I hope that this book contributes to the achievement of that future.

Salvatore Battaglia
1995

How to Use this Book

The Complete Guide to Aromatherapy is a comprehensive and practical guide to aromatherapy. It will provide all the information needed to develop your skills and knowledge as an aromatherapist. However, the book is not intended to replace formal aromatherapy training for those interested in pursing a career in aromatherapy. For information regarding aromatherapy training please refer to *Appendix 8*, which lists organisations that may advise you of the recommended teaching institutions.

The book is divided into six units:

Unit I: Background

Unit I provides you with the knowledge required to develop a holistic framework for the practice of aromatherapy. This is achieved by:

- examining the holistic role of aromatherapy in promoting health and wellbeing
- tracing the history of aromatherapy
- defining an essential oil and explaining the methods of essential oil extraction
- examining the need to ensure strict quality control and quality assurance.

Unit II: Essential Issues

Essential Issues provides you with the knowledge required to understand how aromatherapy works. This is achieved by:

- reviewing the latest research and clinical trials in aromatherapy
- outlining the pharmacokinetics of essential oils
- outlining the chemistry and pharmacology of essential oils
- reviewing the mechanisms of olfaction and the psychological influence of essential oils
- examining the subtle effects of essential oils
- discussing the guidelines for the safe use of essential oils.

Unit III: The Remedies

Unit III provides you with detailed monographs on an extensive array of essential oils and carrier oils. The essential oil monographs include information on the origins, traditional uses, chemical profile, pharmacological and clinical trials, indications, therapeutic uses, subtle effects, energetics, personality profile, methods of use and safety.

Unit IV: Practical Matters

Practical Matters provides you with the knowledge and skills required for the practice of aromatherapy. This is achieved by:

- outlining the requirements for setting up practice
- examining the procedure for conducting a consultation
- outlining a step by step description of the Micheline Arcier aromatherapy massage
- developing guidelines for developing a treatment strategy
- developing guidelines for blending essential oils
- examining the role of aromatherapy in hospitals and nursing homes.

Unit V: Clinical Index

Clinical Index provides you with a clear and detailed guide to the treatment of a wide range of conditions. Each condition is listed with a description of cause and symptoms and followed by the recommended treatment — the essential oils used, their application, as well as suggestions with regards to diet, herbs, acupressure and additional holistic therapies. The following body systems are reviewed:

- the cardiovascular system
- the respiratory system
- the musculoskeletal system
- the reproductive system
- the integumentary system
- the nervous system
- the lymphatic system
- the digestive system
- the immune system.

Unit VI: Aesthetic Aromatherapy

Aesthetic Aromatherapy provides you with the knowledge and skills required to use aromatherapy in skin care and a day spa.

Unit I

Background

Unit I provides you with the basic knowledge of aromatherapy. We will:

- Outline the history of aromatherapy.
- Identify the role of aromatherapy in healing.
- Investigate the biological role of essential oils in plants.
- Examine the methods by which essential oils are extracted.
- Identify the factors that determine the quality of essential oils.

Unit I includes the following chapters:

Developing a Holistic Framework for the Practice of Aromatherapy

Objectives

After careful study of this chapter, you should be able to:

- define aromatherapy
- outline the role of aromatherapy as a healing art
- explain the need to develop standards for the quality of essential oils
- explain the need to develop standards for the training of professional aromatherapists
- explain the need for research into aromatherapy.

Introduction

Aromatherapy has emerged as one of the most popular complementary therapies in the 21st century. Throughout the world, there has been a dramatic rise in aromatherapy's popularity. Many factors have contributed to aromatherapy's popularity:

- The ease in which essential oils can be incorporated into so many different products, whether they be products to scent the home, skin care products or bath products just to name a few.
- Essential oils are readily available to the general public.
- Aromatherapy is very much associated with a feel-good therapy.
- The aesthetic appeal of aromatherapy, which involves two senses that are often neglected in today's society — touch and smell.
- Essential oils have potent proven therapeutic properties.

However, it has been the failure to clearly define the term that has led to a misunderstanding and abuse of the term 'aromatherapy'. There is no doubt that the use of the term has given commercial advantage as the therapeutic implication of aromatherapy has been used to provide credibility for frivolous products.

We see, for example, skin and hair care products all promising to introduce the user to the benefits of aromatherapy. The fact that these products contain essential oils does not mean they will have the efficacy of essential oils used by a professional aromatherapist.

The plethora of self-help aromatherapy books available for the general public has also undermined the role of the professional aromatherapist. The ease with which aromatherapy can be administered makes it possible for the layperson to attempt self-therapy.

For aromatherapy to develop as a holistic health care modality, several issues need to be addressed:

- Clearly definine the term 'aromatherapy'.
- Understand the 'healing art' aspect of aromatherapy.
- Develop standards for the quality of essential oils.
- Develop education standards for the training of professional aromatherapists.
- Develop guidelines for research into aromatherapy.

Defining Aromatherapy

The English word 'aromatherapy' is derived from the French word 'aromatherapie', which was first coined by French chemist Gattefosse in the 1930s.

Gattefosse created a system of aromatherapy that was based on modern scientific thought and experimentation. He developed aromatherapy as a medically based therapy utilising essential oils. The properties of essential oils were proven and researched and could be seen as equal to conventional drugs of the time.

As Gattefosse understood, aromatherapy was a classic allopathic therapy within the framework of conventional medicine in which the essential oils are used to treat disease.

In 1977, the first aromatherapy book was published in the English language. This was *The Art of Aromatherapy,* written by Robert Tisserand. It combined medical applications with a holistic and esoteric view of essential oils. Many other interpretations of aromatherapy have since developed; some of these interpretations have been esoteric, while others began to focus on the fragrance aspect.[1]

Aromatherapy has diversified into four basic strands:

- medical aromatherapy
- popular and esoteric aromatherapy
- holistic aromatherapy and
- the scientific study of fragrance.[1]

Whatever our concept or method of practice is, we need to realise the complexity of aromatherapy. While we can remain true to our own concept of aromatherapy, we should also be exploring other aspects of aromatherapy and respect our colleagues who may have a different approach.

Medical Aromatherapy

While there is no approved definition for the term 'medical aromatherapy', for the purpose of this book I will refer to medical aromatherapy as the style of aromatherapy practised by doctors in France. French doctors have pioneered the clinical treatment of infectious diseases using essential oils.

Asked to comment on the internal use of essential oils, Dr Lapraz, a French doctor who uses essential oils and phytotherapy extensively in the treatment of cancer, says:

> *Our position with regards to the internal use of aromatherapy is very clear. As essential oils are extremely active agents having some demonstrable effects on the different organs of the body, they need to be administered under medical supervision.*[2]

Dr Pénoël, a prominent French medical practitioner who uses aromatherapy, suggests that in the case of serious infections, the only way that aromatherapy can help is an internal, massive and repetitive aromatic treatment involving strong antimicrobial essential oils taken by oral ingestion every 20 minutes! He suggests that within three days such an infection can be completely eliminated by such a treatment.[3]

However, as Pénoël points out, the French patient in a stressful situation cannot easily make an appointment to receive an aromatherapy treatment 'in the English way', which he claims to be a delightful and highly efficacious treatment. The French doctor trained in aromatherapy is also not likely to include lifestyle changes which are necessary as part of a holistic aromatherapy treatment.[3]

Holistic Aromatherapy

In orthodox medicine, the word 'body' indicates the physical aspect, whereas in a holistic approach the 'body' implies a complex of physical, emotional, mental and spiritual aspects. Aromatherapy works on a holistic level by addressing the:

- physical body
- mind
- soul.

A holistic aromatherapy treatment aims at treating the whole person. A holistic approach may include identification and treatment of the disease but it does not focus exclusively on symptoms. It focuses, instead, on the development of wellbeing and enjoyment of life in a system of self-responsibility.

Therefore, holistic aromatherapy utilises the pharmacological, psychotherapeutic and metaphysical properties of essential oils.

The real significance of aromatherapy is using these elements in a holistic manner. Often the main benefits of an aromatherapy treatment come from the pleasant smells of the essential oils, which have a predominantly psychological effect. The essential oils are usually administered by massage, in an oil vaporiser or added to baths. Used in these ways, essential oils add a sense of luxury to the treatment and often have a relaxing effect.

Many people view natural therapies such as aromatherapy as 'magic potions'. However, you cannot just 'zap' people with the essential oils and expect them to get better overnight. It's to do with somebody to talk to, someone who can listen and respond to you, it's about having a hands-on treatment. There is more to holistic aromatherapy than essential oils and massage — it is a healing process.

Aromatherapy as a Healing Art

One of the aspects that makes aromatherapy so intriguing is the range of principles involved. At one end of the spectrum the essential oils are used for their pharmacological action, similar to allopathic medicine, and at the other end is the psychotherapeutic use of the essential oils, where the scent of the essential oils is considered the most important agent to bring about healing.

The distinctive strength of holistic aromatherapy as a healing art is dependent upon:

- the pharmacology of essential oils
- incorporating holistic principles to the use of the essential oils
- the massage
- the therapist–client relationship
- the realisation of the complexity of the problem of illness and ill health
- the role of olfaction.

Pharmacology

Mills describes conventional pharmacology as being entirely pragmatic and an unprincipled science because it suppresses inflammation, kills pathogens, blocks pathological deteriorations and potentially damages physiological responses.[4]

In pharmacology, nature is effectively disintegrated so that the actions of isolated chemicals on isolated pieces or functions of the body can be observed as precisely as possible in a variable world. These observations are then stuck together to make a jigsaw picture of the effect of that substance on the body. On that basis drugs are given to real people.[4]

Most pharmacological research has focused on finding the 'active' principle or constituent. The trace constituents are often seen as a problem that has to be removed. This is the case with eucalyptus oil. Eucalyptus oil is commonly redistilled or rectified.

The 'active' principle in eucalyptus oil is 1,8-cineole. 1,8-cineole has excellent expectorant properties. However, Pénoël says that the residue removed in the redistillation of eucalyptus oil contains precious molecules such as the rare phenol, australol. Even though the amount of australol is low, it works in synergy with the main components and should not be removed if we wish to utilise the essential oil's full healing potential.[5]

My biggest concern is that if we focus exclusively on the pharmacology of essential oils, there will be a tendency for biochemical standardisation of essential oils. This would lead to a loss of the natural biodiversity that exists.

Therefore any pharmacology suited to aromatherapy must be different. At no time must the view of the whole be lost. Traditional pharmacology's role is to draw from human experience and the effects of the mind and body to enable the aromatherapist to better predict the action of each essential oil in the infinitely variable circumstances that will be encountered in practice.

Holmes is also wary of any attempt to validate aromatherapy in terms of chemistry or pharmacology. He says that aromatherapy is essentially an 'energy medicine'. Therefore we need a holistic model of pharmacology for understanding the essential oil functions.[6]

Holistic Principles

The main difference between orthodox medicine and systems based on traditional healing systems is a philosophical understanding of health, disease, the healing process and the interaction of these factors with the individual. However, it has been said that the philosophical basis of aromatherapy is lacking when compared to traditional systems such as traditional Chinese medicine (TCM) or Ayurveda.

Therefore, a holistic model for the practice of aromatherapy could draw on the:

- holistic principles of traditional systems such as TCM and Ayurveda
- empirical context which draws on centuries of traditional use
- analytical scientific research based on the chemistry of the essential oil
- 'signature' of the essential oils — the personality profile.

Massage

The effect of touch clearly has a profound psychological and physical impact. Massage is possibly the only situation in which we can be touched in a caring way by someone who is not close to us, and not feel uncomfortable.

> *Touch is a basic behavioural need, in much the same way as breathing is a basic physical need. When the need for touch remains unsatisfied abnormal behaviour will result.*[7]

Babies will distinguish by movements and feeding behaviour between a stranger and their mother. Premature babies held in a sling between the mother's breasts have improved growth compared with incubator-managed babies.

In animal experiments, deprivation of contact at this early stage is associated with failure to thrive, and slowing of development with neuroanatomical brain changes. It should be no surprise that early deprivation in humans leads to neuropsychological disturbances.

Dr James Prescot, an American neuropsychologist, states:

> *The absence or withdrawal of physical affection in early life, and even as an adult, may be responsible for many types of disturbed behaviour such as depression, violence, aggression and hyperactivity.*[8]

Hooper states:

> *In one hospital, disturbed teenagers go through an intensive course of physical treatment, learning to appreciate the significance of touching and being touched. Since this kind of therapy has been introduced violence at the hospital has noticeably abated.*[9]

The physical benefits of massage are also comprehensive. It stimulates the circulation of the blood and lymph, reduces high blood pressure, stimulates the immune system, reduces muscular tension and relieves pain in muscles and joints.

The healing process in massage has often been underrated. Massage is one of the truly preventative holistic therapies, as it is able to effectively induce a state of relaxation by easing muscular tension. Not only is muscular tension directly related to physical pain, but often relates to psychological tension and repressed emotions. The act of soothing the physical tension has a reflex effect on psychological tension.

Massage can alleviate stress and by doing so enables the patients to utilise their own healing energies. Massage has already been incorporated in some hospitals to relieve muscular tension, promote sleep, relieve pain, reduce high blood pressure, and for its comforting effect.

Field discusses the benefits of using massage to reduce anxiety in children and adolescent psychiatric patients:

> *Fifty two children and adolescents hospitalised for depression or adjustment disorder participated in the study, receiving a thirty minute back massage daily for five days. Self and staff reports of anxiety and depression, behavioural observations, saliva and urine samples, and time-lapse video of night sleep sessions were included in the assessment protocol.*
>
> *When compared to the control group who watched relaxing video tapes, the massage group were less depressed and anxious, and had lower salivary cortisol levels. Their night sleep improved and the staff reported them as being more cooperative and less anxious. Those subjects who were depressed also demonstrated a reduction in urinary cortisol and norepinephrine levels, indicating the longer term effects were more pronounced for depressed patients than the adjustment disorder patients.*[10]

Therapist–client Relationship

People are increasingly dissatisfied with having had their responsibility and involvement in their own treatment and healing taken away. Conventional medicine is often very prescriptive and excludes the patient from understanding their condition. This has led to a major gap between therapist and client, and has meant that people are looking to natural therapies, which consider physical, emotional and psychological aspects of wellbeing.

Bell says that a growing number of doctors are turning to alternative therapies because modern medicine is concerned only with getting rid of the disease and does not deal with wellbeing.[11]

The empathy of the therapist is an important ingredient in the success of a treatment. A trial with pain killers and dental pain showed that identical tablets had widely differing effects when one group was given the tablets impersonally, and the other had a smiling nurse who briefly touched each patient's shoulder and expressed care. If such brief interventions are of value, the influence of personality of the individual administering the treatment is enormous.

Sapira believes that confidence in the therapist is of utmost importance both for the wellbeing of the patient and for the therapist's success. Confidence is initially gained through the impression created by the therapist during the consultation.

> *A physician should appear to be pleased to see the patient; to think nothing but the complaint; to be sympathetic and understanding; to be confident of effecting a cure, and if not, to take a cheerful note and inspire hope; to feel privileged to treat the patient; to be courteous and considerate; and be glad to take the time to hear the patient's problems.*[12]

Many patients of aromatherapy may have experienced physical and verbal isolation and the contact with a caring practitioner will itself be therapeutic. A holistic approach acknowledges that the therapist and the client each play an essential part in the healing process.

Complexity of the 'Problem of Illness' and 'Ill Health'

There has been a growing realisation of the inherent complexity of the 'problem of illness and ill-health' — moving away from the orthodox approach of separating the ailments and symptoms towards an acknowledgment that these symptoms commonly result from inherent imbalances within the person as a whole.

The concept of health today has come to mean a lot more than just a lack of disease or infection at a purely physical level. Rather, it is based on the notion of physical, emotional and psychological wellbeing and an ability to cope positively with a variety of pressures and stresses placed on us by our modern lifestyle and expectations.

Husband says that there is now considerable anecdotal evidence that immunity and resistance to disease are linked to attitude and behaviour.[13]

Meares had for many years suggested that positive thinking and imagery are useful in the treatment of cancer.[14]

Olfaction and the Brain

Research into olfactory perception indicates that only a few molecules are needed to have a substantial effect, such as the recreation of memories and associations.

The effect of smell alone has a powerful influence on the central nervous system. Fragrance researchers are discovering that odours can and do influence mood, evoke emotions, counteract stress and reduce high blood pressure. To explain how essential oils can affect us in this way we must explore the connection between the sense of smell and the brain.

Smell is the only sense in which the receptor nerve endings are in direct contact with the outside world. It is also interesting to know that the olfactory nerve cells are the only type of nerve cell in the body that can repair themselves if damaged.

Essential oils may also have an influence on hormonal response due to the influence on the hypothalamus and they may also influence the cortical areas of the brain that are associated with memory and learning.

Developing Standards for the Quality of Essential Oils

Before developing guidelines for the quality of essential oils we need to define the user groups. It must be remembered that only 5% of all essential oils produced in the world are actually used for aromatherapy. The largest users of essential oils are the:

- food flavouring industry
- perfume industry
- pharmaceutical industry
- chemical manufacturing industry.

The problem that this creates is that the term 'quality of a pure essential oil' has a different interpretation for each of the above users. The food flavouring and perfume industry are only interested in consistency of odour, so are more inclined to prefer 'nature-identical' essential oils. *Nature-identical* essential oils are often reconstituted from other essential oil constituents to create an oil which is similar to that found in nature.

The pharmaceutical industry is only interested in the 'active constituent', so they prefer rectified essential oils.

If we follow the Therapeutic Goods Act of Australia, as a guide for the manufacture of therapeutic goods then essential oils should:

- be correctly identified
- be pure
- be safe for use
- have proven efficacy.

Any essential oil that does not have these fundamental qualities should be deemed to present a potential risk to the health and wellbeing of the end user and should not be used in aromatherapy.

Developing Education Standards for Aromatherapists

There is a need to set standards for training and identification of aromatherapists. Professional aromatherapists may come from different backgrounds, but all should have several qualities in common.

- They have a sound knowledge of the essential oils they use.
- They have a sound knowledge of botany, chemistry and pharmacology of essential oils.
- They have a sound theoretical and practical knowledge of the therapeutic application of essential oils.
- They have a solid grounding in anatomy and physiology, pathophysiology and differential diagnosis.
- They can maintain a sensible balance between the intellectual and intuitive approaches to their work.
- They are, above all else, concerned for the wellbeing of their clients.
- They should belong to a professional organization, representing aromatherapy.

Developing Guidelines for Research into Aromatherapy

While some research has confirmed the pharmacology of essentials oils, the demand for clinical research and validation of aromatherapy has never been greater.

The aromatherapy industry in Australia has eagerly adopted the Good Manufacturing Practices (GMP) as outlined by the Therapeutic Goods Act. However there is still concern over the level of pharmacological and clinical validation for herbal medicines in general. Currently, essential oil suppliers are able to make restrictive therapeutic claims only for the treatment of self-limiting disorders. However, if we wish to market an essential oil for what might be considered a moderate to severe ailment, then it would be subject to clinical evidence based on double-blind clinical trials and experiments on animals.

This is a concern, as there is now considerable doubt that conventional, technological and scientific analysis used in current medical research is suitable for aromatherapy as it fails to acknowledge the human element involved in aromatherapy.

Conclusion

A change is now occurring in health care worldwide and I am pleased to say that aromatherapy is playing a very important role in the shift towards complementary therapies.

However, let us never forget our grassroots origins — to treat the whole person with the focus on empathy, personal care, prevention, health and wellbeing.

References

1. Schnaubelt K. *Essential Oils — Viable wholistic pharmaceuticals for the future.* In Conference Proceedings of the 13th International Congress of Flavours, Fragrances and Essential Oils. 15–19 Oct 1995, Istanbul, 1995; (3): 269–281.
2. Lapraz J. *In profile.* International Journal of Aromatherapy, 1991; 3(4): 12–14.
3. Penoel D. *This is also aromatherapy.* The International Journal of Aromatherapy, 1991; 3(3): 14–16.
4. Mills S. *The essential book of herbal medicine.* Arkana Penguin Books, England, 1991.
5. Penoel D. *Winter shield.* The International Journal of Aromatherapy, 1992; 4(4): 10–12.
6. Holmes P. *Energy medicine.* The International Journal of Aromatherapy, 1998–1999; 9(2): 53–56.
7. Montague A. *Touching — The human significance of the skin.* Harper and Row, New York, 1986.
8. Prescot J. cited in Montague A. *Touching — The human significance of the skin.* Harper and Row, New York, 1986.
9. Hooper A. *Massage and loving.* Unwin Hyman Ltd, London, 1988.
10. Field T, et al. *Massage reduces anxiety in children and adolescent psychiatric patients.* International Journal Alternative and Complementary Medicine 1993; 11(7): 22–27.

11. Bell G. *The new healers*. The Independent, April 1994; 38–42.

12. Shapiro J. *The art and science of bedside diagnosis*. Williams & Wilkins, USA, 1990.

13. Husband A. *Stress, behaviour and the immune system.* Current Affairs Bulletin, Aug–Sept 1994; 25–31.

14. Meares A. *A way of doctoring*. Hill of Content Publishers, Australia, 1985.

History of Aromatherapy

Objectives

After careful study of this chapter, you should be able to:

- identify the role of aromatic materials in ancient civilisations
- trace the development of aromatherapy during the Middle Ages
- examine the origins of aromatherapy in the 20th century
- discuss the future of aromatherapy.

Introduction

When discussing the history of aromatherapy we need to remember that the term aromatherapy was coined only in the 1930s. However, the use of aromatics is as old as civilisation itself.

Even though herbalism involves the use of the entire plant we need to begin our study of the history of aromatherapy by tracing the use of aromatic plant extracts to the origins of herbalism.

Egypt

Egypt was the cradle of the sciences, including medicine, perfumery and cosmetology. Throughout the ancient world Egypt was famous for the use of aromatic substances. In their religious cults, the Egyptians consumed great quantities of *Boswellia papyrifera* (frankincense), and *Commiphora erythraea* (myrrh resin).

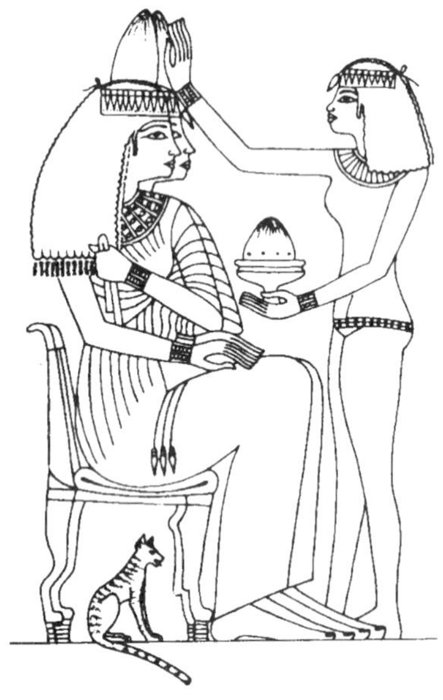

The maidservant adds a few dabs of essential oils to the perfumed cones of aristocratic Egyptian women. (Theban wall painting)

This was not the same frankincense and myrrh presented at the birth of Christ or burned in great abundance by the Romans. That was from another species, not yet known to the Egyptians, which was found in Arabia. The Egyptians sourced frankincense and myrrh from the land called Punt, which is believed to be in the region of Somalia.

Incense was always burned before the opening of a shrine, at the coronation of the pharaoh and for national celebrations. The souls of the dead were thought to ascend above as a cloud of smoke and incense was burned to avert baneful spirits from the bodies of the deceased.

The Egyptians believed in the transmigration of souls. They believed that the soul, after leaving the body, entered the body of some other animal and, having successively passed through all the creatures of the earth, water and air, it again assumed a human shape. The journey was to be accomplished in 3,000 years. This belief accounted for the great care they took in embalming the bodies of their dead, so that after the long journey, the souls might find their original body in a tolerable state of preservation.

The embalming process involved eviscerating the dead body, which was then washed with natron (sodium nitrate salts) from the Wadi el natrum, and stuffing the cavities with myrrh, pine resin and oakmoss.

As distillation had not yet been discovered the main method of extracting the essential oils was by enfleurage and maceration. This was done by steeping the resins, flowers or splinters of wood in oil. The materials were placed in a cloth which was wrung until every last drop of fragrance had been retrieved.

Alternatively, maceration involved boiling of the aromatic substances in the oil. The oils most commonly used were moringa, balanos, castor oil, linseed, sesame, safflower, olive and sweet almond.

The human body also became an object of esteem to be anointed with perfumed oils. Most cosmetics used included aromatic substance, such as frankincense, myrrh, lilies, pine, cedar of Lebanon, gum mastic, mints and other herbs.

One of the best-known perfumes was kyphi. Kyphi was burnt in the temples. A recipe for making kyphi was as follows:[1]

1. Take 270 gm each of: Acorus calamus, mastic, cassia, cinnamon. Grind and sieve. Only the powder is to be used.
2. Take 270 gm each of juniper berries; an unidentified plant; *Cyperus slongus*. Grind. Add to this 2,250 gm of wine. Leave until the next morning. Half the wine will be absorbed by the herbs. The rest will be discarded.
3. Take 1,800 gm raisins and 2,250 gm oasis wine. Grind together well. Remove the rind and pips of the raisins. Place the rest in a pot with the herbs. Leave for five days.
4. Mix 1,200 gm frankincense and 3,000 gm honey in a vessel. Boil gently until it thickens and reduce by 1/5. Mix the other ingredients and leave for five days.
5. Add to this 1,143 gm of finely ground myrrh and you have kyphi.

Classens cites Greek historian Plutarch, who says that kyphi had the ability to relieve anxiety, brighten dreams and heal the soul.[2]

One of the ingredients of kyphi was calamus, which Tisserand describes as having potent narcotic and sedative properties. Calamus contains up to 80% asorone, a toxic phenol, which is a precursor of TMA-2, a phenylethylamine capable of powerful narcotic effects.[3]

Greece and Rome

The ancient Greeks further advanced the use of aromatics. The first treatise on scent was the study *Concerning Odours*, by Theophrastus. Not only did he take an elaborate inventory of Greek and imported aromatics, but he discussed ways in which they could be used. Theophrastus commented on the therapeutic nature of perfumes, saying:

> *It is to be expected that perfumes should have medicinal properties in view of the virtues of their spices. The effect of plasters and of what some may call poultices prove these virtues, since they disperse tumours and abscesses and produce a distinct effect on the body and its interior parts.*[4]

Here he has observed one of the fundamentals of holistic aromatherapy, that essential oils applied externally affect the internal organs and tissues.

While Hippocrates is referred to as the father of modern medicine, it would be more fitting to dub him the father of holistic medicine. Tisserand cites Hippocrates who promoted the benefits of massage:

> *The physician must be experienced in many things, but assuredly in rubbing ... for rubbing can bind a joint that is too loose, and loosen a joint that is too rigid.*[5]

Greek medicine as developed by Hippocrates was based on the four elements — Air, Earth, Fire and Water, and the four humours corresponding to the chief fluids in the body — choleric (yellow bile), sanguine (blood), phlegmatic (phlegm) and melancholic (black bile). The properties of the herbs corresponded to one or more of the four elements — Air, Earth, Fire or Water. The cornerstone of Greek medicine was the concept of mental, emotional and physical balance. Disease was a disturbance of this balance, and it was the duty of the physician to restore and assist the patient's own natural healing powers. Hippocratic teaching emphasised that a healthy body was one in which the four 'humours' of blood, bile, phlegm and choler were equally balanced.[6]

Four centuries later, Galen adopted the Hippocratic teachings of the four humours and made it the cornerstone of an elaborate and rigid system of medicine which would remain unchallenged for the next 1,500 years.[6]

Galen believed that it was not the nose which perceived smell, but the brain. Proof of this, he held, lay in the way in which different odours were known to affect the brain.

According to Tisserand, Pedanius Dioscorides, of Anazarba in Asia Minor, wrote a magnificent treatise on herbal medicine during the 1st century AD. His book remained the medical reference work in Western medicine for over 1,000 years after his death, and much of our present knowledge of medicinal herbs originates from Dioscorides.[5]

His book contains five sections, one of which deals with aromatics. Many of the remedies he discusses are still used today in aromatherapy:[5]

- *Myrrh* — strengthens the teeth and gums and is soporiferous.
- *Juniper* — is described as a diuretic.
- *Marjoram* — is described as soporific.
- *Cypress* — the lux of the belly (diarrhoea). It doth also stanch the blood.
- *Costus* — provokes venerie.

Aromatherapists are aware of the sedative properties of marjoram, that juniper is a diuretic, and that the astringent properties of cypress are beneficial in cases of diarrhoea. Costus, traditionally used as an aphrodisiac, is now wisely avoided, since it can cause allergic reactions.[5]

Some 300 years after Hippocrates, Asclepiades, a Greek physician who was perhaps closer to our concept of an aromatherapist than Hippocrates or Dioscorides, was a great believer in massage. He practised in Greece and Rome, believed in curing his patients with as little discomfort as possible for them, and was against the excessive use of purgatives and emetics, which were then so much an integral part of medicine. Instead, he advocated the use of massage, music and perfume as soothing and healing agents.[5]

The Roman armies helped spread the knowledge of Mediterranean healing plants around Europe. The Romans took good care of their armies, especially when they were posted in distant countries. The legions travelled with their own doctors and surgeons, and when good local doctors could be found, they too were consulted and often enlisted.[6]

In the case of wounds, a lotion of wine and myrrh was prescribed for burns and for relieving inflammations. Roman physician Pliny suggested rue infused in vinegar for comatosed patients to be used as a kind of smelling salts, while the scent of pennyroyal was used to protect from cold or heat and to lessen thirst.[2]

Rome had an insatiable appetite for incense. According to Classen, Nero is said to have burnt more incense than Arabia could produce in a year at his wife Poppeae's funeral.[2] Of all the aromatic substances, Romans loved rose the most. They adorned themselves with it at banquets, decorated their homes with it and, on the occasion of a victory, they strew roses through the street. At one of Nero's feasts, guests were asphyxiated by showers of roses.[4]

China and India

No other region in the world possesses such a wealth of aromatic plants. One Sanskrit author describes the pleasures which the ritual necessity of the daily bath could give to the ruler, followed by a massage with a massage oil in a base of sesame seed oil perfumed with jasmine, coriander, cardamom, basil, costus, pandanus, agarwood, pine, saffron, champaka and clove. Once this rub-down was complete, the king would be dressed in a clean cotton garment and, fully refreshed, emerged to face the day.[4]

Just as Greece had a zone of influence beyond her borders, known as Magna Graecia, the term greater India refers to those countries to the south and east — Sri Lanka, Thailand, Cambodia, Burma, Sumatra, Java and Malaysia. Indian culture percolated down to these areas through numerous traders from India who came in search of materials not found at home.

The list of aromatics originating from India is extensive. Cardamom was first mentioned in the Ayurvedic texts of the 4th century BC. Another highly prized Indian aromatic is Tulsi basil, the herb sacred to Krishna. Exquisite floral aromatics such as jasmine, champaka (a close relative of our garden magnolias) and lotus are believed to have originated from India.[4]

The greatest contribution from India must be sandalwood, whose soft scent was said to induce the calm sought by all the spiritualities of India. Other well-known essential oils whose origins are from India are vetiver and patchouli. Patchouli is a tropical member of the mint family. It was initially used to ward off moths from carpets and fine woven goods such as shawls and jackets. The leaves and stems, which turned brown upon drying, were chopped up and sprinkled among the fabrics.[4]

China's most important contribution to aromatherapy was the citrus species. Almost all the citrus species are believed to have originated from China. *Citrus aurantium,* originating in China, first reached the Mediterranean world in the 10th century (through the Arabs). It is hard to imagine that all of these common fruits were completely unknown to the Greeks and Romans.[4]

The camphor tree was also a very important part of Chinese civilisation. It was extensively used in perfumery, medical and building applications.

The Middle East

The writings of Dioscorides, Galen, Pliny and Zosimus, which were translated into Arabic, fuelled the birth of a purely Islamic body of knowledge.

Westerners are accustomed to the belief that when Europe went through the Dark Ages, the rest of the world did so as well. Islamic culture is so often disregarded in Western culture, yet it is during this period that the use of aromatics flourished in the Middle East, and indeed gave rise to many of the skills and techniques which are still used today.[4]

It is the Persians who are credited with having perfected the art of distillation. Ibn-Sina (980–1037) was known as the 'Prince of Physicians'. Attar of rose was his cure for ailments of the digestive tract. In the West he was known as Avicenna.[4]

It was in the Middle East that glassware was perfected, including pieces that could withstand the heat of distilling. Unlike Christianity, Islam was relatively relaxed as far as the comforts of life were concerned. Muhammad is said to have loved perfumes above all else.[4]

The Arab traders also established trading colonies in India. Soon they had expanded into the Malay Archipelago, where nutmeg, mace and cloves were produced. By 800AD traders from Persia had reached China.[4]

Of all the aromatics in the Arabic treasury, pride must be given to the attar of rose. Legend also holds that when Mohammad rose to heaven, his sweat fell to earth and he said, *'whoever would smell my scent would smell the rose'*.[4]

Islamic culture not only forged a solid bridge between the ancient world and medieval Europe, but it also laid great foundations upon which plant-based holistic medicine could flourish.

The Middle Ages

The decline of the Roman Empire signalled a general decline in the level of civilisation in Europe and most of the knowledge on aromatics was lost for some time.

Personal use of fragrances was considered a frivolous luxury tending towards debauchery by Church leaders. Many early Christians even ceased washing themselves and were proud to reek of 'honest' dirt and sweat.[2]

It was a time of great superstition; the plagues had become an unavoidable part of life in medieval Europe. While science now recognises that the plague had been spread primarily by rat fleas carrying the plague germs, at the time more dramatic agents were put forward as being responsible for the deadly sin.

One of the most popular beliefs of the time was that foul odour was considered one of the most common causes of many diseases. Anthropologist Constance Classen describes a typical European city:

> *European cities were then the most filthy places. Food remains, human and animal waste, blood and entrails of slaughtered animals, dead cats and dogs — to name some. Even blood let from patients by barber–surgeons would be cast into the street as often as not.*[2]

It is not surprising that people generally tended to the strongly aromatic herbs and oils to mask the foul odours which were believed to be the cause of most diseases.[2]

Aromatics were considered not only useful for preventing disease, but for curing it. Medical theory of the time suggested that the nose gave direct access to the brain and that any medication inhaled through the nose would act directly on the brain, hence the spirit. It was also imagined that the spirit, or the life force, was similar in nature to odour, hence making smell the best means of correcting its disorders.[2]

It was here that we find that measures against the plague were directed in controlling and combating corrupt air. Municipal authorities lit bonfires of aromatic woods in the streets to purify the atmosphere. A popular device of the time was a pomander: an orange stuck full of cloves. Physicians recommended that the sickrooms have herbs at the window, an aromatic fire burning in the fireplace, and rosewater and vinegar sprinkled on the floor. Doctors often wore a nose-bag as shown in the picture on the next page. The use of such smells was not without medical value as the essential oils used are now known to be considered powerful germicides.

Many books on distillation were written during the 16th century, especially in Germany, which seems to have been the centre of this aromatherapy renaissance. The books also referred to alchemical practices.

Alchemy was very popular at this time and the distillation of all kinds of substances was one of the alchemists' favourite pastimes in their pursuit of the *quintessence* of matter.

Distillation was still not perfected, but in the early 15th century the *Libellus de distallatione Philosophia* noted that tinctures of herbs in alcohol were impervious to decay and it gave the advice that herbs should not be distilled in vessels of lead.[5]

In Germany, Hieronymus Braunschweig, often referred to as Jerome of Brunswick, who was a physician, wrote several books on distillation. His last great work, the new *Vollkomen Distillierbuch,* was published in 1597. It includes reference to 25 essential oils including rosemary, lavender, clove, cinnamon, myrrh and nutmeg. According to Tisserand, Braunschweig's books on distillation went through 680 editions, appearing in every European language.[5]

Other contributions to the development of aromatherapy were made by Conrad Gesner, and by Ryff, a Strasburg physician, who published *Neu Gross Destillierbuch* in 1545.

In *The Treasure of Euonymus*, published in 1559, Conrad Gesner speaks of essential oils having the power to conserve all strengths, and to prolong life. Tisserand says that his findings on the properties of rosemary oil are remarkably perceptive:

> *It strengtheneth the harte, the braine, the sinews [muscles] and the hoole bodye ... members [limbs] sick of the palsy it heateth them for moste parte, and healeth them sometimes. Fistulaes and Cancars that give not place to other medicines, it healeth them throughlye.*[5]

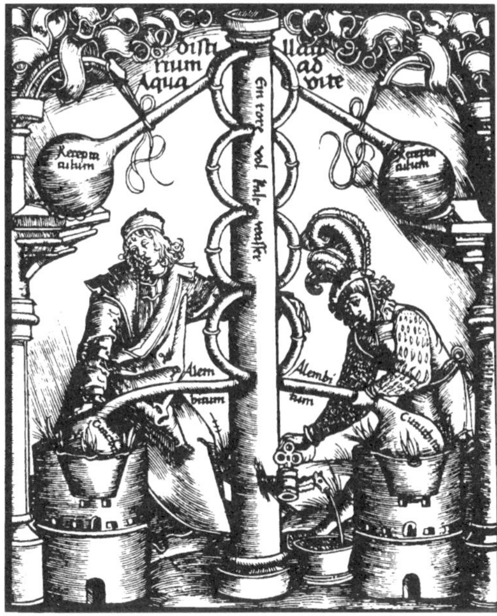

16th century distillation apparatus.

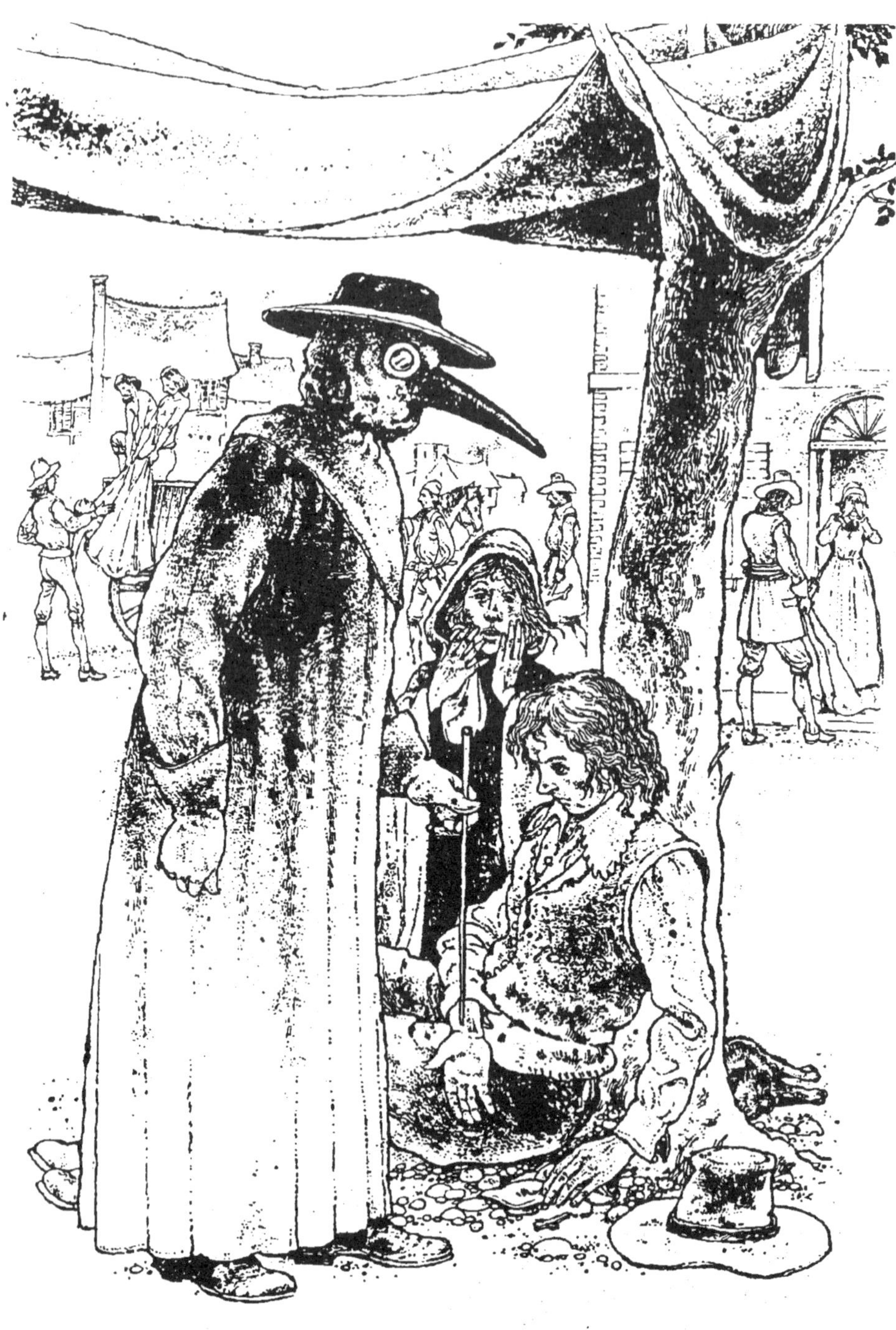

A 17th century doctor is wearing the protective clothing of his profession. The beak through which he breathes is filled with cinnamon, cloves and aromatic herbs.

Many of these comments, especially the properties ascribed to rosemary oil, would be regarded as valid by aromatherapists today.

The Rise of Modern Medicine

Griggs says that Philippus Theophrastus Bombastus von Hohenheim (1493–1541) (commonly known as Paracelsus) was credited with revolutionising medicine, he lay the foundations of both modern and alternative medicine. However, modern medicine would become more interested in active constituents and chemicals rather than the entire plant.[6]

He castigated those in the medical profession who merely followed the texts of ancient Greek and Roman herbalists and would not test their materials and processes by experiences.[6]

The Medical Act of 1511 saw the formalisation of training for physicians. The Royal College of Physicians was given the power to fine unauthorised practitioners. In 1540 barbers and surgeons were given similar powers, when the king had approved their company. Without hesitation the barbers–surgeons began a rampage of prosecuting 'unauthorised practitioners'. These 'quacks' were healers who relied on traditional knowledge of herbs and healing. Most were poor and served the poor.[6]

So ruthless was the persecution that within two years there were insufficient healers. So in 1542 King Henry enacted the Quack's Charter which exempted many unauthorised practitioners from the 1511 Act. The medical elite were outraged, so their target then shifted from the 'quacks' to women, when the King passed the first penal law against witches. Witches had become a convenient scapegoat for the medical establishment.[6]

The 17th century was known as the 'golden age' of English herbalists, notably Nicholas Culpeper, John Parkinson and John Gerardes. Essential oils had become a regular part of the herbalist's repertoire.[5] For instance, Culpeper says of rosemary:

> *The chemical drawn from the leaves and flowers is a sovereign help ... to touch the temples and nostrils with two or three drops for all diseases of the head and brain spoken of before, as also to take one drop, two or three, as the case requires, for inward diseases; yet it must be done with discretion, for it is very quick and piercing.*[7]

Of lavender, Culpeper says:

> *It is of especial use for pains in the head and brain, following cold, apoplexy, falling-sickness, the dropsy or sluggish malady, cramps, convulsions, palsies and faintings. It provokes women's courses, and expels the dead child and afterbirth.*[7]

It is apparant that essential oils were successfully being used for a variety of internal and external problems. Both doctors and herbalists used them, a trend that would continue until the end of the 19th century. By this stage dosages had been established and the need for dilution and suitable vehicles for internal use had become clear.

A gradual division between the physicians who used chemical drugs and those that remained faithful to herbs occurred. Over time the medical establishment became obsessed with science and chemistry and plant-based therapies began to fall out of favour, especially when it was believed that the 'active constituents' could be extracted from the plant, or even better, synthetically derived.

For example, willow (*Salix alba*) is used in herbal medicine for the relief of aches, fevers and rheumatic pain. However, in 1852, salicylic acid, the active constituent in willow, was synthetically derived. The laboratory was now replacing the herb garden as a source of principal materia medica.

Aromatherapy in France

In the 19th century the role of micro-organisms had been identified as the cause of many diseases and it was in France, in the late 1800s, that it was realised that some essential oils were highly antimicrobial.

Somebody drew attention to the low incidence of tuberculosis in the flower-growing districts of France, especially in the south. Tuberculosis was a very common illness at the time; however, it had been noted that most of the workers who processed the flowers and herbs remained free of respiratory diseases. The most likely cause of this was believed to have been the essential oils contained in these plants. This led, in 1887, to the first recorded laboratory test on the antibacterial properties of the essential oils.

In the 1880s, Chamberland, Cadeac and Meunier published similar studies that showed that the micro-organisms of glandular and yellow fever were easily killed by essential oils. They noted the active properties of oregano, Chinese cinnamon, angelica and geranium.

In July 1910 Rene-Maurice Gattefosse discovered the healing properties of lavender oil after severely burning his hands in a laboratory explosion. While he was not the first person to use essential oils therapeutically, he has been given credit for having coined the term *aromatherapie* in 1937.

Gattefosse used essential oils for the treatment of soldiers in military hospitals during the first World War. Some of his observations included:

> *Wounds to the scalp: healed in 10 days Firearm wounds: healed in 15 days Crushing of the thigh, open leg fracture; varices becoming ulcerated; delayed healing*

> *of an amputation stump of the thigh: healed in 21 days after failing with all other medications.*[8]

He concluded by saying;

> *It must be conceded that, while the antiseptic power of essences is of enormous interest, especially since it is not attended by any of the disadvantages found to such a large degree with all the other antiseptics used hitherto, greater attention needs to be devoted to the power they have of revitalising tissue.*[8]

Gattefosse is to be commended for having the insight to see that the therapeutic application of essential oils constituted a discipline in its own right. He was a chemist, so while he did not have much to do with the holistic approach to aromatherapy, he knew the importance of the chemical understanding of the essential oils and as a perfumer he recognised the psychotherapeutic benefits of the fragrance of the essential oils.

Although Gattefosse deserves full credit for his vision of aromatherapy, he was not the only person at the time to recognise the benefits of essential oils. In 1939 another Frenchman, Albert Couvreur, published a book on the medicinal properties of the essential oils.

Griggs says that Dr Jean Valnet is also credited with the further development of aromatherapy. As an army surgeon, he began to use, with great success, essential oils as antiseptics in the treatment of war wounds during the Indochina war from 1948–1959. After the war he continued using essential oils in his capacity as a doctor, and in 1964 published a comprehensive text entitled *Aromatherapie* (also available in English), which has since earned him global recognition.

Valnet describes the benefits of using essential oils:

> *Essential oils are especially valuable as antiseptics because of their aggression towards microbial germs and their harmlessness to tissue — one of the chief defects of chemical antiseptics is that they are likely to be as harmful to the cells of the organisms as to the cause of the disease.*[9]

Herbs, essential oils and careful attention to diet formed an integral approach of Dr Valnet's therapeutic strategy. The prescription his patients were likely to take with them usually combined a mixture of herbs and essential oils in an alcohol base, to be taken in a glass of lukewarm water before meals.[6]

However according to Griggs, for most French doctors of the time, plants were yesterday's medicine. Scientifically clinically tested synthetic drugs had become the norm of the day. In 1972, three doctors, Lapraz, Duraffourd and Belaiche, gathered round Valnet to form the nucleus of a new organisation devoted to the study and promotion of phytotherapy.[6]

While they realised that Valnet's empiric approach was effective, to give aromatherapy credibility they had to work within the framework of modern medicine, not outside it. Belaiche developed a scientifically based medical application of essential oils based on scientific research.

However, the very success of phytotherapy was its own undoing.

> *There was obvious dangers in much of this self-medication by legion of largely amateur herbal enthusiasts, but the herbs and essential oils available for over-the-counter sale were severely limited by French law. Far more of a threat to the public health were the growing legions of doctors armed with a prescription pad, and just enough of a sketchy training to allow them to impress patients with their mastery of phytotherapy.*[6]

Griggs cites Valnet, who was horrified with the irresponsible prescribing of essential oils:

> *On one occasion, a pharmacist rang to ask his opinion of prescription: it consisted of a mix of essential oils and tinctures in capsule form, a cream, an ointment and a liquid preparation, in total, thirty essential oils — including hyssop, sage and rosemary — and seventeen plant tinctures.*[6]

It was the over-commercialisation and charlatanism rampant in the French herbal world that led to its downfall. The cost of essential oils dispensed by pharmacists was reimbursed by the French National Health Scheme. However, to a drug budget already escalating out of control, in 1989, the French Ministry of Health ceased to reimburse herbal prescriptions. Doctors whose consulting rooms had been crammed with patients eager for the new plant medicines saw them empty dramatically once patients knew that they would have to foot the prescription bill themselves.[6]

Holistic Aromatherapy

It was Marguerite Maury, a French biochemist and beautician, who is often given much credit to the development of holistic aromatherapy as it is practised today. While her book, now published in English, *The Secret of Life and Youth*, does not give much practical information on the essential oils, she emphasised the importance of the essential oils not only in massage, but also as psychotherapeutic substances capable of bringing about changes in one's mood:

> *The greatest interest is the effect of fragrance on the psyche and mental state of the individual. Powers of perception become clearer and more accurate and there is a feeling of having, to a certain extent, outstripped*

events. They are seen more objectively, and therefore in truer perspective.[10]

Maury emphasised the importance of applying the essential oils externally, diluted in vegetable oil, in combination with massage:

> *Massage of the conjunctive, neuro-muscular or soft tissues pave the way admirably for the penetration of odoriferous substances, and the resultant rejuvenation ... It is therefore clear that preparations with a basis of essential oils with vegetable oils used as carriers, will be of great assistance.*[10]

It is at this point that we see a clear shift in the original meaning of the French word *aromatherapie*. Maury, who became Chairperson for CIDESCO (Pour le Comite International D'esthetique et de Cosmetologie), forged a link between aromatherapy and the beauty industry. As a result, beauty therapists who were already working in the context of wellbeing were able to introduce additional benefits, such as massage and the essential oils, to their treatment.

At a beauty therapy conference in 1959, Micheline Arcier met Marguerite Maury. This led to Micheline Arcier's lifelong devotion to aromatherapy. She trained with Marguerite Maury and Dr Jean Valnet.[11] Micheline Arcier has developed some of the most effective aromatherapy techniques being used today.

Robert Tisserand is also attributed to the development of holistic aromatherapy. Tisserand's book *The Art of Aromatherapy*, published in 1977, was the first to leave the purely medical approach of aromatherapy, combining medical applications with a more holistic and esoteric view of essential oils.[12]

It is at this point that aromatherapy became an intriguing, semi-medical modality which allowed the layperson to attempt self-therapy for many common ailments. Many other interpretations of aromatherapy began to develop; some of these interpretations were esoteric, while others began to focus on the fragrance aspect.[12]

The development of aromatherapy after 1980 diversified into four basic strands:

- medical aromatherapy
- popular and esoteric aromatherapy
- holistic aromatherapy and
- the scientific study of fragrance.[12]

The Future of Aromatherapy

It has been said that there is no consensus on the ultimate direction of aromatherapy. There are those who suggest that if the aromatherapy profession wants to be respected and acknowledged by conventional Western medicine, then, whether we like it or not, we have to show substantial and replicable clinical evidence of our claims.[13]

While scientific research may help us to identify and validate the active constituents, aromatherapy is inherently a vitalistic modality and the current scientific approach may not be the most appropriate platform for aromatherapy to develop in the future.

What is needed for the future is a framework that provides a platform that will allow aromatherapy to develop in a viable, holistic and confident therapy.

This can be achieved by clarification of the relationship aromatherapy has with science. The scientific exploration of essential oil constituents contributes to the knowledge about the pharmacology of essential oils and their quasi-medicinal application. However, it does not explain the living nature of essential oils from plants.[13]

We also need to understand the role of olfaction and fragrance and its inherent problems. How does one account for the hedonistic qualities of odour? Schnaubelt asks — How can liking or disliking a fragrance be eliminated? It is not surprising that scientific methods run into problems when dealing with the interconnected phenomena such as fragrance, feelings and culture. He says that science will be unable to make meaningful statements in this field as long as it is dependent on measuring the changes of only one variable.[13]

It is also important to recognise that the interaction of aromatherapy with humans cannot be reduced to a single variable experiment. Essential oils are made up of hundreds of different chemical constituents, which initiate different processes all happening simultaneously. Essential oils can elicit complex responses from the psychosomatic networks of any one person. [13]

Schnaubelt says there is also a need for new sciences which understand and allow the existence of psychosomatic networks of the mind and body. These new sciences may give us an insight into the interaction of highly effective sesquiterpene compounds found in essential oils and receptor systems.[13]

A holistic approach acknowledges that aromatherapy connects to the phenomena of life much more closely and intimately than conventional medicine. Schnaubelt beautifully describes the role of essential oils:

> *Essential oils reawaken odour awareness and the connection to individuality, and greater independence improves the ability to take responsibility for ones own health. Self confidence and wellbeing are influenced, providing an improved flow of biological information through the psychosomatic network of body and mind.*[13]

I believe the future of aromatherapy is a very promising one, in which essential oils are integrated into all aspects of life.

References

1. Manniche L. *An ancient Egyptian herbal.* British Museum Press, London, 1993.
2. Classen C. *Aroma: The cultural history of smell.* Routledge, UK, 1994.
3. Tisserand R. *Essential oils as psychotherapeutic agents.* In Proceedings of Perfumery: The Psychology and Biology of Fragrance. Chapman & Hall, UK, 1987.
4. Morris E. *Fragrance: The story of perfume from Cleopatra to Chanel.* Product of Nature and of Art, USA, 1984.
5. Tisserand R. *Aromatherapy for everyone.* Penguin Books, UK, 1988.
6. Griggs B. *Green pharmacy.* 2nd edn. Healing Art Press, USA, 1997.
7. Potterton D. *Culpeper's colour herbal.* W. Foulsham & Company Limited, UK, 1983.
8. Gattefosse R. *Gattefosse's aromatherapy.* From the original French text *Aromatherapie; Les huiles essentialles hormones vegetales.* First published in 1937, English version published by The C.W. Daniel Company Limited, Great Britain, 1993.
9. Valnet J. *The Practice of Aromatherapy.* The C.W. Daniel Company Limited, Great Britain, 1980.
10. Maury M. *Marguerite Maury's guide to aromatherapy: The secret of life and youth.* First published in French as *Le Capital Jeunesse* in 1961. English version published by The C.W. Daniel Company Limited, Great Britain, 1964.
11. Arcier M. *Aromatherapy.* The Hamlyn Publishing Group Ltd, London, 1990.
12. Schnaubelt K. *Essential Oils — Viable wholistic pharmaceutical for the future.* In Proceedings of the 13th International Congress of Flavours, Fragrances and Essential Oils. Istanbul, 1995; 269–279.
13. Schnaubelt K. *Medial aromatherapy.* Frog Ltd, USA, 1999.

What are Essential Oils?

Objectives

After careful study of this chapter, you should be able to:

- define an essential oil
- explain the origin of essential oils
- describe the photosynthesis process
- define the biological role of essential oils
- identify the botanical factors that influence the quality of an essential oil
- define the term chemotype.

Defining an Essential Oil

An essential oil is described as a volatile material derived by a physical process from an odorous plant material of a single botanical form and species.[1]

The ISO (International Standards Organisation) defines an essential oil as follows:

> *An essential oil is a product obtained from natural raw material, either by distillation with water or steam, or from the epicarp of citrus fruits by mechanical processing, or by dry distillation. The essential oil is subsequently separated from the aqueous phase by physical means.*[2]

While this description clearly describes how essential oils are extracted, it does not provide us with an explanation of their origins or purpose.

Drs Franchomme and Pénëol describe an essential oil in terms of the photosynthesis process:

> *Plant essences, in the physiological meaning of the term are most certainly true life essences, elaborated by the secretory cells of the plants that have tapped the photo-electro-magnetic energy of the sun and have converted it, with the intervention of enzymes, into biochemical energy under the form of highly diversified aromatic molecules.*[3]

Price describes essential oils in terms of their biological, commercial and therapeutic significance:

> *... of these secondary metabolites the essential oils have the greatest commercial significance ... whatever else they may do, they give the plant its aroma and flavour and often have a significant physiological effect on people.*[4]

Jean Rose's description of an essential oil gives us an insight into the physiological role of an essential oil in a plant:

> *... but what is this elusive essence of plant material called essential oil? It is the heart and soul of the plant. It is the essence that deters bugs from eating the plant. It is the fragrant aromatic heart of the plant that attracts bees and pollinating insects. It is the chemical component contained in the tiny plant cells that are liberated during the extraction process.*[5]

Lavabre adopts a more esoteric approach in describing essential oils:

> *Essential oils are the fragrant principle of the plant. They are the chemical components that give a plant its characteristic fragrance. In the spiritual approach to aromatherapy, essential oils are considered the life force, the energy of the plant. Alchemists regard them as the quintessence, the soul, the spirit of the plant.*[6]

The term *essential* is believed to have been derived by Bombastus Paracelsus von Hohenheim (1493–1541), who coined the term *quinta essentia* (quintessence). His theory was that it was the last possible and most sublime extract of the plant, which represents the efficient part of every drug and that the isolation of the *quinta essentia* should be the goal of every pharmacist.[7]

Where are Essential Oils Found?

Essential oils occur widely in the plant kingdom, not only in the flowers, leaves and fruit but also in the roots, stems and in other parts of the plants. Often a plant that produces an essential oil may do so in only one of its parts, such as jasmine from the flowers.

However, in the case of the bitter orange tree, three different essential oils may be produced — from the leaves we obtain petitgrain essential oil, from the flowers we obtain neroli essential oil and from the fruit peel we obtain bitter orange essential oil.

Examples of the distribution of essential oils in plants are:

Part of Plant	Examples of Essential Oils
Flowers	Jasmine, orange blossom, rose, ylang ylang
Leaves	Citronella, lemongrass, petitgrain, palmarosa, patchouli
Bark	Cinnamon
Wood	Cedarwood, sandalwood, rosewood
Roots	Ginger, vetiver
Entire plant	Geranium, lavender, rosemary, spike lavender
Fruit peel	Bergamot, lemon, lime, orange, tangerine, mandarin

The more oil glands or ducts present in the plant, the higher the yield of essential oil, thus the less expensive the cost of the oil.

Gattefosse believed that all plants have a smell and hence contain essential oils.[8] However, it is now known that only 15% of flowering plants contain volatile oils:

> *Furthermore the distribution of essential oil producing species in higher plants is rather scattered, often being restricted to specific plant families or genera. Overall about 15% of flowering plants produce essential oils in any significant quantity.*[8]

Essential oils can be found in specialised secretory structures, either on the surface of the plant or within the plant tissue.[9] The type of structure is generally family or species specific. Some examples include:

Glandular Trichomes

These are modified epidermal hairs and can be found covering leaves, stems and parts of flowers in

many plants from the *Lamiaceae* family such as basil, lavender, marjoram, mint and thyme.[9]

Epidermal Cells

Essential oils obtained from flowers such as rose and jasmine are not usually secreted by glandular hairs, but diffuse through the cytoplasm and cell walls of the plant to the outside. The yield of essential oil from these plants is usually very low.[9]

Secretory Cavities and Ducts

These structures can be found throughout the entire plant. They are large intercellular spaces that are formed by the separation of walls of neighbouring cells, or by the disintegration of cells. Spherical spaces are called cavities and these are found in plants from the *Myrtaceae* and *Rutaceae* plant families.[26]

Ducts are elongated spaces and can be found in plants from the *Apiaceae*, *Pinaceae* and *Asteraceae* plant families. Resin ducts are common in the *Coniferae* family and are present in both the needles and the wood.[26]

Oil Cells

These are cells that occur within the plant tissue and differ from the cells adjacent to them, both in the content and their size. Oil cells can be found throughout the whole plant. They can be found in plants from the *Lauraceae, Magnoliaceae, Piperaceae, Valerianaceae* and *Gramineae* plant families.[26]

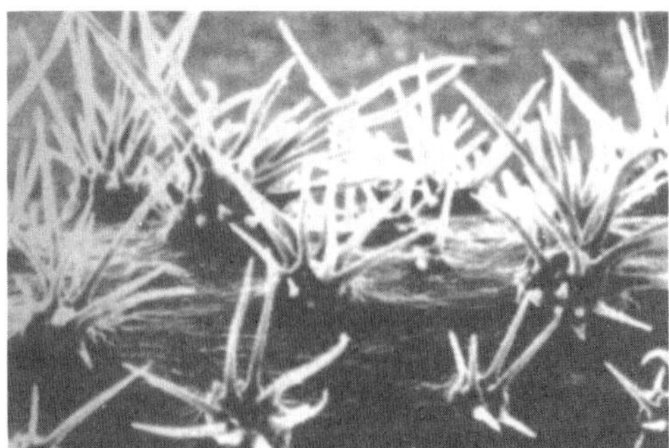

A scanning electron micrograph of the leaf surface of a eucalyptus leaf showing the stellate hairs associated with the oil glands. (Picture courtesy of the Australian Centre for International Agricultural Research)

Origin of Essential Oils

While the exact origin of essential oils is not known, biochemical experiments suggest that essential oils are synthesised in the region of photosynthetic activity in the cells surrounding the oil glands. They then pass through the cell wall into the interior of the gland.[11]

The physiological rationale for the specific aspect of the relationship between photosynthesis and essential oil production is poorly known at present. Monoterpenes have been demonstrated to utilise sugars as a carbon source.[12]

Research has confirmed the possible influence of photosynthesis and photorespiration on the terpene metabolism of peppermint oil.[13] It was found that photosynthesis inhibition by the use of herbicides caused a decline in the content of monoterpene alcohols.

Photosynthesis

The photosynthesis process involves chloroplasts of plants capturing light from the sun and converting it to chemical energy which is then stored in the bonds of sugar and other organic molecules made from water and carbon dioxide.

Cells cannot create their own energy, but as open systems they are able to absorb energy from their surroundings. Photosynthetic cells acquire their energy in the form of light, which they use to make the organic compounds that provide energy to other cells. Hence photosynthesis nourishes almost all the living world directly or indirectly.

The energy-collecting cells of plants are called chloroplasts. The leaves are the major sites of photosynthesis in most plants. The colour of the leaf is due to a green substance known as chlorophyll.

Photosynthesis can be summarised with this chemical equation:[14]

$$6CO_2 + 12\ H_2O + \text{light energy} = C_6H_{12}O_6 + 6O_2 + 6H_2O$$

The carbohydrate $C_6H_{12}O_6$ is glucose, a major product of photosynthesis. The free energy from the sun has therefore been stored in the form of a complex molecule, glucose. This stored energy can then be released to provide energy for other chemical reactions within the plast. Terpenes, the major group of compounds found in essential oils, are devised from mevalonic acid, which is formed from photosynthates. There is evidence which suggests the formation of essential oils in the region of photosynthetic activity in the cells surrounding the oil glands.[7]

Biological Activity of Essential Oils in Plants

The reason why so little is known about the biological role of essential oils is that only small amounts of essential oil are generally present in the plant at any one time.

It is known that the plant will not reabsorb the essential oils that have formed in a leaf before shedding it in winter. Sugar and starches, however, are returned to the main body of the plant prior to the shedding of the leaf, therefore it was not surprising that many botanists concluded that essential oils were merely 'waste products' of the plant's metabolism.[7]

However, modern research rejects this conclusion. There is now evidence for the biological role of essential oils such as:

- a form of attraction of pollinators such as insects
- plant–plant competition, or allopathic interaction
- defence compounds against insects and animals
- antimicrobial properties
- antitranspirant action
- wound healing.[10]

Attraction of Pollinators

There are three main attractants; odour (produced by the volatile essential oil), colour and morphology. Many of the compounds found in the odour glands of insects are also found in flower fragrances and plant volatiles.[10]

Odour is important for night-flying insects and other animals where visual stimulus is practically absent. Bat-pollinated flowers, for example, may have a fruity or cabbagy scent, while moth-pollinated flowers are generally very strongly and sweetly scented. Bird-pollinated flowers generally have no scent, as birds do not respond to scent.[10]

Insects are very sensitive to small concentrations of volatile chemicals. This means that flowers which do not have a strong odour to human senses may still produce enough odour to attract insects.[10]

The maximum scent production coincides with the time when the pollen is ripe and the flower is ready for pollination. Scent is also generally at its peak at the time of the day when the pollinator is around.

Allelopathy

Monoterpenes, the most abundant class of terpenoid compounds found in essential oils, are known to be cytotoxic to plant tissues, impairing respiration and photosynthesis and decreasing cell membrane permeability. Allelopathy refers to compounds that prevent the growth of competing vegetation near established plants by inhibiting germination.[10]

Defence Mechanism

The terpenoid compounds have a wide range of functions in plant interactions with insects and animals. Studies confirm the role of terpenes in the defence of the plant against herbivores and microbial pathogens. There is evidence that indicates that terpenes can be toxic or repulsive to mammals.[10]

The goats that scourge the forest around the Mediterranean normally spare many of the pungent herbs such as wild thyme and wild marjoram. Citronella and camphor oil repel certain insects and sandalwood is impervious to termites. Sage, wormwood, tansy and thuja all contain thujone, which is so powerful against parasites that it has been used as vermifuges in traditional medicine.

Antimicrobial Compounds

Some terpenoid compounds produced by plants have been identified as having antimicrobial activity. These compounds protect the plant from fungal attacks and other microbes.[10]

Antitranspirant Action

The essential oils found on the surface of a leaf have been found to reduce the rate of water loss through transpiration.[10]

Factors Affecting the Quality of Essential Oils

Many factors can affect the quality of the essential oil:

- ecological variables, e.g., soil type, climate and the use of fertilisers and other chemicals
- harvesting time
- genetics and chemotypes
- type and age of the leaf.[7]

These factors must be considered when comparing the essential oil status.

Ecological Variables

Of particular interest are the essential oils produced from plants belonging to the Lamiaceae plant family. These are predominantly all the herbs which are traditionally found around the Mediterranean region.

For example, mild and moderate water stress increases *Ocimum basilicum's* essential oil content and alters the oil composition. Linalool and methyl chavicol increase as water stress increases, while the relative proportion of sesquiterpenes decreases.[15]

Experiments conducted to study the response pattern of *Pelargonium graveolens* to fertilisers and the variation of essential oil constituents under varied agroclimatic regions found that the essential oil yields were greater at lower altitudes than at higher altitudes. The oil produced at higher altitude locations was richer in menthone, citronellol, nerol and geraniol, while the oil produced from plants grown at lower altitude locations was richer in isomenthone, linalool and citronellyl formate. The variations in these growing conditions bring about a change in the quantity and quality of the essential oil produced.[16]

The effect of mineral fertilisers was evaluated on the basis of the fresh plant and essential oil yields. A study involving *Salvia officinalis* found that the concentrations of various chemical constituents were significantly affected by the various concentrations of fertilisers. An increase in fertilisers caused a reduction in the ratio of oxygenated components to hydrocarbons.[17]

Harvesting Time

Many studies have been conducted to determine the optimum time for harvesting. The conclusions are:

- The volatile oil content of the leaf increases with time and also with leaf size.
- The maximum leaf yield was measured at the same time for most species: late summer, but the maximum oil yield varied from species to species. Thus it is important to know at what time in the plant's cycle the plant matter has been harvested.[18]

Investigations into the chemical profile of *Chamomilla recutita* found that several extrinsic factors such as amount of daylight, temperature, air and soil humidity, sowing and harvesting times all affected the quantity and quality of the essential oil produced. It was found that the essential oil content was significantly higher if it were sown in spring rather than autumn.[19]

Another example is *Salvia officinalis*, which contains varying amounts of α-thujone depending on when it is harvested. It contains more after it has flowered, so it is better harvested before it flowers as the α-thujone is one of the more toxic constituents found in the oil.[17]

It was found that *Ocimum basilicum* essential oil distilled from the whole plant gave an oil with a higher percentage of methyl chavicol whereas the flower spikes produced an oil richer in linalool. For aromatherapy purposes it is better to use basil with the least amount of methyl chavicol as this constituent is considered a skin irritant and has possible carcinogenic effects.[20]

There was a marked difference in the menthol/menthone and pulegone ratio of peppermint oil according to the harvesting time. It was concluded that the late harvesting of peppermint before flowering yielded an oil rich in menthone and pulegone, two undesirable constituents, while harvesting the peppermint after flowering yielded an oil richer in menthol.[21]

It was also noted that drying peppermint leaves before distillation did not affect the chemical composition of the essential oil, but was commercially more viable as it allowed larger amounts of plant material to be distilled.[22]

Genetics

Plants belonging to the Lamiaceae family are prone to hybridisation, which makes defining species and subspecies a difficult task. Hybridisation is when two different species cross-pollinate and the offspring is usually sterile.

Of particular interest is thyme. There are over 150 subspecies of the genus *Thymus*. A subspecies occurs when a particular plant produces others like itself, usually with some marked differences between it and the parent species.[23]

Some of the different *Thymus* species investigated include the following:[23]

Thymus Species	Main Constituent
Thymus. vulgaris	Thymol, carvacrol, p-cymene, linalool
Thymus. zygis	Thymol, carvacrol
Thymus. capitatus	Carvacrol, thymol
Thymus. satureoides	Borneol, camphene, γ-terpineol
Thymus. mastichina	Linalool, 1,8-cineole

Chemotypes

A chemotype is referred to an essential oil which is produced from a plant of one botanical species in which the essential oils produced from different locations are of distinctly different chemical composition.

This phenomenon that chemical differences exist in morphologically identical species is widespread among the Lamiaceae family. Two examples in which chemotypes exist are thyme and rosemary. There are six chemotypes of *Thymus vulgaris*:

thymol
carvacrol
linalool
geraniol
α-terpinyl acetate
thuyan-4-ol.[24]

It was found that there was a correlation between chemotype, sexual polymorphism and the environment. It was noticed that the phenol-containing species of thyme often showed two chemotypes, a thymol type as well as a carvacrol type. Their common precursor p-cymene leads to either thymol or carvacrol, even though both substances can be found in many phenol-containing species, usually one dominating.

Rosemary essential oil from *Rosmarinus officinalis* has three main chemotypes:

camphor
1,8-cineole
verbenone.[25]

More information on the difference between the various chemotypes of rosemary can be found in Chapter 5.

When purchasing certain essential oils it is important to know which chemotype you are buying, as the differences in the composition of the oil will affect the therapeutic properties of the oil. It is useful to know the geographic and ecological origin of the essential oil, as this will give you information about its chemotype.

When such a difference occurs it has become a standard practice to identify the oil by the Latin name of the plant followed by the predominant chemical component:

Rosmarinus officinalis c.t *camphor*

Conclusion

The factors affecting the quality of essential oil highlight some of the qualitative and quantitative variations found in essential oils and draw attention to some of the principal sources of this variation. The essential oil industry and aromatherapists would benefit from more carefully controlled experiments aimed at pinpointing these key factors.

References

1. Arctander S. *Perfume and flavour materials of natural origin.* Allured Publishing, USA, 1994.
2. Brud W. *Blending and compounding: Where is the true essential oil?* AROMA '93 Conference Proceedings, Aromatherapy Publications, UK, 1993.
3. Franchomme P. *Phytoguide no.1: Aromatherapy, advanced therapy for infectious illnesses.* La Courete, France, International Phytomedical Foundation, 1985.
4. Price S, Price L. *Aromatherapy for health professionals.* Churchill Livingstone, UK, 1995.
5. Rose J. *The aromatherapy book.* Herbal Studies Course, California, 1992.
6. Lavabre M. *Aromatherapy workbook.* Healing Art Press, USA, 1990.
7. Boland D, Brophy J, House A. eds. *Eucalyptus leaf oils.* Inkata Press, Australia, 1991.
8. Gattefosse R. *Gattefosse's aromatherapy.* The C.W. Daniel Company Limited, Great Britain, 1993. First published in France in 1937.
9. Svoboda K, Hampson J, Hunter T. *Secretory tissues.* The International Journal of Aromatherapy. 1998/1999 9(3); 124–131.
10. Shawe K. *Essential oils and their biological roles.* Aromatherapy Quarterly 1996; 50: 23–28.
11. Guenther E. *The essential oils Vol. 1.* D. Van Nostrand Company Inc. USA, 1953.
12. Sing N, Luthra R. *Sucrose metabolism and essential oil accumulation during lemongrass leaf development.* Plant Science 1987; 54: 127–133.
13. Mafei M. *Photosynthesis, photorespiration and herbicide effect on terpene production in peppermint.* The Journal of Essential Oil Research 1990; 2(6): 275–286.
14. Bettelheim F, March J. *Introduction to General, Organic and Biochemistry.* Saunders College Publishing, USA, 1984.
15. Simon J, et al. *Water stress-induced alterations in essential oil content and composition of sweet basil.* The Journal of Essential Oil Research 1992; 4(1): 71–75.
16. Bhaskaruni R. *Variations in yields and quality of geranium under varied climatic and fertility conditions.* The Journal of Essential Oil Research 1990; 2(2): 73–79.
17. Piccaglia R. *Effect of mineral fertilisers on the composition of Salvia officinalis oil.* The Journal of Essential Oil Research 1995; 7(2): 73.
18. Basker D, Putievsky E. *Seasonal variation in the yields of leaf and essential oil in some Labiatae species.* Journal of Horticultural Science 1978; 53(3): 179–183.
19. Gasic O. *The influence of sowing and harvesting time on the essential oils of Chamomilla recutita.* The Journal of Essential Oil Research 1991; 3(5): 295–302.
20. Bonnardeaux J. *The effect of different harvesting methods on the yield and quality of basil oil in the Ord River irrigation area.* The Journal of Essential Oil Research 1992; 4(1): 65–69.
21. Chalchat J. *Variation of the composition of essential oil of Mentha piperita L. during the growing time.* The Journal of Essential Oil Research 1997; 9(4): 463–465.
22. Perrin, Colson. *Timing of the harvest date for mentha piperita based on observations of the floral development.* The Journal of Essential Oil Research 1991; 3(1): 17–25.
23. Stahl-Biskup E. *The chemical composition of Thymus oils.* The Journal of Essential Oil Research 1991; 3(2): 61–82.
24. Soulier J. *The Thymus Genus.* Aromatherapy Records 1995; 1: 38–49.
25. Lawrence B. *Rosemary oil.* Essential Oils 1981–1987, Allured Publishing, USA, 1989; 60–62.
26. Svobada K. *The biology of fragrance.* Aromatherapy Quarterly, 1996; 49: 25–28.

Methods of Essential Oil Extraction

Objectives

After careful study of this chapter, you should be able to:

- identify the methods of extracting essential oils
- explain the methods of extracting essential oils
- discuss the advantages and disadvantages of each method of extraction.

Introduction

Methods of extracting aromatic substances were developed by alchemists in the early civilisations of the Middle East and ancient Egypt.

The philosophy of the alchemists was that the spark of divinity could be discovered in matter and by subjecting botanical and mineral substances to heating in water baths and stills, the divine eternal spirit would be extracted. While they did not succeed in extracting the divine eternal spirit, we must be grateful to the practitioners of alchemy for what we know of essential oil extraction today.

While it is Maria the Jewess who is credited for inventing the still, it is the famous Arab physician and philosopher Ibn-Sina (980–1037) who is credited with inventing the cooling condenser which he used to produce pure essential oils and aromatic waters.[1]

However, this has been challenged. An archaeological expedition to Pakistan found a perfectly preserved terracotta distillation apparatus from the Indus Valley civilisation from about 3000 BC. This discovery suggests that the Arabs may have obtained their basic knowledge of distillation from this region.[1]

Methods of Essential Oil Extraction

While distillation is the most common method of extraction, special oils and absolutes may require more advanced equipment. The basic methods of extraction are:

- Expression processes
  - compression — sponge
  - écuelle à piquer
  - machine abrasion
- Distillation processes
  - water
  - steam
  - water and steam
  - hydro-diffusion
- Extraction with volatile solvents
  - enfleurage
  - solvent
  - hypercritical CO_2

Expression

Expression is used to extract essential oils contained in the large cells of the flavedo. These, being close to the surface of the citrus peel, are readily ruptured by lateral compression of the peel or puncturing by scarification or grating. Only essential oils from citrus fruits are extracted by expression.

The Sponge Process

The sponge process was one of the original methods used to obtain citrus essential oils. It has been reported that essential oils produced by the sponge process are different to essential oils which have been mechanically extracted.[2]

The fruit is cut transversely into halves, from which the pulp is then removed. The fruit is then soaked in warm water for a short time to allow the pith to absorb a proportion of the water, which softens it and renders it more elastic. The softening process is completed by exposing the peel to the air for several hours, after which it is ready for the removal of essential oil.[3]

The peel is everted by the sponge, so that the flavedo is now on the inside of the hemisphere and is laterally compressed. This causes the rupture of many of the oil cells and the consequent release of the oil, which is absorbed by the sponge.[3]

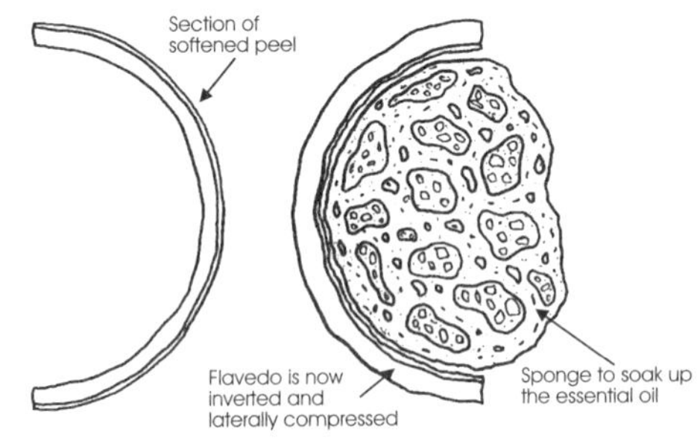

Eversion of fruit in sponge method

The sponge is periodically squeezed into a collecting vessel, from which the essential oil is decanted.

The écuelle à piquer Process

The whole fruit is rotated against the spikes around the rim in order to puncture the oil cells. These cells contain not only essential oil, but also cell sap and protoplasm. The essential oil released is mixed with cell contents from these and surrounding cells which are punctured in the process. The mixture of essential oil and other cell contents, including pigment, is then emptied into a collecting vessel, from which the oil is decanted after separation from the aqueous layer.[3]

Machine Abrasion

The principle of the machine abrasion used for the production of citrus oils is no different from that of the écuelle à piquer process.

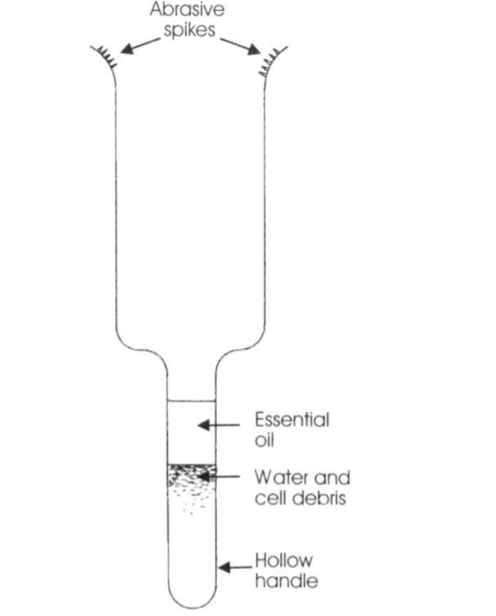

The écuelle à piquer process

The whole fruits are fed from a hopper into a rotating drum within which are rows of spikes. As the fruit tumbles over the spikes, they are stripped of their outer peel, which, in the form of a finely divided mixture of cell debris, essential oil and other cell contents, is washed away by running water into a centrifugal separator which performs a very rapid separation of the essential oil from the aqueous matter.[3]

It should be noted, however, that in this process the essential oil is mixed with other cell contents so that the chance of alteration of the quality of the oil by enzyme action is higher.[3]

The Advantages of Expression Processes

The benefit of the expression processes is that the essential oils are not subjected to heat. Heat may under certain conditions cause decomposition or damage the essential oil. Unfortunately the process is available only for the extraction of citrus oils.

Distillation Processes

The distillation process has remained relatively unchanged in the last 1,000 years. Today, many essential oils are produced by distillation utilising the same technology, whether this is a simple 'backyard' still found in some of the developing countries or a modern distillation plant.

However, many of the primitive 'backyard' stills tend to produce poor-quality essential oil with a minimal return for the effort.[1,4]

The modern distillation plants utilise the latest technology and are usually computer-operated so that the composition of the essential oil can be accurately controlled.[1]

Distillation involves heating a liquid or solid material to a temperature sufficiently high to produce a vapour and then cooling the vapour to cause it to condense to a liquid or solid distillate.

Water Distillation

In water distillation the plant material is completely covered with water. The still is brought to boil. If the air pressure in the still is reduced (e.g., by creating a vacuum), there will be a reduced crowding of molecules of the gases of air at the liquid surface, making it easier for molecules of the liquid to escape. By water distilling under a vacuum it is possible to increase the speed of evaporation of any volatile liquid. Similarly, the boiling point of water or any other volatile liquid is reduced by reducing the pressure at its surface.[3]

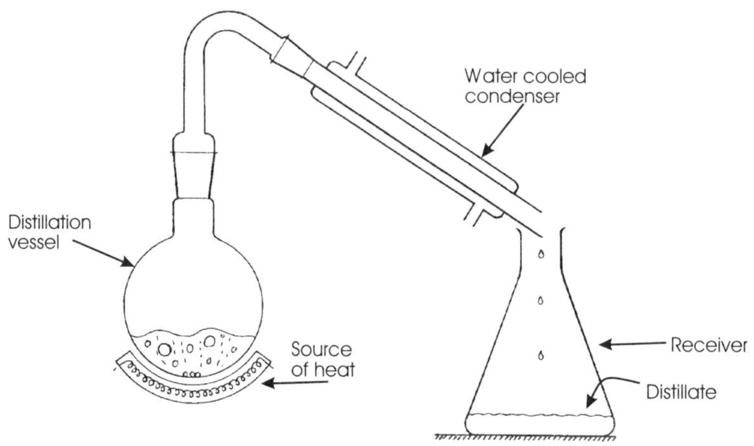

Simple water distillation process

Air pressure decreases with increased altitude, therefore water distillation conducted above sea level will ensue at temperatures below 100°C. A reduced distillation temperature can improve the quality of an essential oil.[3]

To ensure that the plant material can easily release the essential oil contained in the oil gland, hard fruits, seeds and woods are comminuted, that is, reduced to small pieces or powder, before distillation to render their essential oil cells accessible to the boiling water. Other materials such as patchouli are allowed to soak for a period before distillation, to allow fermentation to break down the cell walls to release the essential oil.[5]

This method of distillation is a slow process that favours those essential oils which are not damaged by extensive contact with hot water, which is particularly aggressive towards essential oils containing a high percentage of esters, breaking them down to the corresponding alcohols and carboxylic acids. Because of this, many essential oils require the much faster process of steam distillation.[3,5]

Steam Distillation

In steam distillation, steam from a separate boiler is injected into the distillation vessel. The essential oil is extracted at a much faster rate than water distillation.

The steam is under pressure greater than that of the atmosphere, thus water from which it is produced is boiling at a temperature above 100°C. The object of steam distillation is to complete the process as quickly as possible, as certain essential oil components are thermolabile or heat-sensitive. Therefore, damage to the essential oil through the effect of the steam is minimised.[3,5]

Constituents such as linalyl acetate found in lavender will decompose to linalool and acetic acid and the matricin found in German chamomile will decompose into the intensely blue chamazulene.

The advantage of steam distillation over water distillation is that the essential oil is exposed to the risk of hydrolysis for a relatively shorter period.

Cohobation

Rose otto contains phenyl ethyl alcohol, a colourless, rose-smelling constituent that is water-soluble. When rose is distilled much of the phenyl ethyl alcohol is dissolved in the distilled water. In cohobation, the distilled water is collected and returned to the distillation vessel to be redistilled so that the phenyl ethyl alcohol can be recovered.

The separated phenyl ethyl alcohol is then returned to the original distillate in the correct proportion to form rose otto oil.

Water and Steam Distillation

In the water and steam distillation process, live steam is generated in a separate apparatus and then led through the still, which is filled with plant material and water. This method is a compromise between water distillation and pure steam distillation.[3]

Fractional Distillation

The process is conducted as per normal distillation. However, the essential oil is collected in batches as distillation proceeds, instead of being continuously collected. These batches of the essential oil are called fractions.

Ylang ylang essential oil is produced by fractional distillation. In this process the distillation is stopped and restarted up to four times. The receiver

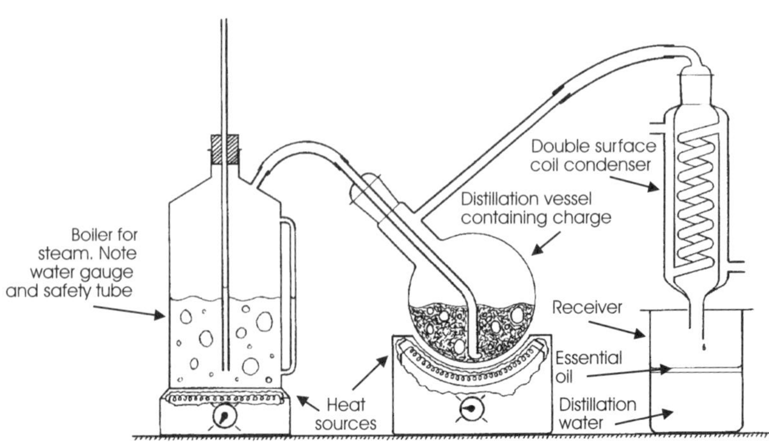

Water and steam distillation process

is changed on each occasion. The first fraction is referred to as ylang ylang 'extra', and the subsequent fractions are referred to as 1st, 2nd and 3rd grade.[3]

The first fraction, ylang ylang extra, contains the most volatile constituents of the essential oil, along with a proportion of constituents of lower volatility. The second and third fractions contain larger quantities of less volatile constituents, while the final fraction is composed of the least volatile constituents of the oil.[3]

Dry Distillation

It is not usual to distil essential oils without the use of water or steam. However, Peru balsam and copaiba are both produced by dry distillation. This is possible by distilling the plant matter in a vacuum, which lowers the boiling point sufficiently for distillation.[3] These two oils are not commonly used in aromatherapy.

Destructive Distillation

If vegetable matter is heated to a high temperature in a distillation apparatus, moisture evaporates from the charge as steam. This displaces all the air from the distillation vessel so that all the oxygen is depleted. The cells of the plant matter begin to char and brown smoky fumes are emitted, the density of which increases as the temperature rises. Eventually, a pale brown, mobile liquid and a black, viscous tarry mass distil over and the 'smell of smoke' pervades the atmosphere. Birch tar and cade oil are both produced by this method.[3]

These two oils are not commonly used in aromatherapy. While rectified cade oil does have therapeutic value, unrectified cade oil is considered a hazardous essential oil.

Rectification

Any essential oil containing 'impurities' which are non-volatiles or of a very low volatility, may be purified by redistillation, either in a vacuum or in steam. Any such redistillation is known as rectification. Eucalyptus essential oil is one such oil that is often subjected to rectification.

The reason is that the standard for eucalyptus oil requires it to have a minimum of 70% cineole. If the distilled oil does not reach these high cineole levels the essential oil will be redistilled so that impurities can be removed, hence increasing the cineole level.[6]

Hydro-diffusion

Hydro-diffusion is a variation on direct steam distillation. The main difference is that the steam is introduced at the top of the still and not at the base.

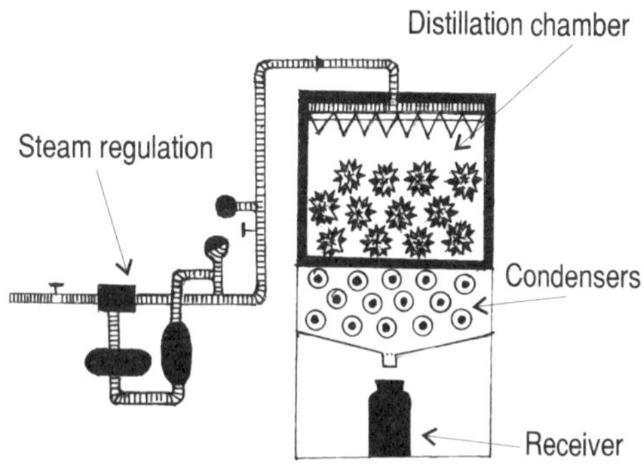

Hydro-diffusion process

Condensation of the oil/steam mixture occurs inside the still directly below the grille or perforated tray supporting the material being processed. The advantages over direct steam distillation are lower steam consumption and shorter processing time, which increases the essential oil yield.

Vacuum Distillation

Vacuum distillation obtains oil from a still under a vacuum. This technique allows for very accurate control of the distillate since it can be adjusted according to the boiling points of the various essential oil constituents.[1]

Molecular Distillation

This process is used to produce volatile essential oils from delicate materials containing some proportion of non-volatile matter, such as the absolutes often used in perfumery. The basic principle involves gentle evaporation of a thin film of material to be treated from a surface over which the film is continuously replenished, under vacuum conditions. Molecules of evaporating volatiles have only a short distance to travel before encountering a cooled surface on which to condense. The essential oil molecules can pass freely to this surface under vacuum conditions.

Very little heat is used to cause the evaporation of the volatiles and most molecules remain intact during the process.

Advantages of the Distillation Processes

It is important to remember that an essential oil produced by distillation will suffer some adulteration in its composition during the distillation process.

This occurs because of the hydrolysis of volatile esters and the hydrolysis of non-volatile constituents of the protoplasm known as glycosides.[5]

A glycoside that has undergone hydrolysis may be partially decomposed to form a sugar such as glucose, which is non-volatile, or it may form a compound called aglycone. The aglycones of certain glycosides present in essential oil-yielding plant matter are volatile and end up forming part of the essential oil. Examples of such volatiles released during distillation include the rose alcohols, geraniol and citronellol.[5]

Williams suggests that it is inaccurate to refer to distilled essential oils as natural products, but more accurate to describe them as products prepared from their natural sources by distillation.[5]

Another reaction which takes place during distillation is the partial hydrolysis of protein forming the living matter of the cells. Weakly bonded fragments of the molecules split off to form highly odorous, sulphur-containing molecules which distil over with the vapours of the essential oil, imparting an obnoxious odour, referred to as a *still note*.[5]

Still notes present in essential oil can be eliminated by exposing the oil to air for several hours or by blowing air into the oil for a short period. This promotes the evaporation of the responsible compounds.[5]

Solvent Extraction Processes

Solvent extraction is applied to those plants whose essential oils would be degraded by distillation. The methods of extraction with volatile solvents are:

- maceration
- extraction with volatile hydrocarbons
- enfleurage
- CO_2 extraction.

For raw materials with a very low concentration of essential oils such as jasmine and tuberose, extraction with volatile solvents is the most efficient way of extracting the essential oil.

Solvent extraction is a very gentle process which tends to create less 'rearrangement' of the essential oil compounds compared with distillation methods.

Compared with steam-distilled essential oils, solvent-extracted oils have a richer fragrance. The disadvantage with this process is that not only the essential oil components of the plant but also the non-volatile constituents such as waxes and plant dyes are extracted.

Maceration

Maceration is the simplest form of solvent extraction. Maceration in hot fat was one of the original

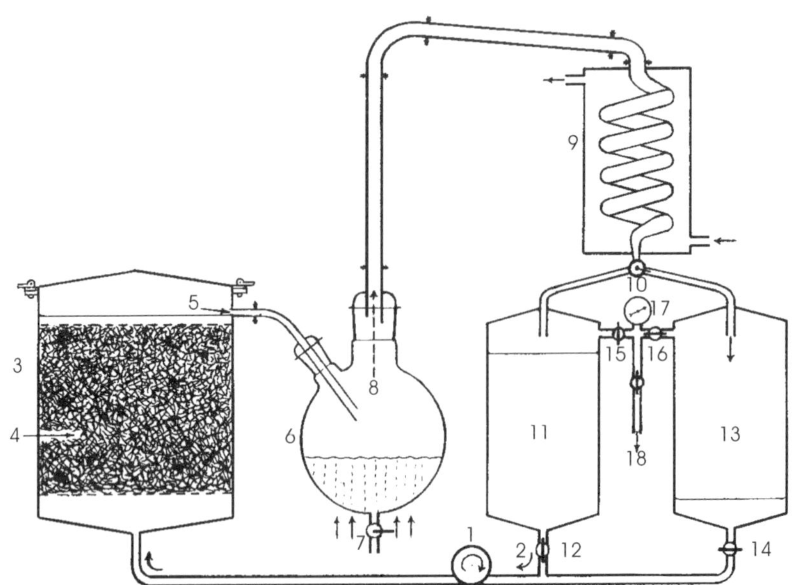

This diagram shows the basic equipment required for the extraction of essential oils with a volatile solvent, coupled with a vacuum still for recovery of the solvent after extraction.

1: Solvent pump; 2: Solvent to extraction vessel; 3 Extraction vessel; 4: Material for extraction; 5: Extract solution to distillation vessel; 6: Distillation vessel; 7: Drainage tap for recovery of concrete after extraction 8: Solvent vapour to condenser; 9: Water-cooler condenser; 10: Two-way tap; Receiver containing recovered solvent being recirculated to extraction vessel; 12: Solvent outlet tap; 13: Receiver being filled with recovered solvent 14: Solvent outlet tap; 15 & 16: Vacuum taps; 17: Vacuum gauge; 18: To vacuum pump.

processes of extracting the essential oils. This process is now almost obsolete. Maceration can be done using hot fat, alcohol, volatile solvents or cold fats. The process involving cold fats is referred to as enfleurage.

Scented flowers are immersed in highly purified melted fat, or mixture of fats, for a sufficient period of time so that the essential oil dissolves in the fat. Other constituents that would dissolve into the fat include natural waxes and plant pigments. The mixture is then strained to remove the exhausted flowers and other debris, and the process is then repeated several times using fresh flowers and the same fat.[3]

The result is that you have a fatty extract solution that is highly fragrant. Once solidified, this product is referred to as the pomade. The essential oil may then be extracted from the pomade with alcohol by the procedure described for the extraction of concretes.[3]

Extraction with Volatile Solvents

This complex mixture of volatile and non-volatile substances dissolved out by the solvent, usually an ether or hydrocarbon, comprises the 'extract'. The extract solution is then placed into a distillation vessel to which very gentle heat is applied, just enough to boil off the solvent, but insufficient to drive off the more volatile constituents from the essential oil contained in the extract.[3]

The concentrated extract solution removed from the distillation vessel is known as a *concrete* if it is not resinous and a resinoid if it is resinous. Concretes contain large quantities of wax or fat, and are only partially soluble in alcohol. The preparation of absolutes from concretes follows the *Principles of the Distribution Law*. The essential oil present in the concrete is soluble in the non-volatile material of the concrete and in alcohol.[3]

The concrete is warmed with some alcohol to a temperature just sufficient to melt it, and the mixture is then stirred. Essential oil from the molten concrete will dissolve into the alcohol as will a small amount of the waxes, fats and fixed oils found in the concrete.

The alcoholic solution is chilled and this precipitates much of the poorly soluble, non-volatile matter. The alcoholic solution is then filtered and the alcohol removed by distillation in a vacuum still at the lowest possible temperature.

There are many liquid solvents used by industry, especially petroleum ether, hexane, toluene, methanol and ethanol.

Ether — Diethyl Ether

While ether is immiscible, it does have the problem of being extremely flammable and the toxicity of the vapours requires most careful handling.[3]

Alcohol — Ethanol

The problem with alcohol is that being a polar solvent it will not only dissolve the essential oils, but also mix the water naturally present in the plant matter, thus dissolving many vegetable pigments. For this reason alcohol is not regularly used for the extraction of aromatic materials, and is used only for certain resinous materials.

Volatile Hydrocarbons

The hydrocarbons that are used or have been used include liquefied butane gas, benzene and hexane. Benzene is no longer used as it is carcinogenic. The hydrocarbons are extremely useful solvents for the extraction of aromatic substances from their natural sources. They have a very low viscosity and readily penetrate plant matter provided it is not too compact. Because of their volatility they are readily distilled off from the extract solutions, especially under pressure.[3]

Concerns about Using Volatile Hydrocarbons

Because the hydrocarbons used as solvents are highly volatile, they do present the risk of being highly flammable. The high volatility, however, means that they can be easily distilled off at relatively low temperatures under a vacuum.

While solvents such as benzene used in the past were considered to be extremely hazardous, solvents used today such as hexane are considered safer. The concern about the use of solvents has focused on several issues:

- solvent residues left in the oil
- the destruction of the life force
- many of the solvent-extracted products are used in food flavouring and many countries have introduced strict regulations controlling the use and type of solvents.[1]

Holmes refers to the solvent extraction process as 'dry-cleaning' the plant. Solvent extraction produces a more complete plant extract. However, he says that contact with the solvent, which is usually a petroleum ether, may result in minute traces of solvent in the final absolute. He suggests that from an energetic perspective that this may devitalise the essential oil through contact with a 'dead chemical substance'.[7]

The whole idea of solvent extraction is that it is done at relatively low temperature compared to traditional distillation techniques. I would suggest that the higher temperature of distillation is more likely to damage the life force than the solvent extraction method.

However, in comparing rose absolute with rose otto, Wabner says that rose otto contains synthetic constituents that are not found in nature.[8]

A headspace analysis of a live rose was compared with that of rose absolute of the same flower and rose otto of the same flower. While the chemical constituents of the rose absolute and live rose were similar, rose otto oil contained several constituents such as rose oxide and damascenone that were a by-product of distillation.[8]

Wabner also dispels the long-held belief that rose absolute should not be used in aromatherapy. To support his argument he makes the following comments:[8]

- Water is not more alive than other chemicals (unfortunately).
- Absolutes can be prepared residue controlled and even residue free.
- Most important is that you can lose up to 50% of the constituents found in the living flower. All the water-soluble components remain in the flower water.

Enfleurage

Jasmine season began at the end of July, August was for tuberoses. The perfume of these two flowers was both so exquisite and so fragile that not only did the blossoms have to be picked before sunrise, but they also demanded the most gentle and special handling. Warmth diminished their scent; suddenly to plunge them into hot macerating oil would have completely destroyed it. The souls of these noblest of blossoms could not be simply ripped from them, they had to be methodically coaxed away. In a special impregnated room, the flowers were strewn on glass plates smeared with cool oil or wrapped in oil-soaked clothes. There they would die slowly in their sleep. It took three or four days for them to wither and exhale their scent into the adhering oil. Then they were carefully plucked off and new blossoms spread out.

This procedure was repeated a good, ten, twenty times, and it was September before the pomade had drunk its fill and the fragrant oil could be pressed from the clothes. The yield was considerably less than with maceration.

But in purity, it was unequalled, the jasmine oil radiated the sticky sweet, erotic scent of the blossoms with lifelike fidelity.[9]

Suskind has eloquently described the enfleurage extraction process in which the essential oil naturally released by fragrant flowers is absorbed by highly purified and odourless solid fat or oil.

Fresh blossoms, gathered in the early morning, are placed upon a thin layer of fat spread on a sheet of glass surrounded by a wooden frame known as a chassis. Within 24 to 48 hours, depending on the nature of the flowers being processed, essential oil is transferred from the flowers to the fat, which absorbs it.

After a period of time the flowers are removed from the chassis and are replaced by fresh, recently picked blossoms. This process is repeated until the enfleurage fat is saturated with the essential oil. This product is called an enfleurage pomade, and consists of the original fat and the absorbed essential oil.

Hypercritical Carbon Dioxide

This process produces essential oils of such a unique quality and purity that they differ immensely from the essential oils produced by steam distillation.

Unfortunately, the hypercritical pressure for carbon dioxide is over 200 atmospheres. This is 200 times that of regular atmospheric pressure. This requires very expensive equipment.[10]

The principle of CO_2 extraction is that any substance can exist in three different states: gas,

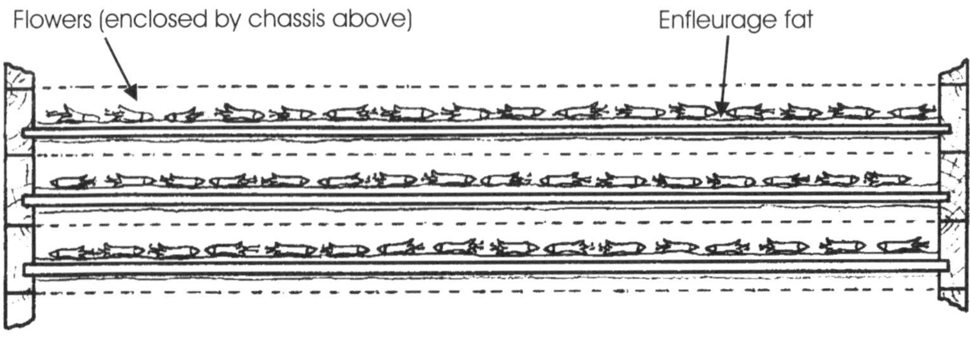

Enfleurage

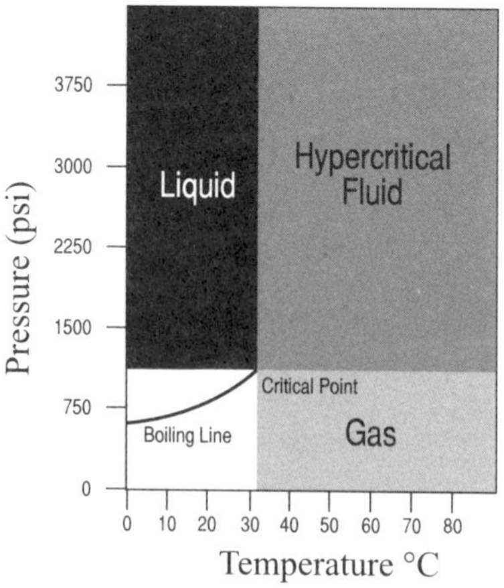

Physical states of carbon dioxide

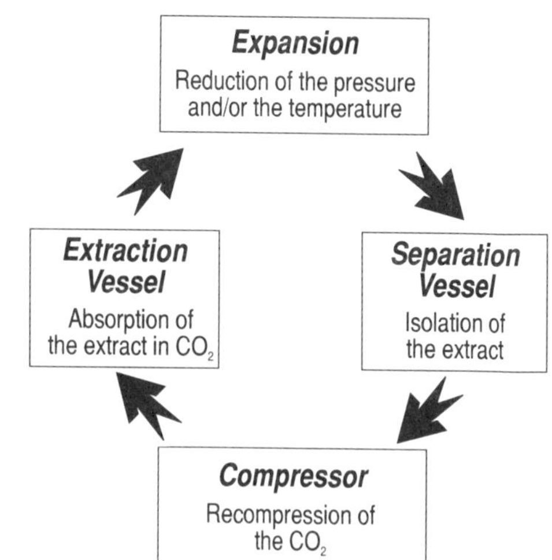

Hypercritical CO_2 extraction process

liquid and solid, depending on its temperature and pressure. In addition, certain substances can be found in the hypercritical state. They are neither liquid nor gas, but rather they are both. The hypercritical fluids disperse as readily as gases and also have solvent properties.

Carbon dioxide is one gas that becomes hypercritical. Its hypercritical temperature is 33°C. Hypercritical carbon dioxide then becomes an excellent solvent of essential oils. The advantage is that the whole operation takes place at a low temperature, and therefore the essential oil is not affected by heat, as may occur in the distillation process.

The extraction process is almost instantaneous and, because the carbon dioxide is inert, there is no chemical reaction between carbon dioxide and the essential oil. Carbon dioxide can then be removed by simply releasing the pressure. The whole process takes place in a closed chamber.

Some of the advantages of carbon dioxide extracts are as follows.[1]

- No organic solvents are employed.
- At low temperatures thermally labile compounds are undamaged.
- There are no off notes, more top notes and more back notes.
- Better solubility because no extra water insoluble monoterpene hydrocarbons are generated during processing.
- No degradation products are formed and the true natural odour and flavour profile is obtained.

The steam-distilled ginger does not contain the non-volatile pungent principles for which ginger is highly esteemed. These constituents are found in the CO_2 extracted oil. This gives the CO_2 extract a more pungent and warming oil which is said to contain up to 20% gingerol and 4% shogaol.[11]

References

1. Weiss E.A. *Essential oil crops.* CAB International, UK, 1997.
2. Guenther E. *The essential oils.* Robert E. Krieger Publishing Company, USA, 1982.
3. Diploma in Perfumery Correspondence Course Notes, Part 2: *Aromatic materials from natural sources.* Perfume Education Centre, Great Britain, 1980.
4. Kerr J. *Steam distillation of essential oils.* Aromatherapy Today, 1999; 11:44–46.
5. Williams D. *The chemistry of essential oils.* Michelle Press, England, 1996.
6. Boland D., Brophy J., House A. eds. *Eucalyptus leaf oils.* Inkata Press, Australia, 1991.
7. Holmes P. *Rose — The Water Goddess.* The International Journal of Aromatherapy, 1994; 6(2): 8.
8. Wabner D. *A rose is a rose is a rose oil.* 2nd Australasian Aromatherapy Conference, Sydney, 1998.
9. Suskind P. *Perfume.* Penguin Books, Great Britain, 1986.
10. Lavabre M. *Aromatherapy workbook.* Healing Art Press, USA, 1997.
11. Arthur D. *Ginger.* The International Journal of Aromatherapy, 1996; (7)4: 20–23.

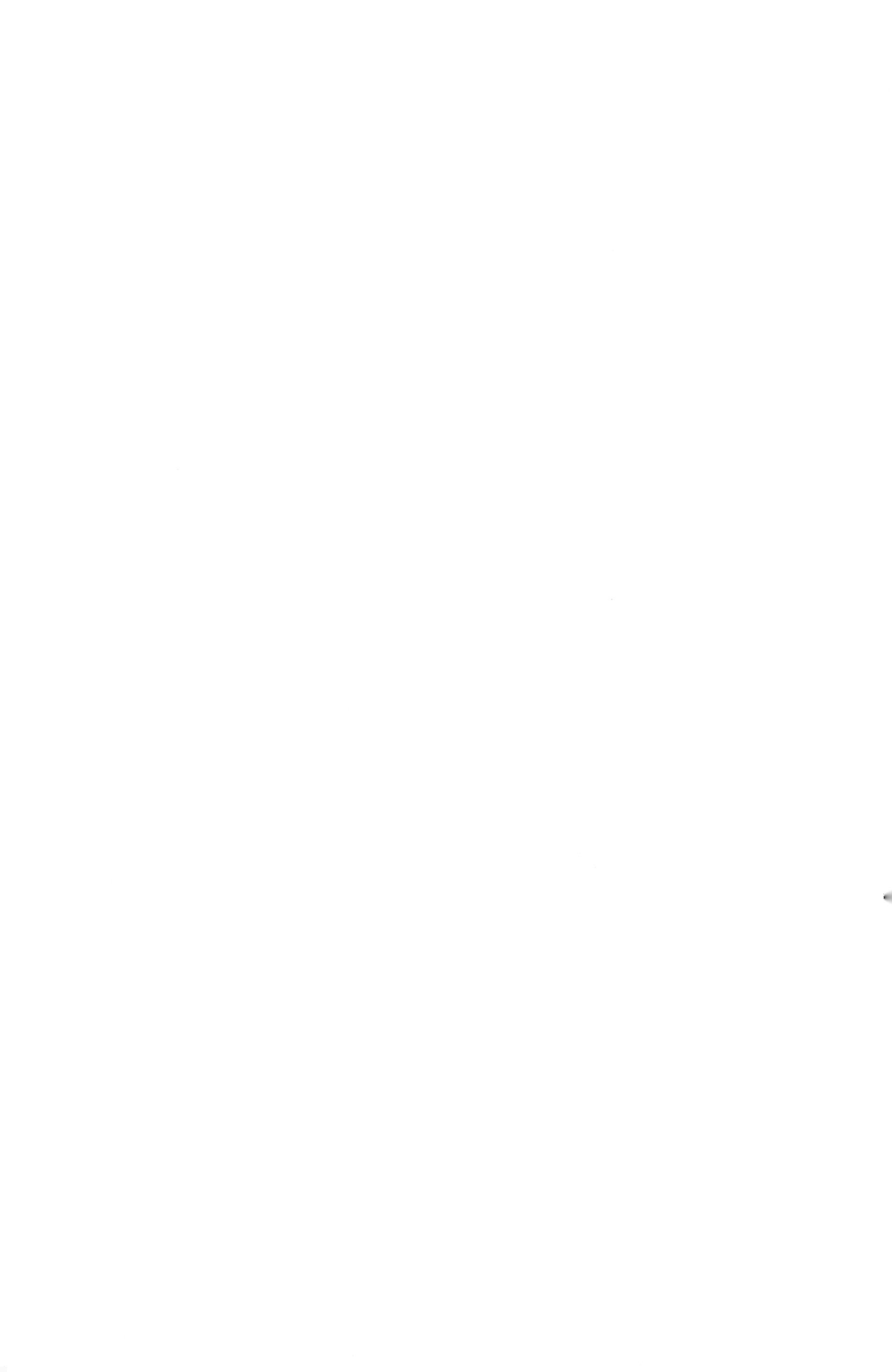

Quality Control and Quality Assurance

Objectives

After careful study of this chapter, you should be able to:

- outline the need for quality control and assurance for essential oils in aromatherapy
- identify the factors influencing the quality of essential oils
- describe the methods used for testing the quality of essential oils
- differentiate between natural and synthetic essential oils.

Introduction

Whether for professional or home aromatherapy use, essential oils of the highest quality should be used. With approximately 5% of the essential oils produced in the world being used for aromatherapy, most essential oils are used for the following purposes:

- food flavouring
- perfumery and fragrances
- pharmaceutical preparations
- chemical manufacturing.

While essential oils produced for each of the above applications are required to be pure, the problem is that the term 'pure' has a different interpretation for each of the users.

The perfume and fragrance industry is interested in consistency of odour and flavour, so they are more inclined to prefer *nature identical* essential oils. *Nature identical* essential oils are often reconstituted from other essential oil constituents to create an essential oil which is similar to that found in nature.

The pharmaceutical industry is interested in the 'active constituent', so they may prefer to use rectified essential oils. To standardise the quality of essential oils it is a common practice to comply with the British Pharmacopoeia (BP), which is often used as an international benchmark.

For example, the BP standard requires a minimum 1,8-cineole content of eucalyptus oil of 70%. If the 1,8-cineole content is less than this the oil must be rectified or redistilled to achieve this standard. From a holistic aromatherapy viewpoint it is recognised that the synergistic action of all the components of an essential oil is far superior to that of the redistilled oil.

The term *pure and natural* used by many suppliers of essential oil simply indicates that no synthetic materials have been added. Essential oils used in aromatherapy must be *genuine and authentic*. This means that the botanical purity of the essential oil should be known and that the oil is unaltered in any way. For an essential oil to be *genuine and authentic,* the following information should be readily available:

- the botanical name
- the part of the plant used
- the country of origin
- the extraction process.

The Botanical Name

If the essential oil is being used for therapeutic purposes, it makes sense that it has been sourced from the proper botanical origins. Often suppliers refer to the essential oils by their common names only. The following examples show that this can be misleading and it is important to specify the true botanical source of the essential oil.

Chamomile

- *Matricaria recutita* — German chamomile
- *Anthemis nobilis* — Roman chamomile
- *Ormensis mixta* — Moroccan chamomile

All three species belong to the *Compositae* (*Asteraceae*) family and are similar in appearance.

Roman Chamomile

A. nobilis or Chamaemelum nobile

Roman chamomile is also known as English chamomile. Roman chamomile oil is predominantly composed of aliphatic esters such as isobutyl angelate and isoamyl angelate. The properties of Roman chamomile are largely influenced by its high ester content. The oil has excellent antispasmodic and sedative properties and it has been used topically to reduce inflammation and accelerate healing.[1]

Roman chamomile oil is generally perceived as having a more pleasing aroma than German chamomile oil and is usually more suitable for its effect upon inhalation, for its sedative and calming properties.

German Chamomile

M. chamomilla, M. recutita

German chamomile is also known as blue chamomile, the major constituents are (-)-α-bisabolol (up to 50%), a sesquiterpene alcohol, and chamazulene, a sesquiterpene hydrocarbon.

The oil has a deep blue colour and a strong, herbaceous medicinal smell. German chamomile oil is well known for its anti-inflammatory properties that have been extensively documented. The α-bisabolol found in German chamomile promotes granulation and tissue regeneration.[2] German chamomile also exhibits antispasmodic, cholagogue and choleretic activity. The essential oil also has demonstrated liver regenerating properties.[3]

Moroccan Chamomile

O. mixta, A. mixta

Moroccan chamomile is a pale-yellow to brownish-yellow oil with a fresh herbaceous, slightly camphoraceous odour. It has antispasmodic, sedative, cholagogue, emmenagogue and relaxing properties and can be used to treat depression, irritability, colitis, amenorrhoea, dysmenorrhoea, liver and spleen congestion.[4]

A typical chemical composition of Moroccan chamomile is:

α-pinene (15.0%), camphene (0.4%), sabinene (0.2%), yomogi alcohol (2.4%), 1,8-cineole (0.5%), limonene (0.8%), santolina alcohol (3.2%), artimesia alcohol (2.3%), trans-pinocarveol (3.0%), borneol (1.0%), bornyl acetate (2.2%), bisabolene (2.5%), germacrene (5.0%), δ-cadinene (0.8%), caryophyllene oxide (0.8%), caryophylladienol (0.7%).[5]

While the properties of Moroccan chamomile overlap with that of German and Roman chamomile, we should refrain from inferring one is better than the other, as each oil is unique.

Cedarwood and Juniper

- *Cedrus atlantica* — Atlas cedarwood
- *Cedrus deodora* — Himalayan cedarwood
- *Juniperus virginiana* — Virginian cedarwood
- *Juniperus mexicana* — Texan cedarwood
- *Juniperus oxycedrus* — Cade
- *Juniperus communis* — Juniper
- *Juniperus sabina* — Savin
- *Thuja occidentalis* — Thuja

There are many more varieties of cedars and juniper trees than are listed above. Some belong to the *Pinaceae* family and others to the *Cupressaceae* family. Both families belong to the conifer class.

Atlas Cedarwood

C. atlantica

The chemical and odour profile of Atlas cedarwood is entirely different from Virginian cedarwood oil. The tree *C. atlantica* is a pine, not a cypress such as the Virginian cedarwood.

It is believed to have originated from the famous Lebanon cedar *(C. libani),* which grows wild in Lebanon and on the island of Cyprus. It is a close botanical relative of the Himalayan cedarwood *(C. deodora),* which produces a very similar essential oil.

The oil is a yellowish to orange-yellow or deep amber-coloured, viscous oil that is occasionally turbid. The odour is described as interesting — with a slightly camphoraceous-cresylic top note and a sweet, tenacious woody undertone.[6]

A typical chemical profile of *C. atlantica* is as follows:

Sesquiterpenes (himachalenes 14.5%, α-himachalene 10%, β-himachalene 42%, cis-bisabolene 1.2%); sesquiterpene alcohols (himachalol 4%, allo-himachalol 2.3%); ketones (α-atlantone 2.65%, γ-atlantone 5%); oxides (himachalene oxide 1%).[7]

Atlas cedarwood is used in aromatherapy for the treatment of acne, dandruff, dermatitis, eczema, bronchitis, catarrh, urinary tract infections, nervous tension and stress-related conditions.[8]

Himalayan Cedarwood

C. deodora

Himalayan cedarwood oil is very similar to Atlas cedarwood oil. It is a yellowish to brownish-yellowish somewhat viscous oil with a rich, herbaceous, camphoraceous, pleasant woody-balsamic undertone reminiscent of Atlas cedarwood.[6]

Virginian Cedarwood

J. virginiana

Virginian cedarwood oil is produced from the distillation of the wood of *J. virginiana*, commonly known as Southern Red Cedarwood.

Virginian cedarwood oil is a pale-yellow to slightly orange-yellow oil that is slightly less viscous than Atlas cedarwood. The odour is at first oily and woody with a sweet balsamic scent typical of cedarwood lumber. The odour becomes drier and more woody, less balsamic as the oil dries out.[6]

A comparative chemical composition of *J. virginiana* and *J. mexicana* is as follows:[9]

Constituent	Virginian cedarwood	Texas cedarwood
α-cedrene	20.0%	21.2%
β-cedrene	6.6%	4.9%
thujopsene	18.9%	29.0%
other sesquiterpenes	13.3%	15.5%
cedrol	31.6%	25.0%
widdrol	4.8%	4.2%

Virginian cedarwood essential oil is traditionally used in aromatherapy for the treatment of respiratory tract infections and for nervous tension and stress-related disorders.[8]

Texan Cedarwood

J. mexicana

The tree has been described as a small and poor-looking relative of the cypress tree. The oil is dark orange to brownish and it has a pleasant, sweet-woody, yet somewhat tar-like or cade-like smoky scent.[6] Texan cedarwood has similar properties to that of Virginian cedarwood.[8]

Cade

J. oxycedrus

The oil of cade is obtained from the destructive distillation from the branches and wood of *J. oxycedrus*, a shrub related to the common juniper.

A rectified oil is then produced by steam or vacuum distillation. Rectified cade oil is an orange-brown to dark-brown, oily liquid with an intense 'tar-like' smoky phenolic odour.[6]

Cade has traditionally been used for the treatment of cutaneous diseases such as chronic eczema, parasites, scalp problems and allergic skin conditions.[8]

Juniper

J. communis

Juniper oil is distilled from the berries, twigs and leaves of *J. communis*. The essential oil from the berries is considered to be the most suitable oil for use in aromatherapy.

It is a clear to pale-yellow oil with a fresh, yet warm, rich-balsamic, woody-sweet and pine-needle-like odour.[6] The oil is traditionally used in aromatherapy for its detoxifying and diuretic properties.[8]

Savin

J. sabina

Native to North America and Europe, it is closely related to common juniper. Savin oil has a high percentage of sabinyl acetate that contributes to savin's toxic properties.

It is considered a powerful emmenagogue and rubefacient, but is an oral and dermal toxin and should not be used in aromatherapy either externally or internally.[8]

Thuja

T. occidentalis

Native to north-eastern America, it is cultivated in France. Thuja is listed in the British Herbal Pharmacopoeia for bronchitis with cardiac weakness and for warts. Thuja essential oil contains over 60% thujone and is considered an oral toxin not to be used in aromatherapy.[8]

Lavender

- *Lavandula angustifolia* — True lavender
- *L. latifolia* — Spike lavender
- *L. x intermedia* — Lavandin
- *L. stoechas* — Maritime lavender

The term 'lavender oil' is meaningless because there are so many species of lavender. The correctly defined name of lavender gives the genus *Lavandula* in Latin, followed by a word which defines the species (e.g., *angustifolia*, *spica*, *stoechas*, *hybrida* etc).

True Lavender

L. officinalis, L. angustifolia

Although lavender has been classified as *L. vera* de Cadolle; *L. officinalis* Chaix or *L. angustifolia* Miller, it is the latter name which is the correct derivation for the most common commercially grown aromatic member of the *Lamiaceae* family.

True lavender is extensively cultivated in Bulgaria and France. It is also produced in smaller quantities in Japan, Morocco, Italy, Algeria, China, Paraguay, Australia and Russia.[10]

Lavender grown and distilled at a higher altitude (from 600 to 1500 m) has a reputation of being the best quality lavender.[6] This is because distilleries located at higher altitudes distil the oil at 92 to 93°C instead of 100°C. This produces an oil with a higher ester content. Even at this small decrease of temperature, hydrolysis of the natural linalyl esters takes place at a much slower rate. A rapid distillation at a slightly reduced pressure will also produce an oil with a higher linalyl ester content.[6]

Spike Lavender

L. spica, L. latifolia

This is a large plant that has close-knit flowerheads with two small side stems. It yields an oil with a camphoraceous scent. The essential oil yield is high, making it an inexpensive oil, and the fact that it grows well at lower altitudes makes farming easier.

Spike lavender has a natural camphor and 1,8-cineole content, making it useful as an inhalation for respiratory infections, for muscular aches and pains and as an insect repellent.[8]

The market demand for spike lavender is much less than that of true lavender or lavandin and it is now produced in much smaller quantities than in the past. Consequently the price of spike lavender is often higher than true lavender.[10]

Lavandin

L. fragrans, L. burnatti

Lavandin plants yield almost twice as much essential oil as true lavender and are easier to grow. Lavandin is a hybrid of true lavender and spike lavender. The lavandin plant is larger and much hardier than that of lavender and is more suitable for large-scale cultivation and harvesting.[10]

Presently, there are three main clones of lavandin:[10]

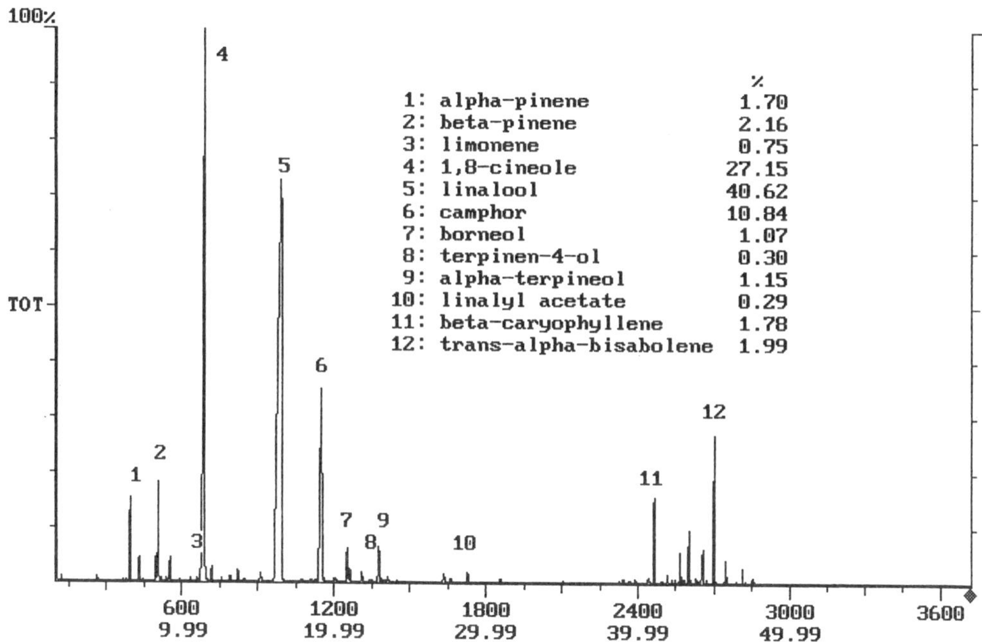

GC-MS analysis of spike lavender — *Lavandula spica*. Courtesy of John Fergeus from Australian Botanical Products.

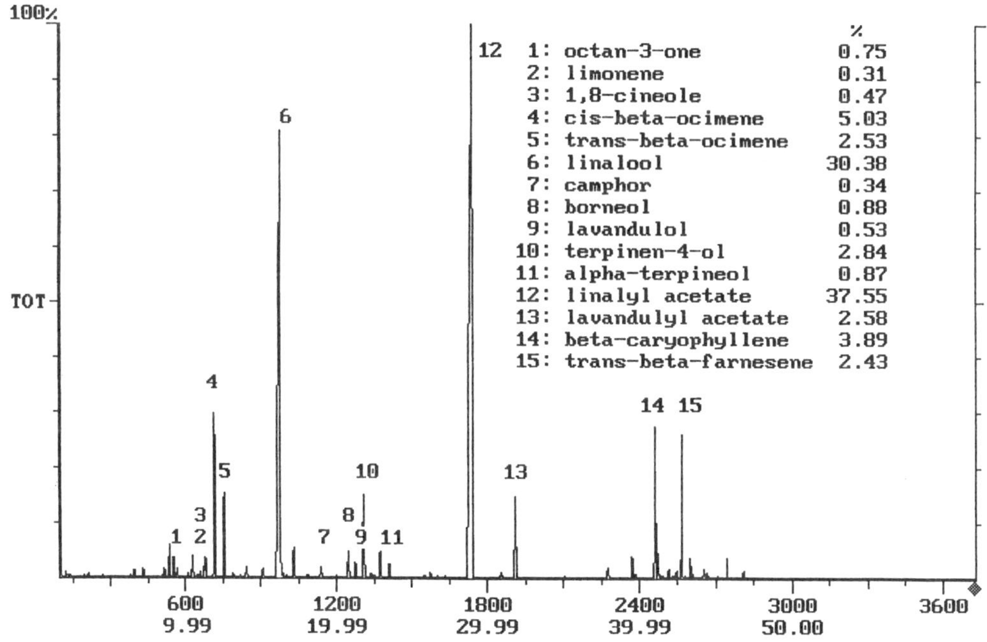

GC-MS analysis of lavender — *Lavandula angustifolia*. Courtesy of John Fergeus from Australian Botanical Products.

- *Abrial* — rich in 1,8-cineole and camphor.
- *Super* — closest in chemistry to *Lavendula angustifolia.*
- *Grosso* — has the highest yield due to bushy habit. It is considered more harsh and terpenic in odour and considered inferior.

Therefore when using lavandin, it is important to specify the particular clone. The Abrial clone is closer to spike lavender in its applications and the Super clone is similar to true lavender. The Grosso clone is rarely used in aromatherapy.[10]

Maritime Lavender

L. stoechas

Maritime lavender is easily recognisable with its two protruding floral bracts.[10] *L. stoechas* is principally used in France for its mucolytic and antimicrobial properties. This is not surprising considering that it has a very high ketone content. It contains approximately 75% camphor and fenchone.[10,11] It is rarely used with children and should be used with caution because of its possible toxicity.[10]

Marjoram

- *Majorana hortensis or Origanum majorana* — Sweet marjoram
- *Thymus mastichina* — Spanish marjoram
- *Thymus capitus* — Spanish oregano

Origanum majorana, also known as *Majorana hortensis*, is the major botanical source of sweet marjoram oil. Sweet marjoram should not be confused with Spanish marjoram (*T. mastichina*) which belongs to the thyme species; oregano (*Origanum vulgare*) which is used to produce oregano oil and with pot marjoram (*O. onites*).[6]

Sweet Marjoram

O. majorana, M. hortensis

Sweet marjoram oil is a pale-yellow or pale-amber coloured, mobile liquid with a warm-spicy, aromatic-camphoraceous and woody odour.[6]

The oil is beneficial for respiratory tract infections, muscular aches, anxiety, depression and insomnia. It can also be used as an emmenagogue for the treatment of amenorrhoea and dysmenorrhea. It is a hypotensive and is used for digestive spasms.[8]

Spanish Marjoram

T. mastichina

This is not a true marjoram and in fact is a species of thyme and is chemically quite different to sweet marjoram oil. It has a high 1,8-cineole content, which gives the oil an aroma reminiscent of eucalyptus.

T. mastichina is recommended for digestive and respiratory spasms because of its antispasmodic properties; for migraines, arthritis and rheumatism because of its analgesic properties and for nervous tension and insomnia because of its sedative properties.[4]

Spanish Oregano

T. capitus

Spanish marjoram is found mainly in Spain, Greece, Portugal, Turkey, Italy and Morocco. Its principal constituent is carvacrol (70–85%) and its composition is similar to that of oregano *(O. vulgare).*

Constituent	Origanum majorana	Thymus mastichina	Thymus capitus
Methyl charvicol	trace	—	—
Terpinen-4-ol	10.7–28.5%	0.7%	0.66%
1,8-cineole	3.7–6.4%	55.0%	—
Linalool	1.0–2.6%	11.1%	2.0%
Sabinene	2.4–4.5%	1.1%	—
Terpinolene	1.9–3.3%	trace	0.07%
α-terpinene	8.4–10.1%	trace	1.2%
Caryophyllene	2.1–4.0%	—	trace
α-terpineol	trace	8.0%	trace
α-pinene	trace	2.6%	0.84%
Cymene	trace	1.3%	15.0%
Myrcene	—	—	2.0%
Thymol	—	—	0.12%
Carvacrol	—	—	62.0%

A typical chemical composition for *Origanum majorana*[12], *Thymus mastichina*[14] and *Thymus capitus.*[13]

Spanish oregano oil is a dark-brownish-red liquid with a strong tar-like herbaceous, but very refreshing odour.[6] The properties of Spanish oregano are similar to *O. vulgare*.[8]

Pine

- *Pinus mugo var. pumilio* — Dwarf pine
- *Pinus palustris* — Longleaf pine
- *Pinus sylvestris* — Scotch pine

There are numerous species of pine that yield an essential oil from their twigs and needles as well as their heartwood.

Scotch Pine

P. sylvestris

The essential oil produced from the Scotch pine is the most widespread variety and commonly used essential oil in aromatherapy. *P. sylvestris* oil is a clear mobile liquid with a characteristic pine, fresh top note with a distinct sweetness.

Longleaf Pine

P. palustris

This species of pine provides the largest source of turpentine essential oils. Turpentine refers to both the crude oleoresin formed as a physiological exudate from the trunk of *P. palustris* or the distilled and rectified essential oil of other *Pinus* species.

Turpentine is recommended as an inhalation for the treatment of chronic diseases of the bronchi with heavy secretion and topically for the relief of rheumatic and neuralgic ailments.[15]

Dwarf Pine

P. mugo var. *pumilio*

Dwarf pine is also known as Swiss mountain pine. This is the favoured pine fragrance for perfumery due to its pleasant balsamic aroma. *Pinus pumilio* has a very pleasant pine-like odour, reminiscent of cypress and juniperberry.[6]

Dwarf pine is often the cause of contact dermatitis, although it is very likely that all pines are potent irritants when oxidised, but not when fresh.[16]

Sage

- *Salvia officinalis* — Dalmatian sage
- *Salvia lavandulaefolia* — Spanish sage

There are several species and cultivars of sage. Mexican sage *(S. azurea grandiflora)* and red sage *(S. colorata)* are used medicinally. Essential oils can also be extracted from Spanish sage *(S. lavendulaefolia)* and clary sage *(S. sclarea)*.[8]

Dalmatian Sage

S. officinalis

The principal source of *S. officinalis* is the Balkans. Dalmatian sage contains thujone, a constituent that is considered toxic in high doses.

S. officinalis essential oil has been used for a variety of disorders such as respiratory infections, menstrual difficulties and digestive complaints.[17] However, *S. officinalis* is not recommended for use in aromatherapy.[8,16]

Spanish Sage

S. lavandulaefolia

Spanish sage is often mistaken for eucalyptus because of its high 1,8-cineole content. It has very little thujone, making it less toxic than true sage, but it should not be used in place of the true sage oil.

Spanish sage is recommended for the relief of muscular aches and pains, arthritis and rheumatism and as an inhalation for asthma and coughs.[8]

Constituent	S. officinalis	S. lavandulaefolia
α-thujone	28.0%	—
β-thujone	8.52%	—
1,8-cineole	11.16%	54%
borneol	13.18%	4.3%
camphene	3.53%	4.0%
caryophyllene	7.15%	—
α-pinene	3.98%	6.0%
β-pinene	trace	7.0%
camphor	0.90%	1.0%
limonene	1.42%	1.5%
terpinen-4-ol	5.09%	—
linalool	—	1.0%

A typical chemical composition of *S. officinalis*[18] and *S. lavandulaefolia*.[19]

Sandalwood

- *Santalum album* — True sandalwood
- *Santalum spicatum* — Australian sandalwood
- *Amyris balsamifera* — West Indian sandalwood

Sandalwood is produced from various species of *Santalum* genus but the oil from *S. album* is the most sought after of the sandalwood oils.

True Sandalwood

S. album

S. album is a small evergreen tree up to 9 m. It is native to and cultivated in the tropical regions of Asia such as India, Sri Lanka, Malaysia, Indonesia and Taiwan. India is the main producer of sandalwood oil.[20]

The oil is a pale-yellow to yellow, viscous liquid with an extremely soft, sweet-woody and almost animal-balsamic odour, presenting little or no particular top note, and remaining uniform for a considerable length of time due to its outstanding tenacity.[6] The quality of *S. album* is determined by its total alcohol content as santalol.

Australian Sandalwood

S. spicatum

Australian sandalwood oil is a pale-yellow to yellow, viscous liquid with a soft, sweet-woody and extremely tenacious odour. It differs from *S. album* in having a rather bitter, sweet top note, and being very resinous.[20]

While *S. spicatum* oil contains less santalols, it contains bisabolols, which indicates that the oil has an excellent anti-inflammatory effect.[21] Anecdotal evidence and clinical studies suggest that the properties of *S. spicatum* are similar to that of *S. album*. Therefore the role of *S. spicatum* in aromatherapy looks very promising considering that the supply of *S. album* has become more restricted.[21]

West Indian Sandalwood

Amyris balsamifera

West Indian sandalwood bears no botanical relationship to true sandalwood or the Australian sandalwood. It grows on the Caribbean islands and neighbouring countries of South America. It is often referred to as amyris oil and it belongs to the *Rutaceae* family. It is a yellow to dark-yellow viscous oil which has been described as having a faintly woody note. It has a mild oily-sweet, balsamic odour which is reminiscent of Guaiacwood.[6] It is considerably different from that of true sandalwood.

It is mainly used as a perfume fixative, in soaps and inexpensive cosmetics.[6,8]

Thyme

- *Thymus vulgaris* — Red thyme
- *Thymus zygis* — Spanish thyme
- *Thymus serpyllum* — Wild thyme
- *Thymus capitus* — Spanish oregano
- *Thymus mastichina* — Spanish marjoram

There are many species and varieties of thyme. It is estimated that there are between 100 and 400 species. The most commonly used species is *T. vulgaris*.

Thyme oil is derived from *T. vulgaris* and *T. zygis*. Two types of thyme oil are produced, red thyme oil and white thyme oil. White thyme oil is obtained from rectifying red thyme oil.[22]

Red Thyme

T. vulgaris

The predominant species is *T. vulgaris*, of which there are up to seven different chemotypes, the most common being:

thymol type
linalool type
carvacrol type
geraniol type
thujanol-4 type[24]

The thymol and carvacrol are located close to the Mediterranean Sea, at a low altitude.[25] The phenol content peaks at the onset of flowering or when the plant is in full bloom.[23]

At higher altitudes between 1,000 and 1,200 m the linalool chemotype is found. Of all the species of thyme, only five have been found with linalool content greater than 50%. These oils smell quite different from the phenol-containing oils. The linalool-rich thyme oils have antibacterial properties, are reputed to be immunostimulants and tonic to the nervous system and are not considered dermal irritants or sensitisers. The geraniol and the thuyan-4-ol chemotypes are considered very rare.[26]

Wild Thyme

T. serpyllum

T. serpyllum is called Mother-of-thyme. There are numerous species and subspecies of *T. serpyllum*. The thymol content of alcohols and monoterpene hydrocarbons in wild thyme is highly variable (47–74%).[22]

Spanish Thyme

T. zygis

Spain produces great quantities of *T. zygis*, which has a high thymol content (50–75%). Various chemotypes of this species also exist: thymol, carvacrol, linalool, geraniol, α-terpinyl acetate and α-terpineol.[25] The thymol chemotype is the most commonly found and commercially available thyme oil from Spain.[25]

Spanish Oregano

T. capitus

Spanish oregano is found in Spain, Greece, Portugal, Turkey, Israel, Italy and Morocco. It has a high carvacrol content (70–85%) and its composition is similar to that of *O. vulgare*.[25]

Spanish Marjoram

T. mastichina

T. mastichina is cultivated in Spain, Portugal and Morocco. It contains mostly 1,8-cineole (60–75%) and linalool (5–20%). Its odour is similar to that of

Constituent	T. vulgaris			T. serpyllum
	Thymol Chemotype	Carvacrol Chemotype	Linalool Chemotype	
α-thujone	4.6%	4.9%	0.26%	1.53%
α-pinene	0.75%	4.3%	0.3%	0.7%
Camphene	0.3%	0.8%	0.27%	0.2%
β-pinene	0.34%	0.35%	—	0.17%
p-cymene	26.0%	33.9%	2.0%	25.0%
α-terpinene	24.0%	44.85%	0.28%	4.85%
Linalool	4.2%	4.2%	77.5%	3.4%
Borneol	0.65%	0.8%	0.2%	—
β-caryophyllene	3.55%	2.5%	2.85	2.5%
Thymol	34.0%	5.5%	2.2%	8.3%
Carvacrol	4.7%	24.5%	trace	14.2%
Geraniol	—	—	—	9.0%

The chemical constituents of several varieties of thyme.[23]

1,8-cineole eucalyptus, making it very different from other thyme species.[25]

The Part of the Plant Used

Many essential oils are produced from the entire plant. However, for some oils the part of the plant used must be specified as the essential oil produced varies qualitatively according to the part of the plant used.

Bitter Orange

Citrus aurantium, subspecies *amara*, is a classic example of a tree from which three essential oils are produced:

- neroli oil
- petitgrain oil
- bitter orange oil.

Neroli oil, water-distilled from the flowers, is a pale-yellow mobile oil which tends to become darker and more viscous with age. It has a powerful, light and refreshing floral top note with very little tenacity.[6]

Petitgrain oil, steam-distilled from the leaves, is a pale-yellow or amber-coloured liquid of pleasant, fresh-floral, sweet odour, reminiscent of orange flowers with a slightly woody-herbaceous undertone and very faint but sweet-floral dry-out.[22]

Bitter orange oil, expressed from the fresh peel, is a dark-yellow to olive-yellow liquid with a fresh citrus odour with a rich, sweet, bitter and dry undertone.

Therapeutically, petitgrain oil resembles neroli oil, though it is slightly less sedative. However, it would be misleading to assume that petitgrain is a substitute for neroli oil.

Bitter orange oil and sweet orange exhibit similar pharmacological activities.[8, 22]

Clove

- clove bud
- clove stem
- clove leaf

Clove bud oil is a clear to yellow mobile liquid, becoming brown with a strong, sweet and spicy odour. Adulterants of clove bud oil are usually clove stem or leaf oil, or clove terpenes remaining after eugenol extraction.[20]

Clove leaf oil is a dark-brown mobile liquid with a harsh, woody, phenolic slightly sweet aroma. The leaf oil is often rectified and is usually a pale-yellow colour with a sweeter, less harsh, dry woody odour closer to that of eugenol.[20]

Clove stem oil is a pale-yellow to straw-yellow coloured liquid of a strong spicy, somewhat woody, but quite pleasant odour. The odour is similar to that of eugenol.[20]

A typical composition of the bud, stem and leaf oil can be differentiated as follows:[28]

Compound	Clove leaf	Clove stem	Clove bud
Eugenol	85–90%	87–92%	80–85%
Eugenyl acetate	0–10%	3–3.5%	8–12%
Isoeugenol	—	trace	—
Caryophyllene	10–15%	6–8%	6–10%
Isocaryophyllene	—	—	0–2.0%

The stem and leaf oil are commonly used to adulterate the bud oil which is considered to be of a superior quality.

Cinnamon

Cinnamon oil can be extracted from both the bark and the leaf. Cinnamon bark has a sweet, warm and spicy aroma with approximately 70% cinnamic aldehyde content. Cinnamon leaf oil is warm and spicy, but lacks the depth and body of cinnamon bark oil. It has a eugenol content of about 75%.

A typical chemical composition of cinnamon leaf and bark oil is reported as follows.

Leaf: eugenol (80–96%), eugenol acetate (1.0%), cinnamaldehyde (3%), benzyl benzoate (3%).[29]

Bark: cinnamaldehyde (40-50%), eugenol (4–10%), benzyl benzoate (1.0%), α-pinene (0.2%), 1,8-cineole (1.65%), linalool (2.3%), caryophyllene (1.35%).[29]

Cinnamon leaf oil is primarily used as a source of eugenol and in perfumes and flavours.

Cinnamon bark is listed in The German Commission E Monographs for internal use for the treatment of gastrointestinal problems and for functional asthenia. However, it is not recommended for topical application because it is a dermal irritant and sensitiser.[30]

The Country of Origin

It is well known that essential oils produced from the same botanical species but grown in different countries can have a distinctly different chemical composition. Factors that may contribute to this include:

- prevailing climatic conditions
- soil type
- genetic factors.

Of particular importance are basil and rosemary.

Basil

According to an extensive analysis of over 200 individual basil plants, five chemotypes of basil oil have been identified:

- linalool
- methyl chavicol
- methyl eugenol
- (E)-methyl cinnamate
- eugenol.[31]

The two most commonly available basil oils are:

- The true sweet basil oil, also known as European or Sweet basil. This oil has a higher percentage of linalool. This oil is generally regarded as safe to use in aromatherapy.[22]
- Exotic or Reunion basil, which is distilled in the Comoro Islands, Malagasy Republic, Thailand and occasionally in the Seychelles. This oil has a higher percentage of methyl chavicol.[22]

The methyl chavicol chemotype basil is more pungent and is reputed to have an antispasmodic effect, whereas the linalool chemotype is reputed to be more sedating and relaxing due to the higher percentage of linalool.[30]

Methyl chavicol is mildly irritating and in high doses a possible carcinogen. It is recommended that basil oil with a methyl chavicol content of 5% or less is used in aromatherapy.[16] For this reason it would be safer not to use methyl chavicol basil in aromatherapy.

Constituent	Origin		
	Comoro Is.	France	Egypt
α-pinene	0.18%	0.11%	0.25%
camphene	0.06%	0.02%	0.07%
β-pinene	0.25%	0.07%	0.43%
myrcene	0.12%	0.13%	0.35%
limonene	2.64%	2.04%	4.73%
cis-ocimene	2.52%	0.03%	0.63%
camphor	0.37%	1.43%	0.57%
linalool	1.16%	40.72%	45.55%
methyl chavicol	85.76%	23.79%	26.56%
α-terpineol	0.84%	1.9%	1.09%
citronellol	0.65%	3.57%	1.76%
geraniol	0.03%	0.38%	0.2%
methyl cinnamate	0.05%	0.34%	0.25%
eugenol	0.74%	5.9%	5.9%

A comparative typical chemical composition of the various chemotypes of *Ocimum basilicum* oil.[27]

Rosemary

Rosemary is another plant which has several chemotypes. Three principal chemotypes of *Rosmarinus officinalis* can be found growing in Europe:

- camphor-borneol
- 1,8-cineole
- verbenone.[24]

Due to their different compositions, these oils can be applied for different purposes to achieve maximum efficiency. Chemotypes with a high camphor content are more effective in cases of muscular aches and pain. The 1,8-cineole chemotype is best used for respiratory congestion, while the verbenone chemotype has excellent regenerative properties and is used in skin care preparations.[24]

Constituent	Origin		
	Tunis	Spain	France
α-pinene	17.1%	18.1%	14.7%
borneol	3.0%	3.1%	6.3%
β-pinene	5.5%	4.8%	5.7%
camphor	14.8%	23.2%	13.1%
bornyl acetate	1.3%	3.4%	1.5%
camphene	6.63%	9.4%	3.6%
1,8-cineole	32.5%	19.2%	25.0%
verbenone	0.4%	0.5%	1.5%
limonene	3.7%	4.0%	7.8%

A typical chemical composition of the principal chemotypes of rosemary oil.[32]

Specifying the Extraction Method

The following examples demonstrate the need to specify the method of extraction when using essential oils for aromatherapy.

Ginger

Ginger oil is produced by steam distillation, occasionally by water and steam distillation of the dried, unpeeled, ground rhizomes of *Zingiber officinale*.

A ginger oleoresin is also produced by solvent extraction of the dried and unpeeled rhizome of *Z. officinale*. Distilled ginger oil's main components are sesquiterpene hydrocarbons (50–66%), oxygenated sesquiterpenes (up to 17%), monoterpene hydrocarbons and oxygenated monoterpenes.[22]

Ginger oleoresin contains mainly the pungent principles gingerols and shogaols as well as zingerone. Shogaols and zingerone are dehydration and degradation products of gingerols.[22]

As a medicinal herb, ginger may be prepared by either decocting the fresh root or by preparing an alcoholic tincture or fluid extract with it. The tincture is considered the most complete preparation as it contains the essential oil constituents as well as the pungent alcohols shogaol and gingerol found in the oleoresin.[33]

While it may be tempting to suggest that the essential oil and herbal extract have similar properties, distilled ginger essential oil contains no pungent components. Therefore, it does not have similar properties to that of a herbal extract of ginger.[33]

However, as the oleoresin contains the pungent and warming components found in the herb, we can expect the oleoresin to have similar properties to that of ginger herbal extract.

Rose

Three main products are obtained from roses: an essential oil, a concrète and an absolute. The essential oil is obtained by steam distillation of the whole flowers, the concrète by solvent extraction of the leaves and flowers and an absolute by further extracting the concrète.[20]

The three products vary from different cultivars or species and also vary from the same cultivar or species grown in geographically separate areas.[20]

Rose otto, is generally accepted to apply to the oil distilled from *Rosa damascena* and it is usually prefixed by the country of origin.[20]

Flowers must be promptly transported to the distillery before being distilled. Rose oil is produced by a two-stage distillation process. It is a common practice to redistill the distilled water, a process known as cohobation.[6]

Rose absolute is obtained by solvent extraction. Holmes refers to the solvent extraction process as 'dry-cleaning' the plant. Solvent extraction produces a more complete plant extract. However, Holmes suggests that contact with the solvent, which is usually a petroleum ether, may result in minute traces of solvent in the final absolute. He suggests that from an energetic perspective that this may devitalise the essential oil through contact with a 'dead chemical substance'.[34]

However, Wabner suggests that rose absolute produced by solvent extraction is superior to the rose otto because rose otto actually contains synthetic constituents that are not found in nature.[35]

He did this by doing a headspace analysis of a live rose and comparing the constituents with that of rose absolute of the same flower and rose otto of the same flower. While the chemical constituents of the rose absolute and live rose were the same, the rose otto oil contained several constituents such as rose oxide and damascenone that were a by-product of distillation.[35]

He also dispels the long-held belief that rose absolute should not be used in aromatherapy. To support his argument he makes the following comments:

- Water is not more alive than other chemicals.
- Absolutes can be prepared free.
- Up to 50% of the constituents found in the living flower can be lost during distillation. All the water-soluble components remain in the flower water.[35]

Rose absolute from *R. centifolia* is an orange-yellow to brown-orange viscous liquid with a sweet, deep-rosy, very tenacious odour. The spicy notes are usually less pronounced, while the honey-like notes are similar to that of *R. damascena*.[6]

Rose absolute from *R. damascena* is an orange-yellow to brown-orange viscous liquid with a rich, warm, spicy-floral and very deep rose odour with a pronounced honey undertone.[6]

Rose otto obtained from *R. damascena* from Bulgaria is a pale-yellow or slightly olive-yellow liquid which is warm, deep-floral, slightly spicy and immensely rich with traces of honey.[20]

Rose otto obtained from *R. centifolia* is colourless to pale-yellow, sometimes with a greenish tinge when fresh. It has a deep, sweet, warm, rich, but less spicy odour than Bulgarian or Turkish rose otto oils.[20]

Ylang Ylang

The large flowers of ylang ylang are subjected to fractional steam distillation or fractional steam and water distillation, thus yielding in succession, ylang ylang extra; ylang ylang 1st grade, ylang ylang 2nd grade and ylang ylang 3rd grade. A complete essential oil is available by non-fractional steam distillation of the flowers or by combining the first three fractions.

In the production of ylang ylang the first fraction of the distillate is collected over several hours and becomes the 'extra' fraction. It is rich in oxygenated constituents but is poor in the high boiling point sesquiterpenes.

The operators of the stills producing ylang ylang oils grade the different qualities by specific gravity and by odour. Since there is no agreed standard, the quality of a given grade varies from one producer to another, a fact that has to be borne in mind when ylang ylang is purchased.

Passing from ylang ylang extra to ylang ylang 1st and 2nd and 3rd grade, the following observations may be made:

- There are decreases in specific gravity, volatility, floral odour character, proportion of oxygenated constituents and price.
- There are increases in sesquiterpene content and oiliness of odour character.

From a perfumer's aspect, ylang ylang extra is the best grade and the most highly valued of the four grades. The traditional use of ylang ylang in aromatherapy as a relaxant and antidepressant indicates that the extra or 1st grade would be more suitable than the 3rd grade, as esters are chemical constituents which have such qualities.

Modification of Essential Oils

The main concern for aromatherapists is:

- dilution
- degradation
- adulteration
- rectification.

Dilution

The label of an essential oil must state the contents and the strength as well as the batch number and expiry date. The strength will indicate if the essential oil has been diluted in a carrier oil. This is often the case with expensive oils such as neroli, rose and jasmine. The correct way to represent this on the label is by specifying the mL/mL. Therefore a 100% essential oil should be represented by 1 mL/1 mL, while a 3% dilution would be 0.03 mL/1 mL.

Degradation

Chemical degradation is a process by which the quality of the essential oil is reduced over time. This usually occurs with essential oils because of prolonged storage, or poor storage conditions. The main factors responsible for essential oil degradation are:

- oxygen
- heat
- light.

Constituent	Extra	1st Grade	2nd Grade	3rd Grade
linalool	13.6%	18.6%	2.8%	1.0%
geranyl acetate	5.3%	5.9%	4.1%	3.5%
caryophyllene	1.7%	6.0%	7.5%	9.0%
p-cresyl methyl ether	16.5%	7.6%	1.8%	0.5%
methyl benzoate	8.7%	6.4%	2.3%	1.0%
benzyl acetate	25.1%	17.4%	7.0%	3.7%
benzyl benzoate	2.2%	5.3%	4.7%	4.3%
other sesquiterpenes	7.4%	28.8%	54.5%	97.0%

A typical chemical composition of the various grades of ylang ylang.[36]

As with most organic products, essential oils have a limited shelf life. This should clearly be shown on the bottle as an expiry date.

Degradation of essential oils occurs with prolonged storage and poor storage conditions. Expired essential oils may not only lose their therapeutic properties, but the chemical changes that an aged oil has undergone may make an essential oil more hazardous. An example is oxidised pine oil, which is more likely to cause dermal sensitisation than fresh pine oil.

Adulteration

Typically essential oils may be adulterated by:

- other essential oils and their constituents
- its own main constituent
- a reconstituted oil
- a pure aroma chemical.

Tests such as optical rotation, refractive index and most important Gas Chromatograph/Mass Spectrometry (GC-MS) can all be implemented to ensure an essential oil has not been adulterated.

Brud says that the availability of true, natural steam-distilled oils that are not blended or treated is very scarce. Due to the high level of blending, mixing and adulteration it is difficult to examine and differentiate a true product from a treated product. He cites several examples where essential oils have been blended with inferior oils.[37]

The first example is geranium oil — *Pelargonium graveolens.* The most sought-after geranium oil is Bourbon. However, this oil is often blended with less expensive geranium oils from other countries such as China, Egypt, Morocco and Algeria.[37] Some people refer to Bourbon geranium as rose geranium, because of its 'rosy' aroma. Most essential oils sold as rose geranium, however, are inexpensive geranium oils distilled over roses, or a blend of geranium and rose odorants.[37]

Often patchouli is blended with other oils such as gurjun balsam oil, copaiba balsam oil, cedarwood, castor oil and aroma chemicals such as 8-camphene, menthanol or isobornyl acetate. These adulterants, however are easily detectable by gas chromatography.[37]

The practice of extension or adulteration of the essential oils may present no great problem when the oils are being used merely for the purpose of fragrances. However, these blended essential oils should not be used in aromatherapy.

The only way to obtain true essential oils for aromatherapy purposes is to have reliable suppliers, either by having direct contact with the manufacturer of the oils or by keeping in contact with a dealer who has enough contacts with producers to offer a full range of the best quality oils available.

Rectification

This means that essential oils are distilled a second time to remove trace constituents. For example, the British Pharmacopoeia standard for eucalyptus requires a minimum of 70% 1,8-cineole content. As some eucalyptus oils have a cineole content less than this, the oil must be redistilled.

Dr Penoel best summarises the concerns of most aromatherapists:

> *Most of the products [eucalyptus oils] found on the usual aromatic market have been redistilled, rectified and refined. In reality, the residue left behind in the still from the rectification of the crude oils is rich in precious molecules (like the rare phenol australol). Even if their proportion seems low, they work in synergy with the main components and should be kept in order for the essential oil to express its full healing potential.*[38]

From a holistic aromatherapy perspective it is recognised that the synergistic action of all the constituents of an essential oil are far superior to that of the redistilled oil. As aromatherapists we should therefore insist on using *'Genuine and Authentic'* essential oils.

Natural Versus Synthetic

Essential oils such as eucalyptus and lavender are readily available in sufficient quantities at reasonable prices. These oils are usually not duplicated in the chemical laboratory. The synthetic substitute would be more expensive than the natural essential oil.

The common problem with these oils is adulteration (with even less expensive similar essential oils). However, this situation is reversed in the case of jasmine or rose. It may take one tonne of rose petals to produce 500 g of rose oil.

Given this situation and the demand for these oils in perfumery, it is not surprising that chemical research has succeeded in producing rather good imitations of these oils. Usually these products smell very nice, and may sometimes be even closer to the fragrance of the actual flower than the true oil. The objective of the artificial fragrance is to duplicate the scent of the flower and not that of the essential oil. It has to be emphasised that synthetic fragrances do not have any of the therapeutic qualities of the essential oil.

Tisserand summarises the way most aromatherapists feel about essential oils:

> *Why natural oils? Why not anything that smells nice whether it is natural or synthetic? The answer is simply that synthetic or inorganic substances do not contain any 'life force'; they are not dynamic. Everything is*

made of chemicals, but organic substances like essential oils have a structure which only mother nature can put together. They have a life force, an additional impulse which can only be found in living things.[39]

However, the following comment summarises the perfume industry's attitude towards the use of essential oils:

The nose of the civilised human being has become more fastidious and demanding. All the rose, mint and lavender fields in the world would not be able to fulfil the needs of hygiene and body care industries alone. The extraction of natural fragrances is difficult and expensive ... The nature identical products which are synthetic substances duplicate their natural counterparts completely in terms of chemical structure as well as fragrance.[40]

Dodd suggests that the aromatherapy argument is faulty:

The chief defect is that aromatherapists are not willing to consider the chemical evidence and so remain in ignorance about current concepts of molecular structure and their relationships to cellular dynamics.[41]

He claims that this belief impeded development of biological chemistry until Wohler synthesised urea in 1828, at which stage it became evident that the chemical substances of living tissues were in all physiological respects identical to the same molecules synthesised in the laboratory.[41]

This argument is valid for the purpose of either perfumery or olfactory experiments. It does not matter whether we use linalool from a laboratory synthesis or a sample that has been isolated from lavender oil, provided that sufficient attention has been given to impurities.

However, research has now proven that individual components of a plant do not always behave in the way we expect when they are isolated and they display their therapeutic properties only in synergy with all the other components of the oil.

Organic Essential Oils

In recent years organic agriculture has gained tremendous support. In 2000 there were more than 17 million acres world wide under organic cultivation.[42]

In Australia, the major certifier of organic produce, the Biological Farmers of Australia, says that the aims and benefits of organic agriculture include:

- satisfying the consumer demand for, and confidence in, verified safe, clean food of high nutritional value
- sustaining and increasing the fertility and biological activity of soils
- enhancing energy and biological cycles in farming systems
- balancing productive farming activities within ecological constraints, preventing or reducing on and off-farm pollution.[43]

It is acknowledged that organic foods are significantly superior to those foods grown commercially in the same soil.[44]

There is no doubt that organically grown plants will produce essential oils of excellent therapeutic activity and of an extremely high quality. Unfortunately certified organic essential oils are still quite rare and expensive. However, as the demand for organic produced products increases, the availability and cost of organic oils will hopefully improve.

The Need for Regulations

In Australia, a Therapeutic Goods Act was legislated in 1990 and regulations required to support the Act were passed in February 1991. This Act brought the Australian therapeutic goods industry under the full control of the Therapeutic Goods Administration, thus providing uniform laws throughout Australia for the manufacture of therapeutic goods.[45]

The promotion and use of essential oils and essential oil products as therapeutic substances mean that essential oil suppliers to the aromatherapy industry have to comply with the Therapeutic Goods Act. The Act requires that all manufacturers of therapeutic goods attain and maintain a licence to manufacture according to the Code of Good Manufacturing Practice (GMP).[45]

The Code of GMP will ensure that a manufacturer of therapeutic goods provides a quality product of consistent quality. The 'quality' of product describes the properties which make it fit for use. These properties are that the products must be pure, have the required efficacy, the correct identity and be safe for use by the general population.[45]

Any product which does not have these four fundamental qualities built into its manufacture and testing should be deemed to present a potential risk to the health and wellbeing of the end user and therefore should not be released for sale. GMP focuses on these quality attributes and ensures they are built into the product throughout all stages of manufacture. Inspection and testing (Quality Control) are used only as confirmation of quality.[45]

Quality is built into a product at every stage of manufacture and following GMP ensures that this happens. To build quality into a product, manufacturers must be disciplined to:[45]

- ensure all the staff receive thorough and continuous training in the requirements of GMP
- develop strict specifications for all starting materials and finished products
- ensure all batches of starting materials and finished products are sampled and tested for compliance with their specifications, using sampling and test procedures
- establish approved procedures and operating instructions for manufacturing all products
- ensure all products are manufactured in a controlled-environment laboratory designed and built to the strictest GMP code
- maintain a detailed batch record system. The batch numbers ensure complete accountability and traceability of the starting material — an essential oil can be traced from the time the manufacturer receives it in its bulk container all the way to the final bottle of essential oil which reaches you, the end user
- monitor the product stability of both starting materials and finished products
- maintain an active self-inspection program to maintain compliance with GMP requirements
- create quality systems and follow set procedures
- ensure that goods are produced according to protocols accepted for registration
- have high quality standards
- have a responsibility to the end user of the product.

Testing the Quality of Essential Oils

To certify the authenticity of an essential oil, it must undergo a series of tests such as:

- organoleptic testing
- physical measures
- chemical analysis.

While odour evaluation is purely subjective, it can be a very effective test for someone with an experienced nose.

Various physical measures carried out on essential oils allow them to be compared with official standards. The density, refractive index and optical rotation are specific values of a pure essential oil that can be measured to establish consistency with a corresponding standard. However, adulterations are not easily detected with these physical tests, therefore it is necessary to turn to chemical analysis. Gas chromatography linked to mass spectrometry (GC/MS) remains the most thorough analysis technique available, as it is able to separate, measure and identify chemical constituents found in essential oils.

Organoleptic Testing

Smell is one of the two senses that responds to the presence of certain chemicals in a qualitative way, and for this reason is known as a chemical sense. The other chemical sense is that of taste, which, together with smell, contributes to the complex sensations we know as flavour.

The organoleptic 'odour' test is considered one of the most important control criteria for testing the quality of essential oils. While it is a very subjective test, it is possible to gain much information about the sensory properties and qualities of the essential oil. Careful smelling requires one to adopt and follow strict procedures, which yield the required information.

Here are some guidelines for adopting the correct approach to smelling.

How To Evaluate an Essential Oil

Essential oils should be evaluated in terms of:

- odour quality — what are the notes present?
- odour intensity
- changes of odour on evaporation
- diffusiveness of odour.

A sample of the essential oil is absorbed to a depth of about 1 cm on a labelled smelling strip, and a sample of the standard is similarly taken at the same time. The strips are smelt for several minutes to compare top notes, again, after 20 minutes to compare middle notes and after several hours to compare base notes. At each stage, the aired sample is compared for odour with a fresh dip.

Odour Description and Classification

As there are no instruments where odour can be measured qualitatively to obtain a numerical value, odour description and classifications are matters of opinion based on human judgement, and as such may be subject to all the vagaries of human nature.

When an attempt is made to describe the qualities of an odour, the difficulty immediately arises that there is a lack of words in the English language which are set aside for the sole purpose of naming individual sensations of smell.

Other senses have their own vocabularies of descriptive terms, which are known and understood sufficiently well for the sensations to which they give rise to be put into words and communicated to the majority of people with fair accuracy. Odours alone are nameless and are usually described by reference to the name of their sources, and by the use of terms belonging to the vocabularies of other senses which have been adopted by the English language for the purposes of odour description.

For example, the odour of lemon expressed oil may be described as:

- *citrus* in reference to the nature of its source
- *refreshing* which is suggestive of an invigorating effect
- *sweet* which is truly descriptive of a sensation of taste but borrowed from usage to express a pleasing kind of odour
- *sharp* which is a term associated with the sour taste of lemon juice, but derived from reference to a finely tapering point or edge.[46]

If one defines the odour of lemon oil as 'citrus' without reference to the other qualifiers, then this description has failed to distinguish the odour of lemon oil from those of sweet orange, grapefruit, lime and bergamot, each of which is 'citrus-like' but different from one another.

Another possible way of describing the odour of lemon oil might be to say that it has the smell of 'lemons'. This expression associates odour-sensations with the names of the corresponding odour sources. This is not only stating the obvious, but it has meaning only for those people who are familiar with the odour in question and who associate it with the same source-name.

Arctander acknowledges the challenge of organoleptic testing:

> *Part of the 'romance' or 'thrill' in perfumery work lies in the fact that, not only are all the materials different in odors but hardly ever will two perfumers give identical descriptions of the same material or the same perfume ... An odor is not 'woody' just because someone says so; it will always have a particular print in your mind. Unfortunately, you are more or less unable to translate this print verbally to fellow perfumers, let alone to laymen.*[6]

However, from the vast multitude of different essential oil odours present, a structure or system needs to be established for grouping together similar odours under appropriate class-names. For the purpose of odour description, there are certain terms, which are in common use throughout the essential oil industry, of which there is a fairly uniform agreement among users of essential oils. These terms fall into two categories:

- odour types
- odour characteristics.

Odour Types

Some of the commonly used terms to describe odour types are:

Anisic

The word 'anisic' refers to the odour of the flavour of aniseed. Liquorice confectioneries are still commonly flavoured with aniseed, and there is a belief that aniseed 'tastes', or smells, like liquorice. Liquorice rhizomes have only a slight, pleasant odour and liquorice extract almost none at all when cold.[46] Essential oils with an anisic odour include aniseed, dill seed and fennel.

Balsamic

A balsam is an oily or resinous material exuded by a plant either as a product of its natural life-processes or in response to injury of its tissues. A considerable variety of odours occurs among balsams; they are usually typified as sweet, warm odours reminiscent of natural vanilla. Balsamic materials are soft and sweet and are usually fixatives and base notes.[46] Essential oils with a balsamic odour include balsam of Peru, balsam of tolu, benzoin and styrax.

Camphoraceous

Camphor is a colourless, crystalline solid having an odour frequently said to be characteristic of the odour of camphor.[46] Essential oils with a camphoraceous odour include cajeput, eucalyptus and rosemary.

Citrus

Citrus odours have the characteristic odour of citrus fruits. While the odours of citrus oils are uniquely different, they all partake of the quality of stimulating freshness which forms an essential part of the odour profile of the citrus type of note.[46] Essential oils with a citrus odour include bergamot, lemon and cold-pressed lime.

Conifer

The refreshing, evergreen tang of the pine forest is essentially invigorating.[46] Essential oils with a coniferous odour include fir, pine and spruce.

Earthy

An earthy scent can be best described as the smell that permeates the air whenever sun-baked soil receives the beneficence of rainfall. There is evidence that the clays present in the soil trap molecules of odorous vapours from the air and then release them when the soil is wet. Essential oils with an earthy odour include patchouli, oakmoss and vetiver.[46]

Floral

The word 'floral' signifies the fragrance of a single flower or of a bouquet of flowers. The term may be useful to describe an odour sensation recalling a flower or flowers.[46] Essential oils with a floral odour include jasmine, rose and ylang ylang.

Fruity
The class of fruity notes comprises odours of the kinds given by whole, edible fruits in their natural condition, by crushed fruits and by fruit juices.[46] Among essential constituents, esters are usually classified as having a powerful fruity note. Citrus notes are usually also classified as fruity.

Green
A green scent is described as having the odour of crushed green leaves. These oils have a breath-takingly natural fragrance quality.[46] Essential oils with a green odour include galbanum and violet leaf absolute.

Herbaceous
The word 'herbaceous' refers to plants that wither away after flowering, while 'herbs' are understood to be those plants that are used in medicines or for culinary purposes. They are somewhat pungent, green and very slightly woody in character.[46] Essential oils with a herbaceous odour include lavender, marjoram, rosemary and red thyme.

Minty
Typically associated with the menthol odour of peppermint or spearmint.

Peppery
A peppery odour will have a characteristically warm dry and spicy odour. It displays a certain pleasant freshness, coupled with a woody note and an 'edge' or 'tingle' which makes it delightfully unique among essential oils.[46] Essential oils such as black pepper and elemi have a peppery odour.

Spicy
Spicy odours give the impression of 'warm', 'hot' or 'pungent'. While everyday experience shows that the sensory properties of individual spices are distinctively different from one another, each also has its own, particular applications in the culinary art.[46] Essential oils with a spicy odour include clove bud, cinnamon and ginger.

Woody
Odours described as woody notes are those of woods such as sandalwood or cedarwood. They are usually unobtrusive and long lasting.[46]

Odour Characteristics

Odour characteristics are terms which are used when the odour cannot be clearly defined by use of the odour names and so it is necessary, if further progress is to be made, to extend the scheme of classification to include descriptive terms representing sensations of odour which are recognisable, but which cannot be associated with any particular physical odour source. The terms are referred to as odour characteristics.

Balanced
A balanced fragrance or blend is one in which neither component overrides the other.[46]

Diffusive
An aromatic material is diffusive if when exposed to the air it rapidly permeates the surroundings with its odour. Oils such as geranium, ylang ylang and violet leaves show this property to a certain degree.[46]

Dry
Odours that give the impression of dryness in association with objects or surroundings are physically dry. Patchouli essential oil has a 'dry' odour. A variation of a 'dry' note is a 'powdery' effect.[46]

Flat
A 'flat' odour impression is one which is featureless and without character.[46]

Fresh
The description of fresh is applied to a fragrance implying a stimulating and enlivening effect. Green and citrus notes are suggestive of freshness.[46]

Harsh
A harsh odour is one which is crude, discordant and imbalanced: a rough and raucous smell. Citronella and red thyme are two classic examples.[46]

Heavy
Among odours considered heavy are jasmine absolute, ylang ylang and tuberose. In undiluted concentrations they permeate the air with a heavy, sombre aroma which is often regarded as oppressive.[46]

Light
Of all the fragrance qualities, lightness of effect is the most delicate, with regard to aesthetic appeal. Lightness of odour suggests high volatility. Neroli and a good quality lavender have such a quality.[46]

Musty
The dry smell of old books and papers is typical of what is meant by a 'musty' note.[46] Essential oils such as patchouli and vetiver have a musty smell.

Rich
A rich odour is described as one which is able to flood the mind with sensation beyond the limit of aesthetic endurance. With rich odours the impression is one of concentration of odours.[46] Oils of rose, ylang ylang and clove bud are known for their richness.

Sharp
Sharpness of odour implies a penetrating effect similar to that found in an excellent quality lemon oil.[46]

Sweet

When an odour is described as 'sweet', this is the kind of sensation which describes an experience of pleasure, it may also denote such terms as 'soft', 'fragrant' and 'delicate'.[46] Examples may include rose or aniseed oil.

Smooth

Smoothness of odour is typical of a soft, sweet fragrances having a balsamic effect.[46] Wood oils such as sandalwood or rosewood would fall into this character.

Warm

The term 'warm' is commonly used for many odours which produce an impression of warmth. It may apply to essential oils such as ginger or wintergreen, which have the association of warming liniments.[46] It may also be used to describe jasmine and rose absolute, which impart the qualities of 'life' and 'warmth'.

Physical Measures

- Specific gravity
- Refractive index
- Optical rotation

Specific Gravity

The specific gravity of a substance is defined as the ratio of the mass of a given volume of the substance to the mass of an equal amount of water at a stated temperature.

$$\text{s.g. (at stated temperature)} = \frac{\text{Mass of a given volume of substance}}{\text{Mass of an equal volume of water}}$$

To measure specific gravity a clean, dry specific gravity bottle of a nominal capacity is accurately weighed. Let us assume that the mass of the bottle and stopper is m1 g.

The bottle is then filled with freshly boiled and cooled distilled water (usually at 20°C). The bottle and contents are then accurately weighed (mass = m2 g).

The bottle is then emptied and thoroughly cleaned before it is filled with the test sample material at the same temperature and weighed with its content (mass = m3 g).

$$\text{Then s.g.} = \frac{m3 - m1}{m2 - m1}$$

Nowadays the specific gravity is measured by means of an electronic specific gravity meter.

The specific gravity of an essential oil is specified by an upper and lower limit as shown following:[47]

Essential Oil	Specific Gravity at 20°C
Bergamot oil	0.882–0.886
Clove bud oil	1.047–1.06
Lavender oil	0.883–0.895

The range allows for natural variations that may occur. If the specific gravity measured does not fall within the limits specified, then there is reason for concern of the quality of the oil. It may indicate that the essential oil has been adulterated with an inexpensive chemical constituent.

Refractive Index

When light passes from one medium to a denser medium, the light is partially reflected, but most of it takes a different path by changing direction at the interface and entering the denser medium at a smaller angle to the normal at the point of incidence than the angle of incidence.

The refractive index is therefore defined as the ratio of the sine wave of the angle of incidence to the sine of the angle of refraction, when a ray of light of defined wavelength passes from air into the essential oil kept at a constant temperature.[48]

The refractive index of an essential oil is specified as an upper and lower limit as shown below:[47]

Essential Oil	Refractive Index at 20°C
Bergamot oil	1.464–1.467
Clove bud oil	1.528–1.537
Lavender oil	1.459–1.464

The refractive quality of an essential oil is very responsive to small changes in the composition of the oil, so an essential oil whose refractive index does not fall within the specified range, may indicate possible adulteration or an oil of poor quality.

The refractive index is measured using a refractometer, an instrument looking much like a microscope.

Optical Rotation

The optical rotation of an essential oil refers to the ability of an essential oil to rotate a plane of polarised light. Light waves are analogous to the waves produced when a rope, secured at one end is flicked at the other end and creates a wave, which moves perpendicular to the surface to which the rope is secured. The wave generated is referred to as a transverse wave.[49]

Ordinary white light consists of transverse waves of different wavelengths, corresponding to the colours of the rainbow, together with the shorter and longer wavelengths. The waves comprising rays of ordinary light.[49]

A polarimeter is used to determine the optical activity of the essential oil. It is a filter which is able to select light waves within a narrow range of wavelengths. To ensure that only light travelling in one plane is used, a 'polaroid lens' is used. This light is referred to as polarised light.

Certain substances (including natural essential oils) have the ability to rotate polarised light in either a clockwise or anticlockwise direction. The polarimeter is able to determine the angle at which the essential oil rotates the polarised light.

Those substances which cause anticlockwise rotation are laevorotatory and are symbolised *l*-, and those which cause clockwise rotation are dextrorotatory and are symbolised *d*-.

The optical rotation of an essential oil is specified as an upper and lower limit as shown:[47]

Essential Oil	Optical Rotation at 20°C
Bergamot oil	+12° to +24°
Clove bud oil	−0° 20′ to −2° 30′
Lavender oil	−3° to −10°

Optical activity is conferred upon a substance by the presence in its molecule of a carbon atom, which is bonded to four different atoms or chemical groups. Such a carbon atom is said to be asymmetric.[47]

The optical rotation of an essential oil is the summation of the optical rotation of its constituents in relation to their proportion in the essential oil. Variations of the proportion of optical active constituents will give rise to a change in the optical rotation of the essential oil. Measurement of the optical rotation is an important aid in detecting of synthetic adulterations to the essential oil.[49, 50]

Chemical Analysis

Chemical analysis of essential oils will identify the components present and determine the amount present.

Gas-liquid Chromatography (GC or GLC)

The term chromatography is derived from the Greek words, *kroma*, meaning colour, and *graphien*, to write.

In gas-liquid chromatography (GC or GLC) mixtures of gases and vapours are separated into their constituents. GLC equipment is able to ensure that every single molecule in the oil is vaporised, but not too quickly. A detector is then able to quantify the amount of constituent present and this is recorded on a graph, which is made up of a series of peaks. Each peak represents one component. The area under the peak is then used to help determine the percentage of the constituent making up the essential oil.[51]

While the GLC is extremely accurate, it has still not told us what each peak is. This is the job of either infra-red spectrophotometry or mass spectrometry.

Infra-red Spectrophotometry

The atoms in molecules are not rigidly bonded together, but tend to vibrate relative to one another in accordance with their mass, the distances apart, the proximity of other atoms and the flexibility of the bonds holding the atoms together.

Infra-red spectrophotometry involves measuring the frequencies at which the molecules vibrate in the presence of infra-red radiation. The infra-red spectrum of a material shows the frequencies at which its molecules absorb infra-red radiation. These are the frequencies at which the molecules are induced to resonate, and are therefore the characteristic frequencies of vibration of the different atoms and group of atoms in the molecules.[51]

Knowing these frequencies which are measured by a spectrophotometer, the analyst can:[51]

- determine the chemical nature of the material under investigation
- determine the quality of the material relative to a standard sample.

Mass Spectrometry

Mass spectrometry can determine the molecular mass of each molecule, thus identifying each constituent of the essential oil.[51]

Conclusion

While the GC/MS analysis technique is remarkable in being able to analyse essential oils, any accurate analysis of essential oils should consider all the techniques that have been discussed in this chapter.

References

1. Fleischner AM. *Plant extracts to accelerate healing and reduce inflammation.* Cosmetic Toiletries 1985; 100: 45–58.
2. Carle R et al. *The medicinal use of Matricaria Flos.* British Journal of Phytotherapy 1992; 2(4): 147–153.
3. Gershbein L. *Regeneration of rat liver in the presence of essential oils and their components.* Food, Cosmetic Toxicology 1977; 15(3): 173–182.
4. Lavabre M. *Aromatherapy workbook.* Healing Art Press, USA, 1990.
5. Lawrence B. *Chamomile oil, wild.* Perfumer and Flavorist 1986; 11(2): 75.
6. Arctander S. *Perfume and flavour materials of natural origin.* Allured Publishing, USA, 1994.

7. Collin P. *Cedarwood.* The Aromatherapist 1996; 3(2): 30–33.
8. Lawless J. *The encyclopaedia of essential oils.* Element Books Limited, Great Britain, 1992.
9. Lawrence B. *Virginian and Texan cedarwood oil.* Perfumer & Flavorist 1980; 5(3): 63.
10. Harris R. *Lavenders of Provence.* In Proceedings of The World of Aromatherapy III. NAHA, USA, 1999; 75–81.
11. Price S, Price L. *Aromatherapy for health professionals.* Churchill Livingstone, UK, 1995.
12. Lawrence B. *Marjoram oil.* Perfumer and Flavorist 1981; 6(5): 27.
13. Soulier J. *The thymus genus.* Aromatherapy Records 1995; 1: 38–49.
14. Lawrence B. *Spanish marjoram oil.* Perfumer and Flavorist 1980; 5(3): 63.
15. Blumenthal M et al. *The complete German commission E monographs*: Therapeutic Guide to Herbal Medicine. American Botanical Council USA, 1998.
16. Tisserand R, Balacs T. *Essential Oil Safety.* Churchill Livingstone, UK, 1995.
17. Valnet J. *The Practice of Aromatherapy.* The C.W. Daniel Company Limited, Great Britain, 1980.
18. Lawrence B. *Sage oil.* Perfumer and Flavorist 1980; 5(1): 55.
19. Lawrence B. *Spanish sage oil.* Perfumer and Flavorist 1980; 5(6): 27.
20. Weiss EA. *Essential oil crops.* CAB International, UK, 1997.
21. Kerr J. *Australian sandalwood.* Aromatherapy Today 2000; 15: 8–12.
22. Leung A, Foster S. *Encyclopedia of common natural ingredients used in food, drugs and cosmetics.* John Wiley & Sons, Inc. USA. 1996.
23. Stahl-Biskup E. *The chemical composition of thymus oils.* The Journal of Essential Oil Research 1991; 3(2): 61–65.
24. Schnaubelt K. *Advanced aromatherapy.* Healing Art Press, Canada, 1995.
25. Soulier J. *Thyme folder.* Aromatherapie Records 1995; 1: 38–49.
26. Soulier J. *Properties and indications: Thymus vulgaris.* Aromatherapie Records, 1995; 1: 50–53.
27. Lawrence B. *Basil.* Perfumer and Flavorist, 1980; 4(6): 31.
28. Lawrence, B. *Major tropical spices — Clove.* Essential Oils: 1976–1977. Allured Publishing Corporation, 1979; 84–145.
29. Lawrence B. *Cinnamon leaf and cinnamon bark oil.* Perfumer and Flavorist, 1978; 3(4): 54.
30. Bowles EJ. *The basic chemistry of aromatherapeutic essential oils.* 2nd edn, Good Scents Aromapleasures, Australia, 2000.
31. Lawrence B. *Essential oils: From agriculture to chemistry.* The World of Aromatherapy III Conference Proceedings, NAHA, 2000; 8–26.
32. Lawrence B. *Rosemary oil.* Perfumer and Flavorist 1982/1983; 7(6); 20.
33. Holmes P. *Ginger oil.* The International Journal of Aromatherapy 1996; 7(4): 16.
34. Holmes P. *Rose — The water goddess.* The International Journal of Aromatherapy 1994; 6(2): 8.
35. Wabner D. *A rose is a rose is a rose oil.* 2nd Australasian Aromatherapy Conference, Sydney, 1998.
36. Lawrence B. *Ylang ylang oil.* Perfumer and Flavorist 1986; 11(5): 195.
37. Brud W. *Blending and compounding.* AROMA'93 Conference Proceedings. Aromatherapy Publications, 1993: 44–54.
38. Peneol D. *Winter Shield.* The International Journal of Aromatherapy 1992; 4(4): 10–12.
39. Tisserand R. *The Art of Aromatherapy.* The C.W. Daniel Company Limited, Great Britain, 1985.
40. Muller J et al. *The H&R Book of perfume.* Johnson Publishers, London, 1984.
41. Dodd GH. *Perfume Oils and Aromatherapy.* From Perfumery: The psychology and biology of fragrance, Chapman & Hall, London, 1988: 27–30.
42. Robbins J. *The Food Revolution.* Conari Press, USA, 2001.
43. *BFA Organic Standards*, Version 4, 2001.
44. Cousens G. *Conscious Eating.* North Atlantic Books, USA, 2000.
45. Battaglia S. *GMP, Quality control and quality assurance.* Aromatherapy Today 1996; 3: 1–21.
46. Diploma Perfumery Correspondence Course Notes. *Part 1: Odours and the sense of smell: Odour description and classification.* Perfumery Education Centre, London, 1980.
47. Williams D. *The chemistry of essential oils.* Micelle Press, England, 1996.
48. ISO 280-1976 (E) *Essential oils — Determination of refractive index.* International Organisation of Standardization, Switzerland, 1976.
49. Clarke S. *Essential oil chemistry for safe aromatherapy.* Churchill Livingstone, UK, 2002.
50. ISO 592-1981 (E) *Essential oils — Determination of optical rotation.* International Organisation of Standardization, Switzerland, 1981.
51. Diploma Perfumery Correspondence Course Notes. *Part 9: Quality control and assurance.* Perfumery Education Centre, London, 1980.

Unit II

Essential Issues

Unit II provides you with the knowledge required to understand how aromatherapy works. Topics include:

- The latest research and clinical trials in aromatherapy.
- The pharmacokinetics of essential oils.
- The chemistry and pharmacology of essential oils.
- The mechanisms of olfaction and the psychological influence of essential oils.
- The subtle effects of essential oils.
- Guidelines for the safe use of essential oils.

Unit II includes the following chapters:

Research into Essential Oils

Objectives

After careful study of this chapter, you should be able to:

- explain the role of research and science in aromatherapy
- explain the placebo effect
- develop an aromatherapy research policy
- identify the different types of clinical trials and research methods
- outline guidelines for conducting a clinical trial.

Introduction

It has been claimed that much of the literature on herbal medicines is based on quasi-scientific studies, folklore, exaggerations and imaginative claims. Many herbal medicines have little or no reliable scientific clinical data to back up their claims, and indications are generally based on traditional uses.

Scientific professionals should keep an open mind and accept that although a substance may lack evidence of efficacy, however this does not mean that it is ineffective.[1] There are many reasons why many herbal remedies have not been evaluated; however, tradition, experience, enthusiasm and anecdotes can be misleading when accepted without sufficient critical examination.[1]

It is with this in mind that this chapter investigates:

- the need for scientific validation of aromatherapy
- some of the more recent scientific validation of aromatherapy
- why scientific validation of aromatherapy is difficult and
- the way in which a scientifically valid trial would be conducted.

The Role of Research and Science in Aromatherapy

An ongoing debate amongst many aromatherapists is what role, if any, science has to play in the future of aromatherapy. It has been said that the traditional basis of aromatherapy provides a completely adequate therapy and that scientific research has very little to offer the therapist.

Schnaubelt warns that scientific validation of aromatherapy often robs aromatherapy of its necessary human element.[2] This issue has also been raised by Anthony, who says:

> *... the nature of complementary therapies is such that double-blind randomised controlled trials, as usually conducted, are rarely applicable, ... therapists question the validity of clinical trials in which the patient's will is not fully engaged through lack of information, and of those not asking the patient how they feel.*[3]

Bone suggests that there might be a fear among natural therapists that plant-based medicine will lose its traditional basis, its insight and soul. There is a fear that aromatherapy will end up being used, like many modern drugs, only for superficial symptom control.[4]

Aromatherapy has become increasingly popular with the general public; the number of persons wishing to study aromatherapy is increasing and the use of aromatherapy within hospitals and nursing homes is gaining popularity.

The increased interest of the public and the medical profession in aromatherapy introduces an urgent need for proper assessment of efficacy. This growth in popularity suggests that aromatherapy is effective in some circumstances, but, without objective assessment, neither the public nor the medical profession can be sure. Rigorous scientific assessment is required.

However, Bone warns us not to embrace what he calls pseudo-science. He states that if we are to incorporate scientific knowledge into our therapies, let it be good science.[4]

This is exactly what Lis-Balchin is concerned about. As an example she cites a 'clinical case study' that was presented at an aromatherapy conference, that suggested that aromatherapy was effective in the treatment of arthritis.[5]

While it may have been true that aromatherapy was beneficial, the point that Lis-Balchin is making is that, without proof, the above study will simply be seen as 'quackery' to the orthodox medical establishment. She suggests that no statistical clinical evidence was presented to show that aromatherapy itself had any medically relevant function other than a 'feel-good' factor.[5]

She also suggested that one must not read into the results what is not there. She says that the design and analysis of clinical studies should be left to the scientific experts. While this comment may be patronising, the fact is that very few aromatherapists have identified the need for research in aromatherapy. It is time for valid 'scientific' research into aromatherapy.[5]

The Benefits of Research into Aromatherapy

There are four broad groups who might be interested in the results of research and scientific enquiry:

1. *The public (patients and consumers).* Consultation with complementary practitioners usually occurs because of word of mouth recommendation or information in the media, not because of the reading of scientific journals. However, the public is indirectly influenced by research through report, in the media and with the safety of medicines of all kinds.[6]
2. *Those speaking for the public.* Although various government departments are involved in monitoring the safety of therapeutic products, they rely on expert medical evidence. They must be convinced of the value of complementary therapies, particularly where legislation is concerned.[6] The Therapeutic Goods Act is the

legislation that monitors and controls all therapeutic goods in Australia.

3. *Practitioners of complementary medicine.* Complementary practitioners often decide to participate in research because they need to justify and protect their therapy from critics and those who might legislate against their practice.[6]
4. *Sympathetic orthodox practitioners.* There are doctors and other health professionals, who have an interest in complementary medicine, who may value research in the area and also conduct it. Their interest is usually outcome-based. Their question is, *Will this therapy aid me in the treatment of patients?*[7]

Research into aromatherapy will be beneficial at many levels. It will:

- satisfy the increasing demand for scientific proof from government legislators regarding efficacy and safety
- allow aromatherapists to understand better how aromatherapy works
- ensure that aromatherapists can practise their skills confidently without the fear of being labelled as 'quacks'
- create a closer working relationship between aromatherapists, scientists and the medical establishment
- ensure that current government legislators see aromatherapy as a viable and beneficial form of health care in the community
- promote pharmacological studies into new essential oils.

The Problems in Pursuing Scientific Research

Most complementary therapists enter complementary medicine because of the desire to practise, but there is very little interest in science or research because they do not form part of either the entrance requirements or the syllabus of many complementary training institutions. This means that complementary therapists who are often called upon to justify their claims, do not have the expertise necessary to provide the evidence that is needed. Most importantly, when you are in private practice, it is not easy to give up the substantial time needed to get involved in a research project.

Schnaubelt articulates the problems in pursuing scientific validation:

> *Once we construct a proper scientific experiment where all variables are kept constant and only one is allowed to change we have a scientifically valid set up, alas it does not have much to do with the reality of aromatherapy anymore. Partly because of these differences, there is very little research directly aimed at the aromatherapeutic processes. Most of the research that aromatherapy enthusiasts rely on is conducted in adjacent fields where effects of terpenes and phenol propanoids are studied for other reasons than aromatherapy.*
>
> *With the apparent interaction between humans and aromatic plants, it is no surprise that human ability to use these plants and oils is rooted much deeper in empirical experience rather than in scientific discovery.*[2]

Mills highlights the problems of pursuing good clinical research:

- To produce results carrying sufficient statistical weight is very expensive and laborious. Herbal medicine (and aromatherapy) in the West can boast no teaching hospitals or research institutes, nor funding by a wealthy industrial sector. The necessary infrastructure is lacking.[6]
- Healing involves an element of purely human contact — the aromatherapist stepping outside his or her own position and into the life of the client is not an event assayable by independent observers or cold analysis, nor predicated by the general conclusions which one might be tempted to draw from such an exercise. Current medical research concerns itself only with measuring events and data divorced from the human being.[6]

Other problems include:

- The essential oils are complex pharmacologically active chemicals. The whole essential oil will have different properties from that of any single constituent alone. Most pharmacological studies involve the use of individual chemical constituents.
- Clinically, essential oils are usually used to evoke healing responses in the body rather than attack the symptoms. This makes it more difficult to compare the benefits of aromatherapy with that of conventional medicines.

Anthony also says:

- Holistic treatments often consist of a number of therapeutic components. It is often difficult to isolate the treatment into its various components.[3]
- Blind designs often used in clinical trials are not very practical for use in aromatherapy, as it is impossible to disguise the treatment. Most aromatherapy treatments will involve essential oils whose odour can not be disguised, some physical treatment and instructions.[3]

- Complementary therapists rarely treat patients with life-threatening disease, and survival is an unlikely endpoint in their studies. The aims of an aromatherapy treatment may range from bringing about a reduction in the discomfort experienced from an unchanged pathology to the eradication of the cause of the symptoms.[3]

Avoiding the Use of Pseudo-science

This problem has arisen because we often attempt to explain 'how aromatherapy works' by using what we think is science.

Bone suggests there is a serious risk that poor science or pseudo-science will render natural medicine an ineffective therapy.[4] Typical mistakes made in pseudo-science are:

- Hypotheses presented as undisputed facts, e.g. oestrogenic essential oils should not be given to people during pregnancy or people with oestrogen-dependent cancers or endometriosis.[4]
- Hypotheses which can be neither proved nor disproved.[4]
- Conclusions based on insufficient evidence.[4]
- Extrapolating excessively from a narrow context of results, e.g. extrapolating from in vitro data to clinical situations without consideration of factors such as dose, metabolism, absorption and distribution of active compounds.[4]
- Quoting obscure or old studies, or studies not published in peer review journals (a peer review journal is one where accepted experts review papers for scientific quality prior to their publication).[4]

The Placebo Effect

A placebo is defined as any treatment (including drugs, surgery, psychotherapy and quack therapy) that is used for its ameliorative effect on a symptom or disease but that actually is ineffective or is not specifically effective for the condition being treated. The placebo effect is the nonspecific psychological or psychophysiological therapeutic effect produced by a placebo, but may be the effect of spontaneous improvement attributed to the placebo.[8]

A placebo treatment may be used with or without knowledge that it is a placebo. Included among placebos are treatments that are given in the belief that they are effective but that actually are placebos by objective evaluation. A placebo may be inert (such as a sugar pill) or active (such as an ineffective drug or drug used at an ineffective dosage), and placebos may include, any treatment, no matter how potentially specific and no matter who administers them.[8]

The term 'the placebo effect' is a phrase which embraces a wide variety of ill-understood effects.[7]

> *The therapeutic impact of 'non-specific' or 'incidental treatment' ingredients to distinguish it from those aspects of a patient's response to treatment which can be unequivocally attributed to some characteristic aspect of the treatment and its presumed 'specific action' on the disorder being treated.*[7]

For example, in the case of a drug, the specific placebo component would refer to any other aspect of the treatment that might exert a therapeutic effect.

The use of the term 'placebo' in research refers to agents or procedures used as controls in experimental studies, whether or not the research includes evaluation of a therapy.[8]

The Placebo Effect in Complementary Medicine

People's knowledge, attitudes and beliefs may lead them towards complementary therapies and a number of different facets of the treatment may persuade an individual that the treatment is worthwhile and should be continued. These factors, along with a variety of other psychological and social influences, may influence the outcome of the treatment.[7]

Examples where psychological factors may play a substantial role in determining the patient's responses to orthodox medical treatments are:

- Recovery from surgical operations can be accelerated if patients receive appropriate psychological preparation.[7]
- Survival following life-threatening diseases such as cancer appears to be influenced by the patient's emotional reaction to the original diagnosis as well as their state of mind during the treatment and follow-up.[7]

These influences are often described by the term 'placebo'. In the case of a drug the specific action refers to the pharmacological effect, while the placebo component refers to any other aspect of the treatment that might exert a therapeutic effect. This might include the expectations of the patient (and the therapist), the power and prestige of the therapist and the credibility of the treatment.[7]

However critics of complementary therapy techniques for which there is no scientific evidence attribute all improvements in the patients treated by these techniques to the placebo effect. To them many complementary therapies appear to have much in common with the largely psychotherapeutic aspects of placebo treatments.[7]

Placebo research is very important to our understanding of the psychological impact of all treatments whatever their nature, for the simple reason that all treatments are in this sense capable of generating 'placebo effects'.[7]

However, the placebo should not be seen as a nuisance variable that merely hinders the evaluation of the drug treatment; it should be seen as an essential element of any approach to therapy which claims to be holistic. Many of the most positive and valuable aspects of the therapeutic encounter contribute to the placebo effect.[7]

Studies of the Placebo Effect

Evidence suggests that placebos administered in an orthodox medical context have induced relief from symptoms in an impressively wide array of illnesses, including allergies, angina pectoris, asthma, cancer, cerebral infarction, depression, diabetes, enuresis, epilepsy, insomnia, Meunière's disease, migraine, multiple sclerosis, neurosis, ocular pathology, Parkinsonism, prostatic hyperplasia, schizophrenia, skin diseases, ulcers and warts.[7]

The placebo response rate varies enormously from study to study and may range from 0 to 100% of patients showing improvement even for the same condition. This variability is not surprising if one considers the apparent benefits of the treatment for any complex condition will depend on the symptoms being targeted and the way the symptoms are measured. Each of these may vary from study to study, as will the overall context in which the study is carried out.

As well as the impact of placebos on symptoms, placebo effects have also been demonstrated on objective measures of certain bodily processes such as blood pressure, lung function, postoperative swelling and gastric motility. This type of evidence reduces the likelihood that placebo effects can be attributed simply to a wish on the patient's part to please the therapist by reporting symptom relief.[7]

In addition adverse effects of placebo administration have been noted in many studies. These include dependence, symptom worsening and a multitude of side effects, both subjective (headache, concentration difficulties, nausea etc.) and objectively visible (skin rashes, sweating, vomiting, etc.).

Understanding the Mechanisms of the Placebo Effect

Attempts to understand the placebo effect typically involve one of two strategies:

- to identify which variables make a placebo response more or less likely
- to test hypotheses about presumed mechanisms of the effect.

The first kind of study has typically looked at patient variables, treatment characteristics or aspects of the therapist and therapist–patient interaction.

Differences between placebo responders and non-responders have long been the focus of interest. Attempts to spot such differences on sociodemographic characteristics such as age, gender, ethnicity and education have yielded weak and inconclusive findings.

Why certain treatments provoke a stronger placebo response than others is still unclear. It has been suggested that technically sophisticated treatments often have greater credibility for the patient and hence generate a stronger expectation of a successful outcome.[7]

Patients seeking complementary therapies often perceive them as being highly credible and effective, which in turn enhances the placebo effect. Studies indicate that those therapists who exhibit greater interest in their patients, greater confidence in their treatments and higher professional status all appear to promote stronger placebo effects in their patients.[7]

Studies of therapist–patient communication have demonstrated the influence of certain therapist behaviours on patient satisfaction and adherence to therapeutic advice. There is reason to believe that the holistic approach adopted by most complementary therapists means that the therapist–patient relationship would play a very important role.[7]

The fact that a patient would actively seek a consultation with a complementary therapist implies that there is a high expectation of benefit on the part of the patient. The patient's expectations have been shown to predict the outcome of psychotherapy and of drug treatments and there is some evidence that expectancy manipulations may influence responses to a placebo. Other investigations have found that therapeutic instructions may influence analgesic responses to placebos and to standard painkillers. However, it was also found that verbal expectancy manipulations alone were not effective in reducing pain.[7]

According to the classical conditioning view, many of the standard procedures of effective non-placebo treatments (e.g. syringes, stethoscopes etc.) have the potential to become conditioned stimuli by their repeated association with symptom relief.[7]

For example — after a while, if a drug is routinely administered by syringe for pain relief, that syringe becomes associated with the relief of pain and comes to have pain-relieving properties itself.

Conditioned drug responses have been demonstrated in animals and in humans.[7]

A distinctive feature of complementary therapies is that in most cases the patient will have actively sought them out, thus increasing their self-perceived commitment. Moreover, many complementary therapies require special efforts on the part of the patient.

Implications of Research on Placebo Effects

It has been suggested that the placebo effect is endorphin-mediated, as it can in some cases be reversed with naloxone. Naloxone is a chemical derivative of opium. It has virtually no action of its own, unless a narcotic drug has been used beforehand. In cases of drug overdose, naloxone by injection produces rapid, often dramatic reversal of the symptoms of overdose.[9]

Whatever the reasons for placebo-induced symptom change, it has become evident that the use of a placebo-controlled condition is essential to the proper evaluation of the specific effectiveness of any form of therapeutic treatment. However it would be careless to ask whether this treatment is a placebo or not; it is more pertinent to ask the following question:

> *In what proportion may the effects of this treatment be accounted for by psychologically-mediated as opposed to direct physically-mediated changes?*[7]

However, when the evidence is not clear and the presumed physical mechanisms of a given treatment are poorly defined and understood, it may be prudent to assume that any given treatment works through any one of a variety of known psychological mechanisms rather than through unknown physical ones. This assumption implies that in the absence of direct evidence from placebo-controlled double-blind trials it is right and proper to regard any new or unusual form of treatment as potentially a form of psychotherapy.[4] This is an extreme, though logically defensible, view that illustrates why the controlled trial, the principal subject of the rest of this subject, has assumed such importance in the scientific validation of healing therapies.[7]

Developing an Aromatherapy Research Policy

A major criticism from complementary medicine is that most research does not meet the required methodological criteria. The claims of therapeutic effectiveness will be taken seriously only when they have been subject to the same rigorous tests as those required in orthodox medicine.[10]

The classical way to test efficacy in orthodox medicine is by clinical trials. The experiment has to follow certain methodological 'rules'. It must:[10]

- compare the effect of treatment with the effect of no treatment (or with other forms of treatment)
- ensure that people who receive treatment are not specifically selected for that group (randomisation)
- ensure control of the placebo effect
- identify a clearly diagnosed illness
- identify a standard treatment for selected patients
- provide for a noticeable change in the value of measured variables
- use measures which are precise, valid and reliable.

Therefore, clinical trials with randomisation and blinding provide the strongest evidence for a relationship between intervention and effect. The most common version of a clinical trial which satisfies these 'rules' is the double-blind trial, where neither the patient nor the person using the treatment knows who is receiving the actual treatment.

Problems Encountered in the Assessment of Complementary Therapies

Complementary therapists are faced with a number of problems in designing and conducting clinical trials. These are:

1. The central problem hinges on the conviction that complementary therapists treat each patient as an individual and the testing of a standard treatment for a standard disease would fall so far short of optimal therapy that the results would be irrelevant.[3]
2. Treatment often consists of a number of therapeutic components.[3]
3. 'Blind' designs are rarely possible with respect either to the therapist or the patient. Most complementary therapies involve some physical treatment, instruction or training that cannot be disguised.[3]
4. Complementary therapists recognise their role as an integral part of the treatment. They appreciate the need for evaluating the safety and efficacy of the individual components of the treatment, however they would expect that the overall effectiveness of the treatment be evaluated from the assessment of the whole therapeutic encounter.[3]
5. Complementary therapists are often aware of the interaction of mind and body, and of their

influence on illness and recovery. This is now supported by recent evidence concerning the interaction of the brain and the immune system Some therapists would go so far as to doubt the validity of any trial in which the patient's potential for self-healing is not fully harnessed.[3]

6. Complementary therapists rarely treat patients with life-threatening disease, and survival is an unlikely endpoint in their studies. The aims of treatment often range from eradication of the cause of the symptoms to no more than bringing about a reduction in the discomfort experienced from unchanged pathology. Objective measure of improvement will sometime be available, but often they will not, and in any case the therapist would rarely be satisfied with an objective criterion alone without finding out how the patient rated the improvement. Subjective data and multiple-ended points are generally not preferred in clinical trials.[3]

The problems identified above indicate that the double-blind randomised control trial, in its standard form, is often not applicable to trials in complementary medicine. However, many of the problems evident to complementary therapy practitioners are also problems at times for orthodox medicine and there are doubts about the applicability of standard trial methodology to some treatment situations within orthodox medicine.

One of the greatest concerns is the appropriateness of the type of questions being asked and of the disease model implied. For the model where a potent treatment 'cures' the condition, the simple question *Is treatment A or treatment B more effective in the treatment of patients with this complaint?* is appropriate, provided that it is accompanied by questions about the possible side effects for the treatment.[3]

A randomised, controlled trial is the method of choice in answering this question, as long as the subgroups resulting from randomisation are comparable with respect to important prognostic variables. With this simple model, comparability can be checked by examining the distribution of markers of the severity of the diseases and of standard demographic factors. There are some treatment situations that conform to this simple model, but there are many which do not conform.[3]

The most common model for treatment in complementary therapies includes situations in which recovery is influenced as strongly by the patient as by the treatment. Here the problems of ensuring and demonstrating the comparability of the treatment and control groups (or two treatment groups) are much more difficult; the larger the number of variables that are recognised as influencing the outcome, the greater the chance that some of them will be poorly distributed, even in studies involving a large number of patients.[3]

The Evidence

Individuals vary in their genetic make-up and in experience, habits, housing, personal relationships, food, stress, exercise, attitude and so on. The complementary therapist is likely to use some of these characteristics of an individual in the planning of optimal therapy. While some of these variables have impressive historical support, there is often very little objective evidence.[3]

However, in reality, orthodox doctors are aware of the importance of the individual in the response to treatment. Much of their traditional wisdom has been lost, as doctors have come to rely on potent treatments because it appeared that the treatment did the healing. It is therefore apparent that individual characteristics of the patient will influence the course of the illness and the responses of the patient to the therapy.[3]

Examining Multiple Variables

There is an unwillingness to look at large numbers of variables in clinical trials, and in particular to look for interactions, on the grounds that if you look at enough factors some will appear significant. This can be a problem for single study. However, if overall patterns are looked for, the likelihood of identical patterns occurring by chance alone is surely inversely related to the number of variables forming the pattern, and to the number of parallel groups examined. Also the number of patients needed for significant results should decrease as the variance attributed to chance is reduced by attributing it to other variables which can be included in the analysis.[3]

Excluding Observer Bias

When a 'blind' study cannot be used, other ways of reducing observer bias must be employed. The most important of these is that an independent assessor, who is unaware of the treatment status of the patient, should undertake initial and final assessments.[3]

The inclusion of overlapping assessments, patient's diary records of pain, analgesic use, activities and the views of the patient's relatives or close friends concerning changes in condition should be considered. All these must be included in the analysis, not just the most favourable. These precautions may actually be more effective than a blind strategy, since there are often signs that disclose the treatment to the therapist, if not the patient.[3]

Factors to Consider when Conducting Research in Complementary Therapies

The most important task facing complementary therapists is to define key research questions. This will involve clarification of conceptual systems used in different disciplines into a form which can be evaluated by empirical data.[11]

Does the Treatment Work?

The question here is whether the patients change for the better as a result of the treatment or would they get better if they were simply left alone?

Often in complementary therapies the positive outcomes of the treatment are gradual and relatively intangible — factors such as emotional and physical wellbeing, healthy lifestyle and more satisfying relationships. Though these factors may be more difficult to assess than specific symptom reduction, they must be included in any comprehensive evaluation of treatment outcome and effectiveness.

Patient Deterioration

Do some patients get worse as a result of the treatment? This possibility is often obscured by the use of group averages which do not differentiate between those patients who do particularly well and those who do particularly badly as a result of a particular intervention.[11]

Therapists are often reluctant to examine treatment failures. However, the identification of deterioration in individual patients in response to a treatment is an essential part of mapping out the optimal range of applications for particular treatments and specifying contraindications.

Durability

The temporal aspects of treatment and recovery are often overlooked in comparisons of outcome of patient groups at a particular point in time.

There are real clinical and practical difficulties involved in producing and evaluating long-term effects, but they are an important aspect of comprehensive treatment evaluation. For example, research into addictive disorders has shown relatively good short-term effects following treatment, followed by consistently high relapse rates within three months following the treatment. It would be interesting to determine whether positive lifestyle changes would influence the duration of the treatment.[11]

Comparative Effectiveness

Complementary therapies include a diversity of disciplines that share some basic common features, such as a concern with treating the whole person, as well as unique conceptualisations of human disease and distress and associated interventions.

An important part of comparative research must be the appraisal of the conceptualisations and procedures of each discipline, in their own terms and in relation to each other, to provide a meaningful context within which comparative outcome studies can be designed and interpreted.[11]

Causal Mechanisms

What aspects of treatment are necessary, sufficient or facilitative of therapeutic change? This question can be addressed by identifying the main components of the treatment and assessing the outcome in patient groups receiving the different combinations of these components.[11]

Therapist Factors

The questions here are what influence do the personal qualities of therapists have on the treatment outcome, and do they bear any systematic relation to professional discipline or training?

Psychotherapy research has found that a wide range of practitioner qualities can affect the process and outcome of the therapy, including personality, interpersonal style, belief, values, gender, power, attractiveness, socioeconomic status and length and type of professional experience. [11]

Patient Factors

As with therapists, a wide range of patient characteristics has been shown to affect the treatment outcome. Research has found that patients' perception of the therapist's qualities, such as warmth, empathy and genuineness, are predictive of treatment success or failure in a variety of therapeutic contexts. By contrast, direct measures of therapist verbal and nonverbal behaviour thought to be expressive of these qualities have not shown consistent links with outcome.[11]

Conducting Research in Aromatherapy

Asking the Right Questions

There are three kinds of questions that can be asked when planning research into aromatherapy. It is important that we understand the difference between these questions, as they can often be a source of frustration and confusion to the person conducting the research:[12]

- Is there an effect?
- If there is an effect, how does it work?

- If there is an effect and we have some idea of how it works, then how can we modify things so that the effect can be intensified?

It is important that the questions be addressed in the order presented. It is advisable that people commencing research for the first time deal with questions of the first kind only. This will allow experience and expertise to build up before tackling the more complex questions of the second type.

Question two involves a discussion of whether aromatherapy works by means of pharmacological mechanisms or more psychological processes.

The following fundamental questions for research into complementary therapies must also be asked:[7]

- Does the therapy have a beneficial effect on any individual disease or disorder?
- Does the treatment have any advantage over existing treatments in terms of efficacy, safety, patient preference, cost and availability?
- Is the effect primarily due to the pharmacological action of the remedy or is it a placebo effect?
- What mechanism might underlie the therapy's action?

There is also a range of 'process' questions, primarily of concern to practitioners. These might concern the reliability and validity of diagnosis, the value of individual techniques and approaches in the overall treatment package, the role of the practitioner in the treatment process and perhaps the attitude of the patient.

How Do you Measure an Experience?

Kirk-Smith stresses the importance of using 'objective' observations (e.g., measurement by a device) where possible over 'subjective' observations (i.e., self-reporting by patients or reports by clinical staff about patients).[13]

The reason for using 'objective' measures is that patients and staff may over- or underestimate the changes depending on what they think the study is about.

The Use of Graded Scales

Graded scales can be used by an observer or by the patient. They are useful to assess things such as pain or wellbeing. Grade 1 may be used to indicate 'no pain' while Grade 5 may be used to indicate 'pain as bad as I have ever experienced'. Assessments need to be frequent enough to give adequate data but not so frequent that they cause the patient any unnecessary distress.[14]

These scales can be used by the observer or by the patient. A tick box format is usually used.

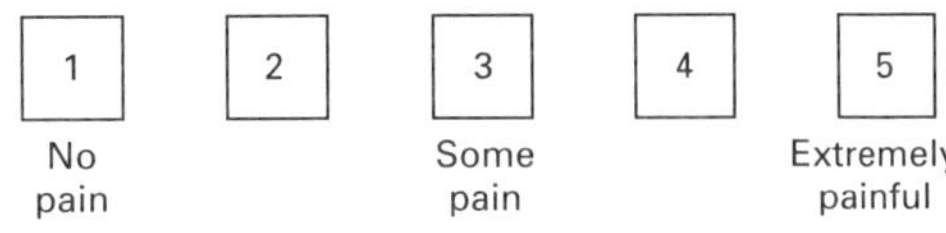

This scale is generally easier to administer and handle statistically. Some say that the analogue scale gives greater accuracy. However, there is evidence that nervous subjects tend to always mark the centre of the visual analogue scales.[14]

The Different Types of Studies

Most studies can be classified as either observational or experimental. In observational studies the researcher simply observes what is happening to a population and has no control over the conditions. In general, observational studies take the form of either surveys or case-control studies.

Experimental studies are generally clinical trials. They are designed to evaluate the effects of various treatments, and the researcher specifies the conditions under which the study is conducted.

The main concern in either type of study is that one uses the results based on a limited sample of participants to make inferences or decisions about the population of interest. How confident we can be about the claims we make on the basis of our sample depends critically on the structure and design of the study.

Single Case Studies

Case studies have always been used as guides to the study of rare clinical situations, for the reporting of new information about side effects of treatment or for introducing views which challenge the existing theories of disease. The clinical account of a single case study was once the primary form of medical knowledge. Unfortunately, it is now dismissed as 'unscientific'.[15]

This is where there is often a split between the clinician and the researcher, the researcher emphasising correlation, generalisation and statistical significance while the clinician emphasises application, specificity and significance to the patient.

However, we must be aware of some of the problems that often arise in single case studies:[13]

1. The patient might have been getting better already.
2. The illness might be in remission.
3. Some unknown external factors might cause improvement e.g., change in the patient's personal situation, diet or even the weather.
4. Some other known internal factor might cause improvement e.g., when the treatment consists of several different elements. (This is often the

case in aromatherapy that involves the oils and the actual massage itself).

5. Some unknown internal factor might cause an improvement e.g., the therapist may give unconscious and subtle cues to the patient; one of many possible 'placebo' effects.
6. The patient may feel obliged to report an improvement to please the clinician.
7. The expectations of the therapist may bias the change in the patient's condition.

The principal feature of single case studies is that they are feasible. The study is not expensive and the results are generally evident. The primary focus of research is upon the treatment benefit for the individual, whereas conventional studies are more concerned with changes in groups of patients. A weakness of single case studies is that, while individual change is specific, it is difficult to argue for a general validity of the treatment.

Simple Comparative Open Trial

A simple comparative open trial is a comparison of treatments in groups of patients by controlling or equalising all variables except the administration itself. In the simplest case there is some form of comparison of one treatment with another.[14]

It is important that patients are selected randomly in each of the groups. This will ensure that bias is eliminated.

Simple Single-blind Comparative Trial

Bias can be reduced by a simple single-blind comparative trial. The investigator knows what treatment the patient has been given, but the patient does not. The use of an independent assessor (i.e., not the therapist) decreases errors due to bias to an even greater extent.[14]

Double-blind Trial

This technique is used for many drug trials. Neither the patient nor the investigator is aware of what treatment the patient is taking. For many forms of complementary medicine this type of design is, unfortunately, impossible to use.[14] How can you disguise the fact that someone is receiving an aromatherapy massage?

Cross-over Versus Non-crossover Design

In a non-crossover trial one group of patients is given the treatment to be tested and the other group some form of dummy treatment or placebo.[14]

The advantages of the non-crossover trial are that there are no carry-over effects from one treatment period to another, and the timing of treatment can be precisely regulated to be the natural history of the disease process.[14]

In a crossover trial one group of patients is initially given the experimental treatment and the other the dummy or standard treatment. Once the effect of these has been established the group given dummy treatment is changed to the active treatment and vice versa.[14]

The advantages of the crossover trial are that fewer patients are required and that variability between patients is lessened.

Experimental Research

Apart from clinical trials already discussed, the questions of research models for studying the action of essential oils are the most difficult. As part of the modern move away from animal experimentation, increasing attention is being paid to techniques for assessing the effects of drugs on cultures of cells, tissues and organs in vitro. Conventional drug research is switching to this direction for preliminary screening in drug discovery programs.

The problems are the limited application of such observations to the in vivo situation and the need to confirm any in vitro findings anyway. It is also impossible to actually know which plant constituents have actually reached internal tissue after absorption. Nevertheless, in vitro techniques may provide valuable supplementary information to other research, as in the following suggested projects:

- The absorption of essential oils on epithelial tissue culture (to reduce the possibility of skin irritation)
- The influence of essential oils on microbiological cultures (much work has already been done in this area, but there are still many questions that remain unanswered)
- Alteration in the migratory behaviour and internal metabolism of macrophages as a result of exposure to essential oils. (There are many claims that the essential oils improve resistance to infection by general enhancement of the defensive mechanism; looking directly at macrophage response is an established screening technique.)
- Using psychophysiological changes such as sweat, saliva, blood and urine to measure emotional responses to the odour of essential oils. This might also include the measurement of electrical potentials generated within the brain which are recorded using an EEG.

There are problems using animals in clinical trials to support research into essential oils. Apart from the difficulty of applying such findings to the human situation, there are extremely strong ethical objections from almost all of those who support the use of aromatherapy. Perhaps we need to develop research along the lines of a therapy system that aims to support the vital functions.[6]

If the intention of any trial was to assess the effects of essential oils applied in therapeutic doses adjusted for body weight and metabolism, there could be little complaint that the animals would be harmed and that they would in fact be likely to benefit. This type of experimentation has already proven to be successful in finding evidence of the sedative properties of neroli when mice were exposed to neroli oil vapours.[16]

Feasible studies might include observing behavioural and social changes after administering the essential oils, and the effects of antimicrobial remedies on the normal resistance of diseases among large populations. These studies would be valuable in veterinary practice.

Stages of a Clinical Trial

While it may be unfeasible to suggest that reading this chapter will provide you with the skills to be a successful researcher, it will provide you with the knowledge required to understand how scientific research is conducted. Furthermore, the information in this chapter may provide a useful foundation for an active collaboration between aromatherapists and researchers.

The following stages are involved in conducting a clinical stage:

- planning (defining the precise purpose of the clinical trial)
- design (how to conduct the clinical trial)
- conduct (doing the clinical trial)
- analysis (making sense of the data)
- interpretation (drawing conclusion).[17]

The following questions should be asked by any prospective researcher:[18]

- Is the project part of an ongoing academic collaboration?
- Is the study model or disease clear and generally accepted?
- Are the planned interventions of demonstrated clinical value?
- Have the therapists' skills been proven?
- Are the remedies of good quality?
- Are the outcome measures clear and have they been previously validated?
- Has bias been eliminated as much as possible?
- Have you obtained ethical consent?
- Have you obtained fully informed patient consent?
- Are your patients suitable?
- Are you planning a publication in a peer review journal?

While the above list may be daunting, it is important that if aromatherapy research is to be taken seriously then it is imperative that they all be addressed before embarking on research.

Presenting a Clinical Trial

The following layout should be used when presenting a research paper.[19]

Title

Summary

This is also referred to as the 'abstract'. It is usually around 250 words and is essentially a very short version of the rest of the document, briefly covering the background, the work already done, the conclusions and ending with the main recommendation.

Introduction

This section provides the background to the research. It should also identify research that has already been done on the subject so that researchers will:

- not repeat what has already been done
- find out the different issues and ways of doing research
- not make mistakes in your research
- identify where the real gaps in knowledge are.

Important statements made must be backed up by references to their sources. Unfortunately, most of the evidence in aromatherapy books and magazines is 'anecdotal' or 'informal'.

Method

It should be detailed enough so that someone else can duplicate the research. Often the following subsections are required:

Subjects
Who was tested, how they were selected and why.

Materials
The oils used, how they were applied, how the treatment was done.

Measures
How the outcomes were measured.

Design
How the overall research was designed. It is important to ensure that a critic cannot say 'This other factor might have caused the results'. If the initial design is faulty no amount of rewriting or re-analysis will correct it.

Procedure

This section should outline practical details of what happened.

Results

The results actually detail what happened in the form of tables, graphs and the results of statistical tests with short descriptive texts drawing out the main points.

Discussion

The discussion gives the interpretation and consequences of the various results sections. The discussion should consider the following:

- Interpretation of the results in terms of previous work referred to in the Introduction.
- Drawing attention to interesting or surprising aspects of the results and their implications.
- Identify improvements that can be made for future studies.
- Suggest future research that should be done.

References

Where the background information came from.

Appendices

Supporting details not needed in the text.

Conclusion

As the momentum for the use of essential oils in aromatherapy grows, it is inevitable that the scientific scrutiny will be greater.

Such scrutiny can be harsh in its requirements for evidence. Aromatherapists need to develop research principles similar to the ones outlined in this chapter or else face the possibility of being denied our rights to treat people holistically using essential oils.

References

1. Rotblatt M, Ziment I. *Evidence-based herbal medicine.* Hanley & Belfus, USA, 2002.
2. Schnaubelt K. *Conference report,* The International Journal of Aromatherapy, 1997; 8(3): 5.
3. Anthony H. *Some methodological problems in the assessment of complementary therapy.* In *Clinical methodology for complementary therapies.* Lewith G, Aldridge D. eds, Hodder & Stoughton, United Kingdom, 1993.
4. Bone K. *Science, "scientism" and pseudo-science.* The Modern Phytotherapist, 1995; 1(3).
5. Lis-Balchin M. *Conference report.* The International Journal of Aromatherapy 1997; 8(1): 4.
6. Mills S. *Out of the earth: The essential book of herbal medicine.* Viking Arkana, England, 1991.
7. Vincent C, Furnham A. *Complementary medicine: A research perspective.* John Wiley & Sons, England, 1997.
8. Shapiro A, Shapiro E. *The powerful placebo.* The Johns Hopkins University Press, USA, 1997.
9. Lewith G. *Every doctor is a walking placebo.* In *Clinical methodology for complementary therapies.* Lewith G, Aldridge D. eds, Hodder & Stoughton, United Kingdom, 1993.
10. Wiegant FA, et al. *The importance of patient selection.* In *Clinical methodology for complementary therapies.* Lewith G, Aldridge D. eds, Hodder & Stoughton, United Kingdom, (1993).
11. Carter D, Nanke L. *Emerging priorities in complementary research.* In *Clinical methodology for complementary therapies.* Lewith G, Aldridge D. eds, Hodder & Stoughton, United Kingdom, 1993.
12. Kirk-Smith M, Stretch D. *Clinical trials II.* The International Journal of Aromatherapy, 1994; 6(1): 32–35.
13. Kirk-Smith M. *Clinical trials IV.* The International Journal of Aromatherapy, 1996; 7(3): 33–39.
14. James I. *Tactics and practicalities.* In *Clinical methodology for complementary therapies.* Lewith G, Aldridge D. eds, Hodder & Stoughton, Great Britain, 1993.
15. Aldridge D. *Single case research designs.* In *Clinical methodology for complementary therapies.* Lewith G, Aldridge D. eds, Hodder & Stoughton, Great Britain, 1993.
16. Jager W, et al. *Evidence of the sedative effect of neroli oil, citronellal and phenylethyl acetate on mice.* Journal of Essential Oil Research, 1992; 4(4): 381–385.
17. Crichton N. *The importance of statistics in research design.* In *Clinical methodology for complementary therapies.* Lewith G, Aldridge D. eds, Hodder & Stoughton, Great Britain, 1993.
18. Monckton J. *Research protocol.* The International Journal of Aromatherapy, 1993; 5(3): 4–5.
19. Kirk-Smith M & Stretch D. *Clinical trials I.* The International Journal of Aromatherapy, 1993; 5(4): 28–32.

Essential Oil Chemistry

Objectives

After careful study of this chapter, you should be able to:

- define organic chemistry
- explain the basic concepts of the chemistry of essential oils
- define the main classes of constituents found in essential oils
- identify the functional groups found in essential oils
- summarise the properties of each main class of essential oil constituents.

Introduction

The purpose of this chapter is to establish basic scientific criteria in which the actions of the essential oils can be identified.

Essential oils consist of an immense array of chemical constituents. However, until recently, very little emphasis has been placed on the chemistry of the essential oils. Most of the knowledge on the therapeutic uses of essential oils has relied on anecdotal evidence handed down over the centuries.

However, the increasing role of science in medicine demands that therapeutic claims be supported by scientific scrutiny.

> *The obvious point to make, of course, is that a great many people have already found herbal medicines effective, and all those using them will have strong anecdotal evidence of their apparent benefits. Compared with the experience of most modern drugs, the human use and approval of most herbal remedies is awesome. The requirement by the medical and scientific establishment for research to 'prove' that herbs are effective is not found among the population at large. It is almost certain that the recourse to herbal remedies as a popular option will outlive the current era of inquiry.*
>
> *Nevertheless, a challenge has been thrown down: "If what you say is so valuable and powerful, then it should stand up for itself in any forum."*[1]

I believe that aromatherapy is able to stand up for itself in any forum and the knowledge and understanding of the chemistry of the essential oils has given aromatherapy scientific credibility.

Organic Chemistry

In the early days of chemistry, scientists said that there were two classes of compounds. One class was produced by living organisms — these substances were called 'organic'. The other class, found in minerals and rocks was called inorganic.

It was also a belief of the time that organic compounds could not be synthesised from inorganic compounds. It was believed that the 'vital force' possessed only by living organisms was necessary to produce organic compounds.

However this theory was disproved in 1828 by Friedrich Wohler. He heated an aqueous solution of two inorganic compounds, ammonium chloride and silver cyanate, and to his surprise obtained urea.[2]

This fits the old definition of 'organic' because urea has been isolated from human urine. This single experiment of Wohler's was enough to disprove the 'doctrine of vital force'. This meant that the words organic and inorganic no longer had real definitions, since, for example, urea could be obtained from both sources. A few years late, Friedrick Kekule assigned the modern definition — organic compounds are those containing carbon.[2]

The chemistry of living organisms is no longer called organic chemistry; today that branch of science is called biochemistry.[2]

Sources of Organic Compounds

With 107 elements other than carbon to choose from, you would expect there to be many more inorganic compounds than organic compounds, but in fact the opposite is true. There are known to be more than three million organic compounds, but only about 200,000 to 300,000 known inorganic compounds. Furthermore thousands of new organic compounds are becoming known each year.[2]

The key to the chemical characteristics of an atom is in its configuration of electrons, which determines the kinds and number of bonds it will form with other atoms. Carbon has a total of six electrons, with two in the first electron shell and four in the second shell. Having four valence electrons in a shell that holds eight, carbon has little tendency to gain or lose electrons to form ionic bonds. It completes its valence shell by sharing electrons with other atoms thus acting as an intersection point from which a molecule branches off in up to four directions.

This electron configuration makes carbon, of all the 108 known chemical elements, unique in the ability of its atoms to catenate; that is, to bond or link up with one another in seemingly endless arrangements of chains, branched chains, rings, multiple rings, combinations of chains and rings and so on.

The possible number of these arrangements that exist in the essential oils is staggering and carbon's ability to form so many compounds is due to:[2]

- Carbon atoms form stable bonds with other carbon atoms, so that both long and short chains of carbon atoms, and even whole networks, are possible.
- Carbon atoms also form stable bonds with certain other atoms, including hydrogen, oxygen, nitrogen, the halogens, and sulphur.
- The valence of carbon is four, which can be made up in many different ways so that many combinations and arrangements of atoms are possible.

Besides carbon atoms, a carbon-based molecule contains hydrogen atoms, and may contain atoms of other elements, such as oxygen, nitrogen and sulphur. The branch of this chemistry that is concerned with the study of carbon-based chemicals is known as organic chemistry, from its original association with substances from living things. Despite this, today innumerable carbon compounds that are known apparently do not occur in plants and animals.[2]

The Structure of Organic Compounds

Organic chemistry molecules are made up of hydrocarbon structures. A hydrocarbon is a compound containing only hydrogen and carbon atoms. Even with only two elements, there are many thousands of known hydrocarbons and a much larger number of possible ones that have not yet been synthesised. There are several families of hydrocarbons:

- Alkanes which have only single bonds.
- Alkenes which have C=C double bonds.
- Alkynes which have a triple bond between two carbon atoms
- Aromatic hydrocarbons which have benzene rings.[3]

When all the carbon atoms in a hydrocarbon molecule are bonded to the maximum number of other atoms (which is 4 other atoms), the molecule is said to be saturated.

Isomers

Variations in the architecture of organic molecules can be seen in the form of isomers. These are compounds that have the same molecular formula but different structures and hence different properties.[2]

Structural Isomers

Structural isomers differ in the covalent arrangement of their atoms. The number of possible isomers increases tremendously as carbon skeletons increase in size. There are only two butanes, but there are 18 variations of C_8H_{18} and 366,319 possible structural isomers of $C_{20}H_{42}$. Structural isomers may also differ in the location of double bonds.

The positioning of the double bond often determines the prefix attached to the name of the molecule (e.g., alpha, beta, gamma or delta — these are often written in Greek letters).

Positional Isomers

Positional isomers differ in the position of the same functional group in their molecules. See example.

$CH_3—CH_2—CH_2—CH_3$

Butane

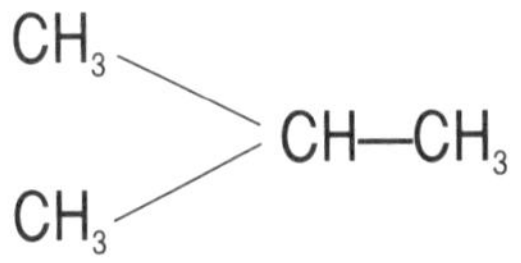

$(CH_3)_2CH—CH_3$

iso-Butane

Example of structural isomers.

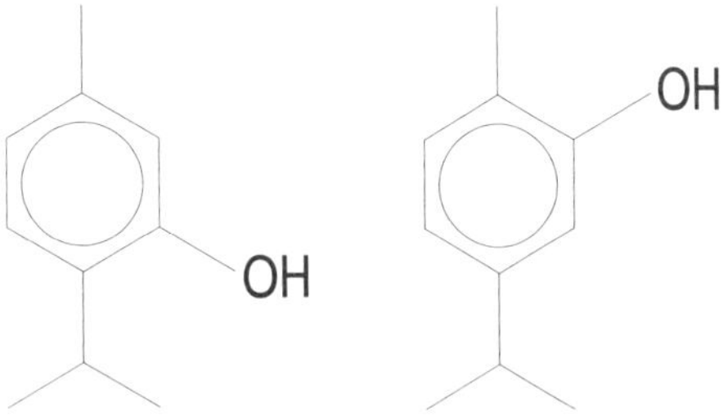

Thymol
(e.g., thyme, ajowan)

Carvacrol
(e.g.,oregano, thyme)

Example of positional isomers.

Functional Group Isomers

Functional group molecules contain the same atoms (as they must to be isomers), but the functional groups are different. For example, the molecular formula for ethyl alcohol is C_2H_6O.

- A molecular formula shows which atoms, and how many of each are present in a molecule.
- A structural formula shows not only all the atoms present in the molecule, but also all the bonds that connect the atoms to each other.

The structural formula for ethyl alcohol is:

```
     H     H
     |     |
H —  C  —  C  —  O  —  H
     |     |
     H     H
```

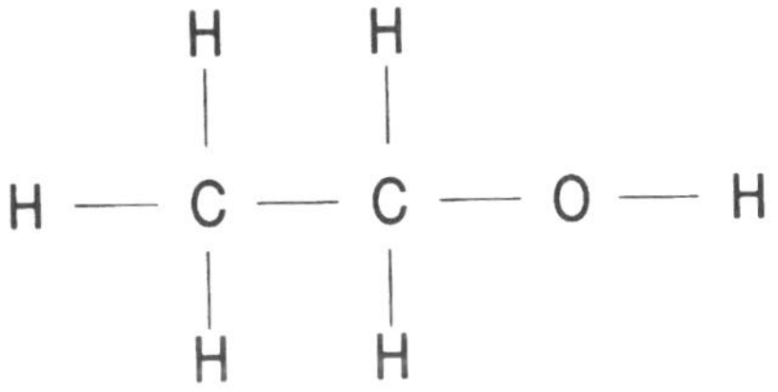

However, ethyl alcohol is not the only compound whose molecular formula is C_2H_60. An entirely different compound, dimethyl ether, is also C_2H_60. The ether functional group is simply an oxygen atom bonded to two hydrocarbons. The structural formula for dimethyl ether is:

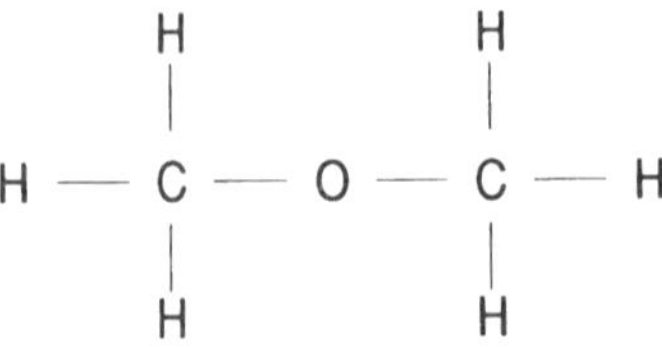

Property	Ethyl Alcohol	Dimethyl Ether
Physical state at room temperature	Liquid	Gas
Boiling point (°C)	78	-23
Melting point (°C)	-117	-138
Reaction with sodium	Yes	No
Poisonous (in moderate amounts)	No	Yes
Anaesthetic (in small amounts)	No	Yes

Comparison of the properties of ethyl alcohol and dimethyl ether.[2]

Geometric Isomers

When a molecule is unsaturated, the double bond does not readily permit rotation around its axis, fixing the different groups into their position. When identical groups are on the same side of the double bond, the isomer is called a *cis*-isomer, when the identical groups are on the opposite sides of the double bond, the isomer is called a *trans*-isomer.

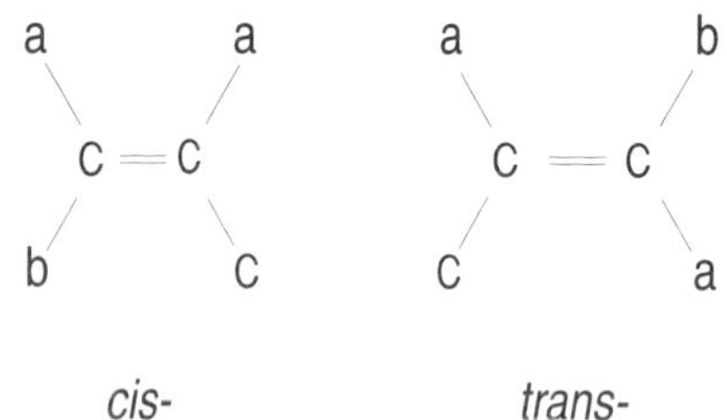

The cis/trans relation is generally used when the attached groups are not identical, but located on opposite sides of the same double bond in different isomers.

Geranial and neral are examples cis/trans isomers found in essential oils. Geranial is also known as α-citral and neral as β-citral.

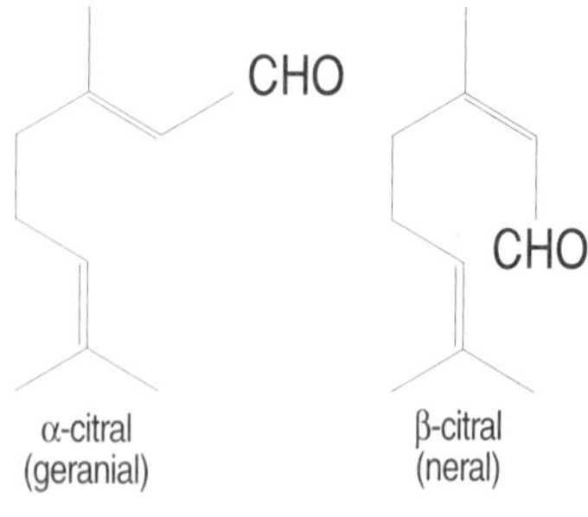

Optical Isomers

Some organic compounds have the power of rotating the plane of polarised light. The molecules which are optically active are those that contain one or more asymmetrical carbon atoms, that is, carbon atoms which are bonded to four different atoms or groups of atoms.

For simplicity, let us consider P, Q, R and S to be four different functional groups. C represents a carbon atom to which these groups are bonded. The compound is represented by the following formula:

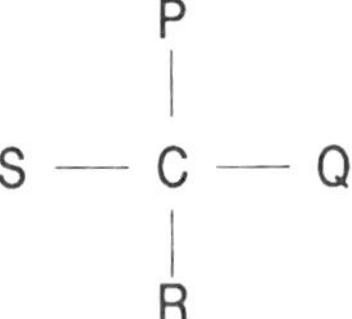

This molecule will be optically active, and can exist in two forms, the molecules of which are mirror images of each other, and cannot be superimposed. The central carbon atom, being bonded to four different atoms or groups, is the asymmetric carbon atom in this molecule.

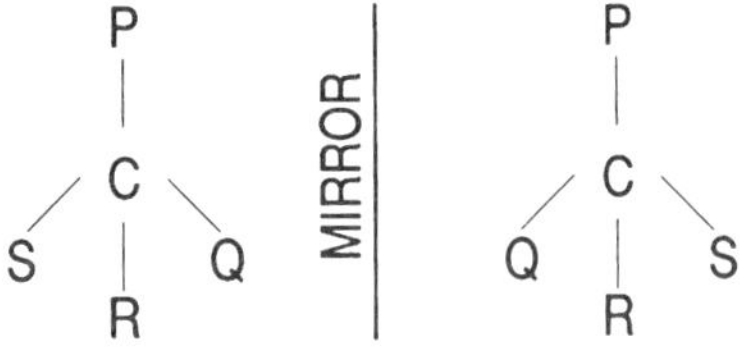

The isomers are usually called the *d*-isomer and *l*-isomer. These molecules will have similar physical properties, but differ in their ability to rotate polarised light. Naturally occurring optically active compounds usually consist of *d*-isomers, whereas those synthesised in a laboratory usually contain equal amounts of *d*- and *l*- isomers. These are refered to as racemic mixtures, which are optically inactive as the two rotations cancel each other out. Most essential oils exhibit optical isomerism. According to Bowles this makes them far more biologically active than synthesised mixtures which contain equal amounts of *d*- and *l*- isomers.[7]

Worse, the inactive isomer may produce harmful side-effects. This may have been the case with thalidomide, the sedative that caused many birth defects in the early 1960s. The drug was a mixture of two optical isomers, only one of which has since been demonstrated to cause birth defects in rats.[3]

Nomenclature

In aromatherapy, the older names for essential oil constituents are used. It would be almost incomprehensible to say, for example, '1-iso-proyl-4-methyl-cylclohexan-2-ol' when 'menthol' is all that is required. The complexity of the essential oils needs not be further complicated by the unnecessary use of long chemical names where short ones will do, provided that the latter are known to, and understood by, all concerned.[2]

The advantage of the I.U.P.A.C (International Union of Pure and Applied Chemistry) nomenclature is, of course, that it is systematic, and can be used to name any molecule, whether or not the substance has a short name.[2] It is not in the scope of this book to discuss the procedure of naming aroma chemicals according to the I.U.P.A.C.

The Chemistry of Common Essential Oil Constituents

Almost all of the molecules found in essential oils are composed of carbon, hydrogen and oxygen. The chemistry of the essential oils is usually determined by two factors:[4]

- the extraction process
- the biosynthesis of the constituent molecules by the plant.

Steam distillation is a process that extracts only volatile and water-insoluble constituents of the plant such as the terpenes and terpenoid compounds and phenyl propane-derived compounds. Many other constituents in the plant do not find their way into the essential oil. Among them are the molecules that are soluble in water, such as acids, sugars and molecules that are too large or too high in polarity to evaporate with steam, such as tannins, flavonoids, carotenoids and polysaccharides.[4]

Schnaubelt says that two basic biosynthetic pathways are responsible for almost all essential oil constituents. Terpenes, sesquiterpenes, diterpenes and triterpenes are all the products of the terpenoid or mevalogenic biosynthesis pathway.[5]

The other large group of constituents belongs to the phenyl propanoid group. They are by-products of the amino acid metabolism and share the amino acid phenyl alanine as the starting point of their synthesis.[5]

Terpenes are biosynthesised from mevalonic acid which itself is formed from the formation of carbon chains from the acetyl groups. The carbon chain of interest is the isoprene unit. Methylbuta-1,3-diene, also known as isoprene, is the molecular structural unit from which all terpenoid molecules are derived.

Terpenoid molecules are made up from the branched 5-carbon units, known as the isoprene unit.

$$CH_2{=}C(CH_3){-}CH{=}CH_2$$

The isoprene unit.

In essential oils we encounter predominantly terpenoid compounds. Terpenoid compounds are chemical compounds whose backbone consists of 10, 15, 20 or 30 carbon atoms. (Multiples of the 5-carbon isoprene unit). While terpenoid molecules with 30 and 40 carbon atoms are found in plants, they are not found in the essential oils. Their molecular weight is too high to allow evaporation with steam.

These terpenoid compounds are present in essential oils as plain hydrocarbons such as monoterpene hydrocarbons or sesquiterpene hydrocarbons or as oxygenated constituents, usually defined by the functional group.

Class of Compounds	No. of Isoprene Units	Occurrence
Monoterpenes	2	Essential oil constituents, iridoids
Sesquiterpenes	3	Essential oil constituents
Diterpenes	4	Components of essential oils and resins, Vitamin A, phytol, gibberellins
Triterpenes	6	Squalene, steroids, heart glycosides
Tetraterpenes	8	Carotenoids, xanthophylls
Polyterpenes	µ	Rubber, gutta-percha

Terpenoid compounds commonly found in nature.[6]

In some essential oils, terpenes are original constituents which are synthesised by the living tissues of the plant and survive the processing of the essential oils; an example is the expressed citrus oils, all of which contain high proportions of natural terpenes.

In some essential oils, such as rose and lavender, the bulk, or the whole, of the terpene content is formed during processing by the action of hot water and steam upon the thermolabile constituents of the essential oil. It has been found that when oils are solvent extracted, instead of distilled, the absolutes obtained are either very low in terpenes or do not contain them at all.

The Major Classes of Molecules Found in Essential Oils

There are three major classes of essential oil constituents:

- monoterpenes and their derivatives (monoterpenoids)
- phenyl propane derivatives
- sesquiterpenes and their derivatives (sesquiterpenoids).[4]

These three groups make up the bulk of practically all the common essential oils. Trace constituents do exist that don't fall into the above categories. Often the trace constituents have unusual chemical structure and many impart a strong overall olfactory impression of a particular oil.

While it would be reasonable to assume that such trace components can have a pronounced influence on the pharmacological action of the essential oil, these shall not be discussed here.

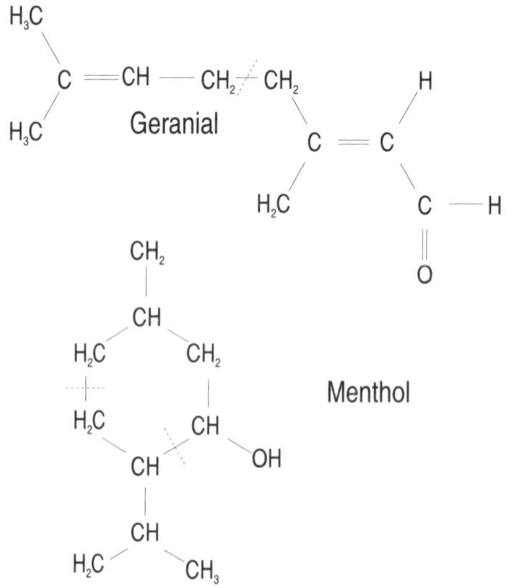

Geranial

Menthol

Two examples of isoprene units joined to form monoterpene compounds. Geranial is a major constituent of geranium and menthol is found in peppermint.

Some of these essential oil constituents include those that have either nitrogen or sulphur atoms included in them. Examples of essential oil constituents containing nitrogen are methyl anthranilate found in neroli oil or indole found in jasmine oil. Essential oil constituents containing sulphur include the sulphides or disulphides found in oils such as asafoetida or garlic oil. These oils tend to have a putrid and pungent odour.

Monoterpene Hydrocarbons

Monoterpenes are found in all essential oils to a greater or lesser degree. Schnaubelt says that the distillation process may influence the concentration of monoterpenes found in an essential oil. Some of the factors are:[6]

- The pH at which the distillation is carried out.
- The pressure and temperature at which the distillation is carried out. High temperature and pressure tend to create a higher concentration of monoterpene hydrocarbons whereas low pressure temperature distillation tends to create an oil richer in alcohol ester and C-15 constituents.

Monoterpenes are known as hydrocarbons, having 10 carbon atoms with at least one double bond. They are classified as either open chain, monocyclic, bicyclic or aromatic. All monoterpene hydrocarbons end in -ene.[7]

Properties

Monoterpenes oxidise rapidly and extensively.[4, 7, 8] The oxidation is said to contribute to the antiseptic properties, and to the skin irritant properties.[7]

Essential oils from citrus rinds and pine needle trees have a proportion of monoterpene hydrocarbons. Monoterpenes are: analgesic[5, 7, 8], antispetic[4, 7, 8], antiviral[4, 5, 8], decongestants[5, 7, 8], general tonics and stimulants[4, 5, 7], hormone-like.[5, 7]

Sesquiterpene Hydrocarbons

Sesquiterpene hydrocarbon molecules have 15 carbon atoms and at least one C = C, and a varying number of hydrogen atoms. All sesquiterpene hydrocarbons end in -ene.

Essential oils produced from plants of the Asteraceae family are relatively high in sesquiterpene hydrocarbons:

Essential Oil	Approximate % of Sesquiterpene Hydrocarbons
Chamomilla recutita	Up to 35%
Helichrysum italicum	Up to 50%
Achillea millefolium	Up to 35%

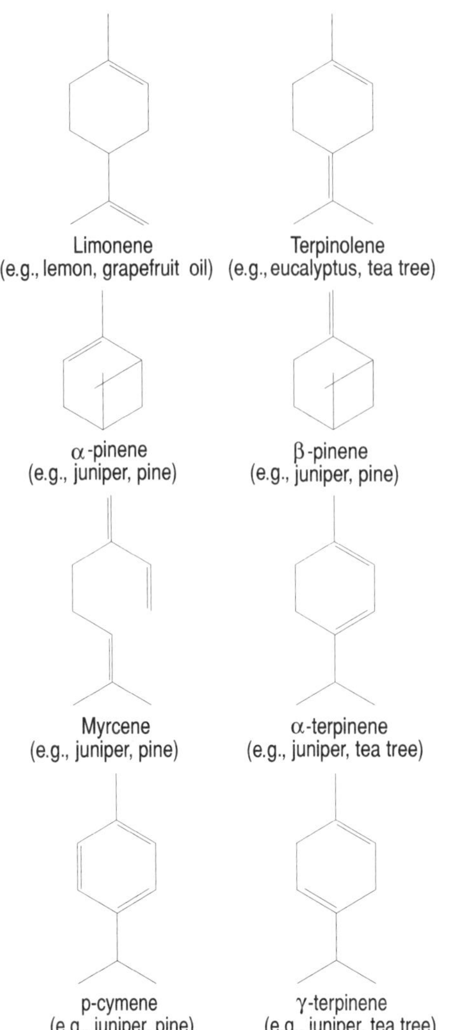

Some monoterpene hydrocarbon structures found in essential oils.

Properties

Schnaubelt says that it is not easy to attach a label of the general effects to this group of compounds.[6] According to Lavabre the influence of the carbon-backbone on the overall character of the molecule can increase with its size. It is not surprising that sesquiterpenes can have such a diverse and individual effect on the overall property of the essential oils.[4]

The sesquiterpene hydrocarbons β-bisabolene and zingiberene, found in ginger oil, are responsible for the oil's anti-inflammatory properties. Clove and black pepper also contain a high percentage of the sesquiterpene hydrocarbon caryophyllene, which contributes to the oil's effectiveness against viruses.[4, 5]

The main properties of sesquiterpenes that have been extensively documented are their anti-inflammatory and antiphlogistic properties.[4, 5, 7, 8]

Functional Groups

A functional group is a small part of an organic molecule consisting of a single atom or group of atoms that substitutes for a hydrogen atom and has a profound influence upon the properties of the molecule as a whole. It is often referred to as the chemically active centre of the molecule.

Many properties of essential oils can be accounted for by the functional groups made up by different combinations of oxygen-containing molecules such as alcohols, aldehydes or ketones. Generalisations can be made, but specific actions of the constituents will be as varied as their structure.

As the physiological properties of molecules are strongly dependent on their functional groups,

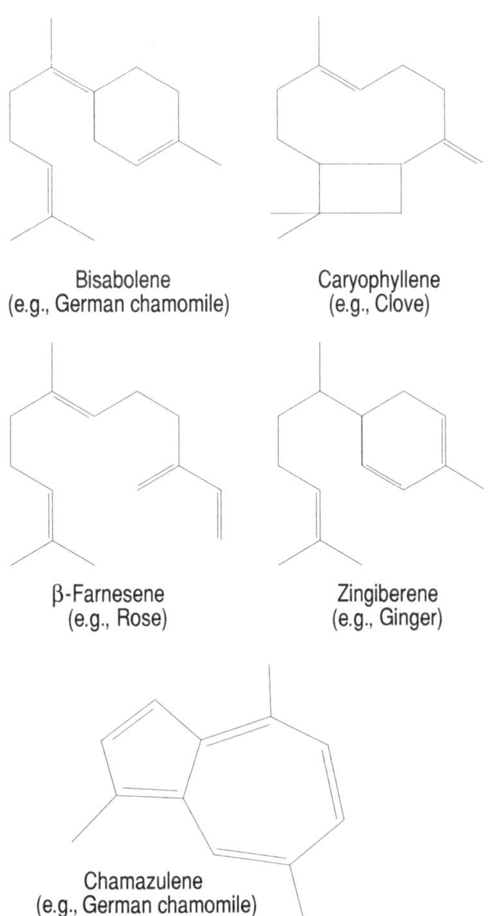

Some sesquiterpene hydrocarbon constituents found in essential oils.

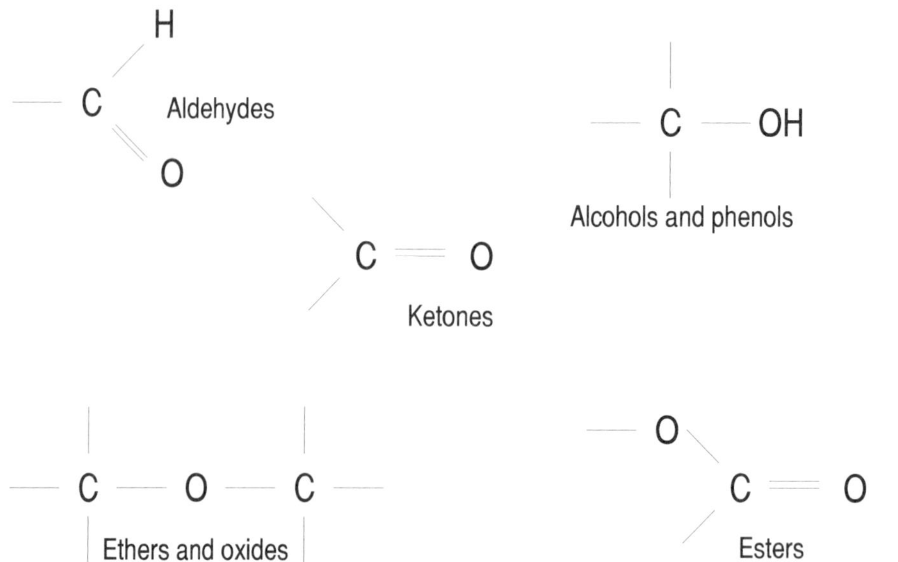

Functional groups found in essential oil constituents.

the different constituents of essential oils will be discussed in these terms.

Alcohols

A molecule which is an alcohol will have a hydroxyl group attached to one of its carbon atoms. A hydroxyl group is also known as an -OH group.

Phenols are also a type of alcohol, but because of their aromatic ring, they are classified differently. Alcohols will all have an ending 'ol'.[7]

Monoterpene Alcohols

Monoterpene alcohols have 10 carbon atoms, and contain a hydroxyl group anywhere along the chain. Monoterpene alcohols are also referred to as monoterpenols.

Properties

Monoterpene alcohols are considered to be the most beneficial and safest of all essential constituents.[4, 6, 7, 8] Lavabre suggests that monoterpene alcohols found in essential oils show a fair degree of diversity with respect to their properties. Most of the essential oils rich in monoterpene alcohols are antiseptic, have a pleasant uplifting fragrance and have a low toxicity.[4]

Properties associated with monoterpene alcohols are as follows:

- strong antibacterial, antifungal and antiviral properties.[4,5,7,8]

OH
OH
Geraniol
(e.g., geranium palmarosa)
Linalool
(e.g., rosewood lavender)
OH
OH
α-terpineol
(e.g., eucalyptus, cajeput)
Terpinen-4-ol
(e.g., tea tree, juniper)
OH
OH
Menthol
(e.g., peppermint)
Citronellol
(e.g., citronella)

Some monoterpene alcohol constituents found in essential oils.

- vasoconstrictive properties — Bowles says that menthol, linalool, α-terpineol and geraniol can make the site of application feel cold.[7]
- tonic and general stimulant properties.[7]
- sedative properties.[7]

While monoterpene alcohols are generally regarded as having a stimulating effect, the pharmacological testing of linalool has shown it to have a distinctly sedative effect. The possible reason for this has been explained by Bowles. She cites work done by Penoel and Franchomme, who suggest that a stressed client will benefit from the tonifying effect of alcohols because their psychoneuroendocrine-immune system is boosted. This induces a state of relaxation.[7]

Essential oils with linalool, include coriander seed, lavender, clary sage, rosewood and the linalool chemotype of thyme.

Sesquiterpene Alcohols

Sesquiterpene alcohols have 15 carbon atoms, and contain a hydroxyl group anywhere along the chain. Sesquiterpene alcohols also end in 'ol'.

Properties

The pharmacological properties of sesquiterpene alcohols are quite varied and it is difficult to generalise them as easily as the monoterpene alcohols. They have been found to have the following properties:

- Anti-inflammatory and antiphlogistic properties[4, 7, 8]
- Antiviral properties — Bowles cites research which found that the sesquiterpenols in sandalwood were effective in inhibiting the *Herpes simplex* virus I and II.[7]
- Anticarcinogenic properties — Bowles cites research that found nerolidol, found in niaouli oil, to be an inhibitor of intestinal carcinogenesis.[7]

Farnesol, a sesquiterpene alcohol found in essential oils such as rose and chamomile, is an excellent bacteriostatic. It is well suited to skin care and deodorant products, as it is known to inhibit, rather than kill, the growth of bacteria.[4]

According to Schnaubelt, sesquiterpene alcohols tonify muscles and nerves, reduce congestion of veins as well as in the lymphatic system, and have moderate antimicrobial effects.[6]

Sesquiterpene alcohols often impart very specific effects that are unique to a given essential oil, for example, vetiver, carrot seed, cedarwood, sandalwood and spikenard.[5]

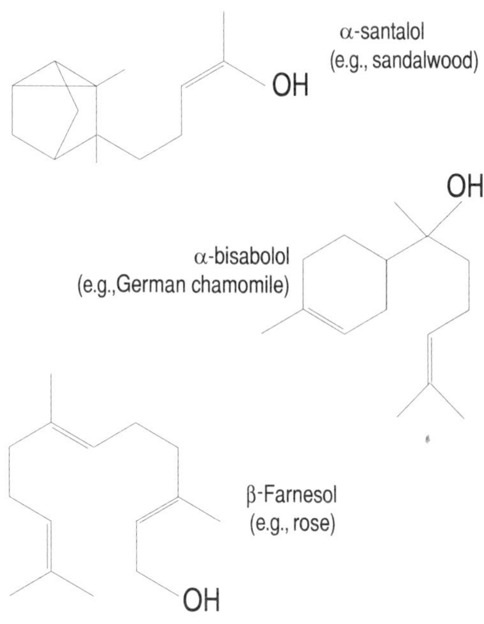

Some sesquiterpene alcohol constituents found in essential oils.

Phenols

The chemical family of phenols is characterised by molecules in which a hydroxy-functional group (-OH) is bonded directly to a benzene ring. The simplest phenol is phenol itself. Phenols, like alcohols, have names which also end in -ol. To discriminate between the two it will be necessary to learn the most important ones or see the structural diagram from which you will immediately be able to differentiate between the two. A phenol is characterised by the fact that it has a (aromatic ring) benzene ring.

Pure phenol is soluble in water, and an aqueous solution of phenol is called carbolic acid. This solution was one of the earliest antiseptics because it is toxic to bacteria. Today it is no longer used directly on patients because it burns the skin. It is, however, used to clean surgical and medical instruments.

A number of phenols appear in essential oils as phenyl propane derivatives. These molecules are made up of an aromatic ring with a propane (3-carbon) side chain. This basic structure of nine carbon atoms is then modified by various groups attached to it.

Essential oils with a high concentration of monoterpene phenols, thymol and carvacrol are ajowan, thyme, summer and winter savory and oregano.

Benzene

Phenol

Representation of the structure of phenol.

Thymol
(e.g., thyme, ajowan)

Carvacrol
(e.g., oregano, thyme)

Some monoterpenoid phenol constituents.

Properties

Some essential oils such as thyme and origanum owe their value in the pharmaceutical field almost entirely to the antiseptic and germicidal properties of their phenolic content. The antiseptic strength of thymol is much greater than that of phenol, yet its toxicity is much lower. Schnaubelt says that there is a slight liver toxicity associated with all phenolic compounds which would become evident if used in high doses for a long period of time.[8]

Bowles cites Penoel and Franchomme who say that the liver has to convert phenols into sulphonates and large internal doses would cause damage to liver cells by depleting them of sulphonates.[8]

Phenols are reactive molecules, which classifies them as 'hazardous chemicals'. Phenols have been classified as being:

- very powerful antimicrobial properties[6, 7, 8]
- skin and mucous membrane irritants[7, 8]
- general tonics and stimulants[7]
- stimulants to the nervous system[8]
- stimulants to the immune system.[8]

Research has found that dietary supplements of thymol and carvacrol significantly reduced the serum cholesterol levels of cockerels.[7]

Ethers

Most ethers occurring in essential oils are phenolic ethers. They are derived from the hydroxyl group of the phenol; the hydrogen is replaced with a short chain, either a methyl group (-CH_3), or 2-carbon ethyl group (-CH_2-CH_3).[7]

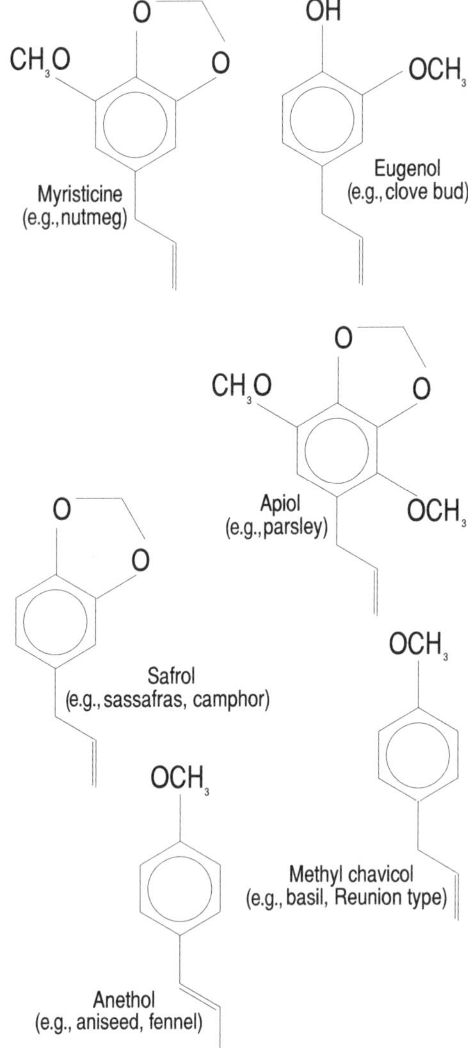

Some ethers found in essential oils.

Ethers are named after the phenol, plus the carbon chain group name and with the word 'ether' attached. Another way of naming ethers is by using the carbon chain name (e.g., methyl, ethyl, propyl) and adding -oxy to indicate the presence of the oxygen group. Some ethers, such as estragole, have an 'ole' ending.[7]

In large doses ethers can have a neurotoxic effect, leading to convulsions and even death.[7,10] Myristicin and elimicin are two ethers found in nutmeg oil, and are psychotropic if ingested in sufficient quantities.[7,9] It appears that myristicin inhibits the monoamine oxidase enzymes in the brain and increases the level of brain serotonin, both of which would induce a state of euphoria.[7] However, Bowles says that topically applied ether-rich oils will not cause psychotropic effects. The ether, safrole is well known for its liver carcinogenic effects.[9]

Properties

The properties of ethers are:

- antispasmodic
- analgesic
- antimicrobial.[7]

Ketones

Ketones have an oxygen atom double-bonded to a carbon atom, but always on a carbon atom that is bonded to two other carbon atoms. Ketones are known by their common name, such as camphor, or usually end in -one.

Properties

There is a certain level of concern regarding the safety of ketones. Certain ketones, notable thujone and camphor, are well known for their neurotoxicity. It is, however, important to note that there are many ketone which are not considered hazardous — for example, jasmone, found in jasmine, and italidone, found in everlasting.

Oils containing the ketone thujone, such as sage, mugwort, wormwood and thuja, should not be used in aromatherapy because of their toxicity.

Lavabre suggests that essential oils rich in ketones are important in aromatherapy because of their ability to ease or increase the flow of mucus and their wound healing properties. Everlasting's excellent wound-healing properties have been attributed to the ketone italidone.[4]

In general ketones are:

- mucolytic agents[4, 5, 6, 7, 8]
- wound healing properties[4, 5, 6, 7, 8]
- neurotoxins[4, 7, 8]
- abortifacients[8]
- analgesic[8]
- Antihaematonal property — in particular the italidones found in everlasting.[7]
- Antiviral — Bowles cites Penoel and Franchomme who say that the papilloma virus and herpes viruses which attack the nervous system can be killed by ketones.[7]

Esters

Esters are made up of an alcohol and an acid and are named after both parent molecules. For example:

Linalool + acetic acid → Linalyl acetate + water

Esters are produced through the reaction of an alcohol and an acid. Typical of the ester group is its reaction with water. Esters contain a double bond between carbon and oxygen (carboxyl group). A second oxygen atom is bonded to the carboxyl group, rendering it an ester group.

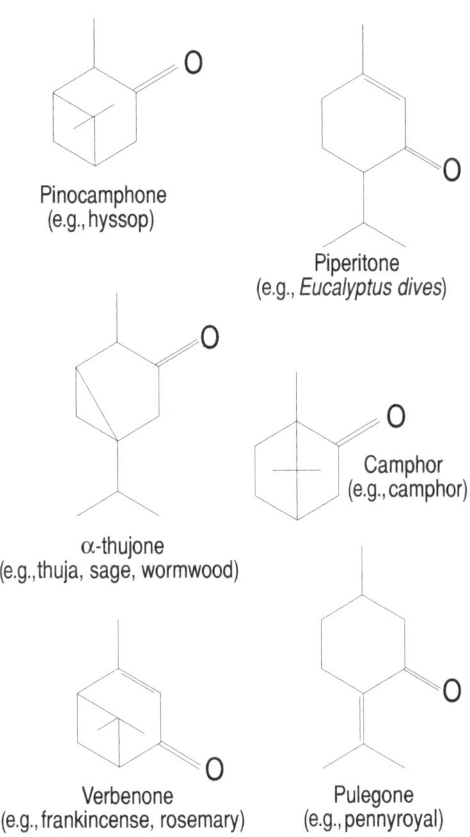

Some monoterpene ketones constituents found in essential oils.

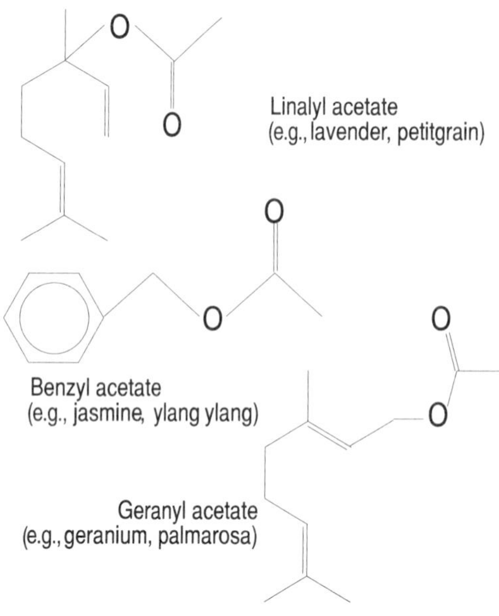

Some common esters constituents found in essential oils.

The naming of esters is as follows: The alcohol drops the -ol and gains a -yl, and the acid drops the -ic, and gains an -ate.

Properties

Esters generally have a fruity and fragrant odour and tend to be used extensively in perfumery. They are well known for their:

- antispasmodic properties[4, 6, 7, 8]
- anti-inflammatory[8]
- calming and tonic to the nervous system[4, 5]
- antifungal[4, 6, 8]
- sedative properties[7]

Esters are generally safe to use and have low toxicity. However the esters methyl salicylate (found in wintergreen) and sabinyl acetate (found in savin) are extremely toxic.

Roman chamomile, well known for its antispasmodic properties, contains a number of esters that are not commonly found in other essential oils. As Lavabre suggested, few essential oils have esters as the main constituent, but often even small amounts of esters are crucial to the finer notes in the fragrance of an essential oil.

Bowles cites Pénoël, who says that esters have a regulatory action on the sympathetic nervous system, and the neuroendocrine system.[7] Schnaubelt cites research which has identified the antifungal properties of esters. Geranium, an oil rich in esters, has excellent effects against candida, while the antimicrobial properties of geranium are quite poor.[6]

Aldehydes

Aldehydes consist of an oxygen atom double-bonded to a carbon atom, at the end of a carbon chain. The fourth bond is always a hydrogen bond. They usually end in -al.

Properties

Aldehydes tend to be very unstable and readily oxidise; therefore it is not surprising that they can be dermal irritants.

It is interesting that aldehydes are often known to have a fresh citrus-like aroma, which would leave you to believe that the aldehyde-rich oils would be more invigorating and stimulating. However, calming and anti-inflammatory properties of aldehydes become apparent when used in very low concentrations.[6]

Generally, aldehydes have the following properties:

- calming to the nervous system[5, 6, 7, 8]
- anti-inflammatory[5, 6, 8]
- vasodilators and hypotensive[8]
- anti-microbial[7, 8]

linalool + acetic acid ⇄ linalyl acetate + water

The formation of esters from an alcohol.

CHO
Citronellal
(e.g., *Eucalyptus citriodora*, citronella)

CHO
CHO
α-citral
(geranial)
β-citral
(neral)
Citrals (e.g., lemongrass, lemon)

Some monoterpene aldehyde constituents found in essential oils.

Lemongrass, an aldehyde-rich essential oil, was found to be particularly effective in inhibiting the *Candida albicans* organism. Repeating the tests with individual constituents of lemongrass showed citral and citronellal were active against the fungi whilst dipentene and myrcene had no activity.[10]

Pharmacological studies have shown that citronellal exhibits its strongest sedative effect at low concentrations and increasing concentration beyond a certain point reduced the sedative effect.

Williams found that *Leptospermum petersonii* (lemon scented tea tree), very high in citral and citronellal, exhibited a much higher antimicrobial effect than *Melaleuca alternifolia* (tea tree). The problem is that the oil has never been commercially successful as both citronellal and citral are not stable, being readily oxidised from exposure to air.[11]

Oxides

Oxides are similar to ethers in that there is an oxygen atom in the carbon chain, which is usually included in the formation of a ring rather than being attached to a short carbon chain. They usually end in 'ole'.

Properties

Oxides are well known for their expectorant properties.[4,5,7,8] However, as Bowles points out, care must be taken with 1,8-cineole in asthmatics as it can set off an asthma attack.[7]

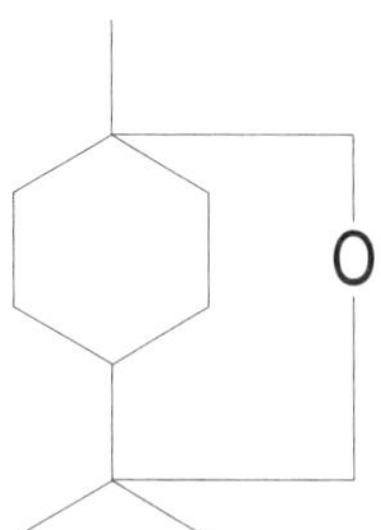

Structural diagram of the most common oxide: 1,8-cineole.

Bowles cites another study which says that 1,8-cineole exhibits anti-inflammatory effects in bronchial asthma by inhibiting the leukotriene B4 and prostaglandin E2 pathways in the blood monocytes of humans with bronchial asthma.[7]

There is also controversy over the antimicrobial effects of 1,8-cineole. In one series of tests it was found to be highly active against gram-positive and gram-negative bacteria, as well as some fungi. There is also some evidence that suggests that 1,8-cineole may be responsible for rosemary's CNS-excitatory properties. Balacs cites studies which state that cineole has been shown to have a similar neurotoxic profile to that of camphor.[12]

According to Penoel, 1,8-cineole has two main pharmacological properties:[13]

- It is an exocrine stimulant for the glands of the respiratory system and digestive organs.
- It is an expectorant because it stimulates mucin-secreting cells and activates the cilia of the respiratory mucous membrane.

Lactones and Coumarins

A lactone contains an ester group, integrated into a carbon-ring system. Coumarins are a type of lactone.[7,8]

Lactones tend to end in 'lactone' but can also end in 'in' or 'ine'. Lactones tend to have similar

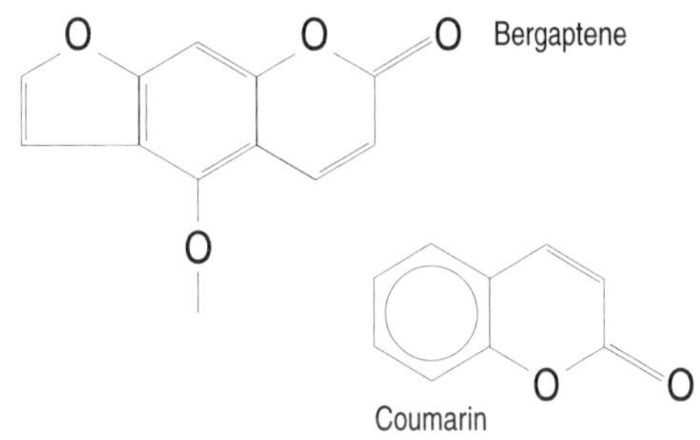

Typical lactone constituents found in essential oils.

neurotoxic effects to ketones and can cause skin allergies, sensitisation and blistering.[7] Lactones are found only in expressed oils and some absolutes, as their molecular weights are too high for them to come over in distillation.[8] The lactone Helenalin, found in *Arnica montana* extracts, is known to be anti-inflammatory.[7] Lactones have a very strong mucolytic effect. Elecampane, rich in the lactones alantolactone and isoalantolactone, is very effective for treating chronic coughs, catarrh and bronchitis.[7]

It has been suggested by Schnaubelt that sesquiterpene lactones have immunostimulant properties. He particularly refers to research done in France on *Inula graveolens*.[6] Properties of lactones include:

- mucolytic and expectorant[7,8]
- analgesic[8]
- temperature reducing.[8]

Coumarins have the distinctive feature of an adjacent benzene ring, which in turn has several different functional groups attached.[7] The properties of coumarins include:

- many are phototoxic and skin sensitising[8]
- anticoagulants[8]
- hypotensives[8]
- sedative effects.[7]

The well-known UV sensitising effect of bergamot oil is due to the presence of a furocoumarin, bergaptene. Coumarins are known to have sedative effects, which is due to the desensitising of the nervous reflex systems.[7]

Conclusion

The many properties of essential oils are a result of the limitless permutations of the essential oil constituents that can be categorised in the basic groups discussed in this chapter.

An understanding of the properties of essential oils according to the essential oil constituent groups has provided us with a scientific framework and rationale for the therapeutic application of essential oils.

While it is possible to predict an essential oil's pharmacological effects based on its main chemical composition, it must be remembered that in some cases, it is the trace constituents that dramatically contribute to the essential oil's pharmacological activity.

Therefore, while such generalisations are useful, it would not be wise to validate aromatherapy only in terms of chemistry, as in holistic aromatherapy the essential oils are capable of working on so many levels.

Highly Recommended Reading

Bowles J. *The basic chemistry of aromatherapeutic essential oils*. Australia, 1993.

Clarke S. *Essential chemistry for safe aromatherapy*. Churchill Livingstone, UK, 2002.

Williams D. *The chemistry of essential oils*. Michelle Press, UK, 1996.

References

1. Mills S. *The essential book of herbal medicine*. Arkana Penguin Books, England, 1991.
2. Bettelheim F, March J. *Introduction to general organic and biochemistry*. Saunders College Publishing, USA, 1984.
3. Williams D. *The chemistry of essential oils*. Michelle Press, UK, 1996.
4. Lavabre M. *Aromatherapy workbook*. Healing Art Press, USA., 1997.
5. Schnaubelt K. *Medical aromatherapy*. Frog Ltd, USA, 1999.
6. Schnaubelt K. *Advanced aromatherapy*. Healing Art Press, Canada, 1995.
7. Bowles J. *The basic chemistry of aromatherapeutic essential oils*. Australia, 1993.
8. Clarke S. *Essential chemistry for safe aromatherapy*. Churchill Livingstone, United Kingdom, 2002.
9. Tisserand R, Balacs T. *Essential oil safety*. Churchill Livingstone, United Kingdom, 1995.
10. Onawunni GO. *Antifungal activity of lemongrass*. International Journal of Crude Drug Research, 1989; 27(2): 121–126.
11. Williams L. *Highly active essential oil blends to combat multi-resistant Staphylococcus aureus*. Australasian Conference Proceedings, Sydney, 1998.
12. Balacs T. *Cineole-rich eucalyptus*. The International Journal of Aromatherapy, 1997; 8(2): 15–21.
13. Penoel D. *Winter shield*. The International Journal of Aromatherapy, 1992; 4(4): 10–12.

Pharmacokinetics

Objectives

After careful study of this chapter, you should be able to:

- explain the permeation of essential oils into the body
- outline the metabolism of essential oils
- outline the excretion of essential oils
- identify the possible interactions that occur between drugs and essential oils.

Introduction

Pharmacokinetics is generally considered under the following headings:

- absorption
- distribution
- metabolism
- excretion.

Absorption

There are several ways in which essential oils are administered for use in aromatherapy:

- dermal
- inhalation
- oral
- rectal.

Dermal

It is often taken for granted that essential oils are absorbed into the skin. It is surprising that very little research has been conducted to address the absorption of essential oils and vegetable oils into the body via the skin. However, the absorption of drugs and cosmetic substances through the skin has been studied in great detail.[1]

Recent studies involving lavender essential oil diluted in peanut oil massaged over the stomach area for 10 minutes indicated that traces of linalool and linalyl acetate were detected in the blood after 20 minutes. After 90 minutes most of the lavender oil has been eliminated from the blood.[2]

Surprisingly, Buchbauer suggests that it is nonsense to apply essential oils by massage.

> *Massage application is wrong because of the high concentration in which the fragrant molecules evoke unspecified effects, in particular irritation by destruction of cell membranes. On the other hand, essential oils reaching cells in very low concentrations as in inhalation where the resultant plasma concentrations of the essential oil compounds are 100- to 10,000 fold smaller, are integrated in special areas of cell membranes and evoke specific effects by influencing the enzymes, carriers, ion channels and receptor proteins which are in these localised areas.*[3]

Whether you agree with Buchbauer's comments on massage application or not, he has been one of the few researchers to determine the amount of essential oil in the blood plasma as a result of inhalation and massage.

Essential oils and vegetable-based carrier oils, being composed of fat-soluble molecules, tend to be easily absorbed into the skin. There are many aspects that need to be addressed to study the factors that will affect absorption of the essential oils into the skin and how they find their way into the circulatory system.

Skin's Structure

It is remarkable that the principal resistance to permeation of most, if not all, substances resides in the paper-thin outer layer of skin called the stratum corneum, or horny layer. This layer is a compact amalgam of dried, dead, elongated cells, the end product of differentiation of the cells produced in the viable epidermis.

Keratin provides the strength and chemical resistance. The horny layer is a rather dry tissue, although the actual moisture content depends on the ambient relative humidity. At low humidity, most of the water associated with keratin and other proteins is tightly bound and oriented so that the tissue has a low effective dielectric constant. Within the cells are low molecular weight hydrophilic substances (such as amino acids and sugars) that are collectively referred to as the natural moisturising factor.[1]

The stratum corneum ranges from about 6 to 15 μm. The uppermost layers tend to flake off, or desquamate, because the biochemical and histological components attaching these cells to each other have deteriorated.[1] The lower layers of the stratum corneum, which are closer to the viable epidermis, are more tightly packed. The intercellular space in the stratum corneum is primarily filled with lamellar layers of skin lipids. The components of this intercellular lipid have been identified, and it has been shown that they differ from those of sebum.[1]

The continuity of the stratum corneum is interrupted by the ducts of the eccrine and apocrine glands and by hair follicles with their sebaceous glands. While these sites account for no more than 1% of the skin's surface area, they are one of the major pathways of essential oils through the skin.[1]

Experimentally, different rates of absorption have been demonstrated depending on the skin location. The permeability of skin at various body sites is rated as follows:[1]

Relatively permeable:	Genitals, head areas such as forehead and scalp, soles and palms, armpits, mucous membranes
Relatively impermeable:	Trunk, abdomen, limbs, buttocks

The viable dermis is at least ten times thicker than the stratum corneum. It tends to possess very little barrier properties to the passage of most substances. However, it tends to absorb permeating

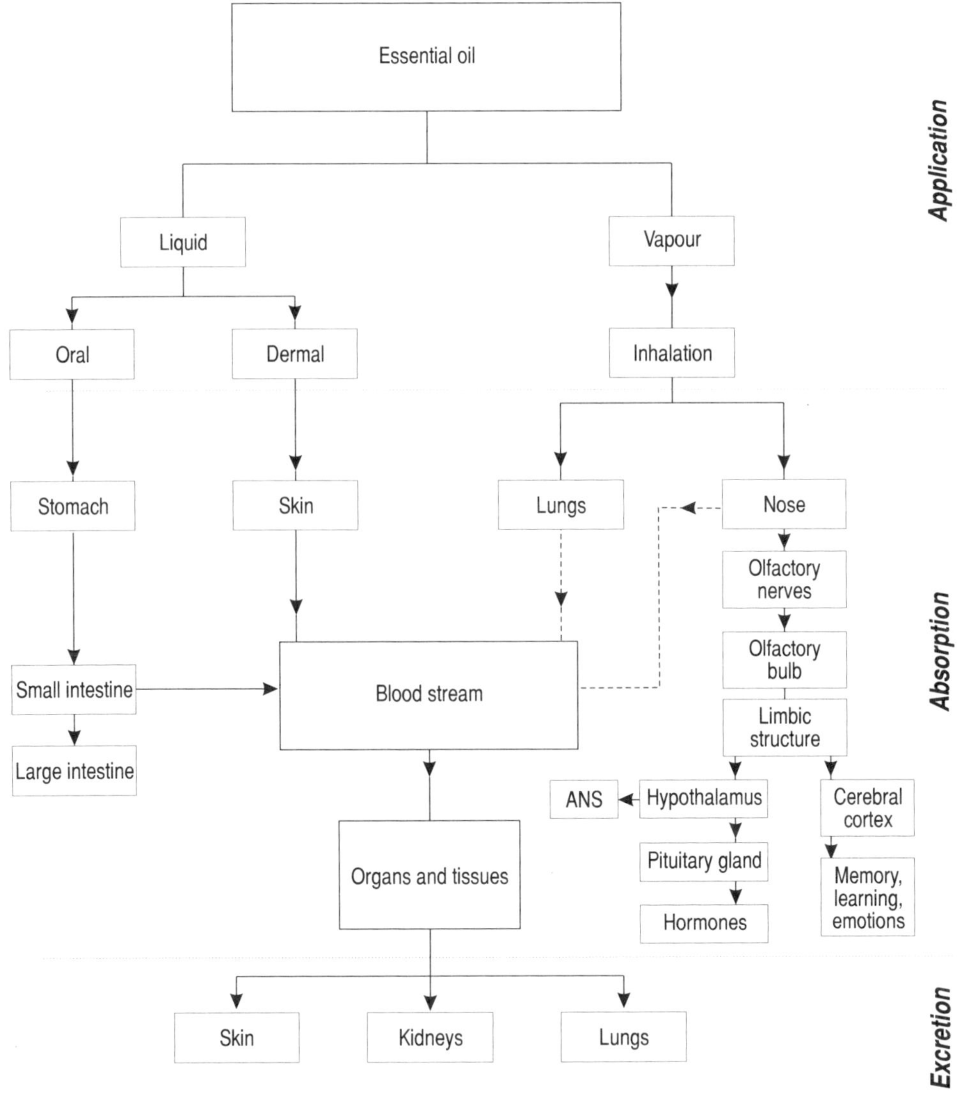

Pathway to illustrate how essential oils are absorbed into the body. The dotted lines indicate only trace amounts of essential oils being absorbed.

substances before they reach the blood vessels of the vascular plexus or the dermis.[1]

The dermis is the lowest skin layer which also plays a role in skin absorption. Whereas the viable dermis is a highly cellular portion of the living skin, the dermis includes a variety of fibrous proteins and the components of the connective tissue in addition to cells. The dermis is believed to offer no barrier to the passage of molecules that reach it, except for molecules that may be substantive to specific dermal components.[1]

Permeation Pathways

For the purpose of clarity the following definitions will apply:[1]

- Substances that have entered the cutaneous capillaries will be defined as being absorbed.
- Substances that have entered the skin but not been absorbed into the capillaries will be considered to have only penetrated the skin.
- Permeation will be the term used to describe a substance that has either been absorbed or penetrated.

When essential oils are applied to the skin, two major pathways exist:[1]

- through the stratum corneum
- via shunts — the hair follicles and sweat glands.

Absorption through the latter is faster than the route across the stratum corneum. However, the stratum corneum is considered to be the major pathway for most substances.[1]

Within the stratum corneum itself, two pathways exist; one crosses the cells and intercellular spaces (polar pathway), while the second involves passage though the intercellular lipid domain (lipid pathway). The polar pathway accommodates primarily water and ions and has a smaller capacity and contributes less to the total penetration while the lipid pathway handles everything else.[1]

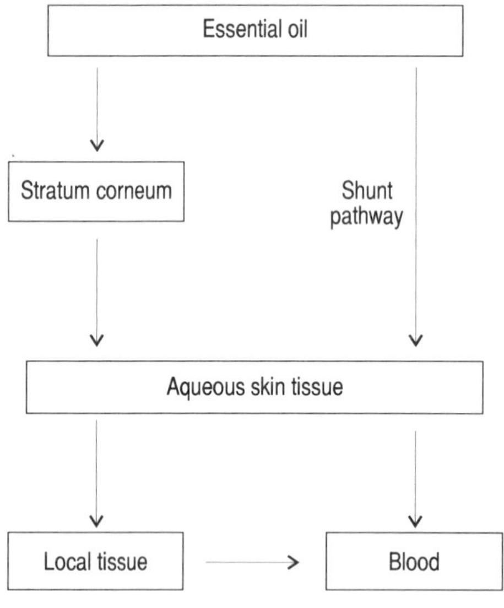

Schematic diagram showing principal absorption pathways.[2]

Factors Affecting Permeation

Factors that influence the rate of essential oil permeation are divided into the following categories:[1]

Biological Factors

integrity of the stratum corneum
skin hydration
cutaneous blood flow
skin biochemistry
hydration

Permeant Factors

molecular weight
partition coefficient solubility
molecular size
use of surfactants

Vehicle Factors

penetration properties
occlusions
pH

Physical Factors

temperature
climate
time

Trauma

mechanical
disease
chemical

Integrity of the Stratum Corneum

Conditions such as eczema, which result in thickened skin, may retard absorption because of the increase in absorptive path length. On the other hand, absorption through psoriatic skin is enhanced.[1] This may be secondary to altered epidermal structure as well as to changes in vascular perfusion.

Systemic disease states could also potentially alter the rate of topical absorption. For example, diabetes is known to alter the structure of the epidermal basement membranes and capillary functions such that compound diffusion out of cutaneous capillaries is enhanced in chronic diabetes.[1]

Skin Hydration

Skin hydration occurs through bathing, sweating, being in an area of high humidity, occlusion or application of a film-forming product such as a moisturiser.

Water influences the barrier performance of the stratum corneum more than any other non-irritating substance and it has been found that skin hydration which results from a bath or shower can enhance essential oil absorption.[1]

Taking a hot bath or shower could also stimulate the blood flow of the dermis, which can increase the absorption of essential oils. Using a massage oil after bathing may be a way of increasing essential oil absorption. Hydration is known to accelerate the absorption of drugs and is the basis of cosmetic skin claims made about moisturisers.

Viscosity of the Oil

Viscosity refers to the thickness of the carrier oil being used. For instance, olive oil, which is viscous, is slowly absorbed through the skin, whereas apricot kernel oil, which is much less viscous, is rapidly absorbed. Because essential oils are highly soluble in vegetable oils it is very likely that the viscosity of the vegetable oil will determine the rate of absorption of the essential oil.[4]

The degree of unsaturation of an oil also affects the rate of cutaneous penetration. Linseed oil, which is rich in polyunsaturates, traverses the skin much better than its low viscosity would lead one to expect; on the other hand olive oil, which is rich in monounsaturated fatty acids, is not easily absorbed by the skin.[4]

Fatty acids such as caprylic, capric, stearic acid, oleic acid and α-linoleic acid are found to be penetration enhancers. All these fatty acids are abundantly found in cold-pressed vegetable oils.[1]

Use of Surfactants

Surfactants are widely used in skin products to serve a variety of functions. It has been found that many surfactants such as soaps and detergents can increase the permeability of the skin.[4]

The mechanisms of action appear to be protein denaturation (permanent), membrane expansion, hole formation and loss of water-binding capacity. It has been demonstrated that the use of surfactants with certain antimicrobial agents has increased the absorption of the antimicrobial agent into the skin.[4]

Occlusions

A common method for increasing skin hydration is by the use of occlusive dressings. Occlusion prevents surface evaporation, resulting in stratum corneum hydration.

Occlusion of the skin can occur from wearing clothes, bandages, plasters, masks and application of products such as petroleum jelly. Not only will the occlusion increase the temperature of the skin but it will also increase the hydration of the skin, and these factors will increase absorption.

Cosmetic face masks are a form of occlusion in which the skin's percutaneous hydration is increased. Fragrances under occlusion have been found to double the percutaneous absorption rate of unoccluded fragrance materials.[1]

Temperature

Either a rise in ambient room temperature or the use of warm oil will lead to an enhanced absorption. Such conditions would also increase vaporisation, thus increasing the amount of essential oil inhaled. No doubt the increased rate of absorption is due to enhanced capillary circulation.[4]

Cutaneous Biotransformation

Apart from the skin's structural role, the skin is a dynamic organ with myriad biological functions such as neurosensory reception, endocrinology, immunological affectors and effector axes, glandular secretions and keratin, collagen, melanin, lipid and carbohydrate metabolism. The skin's complex biological functions may alter the absorption of topically applied substances such as essential oils.

A large percentage of topically applied substances may never penetrate the rate-limiting stratum corneum barrier. If the compound is volatile, as are essential oils, part of it will be lost through evaporation. Topically applied substances may chemically bind to the stratum corneum and thus may be lost due to desquamation.

However, if the substance has entered the stratum corneum, there are three possible fates:[1]

- Complete absorption into the cutaneous microcirculation.
- Formation of a reservoir by binding to the stratum corneum or subcutaneous fat where it subsequently may be slowly released into the capillaries.
- Metabolism by cutaneous enzymes.

In some cases, the route of entry into the skin may be via appendages such as hair follicles or sweat ducts. The ability of the stratum corneum and the lower dermal strata to act as a reservoir for topically applied substances such as essentials oils is well known.[1]

Other physiological activities of the skin are the metabolism of an essential oil and the removal

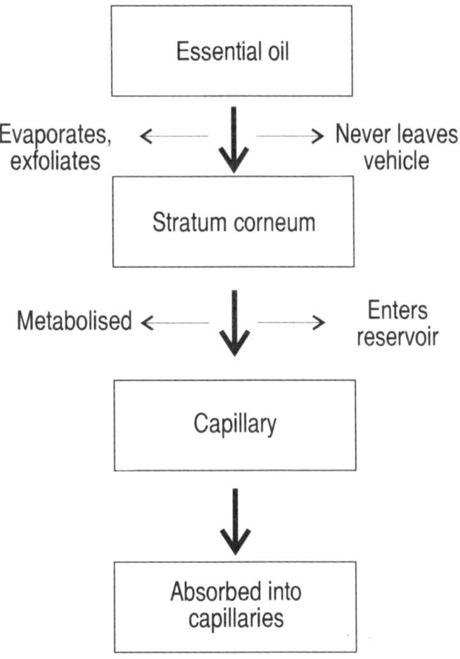

Possible fate of a topically applied essential oil.

of the essential oil from the skin via the vascular and lymphatic pathways or the circulatory system.

The skin is a site of extrahepatic metabolism for certain types of chemicals such as drugs and carcinogens, not to mention carbohydrates, lipids and proteins. Recent studies have indicated that cutaneous metabolism may be an important step in the permeation of some chemicals. It has become clear that various factors will influence the amount of essential oil absorbed, once it has penetrated the stratum corneum.[1]

Some essential oil constituents are believed to be converted into potentially carcinogenic compounds. This seems to be the case with cytochrome P_{450} enzymes which convert essential oil constituents such as safrole and methyl carvacrol into potentially carcinogenic compounds.[5]

It is believed that methyl chavicol-rich essential oils may undergo biotransformation within the skin, being converted to potentially more toxic carcinogenic compounds.[5]

Often, if the essential oil is not metabolised, the vascular and lymphatic systems are still involved in actively clearing it from the surface of the skin.

Metabolism is not the only physiological function of the skin which has a major impact on the absorption of a substance into the skin. Binding of a substance to protein in the skin is critical for the occurrence of certain responses, such as allergic contact dermatitis. Here binding of the penetrant to a cutaneous or serum protein is crucial to the formation of an allergen before induction can begin and cutaneous sensitisation can result.[1]

Entry into the Blood

Molecules which have passed through the epidermis are carried away by the capillary blood circulating in the dermis below. The dermis of the skin has a large network of capillaries which modulate cutaneous blood flow in response to thermoregulatory needs. When the environmental temperature exceeds body temperature, cutaneous blood flow increases so that heat is lost through the skin. In contrast, blood flow is reduced or totally shunted in cold temperatures to prevent surface heat loss.

In vivo topical absorption of methyl salicylate was increased threefold in humans when they were exposed to high ambient temperatures or underwent strenuous exercise. Increased blood flow was presumed to be a major factor, although increased skin hydration or sweating also contributed.[1]

Because the blood flow in the skin is low compared to that in the muscle, it could well be that for easily absorbed substances, cutaneous blood flow will limit the rate of absorption into the bloodstream. In such cases massage can be expected to increase the rate of systemic absorption because it enhances blood flow.

Inhalation

Whenever essential oils are inhaled, the odoriferous molecules may:

- Pass down the trachea into the bronchi, and then the bronchioles and finally into the alveoli, where the essential oil molecules pass into the bloodstream.
- Be absorbed into the bloodstream via the nasal mucosa.
- Bind to the olfactory cilia, thus triggering an olfactory response.

The lipophilic nature of essential oils means that they pass the blood–brain barrier easily. Their affinity for lipid-rich tissues like those of the central nervous system facilitates an exchange of essential oil constituents from the blood into the lipid-rich nervous system.

Studies have shown that essential oils are readily absorbed into the bloodstream through inhalation. They have high solubility in the blood and excellent absorption takes place through the nasal mucosa and pulmonary system.[3,6,7]

Eight healthy people were subjected to short-term inhalation exposure to three concentrations of d-limonene on three separate occasions. The pulmonary intake was almost 70% and it increased proportionally with increased exposure concentrations. A long half-life in the blood indicated an accumulation of d-limonene in adipose tissues.[6]

A correlation was made between peak blood levels of inhaled 1,8-cineole, a constituent of rosemary oil and locomotor activity. The concentration of 1,8-cineole in the blood after inhaling rosemary oil for one hour was similar to that in the breathing air. Inhaled *Rosmarinus officinalis* increased locomotor activity of the brain.[7]

Buchbauer compares inhalation to someone eating a cube of sugar. Not only will they sense a pleasant feeling as they taste the sugar, but the ingested sugar molecules will induce a whole cascade of insulin reactions.[3] Why should the fragrance molecules not act similarly via a molecular interaction as well as producing feelings of wellbeing?

Oral

Oral administration is most popular for drugs which are formulated so that they have little or no taste and gastrointestinal irritation is minimal or non-existent.

Extra care should be taken when administering essential oils orally because a significantly higher percentage of oil would reach the circulation, and the liver would receive a relatively large dose via the portal circulation, which takes blood from the gastrointestinal tract to the liver.[5]

It also needs to be noted that almost all recorded cases of serious poisoning by essential oils have occurred by oral self-dosing of smaller quantities of undiluted essential oil. Other concerns of oral administration include:

- possibility of nausea and vomiting
- irritation of the gastrointestinal tract
- much of the essential oil will be metabolised by the liver
- destruction of the essential oil constituents by stomach acidity or enzymes in the intestines.

Rectal

Suppositories are a common method of essential oil administration by French medical doctors. Some of the advantages of using suppositories include:

- The essential oils can be administered in higher doses than oral administration for the treatment of acute infectious conditions, especially lower respiratory tract conditions.
- There is the absence of the interaction between the essential oil and the gastrointestinal tract or the liver which possibly breaks down the essential oil.[5]
- There is more rapid absorption of essential oil into the body.[5,8]
- They reduce the possible hazardous effects on the liver, especially essential oils containing phenols. In order to excrete phenols the liver has to convert them into sulphonates which may cause damage to the liver by overworking it.[5,8]
- Suppositories are easier to administer than oral ingestion.[5,8]

It needs to be stressed that similar safety issues to those of oral administration need to be considered. Being lined with mucous membrane, the rectum is highly sensitive to irritation and there may be a risk of occasional irritation.

Metabolism

There are three major processes that need to be considered:

- distribution
- biotransformation
- excretion.

It is important to recognise that metabolism of essential oils occurs however essential oils are administered. However, the essential oil components may be metabolised differently depending on the method of administration.

Distribution

Tisserand and Balacs says that fat-soluble substances usually pass readily into the CNS and the liver.[5] Many essential oil constituents, being fat-soluble, can enter the CNS through the blood–brain barrier. The blood–brain barrier is not a physical structure as such, but represents the lack of permeability in cerebral blood capillaries when compared to peripheral capillaries and the presence of cells through which these constituents must pass if they are to reach the brain's nerve tissue. This is to protect the brain from many potentially toxic chemicals.[9]

The brain is very rich in lipids, and so fat-soluble molecules will have a natural affinity for it. Conversely, highly water-soluble molecules will tend to linger in the watery environment of the blood. The essential oils are distributed to the tissue in accordance with the extent of blood flow, the ease of passage across cell membranes and the extent of binding to plasma and tissue proteins.[9]

The body tissue most perfused by blood will also be the tissue most exposed to the action of the essential oil, whilst the tissue with little active circulation will have less chance to respond to treatment. The following list details the different body tissues in decreasing order of blood perfusion:

- endocrine glands, heart, lungs, brain, liver and kidneys
- skin and muscles
- fat tissue
- bone, teeth, ligaments and tendons.[1]

Substances bound to plasma proteins and those with a very low fat solubility do not readily pass through the barrier into the brain.

Molecules with carboxylic acid groups such as phenylacetic acid, ketones, esters and aldehydes tend to hydrogen-bond with plasma albumin. This means that the time that these constituents will remain in the bloodstream is increased, however it also means that the amount of free essential oil constituents available has been reduced.[5]

People with kidney disease or cirrhosis of the liver whose plasma albumin levels are low should use low dosages of essential oils as the concentration of essential oil constituents in the bloodstream will be higher.[5]

When treating pregnant and nursing mothers it should be assumed that the placental membrane is no different from any other tissue and, therefore, essential oils will reach the foetus unhindered. Also, during breastfeeding, the very high perfusion of the lactating mammary glands means that the infant will receive a proportionately high dose of any essential oil that the mother is taking, so care is necessary.[5]

Biotransformation

Many substances which are introduced into the body undergo biotransformation in the liver. If they are pharmacologically active, this process usually results in loss or reduction of their activity. However, some substances are actually activated by biotransformation, often into toxic metabolites.

The types of chemical reactions that are likely to occur in the metabolism of essential oils are known as Phase I and Phase II reactions.[9]

Phase I reactions are those in which a compound is chemically altered to make it water-soluble. This usually involves the following steps:

- oxidation
- reduction
- splitting by hydrolysis.[9]

Most of these reactions are carried out by microsomal enzymes in the liver.

Oxidation (Phase I)

The crucial group of enzymes necessary for oxidation are the cytochromes P_{450}. These enzymes can oxidise a wide range of foreign molecules and have been found to be responsible for metabolising essential oil constituents. Oxidation occurs primarily in the liver and prepares molecules for conjugation.

Glucuronide Conjugation (Phase II)

Phase II reactions are those in which substances that have undergone Phase I are joined to other molecules to make them ready for excretion. This process is known as conjugation.[9]

If the products of transformation are still pharmacologically active, they often undergo a second reaction which will render them inactive. Essential oil constituents containing a hydroxyl group (-OH) such as alcohols and phenols may undergo this second reaction and end up being eliminated from the body as glucuronides.[5]

Glucuronides can be excreted through the urine if the molecular weight of the essential oil constituent is 300 or less. (The molecular weight of monoterpenoids is about 150 and that of sesquiterpenes about 225).[5]

Glutathione Detoxification

The liver contains a chemical called glutathione. Its job is to mop up reactive molecules (e.g., free radicals) before they can damage DNA or protein. Once the liver is exhausted on glutathione, reactive molecules are then able to attack liver cells. It is very unlikely that this could happen when essential oils are applied dermally, but the risk of glutathione depletion could occur from oral administration, especially in the case of accidental ingestion.[5]

In most cases substances introduced to the body undergo transformation which makes them inactive; however, some substances are actually activated by biotransformation.

d-pulegone, found in pennyroyal, is metabolised in the liver to menthofuran via a highly reactive metabolite. This metabolite irreversibly binds to the components of liver cells in which metabolism takes place, quickly destroying the liver tissue.[5]

A similar process of biotransformation is responsible for the hepatotoxicity of methyl chavicol, eugenol and cinnamaldehyde, which may also reduce the level of glutathione in the liver.[5]

Excretion

As soon as an essential oil enters the body, it begins to be excreted. Excretion occurs at the kidneys, via the bile and bowel and to a certain extent through the sweat glands and other body secretions.

The kidneys are the major organs of excretion and many essential oils in the bloodstream will have to be filtered by them. On this basis one would expect the smaller molecules such as aldehydes and alcohols to be filtered out more rapidly than the larger terpene molecules.[9]

Many of the lipid-soluble molecules are known to diffuse passively back through the tubule walls of the kidneys into the bloodstream. Therefore the liver would usually attempt to render fat-soluble substances such as terpenes, terpenoid ketones and ethers into more water-soluble components in readiness for secretion.[9]

Drugs and Essential Oils

We know very little about the physiological and pharmacological drug interaction with essential oils. Tisserand and Balacs suggest that in some cases essential oil constituents may bind to the plasma albumin and displace the drug, thus increasing the concentration of active drug in the plasma.[5]

Some essential oil constituents such as 1,8-cineole increased the activity of microsomal enzyme systems. A study involving inhalation of aerosols and subcutaneous injections of the components was evaluated against the pentabarbitol effect (sleeping time) in rats. The enzymatic activity of three reactions was measured in vitro on liver homogenate of treated and control rats. It was found that 1,8-cineole produced a significant decrease in the pentabarbitol effect by injection and inhalation, and that it was dose-related.[10]

There are to be two main areas of concern:

- Use of salicylate-rich essential oils on the action of warfarin. (Warfarin is an anti-coagulant and is used to prevent the formation of blood clots (or thrombosis) within the blood vessels or within the heart.) It has been found to increase the risk of haemorrhaging.[5] A case is cited by Tisserand and Balacs in which an 85-year-old woman was admitted to hospital with acute cardiovascular problems, and was prescribed heparin, followed by warfarin. Some weeks after leaving hospital she returned, suffering from gross vaginal bleeding, ecchymoses on the left cheek, the right flank and perineum. Her blood haemoglobin had fallen from 117 g/l to 80 g/l. It turned out that the week before she had liberally applied a preparation containing menthol and methyl salicylate to her arthritic joints.[5]
- Myristicin has been found to inhibit monoamine oxidase (MAO). Myristicin is found in essential oils such as nutmeg, parsley seed and mace essential oils. Cases cited by Tisserand suggest that the amount of myristicin found in nutmeg is not very potent as an MAO inhibitor. It is also suggested that topical application is not likely to be a problem.[5]

Conclusion

It is perhaps understandable that very little work has been done on the essential oils as they are made up of so many individual constituents that would make a detailed pharmacokinetic study impossible. However, we need to be able to relate the current knowledge to our practice as aromatherapists, so that we can determine the length of time that the essential oils remain active after application, in what dosage and how often the oils should be applied.

References

1. Zatz J. ed, *Skin permeation: Fundamentals and application.* Allured Publishing Corporation, USA, 1993.
2. Jager W, Buchbauer G, Jirovetz L & Fritzer M. *Percutaneous absorption of lavender from a massage oil.* Journal of the Society of Cosmetic Chemists, 1992; 43(1): 49–54.
3. Buchbauer G. *Molecular interaction.* The International Journal of Aromatherapy 1993; 5(1): 11–14.
4. Balacs T. *Dermal crossing essential issues III.* International Journal of Aromatherapy 1992; 4(2): 23–25.
5. Tisserand R & Balacs T. *Essential oil safety.* Churchill Livingstone, UK, 1995.
6. Falk-Filiipsson A. *d-limonene exposure to humans by inhalation: Uptake, distribution, elimination and effects on the pulmonary system.* Journal of Toxicology and Environmental Health 1993; 38: 77–88. Cited in *The Aromatherapy Database*, by Bob Harris, Essential Oil Resource Consultants, UK, 2000.
7. Kovar KA, Gropper B, Friess D & Svendsen A. *Blood levels of 1,8-cineole and locomotor activity of mice after inhalation and oral administration of rosemary oil.* Planta Medica 1987; 53(4): 315–8. Cited in *The Aromatherapy Database*, by Bob Harris, Essential Oil Resource Consultants, UK, 2000.
8. Azemar J. *Galenic forms for aromatherapy: Suppositories.* Aromatherapy Records 1995; 1: 86–89.
9. Balac T. *Well oiled pathways.* The International Journal of Aromatherapy 1992; 4(3): 14–16.
10. Jori A, Bianchetti A & Prestini PE. *Effect of essential oils on drug metabolism.* Biochemical Pharmacology 1969; 18(9): 2081–5. Cited in *The Aromatherapy Database*, by Bob Harris, Essential Oil Resource Consultants, UK, 2000.

Pharmacology of Essential Oils

Objectives

After careful study of this chapter, you should be able to:

- define pharmacology and pharmacognosy
- examine the problems associated with pharmacology
- redefine the role of pharmacology in aromatherapy
- examine the pharmacological activities of essential oils.

Introduction

As the popularity of aromatherapy grows, members of the medical sector and government legislators will ask more questions regarding the efficacy and safety of aromatherapy. Some of the most common questions asked are:

- Is there any scientific evidence of the therapeutic benefits of the essential oils?
- Have clinical trials been done to prove the properties of essential oils?
- If they have been done, how do we know that the results are no more than a placebo effect?
- Why do the effects of aromatherapy vary from person to person?

As aromatherapists, we may simply argue the fact that we have used the oils in a clinical situation and are satisfied that aromatherapy works. We have seen results (in some cases amazing results!), so any pharmacological investigation into essential oils is only a waste of time and money because all it would do is prove what we already know.

Unfortunately to 'bury your head in the sand' can be quite dangerous in an age where government legislators and powerful orthodox medical establishments are continuously demanding safety, stability and efficacy information on all products claiming to be therapeutic.

Such views are supported by the comments from a spokesperson for the Australian Medical Association:

> *General AMA policy is that if something is scientifically valid, then we will support it.*[1]

He continued by saying:

> *If it hasn't undergone some degree of validation, then we're basically against it, in the patient's interest.*[1]

It is with this in mind that this chapter addresses clinical research that has already been conducted which confirms traditionally held beliefs of aromatherapy.

Pharmacology and Pharmacognosy

The study of the effects of drugs on the body is called pharmacology. Mills describes pharmacology as:

> *...a narrowly fragmentary investigation in which nature is effectively disintegrated so that the action of an isolated chemical on an isolated piece or function of the body can be observed as precisely as it is possible in a variable world. These observations are then stuck together to make a jigsaw picture of the effect of that substance on the body, and it is on the basis of this picture that drugs are given to real people.*[2]

Pharmacognosy is a branch of pharmacology concerned with the study of crude drugs of plant origin. Modern pharmacognosy is concerned with analysing natural medicinal substances and defining their therapeutic activity according to the chemical constituents.

Problems with Pharmacology

Essential oils consist of an immense array of chemical constituents, each liable to be interacting with the others, most with little-known pharmacological action, and worst of all each individual plant has its own unique blend of essential oil constituents.

Mills says that pharmacologists are in search of the 'active principle', which can be ultimately isolated and synthesised. This leads to the standardisation of drugs in which a particular drug is supposed to be designed with the utmost precision and predictability to the symptoms.[2]

From this perspective, Mills says that the claims made by traditional therapists who use plant-based remedies must seem like a quaint but irrational relic from the dark ages.[2] He therefore asks:

> *...how can we justify the use of a constantly changing chemical soup in place of the cleanly extracted, precisely measured active principle?*[2]

However, Mills says that predictability is an illusion to the clinical pharmacologist. He gives the example of digoxin.

> *From any one dose of digoxin, for example, different patients get wildly different responses, and the final prescribed dosage has to be individually tailored.*[2]

Modern pharmacological studies designed for orthodox drugs may not be ideally suited to study the action of essential oils.

While the essential oils have drug-like effects on the mind and body, they differ greatly from drugs because of their:

- chemical complexity
- synergy
- multifaceted actions
- reduced side effects and
- subtle and gentle activity.

Any pharmacology model suited to aromatherapy must take these above factors into consideration.

Lapraz, a medical doctor and leading medical aromatherapist from France, describes the role of pharmacology and modern medicine:

> *Modern medicine chooses to make an in-depth physiological analysis of the human body in order to find a cause for the illness, for example lack of a particular enzyme. Side by side with this very symptom-orientated and analytical approach, the pharmaceutical industry makes a particular drug that is known,*

> *subject to precise analysis, reproducible and always conforms to norms in the context of experimentation. So conventional medicine can now correlate, with utmost precision, the medication to the symptom.*[3]

However, he also goes on to say:

> *We are becoming aware of the limits of such a purely analytical approach as we now understand that disease is multifactorial, with many different aspects that come into play, and we must address all of these causal factors.*[3]

Redefining the Role of Pharmacology for Aromatherapy

Pharmacology will help us define the properties of an essential oil according to its 'action'. This approach, which defines the remedy in accordance with physically quantifiable properties, is mechanistic, reductionist and analytical.

Holmes is wary of such an approach, which results in each essential oil being labelled with a string of qualifiers such as sudorific, hepatic, etc. — which he says are worn-out labels which are meaningless to the practitioner who is unaware of the meaning of its treatment strategies.[4]

Mills suggests that a therapeutic agent should be rated on its ability to provoke a pattern of vital healing responses in the body. He states that any pharmacology suitable for plant-based medicines must become the following:

> *The interpretation of the observed action of the remedy in practice; the process of developing the character of each remedy so that it can be used more creatively and informatively in support of the processes, rather than searching for the actions of the constituents per se.*[2]

If we are to maintain a holistic system of aromatherapy it is necessary to integrate three basic elements:

- The holistic context in which the essential oil is used.
- The empirical context which draws on centuries of traditional use.
- The analytical back-up provided by chemistry and pharmacological studies of the essential oil.

Is Aromatherapy Pharmacologically Based?

In some respects the word 'aromatherapy' can be misleading because it suggests that it is a form of healing which will work exclusively through the sense of smell, and on the emotions. This is not the case, for, apart from the fragrance of the essential oil, each essential oil has a unique combination of constituents which interacts with the body's chemistry in a direct manner and which, in turn, affect certain organs or body systems.

There are two principal approaches to the practice of aromatherapy:

- the medical approach, and
- the holistic approach

As Doctor Peneol states, the medical approach has very little interest in the odour of the essential oil. He gives an example in which he recommends boldo essential oil for a chronic chlamydia infection. Boldo is not a pleasant-smelling oil. In actual fact, it is one of the oils that is not recommended for use in a traditional holistic aromatherapy treatment.[5]

On the other hand, Tisserand states that holistic aromatherapy typically involves an aromatherapy massage with a dilution of 2–3% of essential oil.[6] Tisserand says that the amount of essential oil absorbed into the bloodstream from such a dermal application is likely to be in the range of 0.025 mL to 0.1 mL, some twenty times less than that of oral administration.[6]

Aromatherapy has often been labelled as a relaxing feel-good therapy that is non-specific. One of the special attributes of holistic aromatherapy is that it operates on physiological and psychological levels at the same time.

Buchbauer suggests that the physicochemical properties of essential oil constituents, their molecular size and weight mean that the biological activity of essential oil molecules can be compared with the activity of drugs.[7]

Buchbauer outlines two opposing views that explain the possible mode of action of essential oils. The reflectorial effect theory suggests that the fragrance compounds bring about a desired effect by creating a sensation of a pleasant feeling by having an effect on the limbic system. The limbic system is responsible for all our emotions and sensations like anxiety, fear, feelings of wellbeing and sexual desires.[7]

The systemic theory suggests that the fragrance compounds work by direct molecular interactions, with corresponding receptors in the CNS.[7] I believe that Buchbauer is correct in saying that both theories are correct. He uses the analogy of a person who eats a cube of sugar:

> *One not only senses a sweet and pleasant feeling, but the ingested sugar molecules induce a cascade of insulin reactions also.*[7]

Holistic aromatherapy usually involves massage and inhalations, so the following question needs to be asked:

Are externally applied or inhaled essential oils absorbed into the bloodstream, in sufficient quantities to have a pharmacological effect?

Clinical trials have confirmed that small amounts of essential oil constituents have been detected in the blood within minutes, following massage and inhalation. The amount of essential oil absorbed into the bloodstream from dermal or inhalation application was significantly less than from oral administration, and these same clinical studies confirmed that linalool, the main chemical constituent found in lavender, had a pharmacological sedative affect.

Therefore, if lavender is known to be a sedative pharmacologically then it should always reliably have a sedative effect no matter how it is applied and to whom it is applied.

However, this is not so. It may be impossible to predict the effect of an odour on humans because its effects when inhaled may be subject to the many factors as described:[8]

a) How the odour is applied;
b) The quantity used;
c) The circumstances in which it is applied;
d) The person to whom it is applied (age, sex, personality);
e) The person's mood;
f) Previous memory associations the person may have with the odour;
g) Anosmia.

While factors a), b), and c) can be controlled, the control of d), e), f) and g) is difficult. Therefore the extent to which a psychological effect can override one that is pharmacological, or a pharmacological effect can override its psychological counterpart, has yet to be researched. Some would say that there are no predictable psychological or pharmacological effects at all.[8]

Properties of Essential Oils

This chapter will review the established properties of essential oils. These are:

- alterative
- analgesic
- anti-inflammatory
- antiseptic and antibacterial
- antifungal
- antiviral
- astringent
- carminative
- cholagogue
- diaphoretic
- diuretic
- emmenagogue
- expectorant
- mucolytic
- rubefacient
- sedative
- spasmolytic and
- wound healing — promotion of granulation.

These properties will be discussed in terms of traditional use and current pharmacological studies.

Alterative

An alterative is a remedy that cleanses and purifies the blood. The terms commonly used are detoxifiers or blood purifiers. The concept of blood purification is difficult for a person with a medical or pharmacological background to understand or agree with.

An alterative assists the body's natural eliminatory response by stimulating the liver, lungs, lymphatic system, kidneys, bowels and sweat glands, therefore excreting injurious or toxic matter that may cause irritation such as:

- mucus
- faeces
- urine
- menstrual blood and
- other toxins.

Any essential oil with any of the following properties is classified as an alterative.

- lymphatic — assisting the tissue-cleaning action of the lymphatic system.
- diaphoretic — promoting sweating, thus assisting the excretory functions of the skin.
- expectorant — promoting expulsion of mucus, thus assisting the respiratory system.
- diuretic — promoting urination, thus assisting the kidneys.
- hepatic — enhancing liver function, thus assisting the liver's detoxifying function.
- laxative — promoting bowel movement, thus assisting with the excretory functions of the large intestine.
- emmenagogue — promoting menstruation, thus assisting in the elimination of menstrual blood.

All of the above properties will help promote detoxification for the general treatment of toxaemia.

Analgesic

According to Tyler, pain is an unpleasant sensory experience associated with actual or potential tissue damage.[9] Pain can be defined as acute or chronic in character, and analgesics are used to treat pain. Analgesics used to treat pain can be classified as:

a) narcotics that bind to opioid receptors;

b) non-narcotics that lack an affinity to such receptors.[9]

While substances such as morphine and codeine fall into category a), most essential oils which are applied topically to ease pain fall into category b). In most cases it seems that the analgesic property of the essential oils is due to their ability to inhibit prostaglandin synthesis.

Eugenol, found in clove essential oil, is well known for its local anaesthetic effect. It is well known for its ability to obtain transient relief from a toothache.[9,10,11]

According to Tyler, eugenol, like other phenols, depresses sensory receptors involved in pain perception. The mechanism of action involves, in part, a pronounced inhibition of prostaglandin biosynthesis resulting from a blockage of the cycloxygenase and lipoxygenase pathways.[9]

The anti-inflammatory and analgesic properties of methyl salicylate, found in wintergreen, have traditionally been used in rubs for muscular pain.[9] Menthol has been long employed for the relief of headaches. Other essential oils found to be effective in reducing pain are those containing the ketone, camphor.[9]

Essential oils rich in monoterpene hydrocarbons have been found to have an analgesic effect, especially those essential oils containing para-cymene and myrcene. According to Lorenzetti, myrcene, a component of lemongrass essential oil, was found to have analgesic properties.[12]

The analgesic properties of peppermint oil have also been investigated. Four test preparations were used:

- peppermint oil (10%) and eucalyptus oil (5%);
- peppermint oil (10%) with a trace of eucalyptus oil;
- eucalyptus oil (5%) with a trace of peppermint;
- traces of both peppermint and eucalyptus oils (placebo).[13]

All the preparations were dissolved in ethanol. Thirty-two healthy subjects took part in a double-blind, placebo-controlled randomised study.

Experimental pain sensitivity was significantly reduced only by the peppermint preparation, although the peppermint-eucalyptus mixture and the eucalyptus only mixture increased cognitive performance and was muscle relaxing, but had little analgesic effect.[13]

Anti-inflammatory

Essential oils that are anti-inflammatory are able to decrease swelling and inflammation. There are many reasons for the anti-inflammatory effect of essential oils, and they vary for different essential oils.

The anti-inflammatory property of German chamomile oil is well documented when used topically.[14,15,16] German chamomile is considered an anti-inflammatory due to its chamazulene and the α-bisabolol content.

Professor Della Loggia evaluated the anti-inflammatory activity of essential oils. He states that anti-inflammatory activities have been falsely attributed to many essential oils and their components. Of the 31 essential oils investigated which have traditionally claimed to be anti-inflammatory, only three can be said to have such properties.[15]

The anti-inflammatory effects of (-)-α-bisabolol found in German chamomile have been proven in experiments on adjuvant arthritis in rats.[16] Experiments showed that (-)-α-bisabolol had a greater effect than bisabolol oxides A and B. It was suggested that standardising chamomile preparations of antiphlogistic effectiveness the content of (-)-α-bisabolol was important, but that standardising the amount of oxides present was not necessary.[16]

Balacs cites a German research group that found that chamazulene inhibits the formation of leukotriene B4 in neutrophils in vitro and blocked the artificial peroxidation of arachidonic acid, possibly because of chamazulene's auto-oxidative property.[17] The above research confirms the traditional uses of chamomile.

Balacs also cites a Korean study which confirmed lavender's anti-inflammatory effects. The results of an in-vitro and in-vivo study on the immediate-type allergic reaction in mice found that lavender oil can inhibit immediate-type allergic reactions by inhibiting mast cell degranulation.[18]

A German study has shown extracts of turmeric to have potent anti-inflammatory activity. The researchers suggest that curcumin, found in turmeric essential oil, is responsible for its anti-inflammatory activity.[19]

The anti-inflammatory effect of clove oil has been reported.[10,20] Balacs cites a study which suggests that clove's anti-inflammatory activity is due to β-caryophyllene.[21]

Antimicrobial

The term antimicrobial loosely describes the more specific terms antibacterial, antiviral and antifungal. Before discussing the antimicrobial activities of essential oils, we shall review the methods used to determine the essential oil's antimicrobial activity.

Determining the Antimicrobial Activity of Essential Oils

Hundreds of articles are published each year describing the antimicrobial activity of essential oils. However, according to Williams, the final conclusion is usually along the following lines — 'the activity against a wide range of bacteria, yeasts and fungi'. No scale is given and so the information in this form is of little value if one is to attempt to use the oil in a formulated product.[23]

There are many techniques that can be used to determine the antimicrobial activity of essential oils. The most common method used involves the agar-overlay technique, described by Williams:

> *An agar plate is a circular plastic dish containing a layer of gel that contains the nutrients necessary for the optimum growth of the particular micro-organisms. A layer of the inoculum containing the micro-organism is spread on the surface and the essential oil is added to a paper disc in the middle of the plate.*
>
> *The plate is then placed in an incubator set at the most appropriate temperature for growth of the micro-organism (usually between 37–42° C).*
>
> *Over the period of incubation the essential oils gradually diffuse from the centre through the agar towards the perimeter and as it does so it spreads out and becomes more dilute. While the undiluted oil at the centre may inhibit growth of the micro-organism there comes a stage of dilution when the components of the essential oil are no longer able to inhibit growth. At this radius from the centre there will be a clearly defined zone of inhibition.*[23]

Williams says that there are several ways of controlling the zone of inhibition. Either the concentration of the inoculum can be adjusted or the amount of essential oil added to the paper disc in the centre of the plate can be modified. Therefore if the zone of inhibition can be easily altered, the size of the zone of inhibition has no scientific value unless a standard is established.[23]

Antibacterial Activity

The antibacterial activity of essential oils has been long known. Most of the information regarding the antibacterial properties of essential oils originally came from France.[22]

There is certainly no shortage of research which has proven that many essential oils have bactericidal effects. However, it is most surprising that research has done so little to investigate the actual mechanism/s of the antibacterial property of essential oils.

Schnaubelt says that because essential oils are lipid-soluble they dissolve in the biological membranes. The cell walls of bacteria are such that much of the primary energy metabolism (breathing and consequent formation of ATP) takes place in these membranes.[24]

The effect of essential oils on the primary energy metabolism of bacteria is most likely not the only way in which essential oils affect bacteria. However, it does explain why bacteria can not develop a resistance to essential oils.

The terpenoid constituents have been found to interfere with enzymatic reactions of energy metabolism. Much of the primary energy metabolism takes place in the cell membranes of bacteria. Low concentrations of different terpenoid compounds were able to significantly inhibit oxygen intake and formation of ATP in the cell wall. The oxygen intake was completely inhibited by functional groups such as phenols (thymol and carvacrol); alcohols also revealed the strong inhibitory effects, followed by aldehydes and ketones.[25]

The values of inhibition of oxygen uptake and ATP formation given in the table below were determined by Knobloch using the bacterium *Rhodopseudomonas sphaeroides* as a test organism.[25] This nonpathogenic, gram-negative bacterium was accepted as a test organism for its wide distribution and its ability to grow anaerobically or aerobically on numerous organic compounds.

Compound	% Inhibition of ATP formation	% inhibition of O_2 uptake
Thymol	100	100
Menthol	85	86
Borneol	89	88
Borneol acetate	65	64
Camphor	66	65
Eugenol	90	93
Cymene	24	21

To evaluate the antibacterial activity of essential oils, one has to appraise carefully their penetration through cell walls, their influence on the phospholipid bilayers of cell membranes and the specific interaction with the membrane-integrated enzyme turnover rates represented in nature by the primary energy metabolism of the cell.

Numerous clinical trials have confirmed tea tree oil's antibacterial activity. A case was reported of a woman suffering from anaerobic vaginosis who refused antibiotics and treated herself with tea tree pessaries. Re-examination by her doctor a month later showed normal vaginal secretions and bacterial flora. It was discussed that tea tree oil may be a preferable treatment for the condition rather than nitroimidazoles.[26]

Antifungal Activity

Many essential oils have been reported as having an antifungal effect. Research in India indicated that spikenard oil completely inhibited the growth of *Aspergillus flavus, A. niger* and *Fusarium oxysporum* at 1 ml/L concentration. The oil's action was found to be fungistatic rather than fungicidal. *Nardostachys jatamansi* was also found to be active against a wide range of other fungi.[27]

Further research from India found that coriander was effective in inhibiting *Alternana alternate, Curulana lunata, Pestalotia psidi, Phytophthora parasitica, Trichoderma viride and Collectotricum capsici*. All of the above fungi were inhibited by coriander oil.[28]

A research group from Lahore, Pakistan, studied the inhibitory effects of lemongrass against pathogenic fungi. The sample of lemongrass tested contained between 70% and 80% citral. The samples with the highest citral content were found to be the most active. The following fungi were screened: *Spergillus niger*, *A fumigatus*, *Candida albicans* and *Trichophyten tonsurance* (isolated from patients).[29]

An extensive amount of research has been conducted on the antifungal properties of tea tree oil against *C. albicans*. Carson found the action of tea tree against *C. albicans* was important due to the limited range of topical antifungal agents.[30] Belaiche used tea tree on 28 patients with vaginitis caused by *C. albicans*.[31] They were treated with tea tree pessaries. In another trial, Belaiche found tea tree to be effective against *Versicolor pityriasis* and nail infections (onyxis and perionyxis) caused by *C. albicans*.[32]

Antiviral Activity

Schnaubelt suggests that aromatherapy is ideally suited to the treatment of viral infections because of the connection between the immune system and mind/body connection.[33] He comments on chronic fatigue syndrome:

> *...we must realise that conditions such as CFS breakout when the immune system has been so sufficiently weakened that the opportunistic virus can start to proliferate. We also realise that it is not the long-ago contracted infection with the virus which makes us sick, rather it is the conditions which deplete our immune response ...Considering further that our immune system is tied tightly to our brain and emotions, how could it be that there is not also a philosophical dimension to this: the insanity the corporate culture produces is not at all conducive to mental and emotional health.*[33]

Schnaubelt cites treatments for:

- *Herpes simplex* type I and *Herpes simplex* type II;
- *Herpes zoster* and shingles;
- Epstein-Barr virus (EBV) and chronic fatigue syndrome.[33]

He suggests that immediate application of melissa or other essential oils prevents the herpes viruses from replicating. If this is accomplished, the process is shortened considerably or a new outbreak is completely inhibited. Schnaubelt suggests that the antiviral activity of essential oils is due to their lipophilic nature.[33]

Astringent

Astringents have a firming and healing action on the mucous membranes or exposed tissues. They bring about contraction, they firm and dry up secretions and generally make tissues more dense. Although primarily drying, astringents also prevent moisture loss.

Astringents may be used symptomatically to stop bleeding or to treat diarrhoea. However, it must be remembered that they often do not correct the cause of the problem. According to Holmes, astringents are often classified:[34]

- Those which arrest bleeding (haemostatics) and those which tonify and restore venous circulation — e.g., for the treatment of varicose veins and haemorrhoids. Essential oils which arrest bleeding and restore venous circulation include cypress, frankincense, myrrh, rock rose, sage and sandalwood.
- Those which stop excessive discharge of waste materials — e.g., for the treatment of menorrhagia, diarrhoea, excessive perspiration. Essential oils which stop excessive discharge of waste materials include cypress, frankincense, myrrh, rock rose, sage and sandalwood.
- Those which restrain infection and promote the healing of tissues — vulnerary. Essential oils which promote the healing of wounds and prevent infection and swelling are everlasting, frankincense, myrrh and rock rose.

Carminative

Carminatives relieve intestinal gas, pain and distension. They will settle digestion, increase absorption and promote normal peristalsis, thus promoting digestion and assisting in dispelling accumulation of undigested food materials.

Carminatives' mechanism of action occurs via:[9]

- a reflex that causes a toning of the intestinal walls with resorption and passing through of gases;
- a local irritating effect on the lining of the stomach or the gastric mucosa;
- a spasmolytic effect and relief of flatulence;
- a cholagogue effect.

Many carminatives tend to have warm and dry qualities and are known as digestive stimulants. Carminatives consist mostly of essential oils extracted from the Umbelliferae plant family such as angelica, aniseed, coriander, caraway, fennel and dill.[34]

Tyler suggests that the plants containing volatile oils are the most effective.[9] Weiss says that there are many plants with carminative properties, mainly plants containing volatile oils with specific actions. These include aniseed, caraway, chamomile, fennel, peppermint, melissa and angelica.[35]

The German commission E has found peppermint oil to be an effective carminative.[11] Tyler says that peppermint oil is an effective spasmolytic, stimulant of the flow of bile, an antibacterial and a promoter of gastric secretions.[9]

Cholagogue

Cholagogues are agents producing an increase in the production of bile, while a choleretic causes the bile which has been produced to flow more freely. The two actions overlap to some extent. In researching literature on the cholagogue effect of essential oils it was observed that most essential oils which possessed cholagogue properties also had spasmolytic and carminative properties.

Werbach discusses the effectiveness of a formulation known as Rowachol. Each 100 mg capsule of Rowachol contained the following terpene components:[36]

menthol	0.32 mg
menthone	0.6 mg
pinene	17 mg
borneol	0.5 mg
camphene	0.5 mg
cineole	0.2 mg
olive oil	0.33 mg

In a clinical study involving the above formulation, bile secretion was increased from 1519 mumol/h to 2287 mumol/h. Studies have also shown gallstones to completely disappear within 1 to 2 years.[36] Clinical trials have confirmed that peppermint has significant choleretic activity.[37,39] Other essential oils with choleretic activity included fennel, coriander, German chamomile and lavender.[39]

A clinical trial investigated the choleretic action of essential oil constituents such as menthol, camphene, anethol, borneol and fenchone. In guinea pigs, only menthol caused a increase in bile production, while cholesterol excretion was increased by menthol and camphene. Nerol and anethol increased the production of bile acids. Nerol had a choleretic effect on rats and guinea pigs. It was concluded that the choleretic and cholagogue activity appears to be species-specific.[42]

Diaphoretic

A diaphoretic induces perspiration and by this action restores circulation and dispels fever and chills while eliminating toxins from the body via the skin. Strong diaphoretics are referred to as sudorifics.

Diaphoretics will assist the body in the following ways:

- assist the excretory function of the skin;
- resolve the development of local congestion or inflammation resulting from cold;
- relieve muscular tension and aching joints;
- relieve headaches due to cold and congestion.

Diaphoretics may induce perspiration by:[38]

- Influencing peripheral sensory nerves, which relax and dilate the superficial capillaries and vessels. They influence the surface circulation and then the entire circulation. The increased blood flow results in increased perspiration.
- Influencing the sudoriferous glands indirectly by stimulating the medulla, which controls the action of the sudoriferous glands.
- Entering the circulation, and as they are eliminated by the sudoriferous glands (in the sweat and oil), they stimulate the local nerve fibres, supplying these glands, thereby increasing perspiration.

The initial or acute stages of old and febrile diseases inhibit the circulation of *defensive energy,* which in turn inhibits sweating. Therefore diaphoretic essential oils will stimulate and restore the defensive energy of the body.

In traditional medicine there are two kinds of diaphoretics:

- warming diaphoretics
- cooling diaphoretics.[34]

Warming diaphoretics are used to treat the common cold by dispersing the external pathogenic factors known in Chinese medicine as wind, cold and dampness. Essential oils which are warming diaphoretics include angelica, basil, cardamom, cinnamon, clove bud, eucalyptus, ginger, rosemary and thyme.[34]

Cooling diaphoretics are more effective for treating high fever, sore throats and other inflammatory conditions involving toxins. They are generally also alteratives and may possess diuretic properties. Essential oils which are cooling diaphoretics include German chamomile, everlasting, peppermint, spearmint and yarrow.[34]

Treatment involving diaphoretic remedies should include hot baths, sleeping under a warm blanket and fasting.

Diuretic

The function of the kidneys is to remove waste from the body while maintaining the chemical integrity of its cells and tissues. They work by maintaining the appropriate concentration of electrolytes, amino acids and glucose.[9]

Diuretics increase the volume of urine excreted. This is achieved by:

- stimulating the blood flow to the kidneys, or
- reducing the resorption of water from the filtrate in the kidney's nephrons.[2]

Those that stimulate the blood flow to the kidneys are referred to as circulatory stimulants and cardioactive remedies and include substances such as coffee and tea. Diuretics have the following therapeutic properties:[38]

- they assist in the removal of waste products and toxic materials
- they promote the excretion of waste fluids from the tissues and cavities of the body
- they maintain kidney action by stimulating the normal excretory function
- they help eliminate urine solids, and lessen irritation of the genitourinary tract when the urine contains an excessively high concentration of irritant substances
- they have an antiseptic effect, reducing urinary infection.

Tyler says that the classic botanical diuretics are not diuretics at all, but are more accurately designated as aquaretics. That is, they increase the volume of urine by promoting blood flow in the kidneys, hence increasing the glomerular filtration rate.[9] He says that they do not retard the resorption of Na+ and Cl– in the renal tubes, so quantities of these electrolytes are retained in the body and not excreted along with the water. This means that they are not suited for the treatment of conditions such as oedema or hypertension.[9]

The most active diuretic is juniper berry essential oil. It is known that it is a diuretic as a result of its irritant action. Schilcher suggests that juniper berry oils containing a low ratio of irritating monoterpene hydrocarbons to non-irritating active aquaretic terpinen-4-ol do not exhibit nephrotoxicity. However, Tyler says that this hypothesis requires additional pharmacological testing.[9]

Other essential oils with diuretic properties include black pepper, fennel seed, carrot seed, geranium and parsley seed.

Emmenagogue

Emmenagogues promote and regulate menstruation and are used to treat many special disorders of the female reproductive system such as:

- painful menstruation — dysmenorrhoea
- mucus discharge — leucorrhoea
- absence of menstruation — amenorrhoea

Emmenagogues exhibit several different mechanisms of action. Some act directly on the uterus, myometrium and the vasculature surrounding the reproductive organs. Others affect the uterus and reproductive system indirectly through peripheral systems such as the endocrine, cardiovascular, gastrointestinal and nervous system.[39] Some essential oils help to normalise the menstrual flow by regulating the hormones of the hypothalamus, pituitary and ovaries.[39] Emmenagogues may also be antispasmodic, thus relieving uterine cramps and pain.

Typical emmenagogues include angelica, basil, clary sage, German and roman chamomile, cinnamon, ginger, jasmine, juniper berry, lavender, myrrh, peppermint, rose, rosemary, fennel seed and sweet marjoram.

It needs to be mentioned that emmenagogues are not necessarily abortifacients. Only some are contraindicated during pregnancy. They will be described in *Chapter 12*.

Expectorant

Expectorants promote the discharge of phlegm and mucus from the bronchopulmonary mucous membrane.

The stimulating action on the bronchi makes coughing easier, thus encouraging the natural eliminatory response that brings bronchial secretions and other airborne matter up to the throat. In this cleansing process there are two main problems:[2]

- excessive mucus secretion, which causes an overload of the mucociliary escalator and results in congestion in the lungs.
- an inflammatory response or hypersensitivity, which results in a tight, dry, unstable condition as seen in dry coughs and asthma.

According to Mills there are three categories of expectorants:

- Stimulating and warming expectorants — thus removing mucus by their drying action. These are often referred to as 'stimulating expectorants', because they stimulate activity of the mucociliary escalator leading to a more productive cough.[2] Expectorants that will generate warmth and expel phlegm include aniseed, angelica, basil, cardamom, cinnamon, ginger, hyssop, pine, eucalyptus, fennel, sweet marjoram, rosemary, thyme, myrrh and frankincense.
- Relaxing expectorants. These have a soothing and demulcent effect and are ideal for dry and irritable conditions. They appear to act by reflex to soothe bronchial spasm and loosen mucus secretions.[2] Essential oils for treating dry and irritable conditions include Roman chamomile, cypress, cedarwood and sandalwood.
- Antitussives have cough-relieving actions. They usually have antispasmodic properties.[2] Antitussive essential oils include angelica, eucalyptus, clary sage, cypress, hyssop, myrtle and pine.

It is very important that the cough be identified as either productive or unproductive and that the client be treated with the appropriate essential oils. It is inappropriate to use relaxing expectorants for a congested bronchial condition; conversely, it is contraindicated to use stimulating expectorants for asthmatics.

Tyler says that essential oils such as aniseed, eucalyptus, fennel, peppermint and thyme are used in throat lozenges because they stimulate the formation and secretion of saliva, which produces more frequent swallowing and thereby tends to suppress the cough reflex. He states that volatile oils exert a direct stimulatory effect on the bronchial glands by means of local irritation.[9]

Clinical trials have confirmed the expectorant effect, after inhalation, of some essential oils. As a measure for expectoration the amount and consistency of bronchial liquid was determined. According to clinical trials performed by Boyd the following essential oils and essential oil constituents have been found to be effective expectorants when inhaled: lemon, citral, citronellal, geraniol, limonene and α-pinene.[37]

It was important to note that high concentrations of essential oils dried up respiratory fluids, whereas low concentrations increased fluid, creating an expectorant effect.[37] Boyd's conclusion was that only low concentrations of essential oils should be used in vaporisers for treating lung conditions.[37] Assuming that the results from Boyd from animal experiments can be applied to humans, essential oils can be used for stimulating the secretion of condensed thick mucus in the respiratory tract.

It was also observed that oral application often did not have a pronounced effect whereas inhalation showed good results in very low dosages. A further observation was that the desired effect of the inhaled essential oils was greatly reduced or even absent when dosages were applied which gave a pronounced aroma in the inhaled air. According to Reichelmann, it is advantageous to use concentrations which make the inhaled air only faintly aromatic as the secretion-stimulating effect seems to change to a suppressant effect with higher doses.[37]

Application of essential oils to the skin has also been found to be effective for the treatment of chronic obstructive bronchitis. The expectorant effect of certain essential oils and their constituents has been traditionally utilised in chest rubs and inhalations to improve bronchial secretion and reduce bronchial spasms.[40]

Cineole found in eucalyptus oil is well known for its expectorant properties. It has been postulated that eucalyptus oil has an effect of reducing surface tension between water and air in the lungs, a property which would presumably enhance the effect of the lungs' own surfactant.[41]

Rubefacient

Essential oils with rubefacient properties usually increase local blood circulation, which can be observed by a redness of the skin, but they also influence the inner organs. The local skin irritation, the primary irritation, sets free mediators in the body which in turn cause vasodilation.

The local skin irritation can also have an analgesic influence on the inner organs. The primary irritation also causes humeral reactions, the results of which can be observed as anti-inflammatory effects. Besides an agreeable feeling of warmth and relief of pain, anti-inflammatory effects can be observed.

Essential oils with rubefacient properties include black pepper, cinnamon, clove bud, ginger, lemon, nutmeg, peppermint, pine, rosemary and thyme.

Sedative

Lavender essential oil diluted 1:60 with olive oil was given orally to mice, and the sedative effects observed by performing a number of tests. It was found that a significant interaction existed with pentobarbital; the sleeping time was increased and asleeping time was shortened.[43]

Under standardised experimental conditions lavender significantly decreased motility, and hyperactivity which had been induced by caffeine injection was reduced almost to normal. It was concluded that the effectiveness of the traditional aromatherapy use of lavender as a sedative was proven and that the use of lavender could facilitate and minimise stressful conditions.[44]

The sedative effect of neroli, citronellal and phenyl ethyl acetate was confirmed in a clinical trial. The motility of mice was reduced from an arbitrarily graded 100% for untreated animals to 34.73% by neroli, to 50.15% by citronellal and 54.94% by phenyl ethyl acetate. The method of application was inhalation.[45]

There is much evidence that essential oils, being aromatic lipid-soluble and electrically active compounds, have a profound psychophysiological effect when inhaled.

Spasmolytic

Essential oils with spasmolytic properties are also known as antispasmodics. Some essential oils have been found to relieve smooth muscle spasms, hence their usefulness for the treatment of problems associated with the:

- digestive system
- respiratory system
- reproductive system.

The majority of the research cited investigates the spasmolytic property of essential oils on the digestive system.

The most common and successful essential oil is peppermint. The spasmolytic activity of peppermint has been extensively researched. Hills suggests that peppermint oil reduces the availability of calcium in the gastrointestinal smooth muscle.[44] Evidence for the calcium-antagonistic properties of peppermint oil shows that menthol not only reduced the binding of specific calcium channel ligands in smooth muscles but also inhibited depolarisation-induced calcium uptake into neuronal preparations.[46]

The essential oil of German chamomile is rich in mono- and sesquiterpenes and was found to exert a dose-dependent spasmolytic effect on the smooth muscle of the intestine.[47] Lis-Balchin cites essential oils such as fennel, dill, *Eucalyptus citriodoria* and peppermint as being a few of the essential oils with a spasmolytic action.[48]

The spasmolytic activity for a number of essential oils such as chamomile, caraway seed, fennel, orange and peppermint has been confirmed. According to McKenzie, peppermint oil was used to relax smooth muscles of the bowel for patients with colostomies. This was found to reduce colonic pressure and reduce the frequency of bag changes and postoperative colic.[49]

Leicester found that peppermint oil reduced colonic spasms during endoscopy. Colonic spasms generally cause discomfort and physical hindrance during flexible sigmoidoscopy and intravenous antispasmodic drugs are usually used to counter this. In 20 patients, peppermint oil was injected along the biopsy channel of the colonoscope and in every case colonic spasm was relieved within 30 seconds.[50]

Weiss says that thyme is the remedy of choice for whooping cough. The spasmolytic action on bronchiolar spasm is one of the main characteristics of thyme. He calls it an expectorant with antispasmodic properties. Whenever there are spastic elements in a cough, thyme will benefit.[35]

While Weiss is talking about the whole herb, he does state that the volatile oil in thyme is the principal component that gives thyme its antispasmodic properties.[35]

Wound Healing

Essential oils have traditionally been used to promote the healing of wounds. Perhaps the most notable story is how Rene Gattefosse burnt his hand in a laboratory explosion and utilised pure lavender to heal his wound. He observed the rapid healing and pain-relieving effects of lavender. Gattefosse went on to collaborate with physicians such as Drs Sassard, Meurisse, Forgues and Machand, all of whom worked with essential oils in treating a wide variety of disorders including wounds and burns.[51]

Essential oils which promote wound healing include frankincense, German chamomile, everlasting, lavender, myrrh, neroli, palmarosa, rose, sandalwood and yarrow.

Gattefosse cites work done by Dr P. Sassard, who had the following to say of the wound-healing properties of lavender:

> *...in all cases the following was noted: the rapid disappearance of pus, decrease in the number of bacteria, powerful stimulation of healing, recovery in a very short time.*[51]

Guba has cited everlasting as having wound-healing properties. He has attributed this to the high concentration of the unusual diketonic hydrocarbons known as b-iones (15–20% italidones I, II and III).[52] Ketones generally exhibit excellent wound-healing properties.

A German study tested the therapeutic efficacy of chamomile on wound healing and found that it decreased the wound weeping area.[53]

Bone and Mills say that the wound-healing activity of chamomile is linked to its anti-inflammatory activity. They cite several clinical studies which demonstrate chamomile's wound-healing activity.[53]

Calendula officinalis has been traditionally used for the treatment of skin ailments and to facilitate wound healing.[9,11] Calendula is generally used as an infused oil or an aqueous extract.

Rosehip vegetable oil is a rich source of polyunsaturated fatty acids, linoleic and linolenic acid. Research indicates that topically applied oils containing essential fatty acids will speed the wound-healing process by assisting the formation of prostaglandins.[52]

Guba suggests that prostaglandins may be involved in the wound-healing process by increasing local blood supply, mediating leucocyte emigration into the wound and assisting the synthesis of granulation tissue.[52]

References

1. Long N. *Business is booming for alternative treatments.* The Weekend Independent, Aug 11, 1995: 14.
2. Mills S. *Out of the earth.* Viking Arkana, England, 1991.
3. Scott C. *In profile: Dr Jean Claude Lapraz.* The International Journal of Aromatherapy, 1991; 3(4): 12–14.
4. Holmes P. *The energetics of western herbs — Vol. 1.* Artemis Press, USA, 1986.
5. Peneol D. *This is also aromatherapy.* The International Journal of Aromatherapy, 1991; 3(3): 14–16.
6. Tisserand R. *Aromatherapy as mind–body medicine.* The International Journal of Aromatherapy, 1994; 6(3): 14–19.
7. Buchbauer G. *Molecular interaction.* The International Journal of Aromatherapy, 1993; 5(1): 11–14.
8. Tisserand R. *POP'91 Conference report.* The International Journal of Aromatherapy, 1991; 3(3): 10–12.
9. Tyler V. *Herbs of choice.* Haworth Press, USA, 1994.
10. Bruneton J. *Pharmacognosy.* Lavoisier Publishing Inc, France, 1999.
11. Blumenthal M, et al. *The complete German commission E monographs: Therapeutic guide to herbal medicine.* American Botanical Council USA, 1998.
12. Lorenzetti BB, et al. *Myrcene mimics the peripheral analgesic activity of lemongrass tea.* J. Ethnopharmacol, Aug; 34(I): 43–8 (1991). Cited in *The Aromatherapy Database*, by Bob Harris, Essential Oil Resource Consultants, UK, 2000.
13. Balacs T. *Research reports.* The International Journal of Aromatherapy, 1995; 7(2): 40–42.
14. Fleischer AM. *Plant extracts to accelerate healing and reduce inflammation.* Cosmetic Toilet, 1985; 100: 147–153.
15. Della Loggia R. Paper presented at the 24th International Symposium on Essential Oils. Berlin, 1993.
16. Isaac O. *Pharmacological investigations with compounds of chamomile.* Planta Medica, 1979; 35: 188–194.
17. Balacs T. *Research reports.* The International Journal of Aromatherapy, 1996; 7(2): 40–42.
18. Balacs T. *Research reports.* The International Journal of Aromatherapy, 2000; 10(1/2): 68–71.
19. Balacs T. *Research reports.* The International Journal of Aromatherapy, 2000; 5(1): 24–26.
20. Leung A, Foster S. *Encyclopedia of common natural ingredients used in food, drugs and cosmetics.* John Wiley & Sons Inc, USA, 1996.
21. Balacs T. *Research reports.* The International Journal of Aromatherapy, 1997; 8(2): 43–45.
22. Price S, Price L. *Aromatherapy for health professionals.* Churchill Livingstone, UK, 1995.
23. Williams L. *Ranking antimicrobial activity.* The International Journal of Aromatherapy, 1996; 7(4): 32–35.
24. Schnaubelt K. *Aromatherapy lecture notes.* Pacific Institute of Aromatherapy, USA, 1987.
25. Knobloch K, et al. *Antibacterial and antifungal properties of essential oil components.* The Journal of Essential Oil Research 1989; 1(3): 112–128.
26. Dept. Genito-urinary Medicine, Swansea,. *Tea Tree oil and anaerobic (bacterial) vaginosis.* Lancet, 337(8736): 300. Cited in *Australian Tea Tree*, by C. Dean, The 2nd Australasian Aromatherapy Conference Proceedings, Australia, 1998.
27. Mishra D, et al. *The fungitoxic effect of the essential oil of the herb Nardostachys jatamansi* Dc. Tropical Agriculture 1995; 72(1): 48–52. Cited in *The Aromatherapy Database*, by Bob Harris, Essential Oil Resource Consultants, UK, 2000.
28. Garg SG, Siddigini N. *In vitro antifungal activity of the essential oil of Coriandrum sativum Linn.* J.Res. Ed. In. Med. 1992; II(3) 11–13v
29. Qarier R. et al. *Antifungal activity of lemongrass essential oils.* Pakistan Journal of Scientific and Industrial Research. 1992; 35(6): 246–249.

30. Carson CF. *The antimicrobial activity of tea tree oil.* Medical Journal of Australia, 1994; 160: 236. Cited in *The Aromatherapy Database*, by Bob Harris, Essential Oil Resource Consultants, UK, 2000.

31. Belaiche P. *Treatment of vaginal infections of Candida albicans with essential oils of Melaleuca alternifolia.* Phytotherapie, 1985; 15: 15–17. Cited in *The Aromatherapy Database*, by Bob Harris, Essential Oil Resource Consultants, UK, 2000.

32. Belaiche P. *Treatment of skin infections with the essential oil of Melaleuca alternifolia.* Phytotherapie, 1985; 15: 15–17. Cited in *Australian Tea Tree*, by C. Dean, The 2nd Australasian Aromatherapy Conference Proceedings, Australia, 1998.

33. Schnaubelt K. *Aromatherapy and Chronic Viral Infections.* Aroma '93 conference Proceedings Aromatherapy Publications, East Sussex, England, 1994.

34. Holmes P. *The energetics of western herbs — Vol. 1.* Artemis Press, USA, 1986.

35. Weiss F. *Herbal medicine.* Beaconsfield Publishers, England, 1988.

36. Werbach MR, Murray M. *Botanical influences on illness: A sourcebook of clinical research.* Third Line Press, USA, 1994.

37. Cited from Mediherb Monitor No. 7, December 1993.

38. Willard T. *Textbook of modern herbology.* 2nd ed, Wild Rose College of Natural Healing Ltd, Canada, 1993.

39. McGuffin et al. eds, *American Herbal Products Association's botanical safety handbook.* CRC Press, USA, 1997.

40. Schafer D, Schafer W. Pharmacological studies with an ointment containing menthol, camphene and essential oils for broncholytic and secretolytic effects. Arzeimittelforschung 1981; 31(I): 82–86. Cited in *The Aromatherapy Database*, by Bob Harris, Essential Oil Resource Consultants, UK, 2000.

41. Balacs T. *Cineole-rich eucalyptus.* The International Journal of Aromatherapy, 1997; 8(2): 43–45.

42. Rangelov A, et al. *Experimental study of the cholagogic and choleretic action of some of the basic constituents of essential oils on laboratory animals.* Folia Medica, 1989; 30(4): 30–38. Cited in *The Aromatherapy Database*, by Bob Harris, Essential Oil Resource Consultants, UK, 2000.

43. Guillemain J, et al. *Neurodepressive effects of the essential oil of Lavendula angustifolia mill.* Ann Pharm 1989; 47(6): 337–343. Cited in *The Aromatherapy Database*, by Bob Harris, Essential Oil Resource Consultants, UK, 2000.

44. Buchbauer G, et al. *Aromatherapy: Evidence for sedative effects of the essential oil of lavender after inhalation.* Z Naturforsch, 1991; 46(11/12): 1067–1072. Cited in *The Aromatherapy Database*, by Bob Harris, Essential Oil Resource Consultants, UK, 2000.

45. Jager W, et al. *Evidence of the sedative effect of neroli oil, citronellal and phenyl ethyl acetate on mice.* Journal of Essential Oil Research, 1992; 4(4): 381–385.

46. Hills JM. *The mechanism of action of peppermint oil on gastrointestinal smooth muscle. An analysis using patch clamp electrophysiology and isolated tissue pharmacology in rabbit and guinea pig.* Gastroenterology, 10(1): 55–65. Cited in *The Aromatherapy Database*, by Bob Harris, Essential Oil Resource Consultants, UK, 2000.

47. Acterrath-Tuckermann U. et al. *Pharmacological investigations with the compounds of chamomile.* Planta Medica, 1980; 39: 38–50. Cited in *The Aromatherapy Database*, by Bob Harris, Essential Oil Resource Consultants, UK, 2000.

48. Lis-Balchin M. *The chemistry and bioactivity of essential oils.* Amberwood Publishing Ltd, England, 1995.

49. McKenzie J, Gallacher M. *A sweet smelling success: Use of peppermint oil in helping patients accept their colostomies.* Nursing Times 1989; 85(27): 48–49.

50. Leicester RJ, Hunt RH. *Peppermint oil to reduce colonic spasm during endoscopy.* Lancet, 1982; 2(8305): 989.

51. Gattefosse R. *Gattefosse's aromatherapy.* Translated by Robert Tisserand, England, First published in 1937, English version published by The C.W. Daniel Compant Limited, Great Britain, 1993.

52. Guba R. *Aromatic extracts as wound healing agents.* Aromatherapy Today, 1997:3:

53. Bone K, Mills S. *Principles and practice of phytotherapy.* Churchill Livingstone, UK, 2000.

Biology and Psychology of Essential Oils

Objectives

After careful study of this chapter, you should be able to:

- outline the evolutionary role of olfaction
- explain the role of human body odour
- define anosmia
- describe the olfactory organs and the olfactory pathway
- outline the effects of olfaction on the brain
- examine how human behaviour and mood are affected by olfaction
- discuss the link between olfaction and emotions
- discuss the role of environmental fragrancing.

Olfaction

The Role of Olfaction in Aromatherapy

The term 'aromatherapy' implies that the therapeutic effect is derived from the 'aroma' of the essential oils. It suggests a treatment involving smell. However, many aromatherapy books place very little emphasis on the smell of essential oils and the olfactory processes. While much emphasis is placed on aromatherapy as a 'feel good therapy' in which the pleasant smell of the essential oils contributes to a sense of wellbeing, very little has been understood about the mechanisms of olfaction.

Olfaction and in particular, the way in which we interpret and process odours has been very poorly understood by physiologists. It has only been in the last 10 years that we have started to unravel the mysteries of olfaction.

During the past decade, numerous research groups have conducted research aimed at measuring the effects of odours on the human psyche. Researchers have used a variety of techniques such as measuring changes in the patterns of electromagnetic activity in the brain, changes in physiological parameters such as heart rate and electro-dermal activity, and changes in mental and physical performance and in mood and perceived state of health.

Understanding olfaction is the most exciting aspect of aromatherapy. I believe that olfaction plays a very important role in the efficacy of aromatherapy and an understanding of the mechanisms of olfaction will help us develop clinical skills.

The Evolutionary Role of Olfaction

The sense of smell is highly developed in animals, being used to detect food, identify individuals and enemies, mark territory and identify the opposite sex. Most anatomy and physiology books suggest that olfaction is the least important of the senses because humans do not rely on smell for communicating, finding food or for sexual attraction.

In the animal kingdom, most smells are 'hard-wired in', meaning that they act as a form of communication.[1] Van Toller gives the example of a termite colony where a battle has occurred with another colony. If the soldier termites are depleted when they return, the 'soldier smell' of the colony will be at a low level. Then young termites will turn into soldiers until the level of odour comes back to where it should be. He says that this also occurs with bees, but the trouble is that it leads to stereotypical behaviour, where individuality does not exist.[1]

Stoddart explains the existence of a relationship linking olfactory sense with sex and reproduction.[2] He cites experimental studies in mammals that confirm that sexual attraction and the physiological process of reproduction are controlled by the olfactory system and that if the olfactory system is damaged reproduction does not occur.[2] He then asks whether the same is true for our own species.

Evidence suggests that the evolution of human beings has suppressed our ability to decode the information content of sexual odour signals that emanate from other human beings. The suppression relates to the genetic and sociobiological imperative for a strong pair bond to form between an infant's mother and father. This provides the infant with the best chance of survival in a hostile and competitive world.[2]

The Role of Olfaction in Humans

Youngentob says that the sense of smell is considered less critical to survival of humans, although there are times when detection of odours such as smoke, gas or decaying food can prevent bodily harm. He says that civilised society seems to emphasise the impressive hedonic effect of olfaction. For example, people add seasoning to their foods, perfumes to their bodies and incense to their homes.[3]

Olfaction plays a very important role in flavour perception and the recognition of tastes. Much of what people think they taste, they actually smell. Youngentob cites a study, which asked subjects to identify 21 common food substances placed on the tongue. There was a decrease from the average of 60% correct to 10% correct when the nasal cavity was made inaccessible to any vapours given off by the substance. Even coffee and chocolate, which were correctly identified by over 90% of test subjects when the nose was accessible, were not identified correctly by any subject when the nose was accessible.[3]

Therefore olfaction appears to have a tremendous impact on the quality of life, and anything that interferes with appropriate functioning of olfaction can be profoundly distressing.

The Role of Human Body Odour

It is strange that human beings, who have the most developed scent glands of all primates, generally regard body odours as unpleasant and distasteful and will go to great efforts to eliminate such body odours.

While there is no doubt that the axillary glands of human beings are larger, contain more apocrine glands than any other primate and produce a musky steroid, there is doubt that they have any real pheromonal effect.

The active suppression of body odours in man can be interpreted from ethological and cultural viewpoints.[4,6]

Before the mid-18th century, there was a higher tolerance to odours. People were unavoidably subjected to many stenches such as excrement, refuse, stagnant water and unwashed bodies because of lack of public health infrastructure and hygiene. Bathing was believed to be detrimental since it removed the dirt that obstructed the pores and thereby gave one a 'protective coating' against the penetration of the skin by miasmas. It was also believed that the vigour of the individual was associated with the intensity of the body odour.[5]

The situation soon changed when scientific discoveries identified infection and illness with microorganisms that were associated with putrid odours. This lead to a massive sanitary reform and the fear of disease caused the public to be less tolerant of putrid odours, including body odours, as it usually signified disease.[4]

Therefore it can be said that scientific advances initiated a cultural shift in the perception and significance of odours, leading to a society in which body odour and the sexual significance of animal odours were suppressed.[4]

The Production of Axillary Odours

The axillae have three secretory glands, the eccrine (sweat), the apocrine and the sebaceous glands. The mixing of the waxy eccrine secretion with the sticky apocrine secretion and the continuous excreted sebum helps these secretions to spread over the whole of the axillary skin and hair surfaces.

The axillae are highly vascular, with blood vessels providing heat for evaporation. Axillary hair enhances diffusion of odour and also provides a very large surface area for bacteria, which, with the combination of heat and humidity of the armpit, allows proliferation of selected bacteria. These break down the glandular secretions and produce the characteristic axillary odour.[4]

The function of the apocrine glands is still unknown. However, it is known that their secretions are dependent on endocrine activity, which in turn is sensitive to psychological and emotional stress.[4]

An individual's axillary odours are the result of interactions between genetically influenced factors such as distribution of skin glands and endocrine and metabolic processes and environmental variables such as diet and the enzymatic breakdown of secretions of micro-organisms.[4]

Two odorous steroids present in male axillary sweat are androstenone and androstenol. These compounds are synthesised in the testes and transported to the salivary glands via the general body circulation. It has been suggested that these pheromones have no known physiological function.[4]

These steroids are active in olfactory communication in pigs. The scent of androstenone and androstenol in the saliva of boars induces an immobilisation reflex and the adoption of a mating posture in oestrous sows. Androstenone also enhances the onset of puberty in piglets.[4]

Motherhood and Infancy

Olfactory communication among humans has its origins in our past and present animal nature. Among animals, lasting bonds are immediately established between mother and offspring. Young animals and their mothers exchange odour signals that trigger maternal and nursing instincts and also enables them to identify and locate each other and their home site.[7]

Researchers all agree that humans are able to make the right assessments of odour identification in the recognition of kin. Newborn infants can correctly identify their mother's breast and to the odour of their mother's axilla, and similarly mothers can correctly recognise their own infants by odour.

Olfaction is found to vary dramatically with hormonal change. According to Damian, a woman's sense of smell perception heightens during ovulation while her sense of smell is dulled soon after conception and throughout the first trimester of pregnancy before once again becoming osmatic. During pregnancy many odours, even familiar or favourite scents, can become overwhelming or too strong. This not surprisingly causes food aversions, which happens to be a natural primary child protection mechanism, as is sudden nausea or morning sickness.[7]

Odour Reception and Effects of Androstenone

Humans are very sensitive to androstenone. It has been suggested that women are more sensitive to androstenone than men. The odour is perceived predominantly like urine, perspiration, animal or amine by 40% to 50% of the population. Others perceive the odour as musky or floral.[4]

A study found that women were attracted to sit on an androstenone-treated chair in a dentist's waiting room, whereas men avoided it. It has been suggested that androstenone increases female responsiveness.[4] However, other studies found that androstenone had no significant influence on ratings of physical attraction of the opposite sex.

Anosmia

Anosmia is defined as the lack of or inability to smell. Conditions such as sinusitis, allergies, nasal polyps, tissue damage and head trauma may all lead to anosmia. Surgical or toxic side-effects, exposure to drugs, endocrine disorders and nutritional deficiencies such as a lack of vitamin A or the mineral element zinc and the concurrent zinc–copper imbalance may also contribute to a loss of smell.[8]

There are two main causes of anosmia. The first is head injury and is considered the most common. Road traffic accidents are the cause of most cases of anosmia. Anosmia may also occur in cases where one has received a blow to the head. This may tear fine nerve fibres as they pass to the olfactory bulb.[8]

The second main cause of anosmia is viral infections. In most cases an infection causes temporary nasal obstruction, which leads to a loss of smell, but in some cases when the individual has recovered from the infection and the nasal obstruction clears, the olfaction does not return.[8]

Complete anosmia can result in serious problems. There is usually an element of depression and patients describe the world as dull and colourless. To many patients, the inability to taste food has been the major loss.[8]

When patients have a partial loss of smell, which is referred to as 'hyposmia', or when the smell comes and goes, the olfactory organ is normal and mucous or inflammation may be causing temporary obstruction.

The Anatomy and Physiology of the Primary Olfactory Pathway

The Principles of Olfaction

The olfactory system is a molecular detector of remarkable sensitivity. It has the capacity to discriminate among literally millions of odorants, including those that have never before been experienced. Similarly, the capacity to identify odorants on re-exposure is limited only by the lack of vocabulary that can be used to describe them. Understanding how olfaction works has been an extremely difficult task as there has been a lack of a clear physical energy continuum to define and characterize the odorants. Unlike vision and sound there is no simple quantifiable unit such as a wavelength of colour or frequency of pitch. This is made even more complex by finding that similar chemical components have quite different smells. For example, *d*-carvone smells like caraway, and *l*-carvone smells like spearmint. Both are stereoisomers; their formulas are the same, but the two molecules are mirror images.

The Nasal Cavity and Nasal Mucosa

Olfaction begins in the nasal cavity. The nasal cavity of a human being is comprised of two high-vaulted and laterally compressed spaces on either

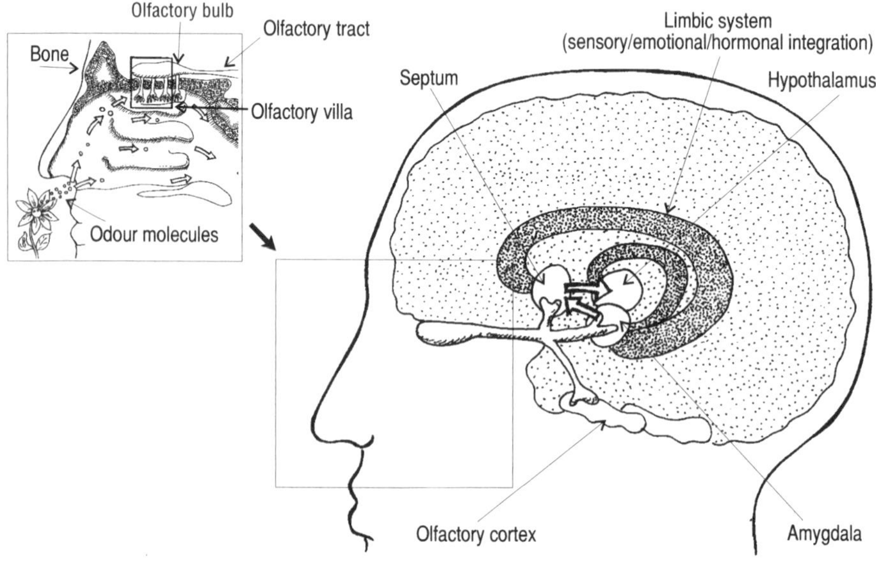

A schematic of the olfactory system with its primary and secondary paths to other regions of the brain.

side of the median nasal septum. The lateral walls of the spaces are thrown into three or four folds, which are all that remain of the complex and scrolled bones in the quadrupedal mammals.[6]

Only the conchae, or folds, highest up in the cavity bear olfactory mucous membrane; the remainder of the cavity is lined with respiratory epithelium whose role it is to clean, warm and humidify inspired air before it reaches the lungs.[6]

The respiratory epithelium is richly supplied with blood vessels and exhibits a periodic cycle of distension and shrinkage, which alternates between the nasal cavities. The airflow into both nasal cavities is not the same. The functional significance of this is not clear but Stoddart suggests it may serve to enhance a degree of perceptive difference between the two parts of the olfactory system, which renders it more acute.[6]

Olfactory Receptor Neurons

The olfactory receptor neurons are found in the olfactory mucosa located in the superior nasal sinuses. Olfactory receptor cells occur at intervals of about 3–5 μm and there are approximately seven million receptor cells in a human being. This is far less than in other mammals.[6]

The cilia that project from the receptor cells at the surface of the mucosa have a relatively thick proximal portion (approx. 0.25 μm diameter) and extends up to 200 μm from the cell. The cilia lack dynein, the substance that contains Mg ATPase that generates force for ciliary motility. Stoddart believes that the cilia are probably immobile. Bowman's cells within the mucosa secrete a layer of mucus, some 10–50 μm deep over the surface, which is kept moving at 10–60 mm per minute by the action of normal motile cilia.[6]

The axons of the receptor cells are amongst the thinnest nerve cells in the body. They gather together in bundles called villa around which is wrapped Schwann cell glia and connective tissue, and project through the cribriform plate of the ethmoid bone at the front of the skull, against which is appressed the olfactory bulb of the brain, and enter the bulb.[6]

Barry says that the olfactory receptor neurons are unique neurons, in that they are the only neurons to be regenerated throughout life.[7] Key says that unlike other regions of the nervous system where neurons are long-lived, in the olfactory system the sensory neurons have a limited life-span. It is generally believed that primary olfactory sensory neurons live for about 30 days, dic, and are replaced by proliferating stem cells located in the basal portion of the sensory epithelium. While the primary olfactory neurons appear to be inaccessible to direct physical perturbations, they can be damaged by head injuries, as well as volatile toxins, noxious chemicals and infectious agents.[9]

It is very interesting that the first synapse in the olfactory pathway occurs in the brain after the olfactory nerve has entered that structure. This is very different to other synapses between receptor cells and the brain in the eyes and the ears. This indicates the structural simplicity and the evolutionary antiquity of olfaction.[6]

Olfactory Transduction — How Do Olfactory Receptor Cells Encode and Decode Olfactory Information?

Transduction is the process by which the events of the physical world become represented as electrical activity in a sensory nerve cell. The odour, which is gaseous substance, reaches the nasal cavities through the nostrils. Sniffing (a reflex as well as a voluntary inspiratory action) increases the airflow through the upper sinuses. In the olfactory mucosa, the odour must first dissolve in the mucous fluid layer before they can activate the receptor cells.

Genetic studies of Buck and Axel suggest that there are about 1,000 different odour receptors and each olfactory receptor neuron expressing one type of receptor. When an odorant molecule binds to a particular receptor a signal cascade is initiated, involving one of two pathways:

- adenosine 3'5-cyclic monophasphate (cAMP)
- inositol 1,4,5-trisphosphate (IP_3).[10]

The membranes of the immobile cilia contain receptor sites to which odours bind. The binding increases cyclic AMP levels (intracellular messenger) within the receptor cells, which serves to amplify the signal and eventually cause membrane depolarisation by increasing permeability to a cation (sodium or calcium).[11]

The resulting receptor potential then induces action potentials in the axon, which are conducted to the olfactory bulb. The sum of receptor potentials of many olfactory neurons produces the electro-olfactogram, which may be recorded from the surface of the olfactory mucosa.[11]

How Do We Distinguish a Particular Odour?

At this stage the mechanism of odour discrimination is poorly understood. It is not known exactly how olfactory cells are triggered by an odorant or how an odorant molecule impressed upon the olfactory epithelium is recognised and transduced into a nerve impulse.

It has been suggested that each odorant molecule has its own molecular geometry, which defines its unique fragrance. However, Turin suggests that it might be the special vibrations of the atoms or atom groups within the molecule that are responsible for olfactory response and that the olfactory neurons behave like a spectroscope.[12]

According to another theory, odours, like taste, can be categorised into a finite set of primary odours (i.e., floral, musky, minty, camphor, putrid, etc.). It has been assumed that a given odorant stimulates a subset of primary receptors, causing a specific neural firing pattern that registers within the olfactory bulb and allows identification of the detected odorant.[3]

Barry describes the selectivity of the olfactory system as exquisite. He says that the sensitivity of the olfactory system is extremely impressive, exceeding the sensitivity of any other neuronal system. We are able to distinguish between at least 10,000 different odorants, with many differently perceived odours only having minor differences in molecular structure. Most common smells represent complex mixtures of odorants.[13]

Like photoreceptors, the olfactory receptor cells work by the action of a stimulus acting on a receptor protein at the receptor's surface. Odorants are small molecules which are light enough to be inhaled into the nose, but is sufficiently complex to be recognised as having a structural characteristic unique to that odorant. The recognition of the odorant is performed by hundreds of unique olfactory receptor proteins.[14]

It is now know that a peculiar feature of the odorant (called an epitope) is recognised by a particular genetically unique receptor, while another feature is recognised by a different unique receptor. A code of 'epitode map', analogous to a bank account personal identity number (PIN), forms from the action of the receptor proteins on the cells in which they are embedded. A cascade of biochemical events in each cell follows the binding of the odorant to the receptor. The resulting ionic disturbance on the cell membrane, if sufficiently large, causes a spike discharge (nerve impulse) to travel down the axon of the olfactory cell to its first synapse with the mitral and tufted cells of the olfactory bulb.[14]

According to Sullivan the field of olfaction has come far in the last few years, and we now have a better understanding of the molecular and cellular bases of olfactory discrimination. Future advances in our knowledge of olfactory perception lie in the anatomical tracing of the axonal projections from the olfactory bulb to the cortex, where the conscious perception of olfaction occurs, and the imaging of cortical responses to odour stimulation.[15]

The Olfactory Bulb

As we have already discussed when an odorant enters the nasal cavity, it binds, to odorant receptors present on the cilia of the olfactory sensory neurons. Binding of odorants to their receptors triggers a cascade of events that ultimately lead to depolarisation of the olfactory neuron receptors and propagation of action potentials along their axons. The unmyelinated olfactory receptor neuron axons gather to form the olfactory nerve, which carries peripheral input to a series of spherical elements in the olfactory bulb, known as glomeruli. Within glomeruli, peripheral axons form synapses with mitral and tufted (M/T) cells, the output cells of the olfactory bulb (known as second order olfactory neurons). Information is then carried via the axons of the M/T cells to higher brain regions where conscious perception of odorants occurs.

The olfactory bulb is where the olfactory messages are initially processed and then sent to the higher olfactory areas of the brain. It is believed that odour identification or mapping of some odorants occurs in the bulb.[6]

The olfactory output from the bulb to the brain has several targets, the main one being the primary olfactory cortex and the higher olfactory association areas. These areas are the sites of olfactory discrimination, perception and memories. The second target is the limbic system structures where olfactory signals activate smell-related emotions and behaviours.[6]

Olfaction and the Brain

The Higher Olfactory Pathways

From the first synapse, in the olfactory bulb, secondary neurons pass via the lateral olfactory tract to form a second synapse in the anterior olfactory nucleus, from where tertiary neurons project to the pyriform cortex, which lies at the anterior end of the hippocampus gyrus. From these neurons, two main pathways have been identified. One is the thalamus, which then projects to the neocortex in the orbitofrontal cortical region, and the other is the preoptic/lateral hypothalamic region.[6]

The neocortical part of the brain is the cognitive part of the brain where sensory processing occurs — it is the neocortical pathway that enables us to perceive the scent of a rose and to correctly identify its specific variety. The preoptic/lateral hypothalamic region is a noncognitive area, which forms part of the 'limbic system'. The hypothalamic centre regulates feeding autonomic responses and hormonal control.[6]

The Limbic System

The anatomical pathways in the brain of the olfactory system converge in an important area of the brain known as the limbic system. Once called the rhinencephalon, the limbic system is the 'nose' brain. The limbic system is a complex system of 122 regions and associated tracts.[16] Van Toller describes the function of the limbic system:

> *In general terms the limbic system makes rapid parallel decisions integrating the necessary parts of the central nervous system and the body required for any decision. Externally the limbic system directs somatic motor output for eating, copulating, fighting. Internally it directs body posture for food, sexual activity or sleep, controlling the internal viscera and hormones. It has specific areas that govern mood and feeling states and, importantly the sense of smell.*[16]

While it is now agreed that the limbic system is heavily committed in the expression of emotion, it is still not known whether it is involved in generating emotion or integrating it.

Together with the hypothalamus, the limbic system initiates and governs primitive and emotional drives — sex, thirst, hunger — and it evokes visceral and behavioural mechanisms such as rage, fear, sorrow, revulsion, physical affection and sexual attraction.

The Brain Hemispheres

The left and right hemispheres of the brain are connected by the *corpus callosum,* a large nerve bundle that allows the two hemispheres to communicate. Although the hemispheres are similar in shape and appearance, they are unequal in function. In most individuals the left hemisphere is dominant (e.g., 90% of people are right-handed).

Damian suggests that recent scientific efforts to distinguish the relative functions and distinctive attributes of the hemispheres have been tainted by trendy pop psychology and romantic new age notions which glorify the right brain and belittle the left brain as being boring, dull, rigidly restricted and predictable. We are also told that the right brain is intuitive and creative.[7]

While the right brain is neither intuitive nor creative, it is actually superior in representational and visuospatial functions, in perception and discrimination of musical tones, speech intonations and in emotional responses. In broad terms the right hemisphere functions are holistic and spatial (hence labelled artistic), whereas the left hemisphere appears to be specialised for logical and analytical operations.[7]

Often the corpus callosum in patients suffering from epileptic seizures is cut. This prevents the spread of seizures from one hemisphere to the other. Careful testing of these patients reveals that each hemisphere not only functions independently but in a different manner.[7]

If a key is placed in the right hand of a blindfolded patient, the sensory signals reach the left hemisphere due to the crossing of sensory pathways. Upon being asked about the nature of the object the patient verbally replies 'a key'. If the key is placed in the left hand, its sensory image would be the right hemisphere. In this case, the patient is not capable of verbally describing the key although he can recognise the object and point to the name or a shape of a key. This implies that the centre for verbal expression is in the left hemisphere and that only the right hemisphere has access to the speech centres via the corpus callosum and that it has full perceptive, cognitive and nonverbal motor competence.[7]

It has been found that the right hemisphere exhibits greater activity during olfactory processing.[33] This is not surprising as the left brain is involved in highly discriminatory functions of rational thought, speech and language, whereas the right brain is less discriminate, more emotional and hedonic.[7]

Damian suggests that the odour response of the left brain makes odour identification possible and easier, while the right brain is involved in the emotional and hedonic response to the odour. They also suggest that essential oils may appeal more to the left or right brain, or that they may actually better harmonise the activities of both.[7]

Essential oils stimulating the right brain evoke emotional responses (feelings, memories, images), whereas those stimulating the left brain affect intellectual processes (mental concentration, reason, judgement, logic). The extent of this effect is highly variable with each individual and depends on many factors such as age of the individual, previous memory associations and surrounding circumstances and influences.[7]

The Hypothalamus

The hypothalamus is the highest brain structure directly concerned with the homeostasis and integration of internal activities. The strategic location of the hypothalamus, in the base of the brain and above the pituitary gland, provides an ideal situation to exert control over the lower autonomic and endocrine systems and to be controlled by the higher forebrain centres.

Together with the limbic system the hypothalamus governs primitive and emotional drives such as sex, thirst and hunger and it is responsible for evoking behavioural mechanisms and 'gut feeling' responses such as rage, fear, sorrow, revulsion, physical attraction and sexual attraction. The pheromonal-sexual-olfactory connection takes place in the limbic-hypothalamic region of the brain.[13]

One of the most important functions of the hypothalamus is the control of the autonomic nervous system and regulation of visceral function: regulation of heart rate, blood pressure, respiration, digestive activity and levels of hormones. Regulation of visceral functions depends on two systems. One is the sympathetic nervous system that prepares the body for fight or flight, raising the heart rate and the blood pressure — and decreasing digestive activity, since the blood flow is needed elsewhere. The parasympathetic nervous system does the reverse, preparing the body for more vegetative activities.

It is possible to now understand that the hypothalamus plays a very important role in regulating body functions and activities during times of stress, and that the essential oils via their influence on the limbic system and hypothalamus can play a very important role in the management of stress.

The Hippocampus

Located deep within the brain, behind the eyes, the hippocampus together with the limbic system has a primary role in processing events and experiences into memories. However it is not the sole processing point, nor the final repository of long-term memory. Memory processing and storage also occur elsewhere in other areas of the brain. The hippocampus serves as a station in which memories linger for an extended but indeterminate period of time in a suspended state between short-term and long-term memory.[7]

Psychotherapeutic Effects of Odours

Mechanisms of Action

According to Jellinek the mechanisms by which odours influence the human psyche are:

- the pharmacological mechanism
- the semantic mechanism
- the hedonic valence mechanism
- the placebo mechanism.[17]

The Pharmacological Mechanism

Many essential oils and their constituents are absorbed into the blood stream when they are inhaled or applied topically. These essential oils and their constituents may have an effect on the mental states via the central nervous system or the endocrine system.

It has also been suggested that the essential oils have the ability to affect nerve cell conductivity by binding with nerve cell membranes and acting as modulators of calcium ion channels. Therefore, one can assume that the essential oils have a direct pharmacological effect. Jellinek believes that the amount of essential oil entering the blood stream by inhalation would be very much less than the usual pharmacological modes of application and that the likelihood of a systemic effect would be correspondingly reduced.[17]

To the pharmacologist, the effects of active agents are the result of their biochemical interaction with bodily organs and physiology. These effects therefore depend upon chemical properties as defined by the chemical properties of the therapeutic substance. If an effect for a particular substance has been clearly identified, one cannot assume that a substance, even one closely related chemically, would have the same effect. Hence, the *pharmacological mechanism* of action implies substance-specificity.

Jellinek suggest that in aromatherapy, the odour of the essential oil is more or less incidental, and one should expect people unable to smell an essential oil to experience the same pharmacological effects as people who perceive it.[17]

The Semantic Mechanism

Jellinek says that odours are experienced within the context of life situations. If the experience of an odour occurs in a situation that is highly charged emotionally, the emotions experienced are stored in memory along with the odour experience. When the odour is experienced at a later time, its memory trace, including the emotional effect, is retrieved. If in a learning situation the emotional impact led to hormonal changes (such as an increase in blood adrenaline levels), these changes take place again, when the odour is smelled again.[17]

According to the *semantic mechanism*, effectiveness is the result of perception and of activating memory traces. Jellinek gives an example of cool freshly squeezed lemonade from your childhood which will gave you a sensation of being refreshed. Smelling lemon oil at later stage will always be associated with the same refreshing sensation.[17]

The Hedonic Valence Mechanism

Jellinek says that according to a current psychological theory, the 'core' experience is what psychologists have called hedonic valence — feelings of pleasure or displeasure, which form a sort of primitive experimental matrix from which all of those affective or emotional states emerge.[17]

Hedonic valence influences a wide range of cognitive and behavioural responses, including memory recall, evaluation of ambiguous stimuli, optimism, helpfulness and a disposition towards flexible and creative thinking. There is considerable experimental evidence that hedonic valence is positively affected by pleasant odours and negatively by unpleasant odours.

According to the *hedonic valence mechanism*, effectiveness depends upon the effect of the stimulus on the subject's affective state. That is, the subject's state of pleasure or displeasure. For example, two odours that please me equally will have the same effect upon me, even if one of them reminds me of lemonade and the other one reminds me of flowers.

The Placebo Mechanism

In medicine the placebo effect is well known. These subjectively experienced, often objectively measured effects are caused not by the therapeutic substance that has been administered but the expectations that the patient has of the medication. For example, a pill containing lactose may relieve pain or promote sleep as a pill of identical appearance and taste that actually contains an active agent, as long as the patient (and the administrating practitioner!) does not know that the active agent is not present.

Experimental evidence indicates that comparable effects also occur with odours. A given odourant, administered at the same concentration to three groups of test subjects, elicited markedly different responses depending on whether the substance had been described as health promoting, neutral or potentially harmful.

Jellinek cites a study by Schiffmann on the mood effects of perfumes, positive effects were registered even with respondents who had received plain alcohol in place of the fragrance they had selected.[17]

According to the *placebo mechanism*, all that matters is how I expect the odour to affect me. The actual nature of the odour is irrelevant. If a therapist manages to convince their client that ylang ylang essential oil will relieve their depressed mood, then it will do just that — irrespective of its chemical composition.

Memory associations are relevant in the sense that you will find it difficult to convince someone of the curative powers of an essential oil that is quite familiar to them and has never shown any beneficial effects in the past.

Experimental Evidence

Can the response of individuals to aromas be monitored, in the same way that the beating of the heart can be recorded? A traditional method that is used to measure psychological responses to odour is the use of psychometric scales in which the subject scales a list of descriptors relating to their psychological state/feelings. One of the problems with this technique is that the response is largely subjective.[10]

A better method should measure covert physiological responses that accompany behavioural changes. Long-term psychophysiological changes can be measured using bodily fluids such as sweat, saliva, blood and urine. Short-term changes can be measured by recording the minute bioelectrical potentials found throughout the body. These may include muscle potentials and heart rate as well as the electrical potentials generated within the brain. The latter are recorded by an EEG.[16]

Techniques recording the electrical activity of the brain are non-invasive, relying on electrodes stuck or firmly held on to the scalp. The electrodes detect minute electrical currents on the surface of the brain and these electrical signals are then amplified by a factor of a million times.[16]

The first study to investigate the effect of fragrance on the brain was conducted by Moncrieff in 1962 using an EEG. An EEG monitors brainwave patterns; an increase in alpha activity indicates a state of relaxation while an increase in beta activity shows stimulation.[16]

This study and others suggest that the measurement of the brainwave activity is an accurate method for assessing the response of the brain to odour, as it was almost independent of the subject's mood, expectations or level of arousal.[16]

Often studies using EEG measurements and essential oils as odorants disagree, concluding that EEG changes are very much subject to cognitive mediation — dependent on the person's expectations and experiences of the odours presented.

Torii describes another technique called *Contingent Negative Variation* (CNV). CNV is described as an upward shift in the brainwaves recorded by electrodes attached to the scalp, occurring in situations where subjects are expecting something to happen. For example, a subject is given a sound stimulus followed by a light stimulus. When the light appears, the subjects are requested to turn it off as quickly as possible. Within the interval between the two stimuli there appears a slow, upward shift from the baseline of the subject's EEG. This shift in the EEG is what is referred to as the CNV. Unfortunately the CNV cannot be determined from a single EEG trace and the EEG must be averaged using between 10 and 20 EEG trials before determining the CNV. The CNV is considered to be a very sensitive measure for determining the effects of odours on brain electrical activity.[18]

Another technique referred to as *Brain electrical activity mapping* (BEAM) is a technique that involves the application of computer technology for on-line analysis of EEG data. The EEG data is subjected to a fast Fourier transformation and displayed as coloured topographical maps. By contrast with older methods of visually inspecting recordings of EEG ink tracings on paper, the technique is very fast, and it allows for rapid observation of real-time cortical activity.[16]

Van Toller says that the BEAM technique allows observation of the two hemispheres of the brain and how the cortex processes information.[16]

However, Jellinek says that the experimental evidence gathered in the 100 or thereabouts studies on odour effects, we are faced with a picture that is both rich and disappointing. Jellinek is referring to the fact that so few studies resolve or even address the following important question:[17]

- By what mechanism did the observed action come about?

Only if we know the mechanism involved can we answer questions such as the following:

- Can we expect this finding also be true for other kinds of people and in other cultures?
- Can we expect similar findings under conditions other than those prevailing in the experiment?
- Is this effect specific to the odorous substance tested or can we expect the same effect for an array of other substances? What about any substance or blend that has the same odour? Alternatively, any substance or blend considered equally pleasant or unpleasant.

The lack of conclusive information about the mechanisms originates from the following facts:

- In actual practice the mechanisms are not clearly separated but often come into play jointly.
- Most experiments were designed with but one of the possible mechanisms in view.

Jellinek says that by not being fully aware of the possibility of the other mechanisms at work, researchers often fail to ask the questions that could have provided clarification or they failed to build safeguards into the experimental design to avoid those alternative mechanisms; or they ignored evidence for such mechanisms if it did emerge from their data.[17]

Therefore, we have much data but we do not know what conclusion we may legitimately draw from them. For example, the researchers who used the CNV technique concluded that 'we are able scientifically to prove the truth of the old adage that jasmine stimulates and lavender relaxes. This statement implies a pharmacological mechanism.[17]

However, other findings using CNV threw doubts upon the pharmacological interpretation. While it was found that food odours led to an increase in the CNV pattern, a similar increase also occurred when the test subjects thought about food without actually smelling it. This suggests the placebo mechanism also was at work.[17]

Odours and Memory Associations

Many studies suggest that long-term odour memory is stronger than long-term visual memory. This is partly because of our primitive self-preservation or species preservation instincts and because the subconscious connection to smell uses far less stimulus discrimination than does conscious sight. It is also known that odours used in aversion therapy and positive reinforcement leave a lasting impression and that odours can be useful to jolt or prompt recall, even in cases of amnesia or comatose conditions.

Experiments have found that students exposed to pleasant smells during a word exercise, and again during testing the next day, remembered their answers better than those who were not offered the scent. In one experiment using a smell association memory exercise, 72 students were presented with a list of 40 common adjectives and asked to write down an antonym for each. They were not informed of the plan to test their answer recall the next day. Some of the students were exposed to scent during the word matching only, some during the later recall test only, some during both sessions and others not at all.[7]

Those students exposed to the aroma for both sessions recalled a considerably higher percentage of their answers than did the other groups. It was concluded that the same odour must be present at the learning and the testing stage for there to be any memory association. It was also concluded that as long as the odour was perceived as being pleasant, it would not matter which odour was used.[7]

Essential Oils and Stress Management

With regard to using aromatic substances in the field of stress management, fragrances have a proven role to play in those individuals who are stressed, but the effects upon non-stressed subjects are more difficult to measure.

Dr Craig Warren chose blood pressure as a measure of stress. Blood pressure is primarily controlled by the sympathetic nervous system, which is responsible for mobilisation of the body during times of stress. He investigated the properties of nutmeg oil that has a rich anecdotal history as an essential oil for reducing the effects of stress.[19] Using traditional psychophysiological stressors such as mental arithmetic and a phrase completion task he found;

> *... that when nutmeg oil was added to a fragrance, our subjects displayed a reduced blood pressure response to stress, compared to the same fragrance without nutmeg oil. We obtained a U.S. Patent for this stress-reducing use of nutmeg as a fragrance. We also found that a nutmeg based fragrance did not have any relaxing or stress reducing properties when the typical subject was sitting quietly at rest, that is, in a non-stressed state.*[19]

The results obtained in these studies have a direct relevance in the field of aromatherapy and it is possible to conclude that:[31]

- The fragrance does not have to be intense in order to be effective. Changes are measurable even in subliminal levels. The more intense the odour, the less pleasant it becomes.
- Odour perception and its subsequent psychophysiological effect are extremely subjective and will vary from person to person.
- As a person's expectation of an odour affects their physiological response, the way in which the odour is presented to them by the therapist is an important consideration.
- The odour should form an important part of the therapy if the full mood benefits of fragrance are to be obtained.
- If a paired emotional response with an odour is desired, the same fragrance should be used until odour conditioning occurs.

The Subliminal Influence of Odours

> *... people could close their eyes to greatness, to horrors, to beauty, and their ears to melodies or deceiving words. But they could not escape scent. For scent was a brother to breath. Together with breath it entered human beings, who could not defend themselves against it, not if they wanted to live. And scent entered the very core, went directly to their hearts, and decided for good and all between affection and contempt, disgust and lust, love and hate. He who ruled scent ruled the heart of men.*[20]

It is not so much the gruesome murders that the central character in Patrick Suskind's novel, *Perfume: The story of a murderer* commits that sends shivers down your spine, but the fact that this man can control people's behaviour by concocting a perfume.

Whether you like it or not odours have the ability to produce psychophysiological responses at levels which are considered to be below the detection threshold. Kirk-Smith demonstrated this effect with musk that was administered below detectable threshold levels.[4]

Knasko found that shoppers lingered longer, without knowing why, in a shop that had a subtle floral fragrance dispersed throughout the air. If you have a retail shop, there is no need to rush out and start your oil burner — she also said sales were not increased.[21]

Hirsh recruited 31 shoppers to act as volunteers, 26 women and 5 men, but did not tell them that the experiment involved olfaction. Each person was asked to examine two identical pairs of shoes, which were placed in two separate rooms which were identical except for one variable, the air in one room was odour-free and the other perfumed with a mixed floral scent.[22]

Immediately after each examination and before leaving the room, each subject completed a questionnaire to evaluate the likelihood of buying the shoes. The results indicated that the scent-filled room was far more conducive to a sale.[23]

Damian cites Dr Charles Wysocki, an olfactory research scientist who says that smell is an intimate, individualistic sense, and that it is very vulnerable and warns that human emotions, with which smell is associated, can be readily exploited through the use of odours, scents and fragrances.[12]

Aromatic mood control could backfire as studies have shown that unidentified odours can make people feel anxious.[7]

Emotion and Olfaction

No other topic in the field of psychology and olfaction is of greater interest to the general public and researchers as the relationship between smell and emotion. The emotional impact of aromatic substances is central to:

- perfumery
- aromatherapy
- product and environmental fragrancing.

When asked *'Why do you wear a perfume or aftershave?'* the answer is usually *'because it makes me feel good'*. Does this mean *'I feel good because I smell good'*?

According to Knasko this may very well be the case. Perception of pleasant or unpleasant (once again subjective) fragrance has been shown to affect creativity, mood and perceived health.[21]

It was a popular belief that emotions are lower-order feelings and behaviour that humans could best do without. This view stems largely from the philosophical school of the rationalists. It was Descartes who said that reason was a specific human attribute as opposed to the emotional, non-rational and instinctive behaviour of the lower animals.[16]

Van Toller says that emotion, to a large extent, is dependent upon individual learning. There appear to be few primary biological emotions, but many secondary or learnt emotions. He also says that emotion is usually ignored in the educational process.[16]

However, Van Toller asks:

> *Does the account by the rationalists present a true picture of emotion and its role in human behaviour? The first point to make is that it is to humans that we look for to see emotion in full flower. By comparison with human emotions animals reveal a pale imitation. It is in humans that we see emotion from its most ugly to its most beautiful.*[16]

Emotion, like olfaction, while a phylogenetic old brain system, was too important to remain as a simple reflex mechanism. Each subsequent development of the brain resulted in the emotional systems being carried through into the developing brain areas. Each stage in the development of the brain changed and modified human emotion.[16]

Human motivational systems of hunger, thirst and sex appear to have undergone similar, though less dramatic change and refinement. According to Van Toller it is in human beings that we find eating and drinking replaced by the rituals of dining and similarly, human sexual activity may take on erotic and deviant forms. The point that Van Toller is making is that although the basic functions of emotion and motivation still have their primary modes of action in their original brain structures, they have come to take on new behavioural dimensions which arise from circuits in the newer areas of the human brain.[16]

Van Toller says that emotion, to a large extent, is dependent upon individual learning. There appear to be few primary biological emotions, but many secondary or learnt emotions. He also says that emotion is usually ignored in the educational process and suggests that this is why we have all witnessed groups of middle-aged people joining 'encounter groups' in attempts to come to terms with their 'emotional' problems.[16]

It is now apparent that the limbic system governs our emotions:

> *The human mind is multidimensional, multifaceted, and consists of several levels. The relatively easily accessible conscious mind resides in the left part of the brain. The right brain is associated with social, emotional, non-linguistic unconscious awareness. The most primitive, relatively inaccessible, almost purely emotional aspect of the mind is referred to simply as the unconscious and is associated with the limbic system.*[22]

Odour and Personality Types

Defining Personality

A clear understanding of the factors that determines our personality is still shrouded in mystery. Some of the factors that are believed to contribute to one's personality include genetics, being male or female — in terms of hormones and socially acceptable behaviour, parental influences, influences from our siblings and our age relative to them, the environment that we grow up in and the people with who we socialise and work with.

Characterology

Classifying people according to their personality and character is quite common. For example, many of us are familiar with the astrological signs — earth, fire, air or water, and how these can be used to interpret ones character.

Worwood cites many other examples of systems used to classify different personality types. The Sufis developed the nine characters of the enneagram, the Chinese use yin/yang and the five elements of water, fire, wood, metal and earth, while Ayurveda uses the principles of vata, pitta and kapha to determine personality types. Jung used the four humours of Greek medicine to develop his psychoanalytical theories.[24]

When Doctor Bach developed the Bach flower remedies in the 1930's, the psychological and emotional characteristics of the individual were central to the remedy being chosen. Dr Bach believed that each person's personality and nature could be matched with a particular remedy, which will be taken for a short-term or long-term basis to deal with the passing problem.[24]

It must be stressed that all the systems of characterology emphasise that no one character is 'better' than the other, and that balance is more important.

Personality Types and Odours

In the past, the significance of psychological and physiological factors in the selection of fragrances was given varying degrees of attention. Representatives of the classical approach felt that the selection of fragrances was made on an irrational basis, and could not be explained on the basis of specific factors, it was held to be a purely random occurrence and thus not psychologically definable.

According to the authors of H&R Fragrance Guide every individual develops a distinct relationship to the areas of odours and fragrances in each developmental stage. These odours and fragrance experiences are linked to feelings, emotions and emotionally coloured experiences, which are stored in the limbic system via a personality-specific stimulus processing step.[25]

Factors Influencing a Person's Odour Preferences

It has been suggested that the following factors may influence the way in which humans respond to odours:

- the influence of age, culture, lifestyle, geography and climate
- memory associations
- emotions and person's mood.[25]

It is often impossible to assess accurately an individual's emotional reaction to a particular odour without taking into account the following:[32]

- how the odour was applied
- how much was applied
- the circumstances in which it was applied
- the person to whom it was applied (e.g., age, sex)
- what mood the person was in when it was applied
- what previous memory associations they may have with the odour
- cultural and social factors
- anosmia or the inability to smell
- expectations or thoughts about the odour

For a person to be drawn towards a particular fragrance it must correspond to the emotional fragrant needs of a person.

Fragrances are often seen as an expression of a desired lifestyle. For example, many people today associate patchouli with an alternative/hippy lifestyle. This lifestyle association is of course influenced by the abundant use of patchouli in the late 60s and early 70s. The lifestyle of a person, which includes attitudes and ideas, can be strongly influenced by intellectual factors.

Essential Oils and Personality Profiling

Mailhebiau points out that in drawing up aromatic character profile that:

> *...we are not claiming to attribute a specific animistic form to a specie of plants. We are, rather, emphasising the laws of interactive affinities between the plant and human kingdoms which, when properly understood, make it possible to make up a remedy specific to each person.*[26]

For example the character profile of lavender according to Mailhebiau is:

> *Lavender is the essence of the soul, magnetic and formative, the perfect symbol of gentleness and maternal love ... tireless, always even-tempered, with unfailing gentleness and devotion, lavendula cares for and calms, listens to and remedies a thousand ills. She takes care of children, adults and the elderly, animals, plants, the earth and sky*[26]

The character profile of lavender according to Worwood is:

> *Lavender could be called the mother, or grandmother of essential oils, able to care for a multiple of physical and psychological problems and like a mother, accomplishing several jobs at the same time ... lavender is completely mothering in its personality — electric, formidable, yet gentle and kind, is direct, pure thought, brave and humble*[24]

Worwood has developed a system, which she refers to as *Aroma-Genera*. She has classified nine personality types according to the following groups — *florals, fruities, herbies, leafies, rsinies, rooties, seedies, spicies* and *woodies*.[24]

Individual Prescription

If an individual is drawn towards a particular essential oil, then is that essential oil defined as having the same personality characteristics? The answer to this is yes and no. There are two interrelated dynamics to take into consideration:

The signature scent: i.e. The essential oil corresponds to the physical, emotional and mental characteristics of the user.

The regulating scent: i.e. The essential oil is needed to balance what is absent in the health or personality of the user.

Suzanne Fischer Rizzi gives an excellent example using ylang ylang. She describes the personality of ylang ylang much like the title character Carmen from George Bizet's opera — fiery, temperamental, passionate and erotic. Although her emotions are deeply felt, she never loses her balance. Aware of her own fascinating radiance, she is capable of casting magical spells. Her wardrobe is bright and colourful and she loves to wear jewellery.[27] However when ylang ylang is used for its regulatory scent it is more suitable for:

> *this second woman who often does not allow herself to live, who hides her femininity, dresses drably, and does not trust her intuitive powers. Extremely frustrated, she appears nervous, depressed and tense.*[27]

What are the factors that determine how the odour of an essential oil corresponds to the physical, emotional and mental characteristics of the user? Is there a rational approach or does the idiosyncratic nature of smell make it virtually impossible to assess the response and personality characteristics of essential oils? It may be impossible to assess accurately an individual's reaction to a particular odour without taking into account the following:[25]

Biological: what effect the odour is likely to have physiologically on the systems of the body, i.e., lavender is generally relaxing while basil is generally stimulating.

Archetypal: what universal associations odours have, i.e., the scent of rose suggests femininity, love, divinity and sweetness in all cultures alike.

Cultural: certain scents take on specific meaning according to the environmental, social and cultural factors involved — the odour of frankincense for example, will be especially significant with the religious ceremonies in many Christian religions.

Individual: personal associations and preferences due to first-hand experience, which may be either positive or negative.

Gender Differences in Olfactory Response

According to Damian, females are generally more adept than men in matters relating to olfaction.[8] Generally females are able to detect odours in lower level concentrations and are better able to identify odours of all kinds. The reasons are as follows:[7]

- Females have an inborn reproductive protective skill whereby the fetus needs to be protected during pregnancy.
- Females tend to be more right brain-oriented and -influenced than men.
- It is also known that women are more readily able to verbalise their feelings because the female corpus callosum allows easier internal cross-talk between brain hemispheres. Men are more apt to use language for communication of ideas and to exchange objective information and knowledge, rather than expressing subjective emotions or impressions.

Environmental Fragrancing

Environmental fragrancing is defined by John Steele as the ambient transformation by scent of personal, work and public spaces.[19] Environmental fragrancing alters our social smell-scape, modifying the aromatic terrain in which we live, work, pray and play.[1]

Burning essential oils or incense is by no means a recent fad or trend; ancient civilisations of Egypt, Persia, Greece, China and India all used the burning of resins, herbs and essences for religious ceremonies and social events.

Knasko conducted a clinical trial that measured the effect of ambient odour on creativity, mood and perceived health:

> *ninety subjects were divided into three groups (of equal sexes) and each group placed in a room for one hour which contained a hidden source of either lavender, or lemon or dimethyl sulphide, questionnaires on mood, health and the environment were then completed, and personality and creativity tests performed.*
>
> *The experiment was repeated a week later with no odour present in the room. It was found that exposure to malodour tended to lower mood ratings but that the pleasant odours had no effect on the mood. Lemon was found to decrease health symptoms reported, possibly to the association with cleanliness and freshness. There was a relationship between personality traits and the effect of odour on mood and performance. It was suggested that associations and expectations regarding odours may be important in the effect of ambient odour on health and mood.*[28]

According to Steele the benefits of environmental fragrancing are:

- improved interior design aesthetics
- reduced sick building syndrome health problems
- optimised performance and creativity in the workplace.[29]

The sick building syndrome has become an issue in many internal building climates that are closed systems regulated by heating, ventilation and air-conditioning. This sealed environment leads to a buildup of toxic emissions which are released from the synthetic textiles, carpets, paints, wallpaper, insulation, solvents, adhesives and copy machines.[19]

Its not surprising that the US Environmental Protection Agency reported that the levels of pollutants inside buildings can be as much as 100 times greater than outdoor levels. To add to this think of all the bacteria, viruses and fungi that breed in the warm stagnant water of humidifiers, filters, condensers, drip pans, ducts and pumps of the air conditioners. According to Steele, absenteeism has increased by nearly 50% in 'sick buildings'.[29]

Japan has been leading the way in the use of environmental fragrancing to improve productivity. Based on brain wave research of Professor Shiziro Torii of Toho University, Shimizu, a Japanese construction company has developed a system for environmental fragrancing that operates by dispersing scents by a pre-timed 'scent plan'. Research has shown that a lemon scent increased productivity and reduced keyboard error rate by 50%.[30]

In general it has been confirmed that pleasant odours tend to:[19]

- enhance creative performance and setting higher goals
- generate more positive evaluation of words and pictures of people
- elicit more happy memories.

References

1. *In Profile: Dr Steve Van Toller*, Interview with Jennie Harding, The International Journal of Aromatherapy 1994; 6(1): 4–7.
2. Stoddart M. *The noselessness of man*. 2nd Australasian Aromatherapy Conference Proceeding. Sydney, Australia, 1998.
3. Youngentob SL. *Introduction to the sense of smell: Understanding odours from the study of human and animal behaviour* from *Tastes & Aromas*, UNSW Press, Australia, 1999: 38–49.
4. Kirk-Smith M. *Human olfactory communication*. AROMA '93 Conference Proceedings, Aromatherapy Publications, Brighton, 1993.
5. Corbin A. *The foul and the fragrant*. Berg Publishing, United Kingdom, 1986.
6. Stoddart M. *The scented ape*. University Press, Great Britain, 1990.
7. Damian P & K. *Aromatherapy; scent and psyche*. Healing Arts Press, USA, 1996.
8. Douek E. *Abnormalities of smell* from *Perfumery: The psychology and biology of fragrance*. Chapman and Hall, Great Britain, 1988.
9. Key B. *Anatomy of the peripheral chemosensory systems: How they grow and age in human*. From Tastes & Aromas. UNSW Press, Australia, 1999: 138–148.
10. Axel R. *The molecular logic of smell*. Scientific American, Oct 1995: 130–137.
11. Barry PH, Balasubramanian S, Lynch JW. *How sensory cells encode information: The processes that underlie sensitivity to chemical stimuli, their quality and their quantity*. From Tastes & Aromas. UNSW Press, Australia, 1999: 120–129.
12. Turin L. A spectroscopic mechanism for primary olfactory reception. Chemical Senses 1996; 21(6): 773–791.
13. Barry PH, et al. *How sensory cells encode information: The processes that underlie sensitivity to chemical stimuli, their quality and their quantity* from *Tastes & Aromas*, UNSW Press, Australia, 1999: 120–129.
14. Bell GA. *Future technologies envisaged from molecular mechanisms of olfactory perception*. From Tastes & Aromas. UNSW Press, Australia, 1999: 149–160.
15. Sullivan SL. *Information coding in the mammalian olfactory system*. From Tastes & Aromas. UNSW Press, Australia, 1999: 130–137.
16. Van Toller, S. *Emotion and the brain* from *Perfumery: The psychology and biology of fragrance*. Published by Chapman and Hall, Great Britain, 1988.
17. Jellinek S. *Psychodynamic Odor Effects and Their Mechanisms*. Perfumer and Flavorist, 1997: 22; 29–41, 1997.
18. Torii S. *Contingent negative variation (CNV) and the psychological effects of odour*. from *Perfumery: The psychology and biology of fragrance*. Published by Chapman and Hall, Great Britain, 1988.
19. Warren C. *Mood benefits of fragrance*. The International Journal of Aromatherapy 1993; 5(2): 12–15.
20. Suskind P. *Perfume: The story of a murderer*. Penguin Books, England, 1985.
21. Knasko S. *Ambient odour effects on human behaviour*. The International Journal of Aromatherapy 1997; 8(3): 28–33.
22. Hirsh A. *Sensory marketing*. The International Journal of Aromatherapy 1993; 5(1): 21–23.
23. Van Toller S. *Olfaction, emotion and cognition*. The International Journal of Aromatherapy 1997; 8(2.): 22–27.
24. Worwood VA. *The fragrant mind*. Transworld Publishers, Australia, 1995.
25. Muller J. *The H & R book of perfume*. Johnson Publications Limited, London, 1994.
26. Mailhebiau P. *Portraits in Oils*. The C.W. Daniel Company Limited, Great Britain, 1995.
27. Fisher Rizzi S. *Complete Aromatherapy Handbook*. Sterling Publishing Company, USA, 1990.
28. Knasko S. *Ambient odor's effect on creativity mood and perceived health*. Chemical Senses 1992; 17(1).
29. Steele J. *Environmental fragrancing*. The International Journal of Aromatherapy 1992; 4(2): 8–11.
30. Tisserand R. *Lemon fragrance increases office efficiency*. The International Journal of Aromatherapy 1988; 1(2): 2.
31. Harris R, Lewis R. Psychophysiological effects of odour — Part 1. JACM, 1994; 12(1): 16.
32. Tisserand R. *POP '91 conference report*. The International Journal of Aromatherapy. 1991 3(3); 10–12.
33. Tortora G, Grabowski S. *Principles of anatomy and physiology*. 10th edn, John Wiley & sons, USA, 2003.

Subtle Aromatherapy

Objectives

After careful study of this chapter, you should be able to:

- define the relationship between spirituality and wellbeing
- explain the term vibrational medicine
- explain the term subtle aromatherapy
- explain the role of plants and aromatics in metaphysical healing
- describe how to use essential oils in subtle aromatherapy
- examine the relationship between colour therapy and aromatherapy
- examine the relationship between chakras and aromatherapy
- explain the role of essential oils during meditation.

The Relationship Between Spirituality and Wellbeing

The health care industry has adopted a humanistic approach that has come to dominate much of Western thinking. It is concerned with human rather than divine or spiritual matters. Such an approach emphasises common human needs and a rational way of solving human problems. People are seen as rational beings whose intellect enables them to act responsibly.[1]

Everything can be reduced to logic, quantifiable and observable evidence, and mind and body are separate and soul denied.

However, Wright and Sayre-Adams remind us that many of the great rationalists such as Descartes and Newton were devoutly religious people.[1] Yet what was subsequently built on their thinking has often turned away from any suggestion of the possibility of a transpersonal human dimension.

Wright and Sayre-Adams say that humanism's recognition of our personal, but finite, existence connecting to others through our interpersonal relationships limits the possibilities of what it is to be fully human.[1]

The tendency for humanism is to arrange life into physical, social and psychological compartments, while spiritual and metaphysical issues tend to be lumped under psychological problems.

Defining Spirituality

Spirituality transcends the limitations of the human mind and body, it assures us that we are not alone, that we do not have to be in control of others — thereby allowing us to trust, to be honest, and therefore vulnerable, and to live in acceptance of ourselves and others and to share faith in a power greater than ourselves.[1] For some people, spirituality simply implies a connection with a deeper meaning and purpose of life, and does not necessarily mean acceptance of the divine.[1]

However, an exclusively humanistic and scientific view suggests that only we can be in control. The reduced world of *'just me and nothing else'* feeds the need to be in control of everything.[1] According to Jones, it is the fear of losing control that is the greatest symptom of our age:

> *Many an ulcer, hypertensive, or anxiety attack begins when contemporary men and women sense their lives slipping out of control and this in turns lies at the root of many illnesses and a close-mindedness about spiritual experience.*[2]

Wright and Sayre-Adams suggest that we are sick or diseased when we are not in a state of complete spiritual wellbeing. They suggest that the need to find meaning in life is not just a feature of those who are sick or close to death. It is a universal trait necessary for the maintenance of life and part of a well-developed personality. Therefore, if we have not deepened our understanding of our place in the scheme of things and our spiritual roots, we may be more prone to ill health.[1]

According to Jones, spirituality is *'tuning the spirit within us to its source'*.[2] Wright and Sayre-Adams cite Kelting, who believes that this desire to be 'attuned' lives in all of us and that we seek a sense of purpose, destiny and value, grounded not only in ourselves, but in the wider nature of things. We also seek comfort and love, not just for and from one another, but for and from the greater realm of being.[1]

Spiritual experiences can be profound and life-transforming. There seems to be a growing hunger for spiritual connection in our culture, a hunger that orthodox religions often seem unable to satisfy.

Vibrational Medicine

Many people may not be familiar with the term 'vibrational medicine'. In actual fact, there are many sceptics who lump vibrational medicine together with mysticism, the occult, supernatural or new age hocus pocus.[3] Dare I say that some of these sceptics may be unaware of the basic fundamental principles of physics.

Vibrations underlie every aspect of nature. The vibrations of atoms create sound and heat. Light is another form of vibrating energy. These are examples of the different types of energy that make up the electromagnetic spectrum, which also includes radio waves, television signals, X rays, ultraviolet radiation, ultrasonic waves and microwaves. The only difference between all these forms of energy is their frequency or rate of vibration.[4]

Albert Einstein's famous equation $E = mc^2$ describes how energy and matter are interrelated. In fact, energy and matter are two different forms of the same thing. It is from here that we can begin to conceptualise human beings as multidimensional energy systems.

Energy

The concept of 'energy' or 'subtle energy' that has been used in alternative and complementary therapies is one that has come under a great deal of criticism.

The concept of energy is used in many cultures; the Chinese use the term *Qi,* while in India the term *prana* is used. These are all labels for the energy that many complementary and alternative practitioners say they work with to precipitate healing.

However, modern science recognises only four forms of energy: gravity, strong and weak nuclear forces and electromagnetic. Wright and Sayre-Adams claim that much of the energy that has been spoken about in the field of complementary therapies is not clearly definable or measurable.[1]

Oschman documents an extensive range of scientific studies that have been able to quantify the subtle energy of the body. He says that all life depends upon molecules interacting through vibrating or oscillating energy fields.[3] This is supported by Gerber, who says:

> *In the living body, each electron, atom, chemical bond, molecule, cell, tissue, organ (and the body as a whole) has its own vibratory character. Since living structure and function are orderly, biological oscillations are organised in meaningful ways, and they contribute information to a dynamic vibratory network that extends throughout the body and into the space around it. Energy medicines and vibrational medicines seek to understand this continuous energetic matrix, and to interact with it to facilitate healing.*[4]

In search of scientific evidence for the existence of the energy field around living beings, Gerber discusses the work of neuroanatomist Harold S. Burr:

> *Burr was studying the shape of energy fields around living plants and animals. Some of Burr's work involved the shape of electrical fields surrounding salamanders. He found that salamanders possessed an energy field roughly shaped like an adult animal. He also discovered that this field contained an electrical axis which was aligned with the brain and spinal cord.*
>
> *Burr wanted to find precisely when this electrical axis first originated in the animal's development. He began mapping the fields in progressively earlier stages of salamander embryogenesis. Burr discovered that the electrical axis originated in the unfertilised egg. This discovery contradicted the conventional biological and genetic theory of his day.*[4]

Recent research has lent further credibility to Burr's theories of bioenergetic fields from experimental work in the areas of electrographic photography, otherwise known as Kirlian photography. This is a technique whereby living objects are photographed in the presence of a high frequency, high voltage, low amp electrical field. This technique was pioneered by the Russian researcher Semyon Kirlian.[5]

Gerber gives us a clear insight into the potential future of energy medicine:

> *Medicine that is directed towards an understanding of energy and vibration, and how they interact with molecular structure and organismic balance, is a slowly evolving field known as vibrational medicine. In a real sense, vibrational medicine is Einsteinian medicine, since it is Einstein's equation which gives us the key insight toward understanding that energy and matter are one and the same thing. The current model of medicine is still Newtonian in character, for pharmacokinetic therapy is based upon a biomolecular/mechanistic approach. Surgery is even cruder approach of Newtonian mechanistic roots. The healing arts must be updated with new insights from the world of physics and other allied sciences.*[5]

He goes on to say:

> *... the recognition of our relationship to these higher frequency energy systems will ultimately lead to a fusion of religion and science as scientists begin to recognise the spiritual dimension of human beings and the laws of expression of the life-force. The trend of 'holism' in medicine will ultimately move physicians towards the recognition that, for human beings to experience health, they must enjoy an integrated relationship between body, mind and spirit.*[5]

Systems Used to Describe the Multidimensional Energy Systems of the Human Body

Throughout history humanity has found different ways of exploring, describing and working with this subtle anatomy.

Much of our knowledge of energy systems, sometimes referred to as 'subtle-energy' systems, comes from sacred and spiritual knowledge of Asia.

The most common systems or models used in vibrational healing today are the meridian system of Traditional Chinese Medicine (TCM), the chakras and the human aura or energy field.

Traditional Chinese Medicine (TCM)

The principles of Chinese medicine are extremely interwoven and complex. It embraces the ideas of *Qi* — the life force or subtle energy which permeates the universe and sustains all living things. It embraces the ideas of the Five Elements, of Yin and Yang and the meridians that are the channels through which *Qi* flows. All of these factors are delicately interrelated.

The greatest difficulty for the Western student of TCM lies in the tremendous difference between Western and Chinese patterns of thought. In the West, the word 'body' indicates the physical aspect — 'the body' as distinct from 'the mind' or 'the spirit'.

In TCM, the word 'body' implies not only the complex of physical, emotional, mental and spiritual aspects, but also the ongoing interaction between this complex and the external environment.

TCM recognises the acupuncture meridian system which consists of a series of channels, known as meridians, that acupuncturists are able to manipulate by inserting fine needles into special points along the meridians. The meridians carry the life force or energy, known as *Qi*, and according to TCM, illness can result from an imbalance of *Qi* energy to the organs and body. Therefore, the goal of acupuncture is to rebalance the flow of *Qi* throughout the body.

Chakras

There is another form of energy that is important to human health that Gerber refers to as 'spiritual energy'. He says that the chakra system is the most important pathway for spiritual energy.[4]

The word *chakra* comes from Sanskrit and means wheel, or vortex. Described as wheels of forces arranged vertically on the trunk and head, chakras are transfer points for our thoughts and feelings and the physical functioning of specific endocrine glands. Chakras appear to be involved in the flow of higher energies via specific subtle energetic channels to the cellular structure of the physical body.[5]

The flow of this energy through our chakra system is influenced by our personality and our emotions, as well as our state of spiritual development. Anatomically, each chakra is associated with a major nerve plexus and a minor endocrine gland. The seven major chakras are located in a vertical line ascending from the base of the spine to the head.[5]

The Human Subtle Bodies — The Auras

In addition to the life energy and the spiritual energies from the acupuncture meridians and the chakras, other energy systems also influence our health and wellbeing.

Surrounding and interpenetrating our physical body is an energy field or structure known as the 'etheric body'. The etheric body is described by Gerber as a kind of duplicate of the physical body that actually occupies the same space as the physical body, but at a higher vibratory rate or frequency. It is actually the first in a series of auras that we call the 'higher spiritual bodies'.[4]

Gerber says that our soul, or our 'true self' expresses itself through a physical body that is influenced by these higher spiritual bodies.[4]

The first of these higher spiritual bodies is known as the etheric body. It is a highly structured energy field that is invisible to the naked eye, but can easily be seen by some psychically gifted people who are able to see auras. Most people working in subtle healing can sense the aura in non-visual ways. It is not difficult to feel with your hands the energy emanations, especially the etheric and astral bodies.[6] Kirlian photography is a technique that can be used to take an image of the etheric body.[4]

Besides the etheric body, there is the astral body, which participates in how we feel and how we express ourselves, and how we are influenced by our emotions. Some clairvoyants refer to the astral body as the emotional body.[4]

While the etheric body is strongly attached to the physical body, the astral body appears to be more mobile and can move about independent from the physical body.[4]

Beyond the etheric and astral bodies resides another spiritual body known as the mental body. The mental body is composed of subtle magnetic energy that vibrates faster than astral energy. The mental body is involved in the energy of thought, creation, invention and inspiration.[4]

Finally, the human energy field extends to an even higher spiritual plane known as the causal body. Gerber says that the causal body might be considered the closest thing to the soul. The record of all that a soul has experienced on the physical earth plane, in its current life as well as past lives, is said to be contained in the causal body.[4]

Gerber cites a number of spiritual philosophies that suggest that the soul lives many different lives through a variety of different physical bodies over the course of the earth's history. He says that to truly understand the causal body, one must believe that the human soul is immortal and that it becomes progressively more spiritually enlightened by returning to earth numerous times in different physical bodies. This is the cornerstone of reincarnation, a belief system shared by millions of people throughout many different cultures of the world.[4]

Gerber says that the causal body retains a memory of our past lives, and unresolved traumas and conflicts may be carried over from one lifetime to affect the body and life patterns of another lifetime. The unique types of health problems, related directly to the causal body, are known as 'karmic illnesses'.[4]

An understanding and appreciation of the high spiritual bodies — our etheric, astral, mental and causal bodies, as well as the chakras and the meridians — gives us a holistic way of looking at concepts of health and wellness from a multidimensional perspective.

Subtle Aromatherapy

It is interesting to look back at some of the rather esoteric definitions of essential oils.

> *Essences are like the blood of a person … the essence is the most ethereal and subtle part of the plant …*[7]

or

> *It is this life force of the plant which we introduce into the body by aromatherapy ... It has been said that essential oils are actually the hormones of the plants.*[8]

By the 1990s aromatherapy was rapidly becoming popular and there was a need to validate it in order to keep legislators satisfied. We began to focus on the science, chemistry and pharmacology to understand how the essential oils worked. Science can even explain how essential oils make a person feel good emotionally through its work in the area of olfaction and brain chemistry. It is interesting to see how science has modified the definition of an essential oil:

> *... of these secondary metabolites the essential oils have the greatest commercial significance ... whatever else they may do, they give the plant its aroma and flavour and often have a significant physiological effect on people.*[9]

or

> *... but what is this elusive essence of plant material called essential oil? It is the heart and soul of the plant. It is the essence that deters bugs from eating the plant. It is the fragrant aromatic heart of the plant that attracts bees and pollinating insects. It is the chemical components contained in the tiny plant cells that are liberated during the extraction process.*[10]

While these definitions are technically accurate, they do not encompass the subtle aspects of essential oils described earlier.

Holmes says that whether we're trying to describe how an essential oil works on the body or soul, or whether we're trying to explain why a particular blend has such miraculous effect on a certain client, we are usually attempting to validate aromatherapy in terms of chemistry or pharmacology, yet aromatherapy is essentially an *energy medicine*.[11]

The chemistry of the essential oils can help us understand the pharmacology of essential oils, olfaction can help us understand the psychological benefits of essential oils and an understanding of the concepts of vibrational medicine can help us understand how essential oils work at a subtle level.

The notion of subtle aromatherapy promoted nowadays implies the use of aromatherapy to purely influence the subtle body, the psyche and the soul. However, it must be emphasised that you cannot practise 'subtle aromatherapy' on its own because holistic aromatherapy includes 'physical aromatherapy', 'emotional aromatherapy' and 'subtle aromatherapy'.

Perhaps Worwood best describes subtle aromatherapy:

> *I daresay there are those who will set up practice as 'energetic' or 'vibrational' aromatherapists on the basis of the idea that 'all illness starts in the etheric'. It does not matter where the illness starts, the point is that it is there — manifesting in the physical, mental, emotional and spiritual, or all four.*
>
> *To treat a person energetically, all aspects of the person must be understood. Energetic therapies cannot make shortcuts by-passing the physical, because vibration is part of essential oils and the physical body. You cannot ignore it. The subtle and physical bodies of a person work together like a colour printer's primary colours — one does not make sense without the other, and you need all the colours, or 'bodies' to see the whole. Vibrational or subtle aromatherapy is aromatherapy.*[12]

The Spiritual Role of Aromatics in Traditional Cultures

Generally, pleasant fragrances are often closely identified with beneficial deities and forces, while foul odours are closely identified with harmful deities and forces. Muslim inhabitants of the United Arab Emirates say that 'a dirty, smelly body is vulnerable to evil; the scented person is surrounded by angels'. The olfactory rites of the UAE reflect this belief. The most efficacious scent for attracting angels and dispelling evil spirits is thought to be frankincense smoke.[13]

Similar beliefs can be found in other Arab cultures. In Morocco, foul odour is closely associated with evil spirits. Classens says that;

> *Sacred rites of smell are common to many peoples. In Mexico, the Tzotzil people dedicate to their deities candles and copal incense, which they refer to as 'cigarettes for the gods'. Hindu temples are redolent with odours of sandalwood and other aromatics. The Nigerian Songhay pour out perfumes on the altars of their gods. The Dakota of the Western plains send up smoke signals of burning sweet grass to their deities.*[13]

The Chewong people of the Malay Peninsula consider odour the fundamental means of interaction with the spirits. Chewong children wear a piece of wild ginger tied around their necks to keep harmful spirits away by the pungent smell. Good spirits, in contrast, are attracted by and 'fed' with an incense of fragrant wood, ritually offered to them every night.[13]

The Chewong shaman takes some of the incense smoke in his fist, puts his fist to his mouth and blows in four directions, after which he prays to the spirits for divine protection. The smoke is believed to carry the shaman's words up to the spirit world. On no account must this incense offering be neglected as this would interrupt the communication with the spirits and endanger the Chewong community.[13]

Classens says that the Batek Negrito believes that the spirits are very sensitive to smell. The Batek

Negrito spirits, the *hala*, are said to live in a perpetually fragrant land of fruit blossoms. The *hala* are exceedingly fond of the scents of flowers and incense and strongly dislike those of blood and burning hair. Batek olfactory rites, therefore, are centred on either propitiating the *hala*, or taking care not to offend their sensibilities with the latter.[13]

In certain cultures odours not only help one communicate with the spirits, but make it possible for one to temporarily become a spirit. In the Afro-Brazilian spirit possession cult, Batuque, incense sets the stage for the arrival of spirits. The act of burning incense serves to purify the ritual space and the participants, thus making them fit for the presence of the spirits.[13]

Evil spirits are often held to be the source of harmful odours and illnesses. The Hausa of Northern Nigeria believe that evil spirits are thought to enter the soul of an individual through the nose, causing mental derangement. Individuals manifesting symptoms of mental illness are therefore commonly treated with hot, peppery medicinal snuff which causes violent sneezing and hence it is thought to expel the offending spirit. As a supplement to this treatment, the afflicted person will be placed in a small room, which is then filled with a thick, disagreeable smoke of burning shrew, mice, scorpions and herbs. It is hoped that the spirit will be made so miserable by this unpleasant fumigation that it will soon depart.[13]

The Role of Incense

Almost all human cultures have used incense in numerous social situations. In ancient times there was very little to distinguish perfumes used to scent the body and incense which was burned on the altars to the gods. The word 'perfume' is derived from Latin 'per fumen' (by smoke).

The earliest recorded use of incense comes from the Chinese who burned various herbs and plant matter such as cassia, cinnamon, styrax and sandalwood. The Hindus absorbed the cult of incense from the Chinese and introduced frankincense, benzoin and cypress into the recipe.[14]

It is believed that the early Hindus opened the first trading routes to the west and in particular to the incense lands of Arabia where the cherished frankincense grew. The ancient Egyptians acquired the incense cult from the Hindu traders some time around 3600 BC.[14]

The significance and importance of incense to the Egyptians was matched only by its value — gold, frankincense and myrrh were the three costliest commodities in the realm and remained so for many centuries. The Egyptians believed that frankincense was the sweat of the gods that had fallen to earth; thus it had the gods' odour. Pliny reminds us that the ancient Egyptians believed that the phoenix — the mythical bird that is supposed to arise from fire — brought incense to Punt in his claws, and the scent of incense was his own scent. The Hebrews thought the phoenix was a god reincarnated, and the Egyptians saw him as the soul of Osiris.[14]

Just as the Egyptians had learned of incense from the traders of the East, so the Greeks acquired the knowledge from the Egyptians. The ancient Greek gods delighted in aromatics and were aromatic themselves. Zeus is described by Homer as being wreathed in a fragrant cloud.[14]

According to Socrates the mind and the soul or life force could themselves be conceived of as 'essences'. Lucretius writes that the soul is part of the body in the same way that scent is part of a lump of frankincense. The acts of emitting and inhaling odour, consequently, were not simply thought of as sensory processes, but as models for the expression and attainment of knowledge and life.

The Healing Energies of Plants

Human beings have always been drawn to the healing power of plants. Plants have always been central to medical and spiritual practices of humanity as far back as we have any evidence. Indeed, in many traditions there is no distinction between medicine and religion: the shaman is both priest and doctor. For example, the American Indian concept of 'medicine' is not limited to the cure of physical ills, but embraces the spiritual wellbeing.

While pharmacological research acknowledges the ability of plants to heal, in subtle aromatherapy we are drawn on less tangible properties of plants to help in healing and transformation.

It is far more difficult to explain the vibrational or subtle energy of plants than it is to describe the physical properties.

So how can we set about discovering the subtle healing properties of plants?

According to Davis, this can be done by:[6]

- researching the ancient use and traditional practices of people who have preserved by shamanistic traditions those of the Native Americans, Maoris and Aborigines
- researching traditional folklore and myths and the symbolism of plants in art, poetry and writing of mystics
- studying the plants themselves. Spend time near plants and be sensitive to them. The shape, texture, colour, habitat and the smell can all tell you something about the plants' healing

energies. This has led to the development of the *Doctrine of the Signatures.*

- Another way of appreciating the plant's energy is to become aware of its aura. The vibration of each plant aura is extremely refined and clearly indicates the particular area of healing to which that plant is best fitted.

Davis says that we should not lose sight of the original intent of offering aromatics to a deity or higher power. If your personal beliefs include a deity or higher consciousness, it can be very beautiful and meaningful to make an offering of your essential oil. If not, you may wish to dedicate the aromatic offering to world peace, to individual or planetary healing, or to your own higher self.[6]

Doctrine of the Signatures

The *Doctrine of the Signatures* proposes that the healing properties of plants are influenced by their physical features and habitat. By contemplating the botanical features of aromatic plants we may discover aspects of the personality or signature of many essential oils.

The *Doctrine of the Signatures* provides us with tangible images to describe the subtle healing properties of particular plants and essential oils. It can be explained in terms of the following:

- the aroma of the essential oil
- the anatomy of the plant
- the habitat of the plant
- the part of the plant used.

Aroma

The unique aroma of each essential oil reveals an aspect of its character and healing potential. We intuitively respond to the signatures of aromatic plants via their scent, which often evokes powerful emotions and memories.

It is well known that individual memory associations influence our response to odours. When these associations are universal they contribute to the signature of an essential oil.

For example, the sweet floral scent of neroli and rose bloom in spring when nature is most abundant and colourful. It is therefore not surprising that essential oils with floral aromas encourage us to be sensual and creative.

Wood oils such as cedarwood and sandalwood remind us of the forest or wood, where time seems to stand still. These essential oils have a serene quality and are often used to heighten spiritual awareness.

The Anatomy of Plants

According to the *Doctrine of the Signatures* the shape, texture and colour of plants often reflect their subtle action.

Shape

One of the most important factors in a plant's signature is its shape. A sturdy tree reaching upwards to the heavens is very different from the delicate appearance of a rose on a thorny vine. In aromatherapy, we must consider the shape of the whole plant that produces the essential oil. For example, the vertical shape of trees imparts a sense of direction and purpose, which is reflected in the signatures of essential oils extracted from the wood of plants.[15]

In contrast, the soft and delicate appearance of many flowers is reflected in the calming nature of most floral oils.[15]

Texture

The texture of plants and their producing organs are sometimes significant aspects of a plant signature. The hard and tough texture of wood suggests the ability of essential oils such as sandalwood and cedarwood to give us strength and endurance to overcome adversity.[15]

In contrast the texture of petals such as rose and chamomile is usually soft and delicate, reflecting the comforting effect that many floral essential oils have on the emotions.[15]

Colour

The colours of plants are often expressions of the unique nature of essential oils. For example; the violet colour of the flowers of *Lavandula angustifolia* reflect its gentle, calming nature and its ability to help us develop our intuition and spiritual awareness.[15]

Yellow is associated with intellect and lemon is clarifying to the mind, helping us to synthesise our thoughts and make decisions, while orange symbolises creativity — similarly the essential oil of sweet orange promotes creative expression and is playfulness.[15]

Habitat

Essential oil producing plants are grown all over the world, in a variety of climates. Each plant requires different growing conditions for its health and survival.

True lavender is a good example. *Lavandula angustifolia* is grown in many countries including Australia and Tasmania. There are distinct differences in the chemical composition, aroma and subtle qualities between Tasmanian lavender and the French lavender.

The French lavender is grown at moderately high altitudes and has a sweet floral scent which is calming and serene, reminiscent of the plant's habitat. In contrast the scent of Australian lavender has a fresh green top note with a subtle floral undertone — it is more uplifting and invigorating, which is reflective of the Australian environment.[15]

The Part of Plant Used

Roots

Roots provide stability by attaching the plant to the earth and absorbing nutrients and water from the surrounding soil, which enable the plant to survive. Therefore essential oils extracted from the roots of plants tend to be stabilising and strengthening. They have an affinity with the Earth element and tend to be grounding.[15]

Lavabre says that essential oils produced in the roots tend to have a very grounding energy and have a food-like quality to them. They are not very refined, but they usually are potent stimulants of the vital functions.[16]

Wood

The strength of wood allows trees to grow to incredible heights and live for hundreds of years. Wood oils reflect the durable nature of trees providing strength and endurance needed to tackle life's challenges.[15]

Lavabre says that wood oils are centring and equilibrating.[16] Wood oils have the power to open our consciousness to high spheres without making us lose control. Hence they are particularly useful in rituals, meditation and yoga.

Flowers

Flowering plants produce the seeds for reproduction within the flower itself. The flower also produces the scent to attract insects for pollination. Many floral oils such as jasmine and rose have an affinity with the reproductive system and are referred to as aphrodisiacs.[15]

Lavabre describes the flower as the plant's ultimate achievement. He suggests that a very strongly scented flower such as rose indicates a spiritually evolved plant and is a sign of intense astral activity.[16]

Leaves

Essential oils produced in the leaves correspond to the lungs of the plant. Lavabre says that the plant's leaf system corresponds to its vital body.[16] Essential oils produced in the leaf have a strong affinity with the respiratory system.[16]

Fruits

The fruits of plants protect and nurture the seeds that will enable new plants to be created. Essential oils derived from the fruits are often associated with nourishment and creativity.[15]

Resin

Many trees and shrubs produce resins. The gum has powerful wound-healing properties. Lavabre says that these essential oils have been extensively used in rituals and religious ceremonies, and that they have a very pronounced soothing, comforting, fortifying and elevating action on the soul and spirit.[16]

Seeds

Lavabre says that essential oils produced in the seed bring us back to the physical world, being less sophisticated, more humble and straightforward. They are generally invigorating and have a strong affinity with the digestive system.[16]

Using Essential Oils in Subtle Aromatherapy

Davis says that you can use essential oils for their subtle effects in any way you like. You do not need to be tied to any conventional method of application.[6]

What matters is the INTENT. Each time you use an essential oil for subtle or spiritual purposes, begin with a clear idea of what you aim to achieve and how you want the oil to help you.

In subtle aromatherapy the therapist may not be required to use massage — in some instances there may not even be a need for a therapist, as in the use of aromatics in diffusers as a meditation aid or in ritual bathing. Davis provides us with the following guidelines:

- Work safely — observe all the safety rules that apply to the normal uses of essential oils.
- Use very little oil — when using essential oils for their subtle properties less is better.
- Use very good quality oils.
- Work ethically.[6]

Worwood suggests that there are three main ways of using essential oils in spiritual healing:

- in the room
- in the auric field of the client
- on yourself, the therapist.[12]

The Room

Worwood suggests using essential oils in the waiting room. The aromas will relax and open the hearts of people, making them more receptive to healing. She states that it is generally not necessary to use blends while giving spiritual healing. The essential oils are being used to facilitate that flow, by creating that space in which healing can take place, and single oils have a simplicity and clarity that is appropriate.[12]

The Auric Field

Disease manifests in the subtle body before any physical symptoms are apparent. The vibration of the aura may be disturbed and the use of appropriate essential oils on the aura will help to restore harmony. To give an auric massage, you do not need to mix essential oils in a carrier oil.[6]

Once you have selected the appropriate essential oil, the following methods of application can be considered:

- Place 1 drop of neat essential oil in the centre of the palm of one hand, rub the hands together, and smooth around the outside of the body. Start on the side of the body, from the feet, working to the top of the head. Then repeat the movement on the front of the body, feet to head; then on the back, feet to head.[6,12]
- Using an essential oil solubiliser, dissolve the essential oil in water and store in a spray/mister bottle. Spray around the body and over the top of the head.[12]

The Therapist

Therapists can use essential oils to open their energy channels. Worwood suggests applying the essential oil to the soles of the feet. You can do this by placing a small smear of essential oil on each foot, at the uppermost point of the arch of the foot. She says that this will have an effect along the whole spine, and on the chakras, and will help to clear your energetic field.[12]

Colour Therapy and Aromatherapy

Colour therapy is not new to vibrational healing. Colour therapy has been used in the healing temples in Egypt, Greece, China and India.

Colour therapy utilises the vibrational frequency of the colours of the spectrum to correct the imbalances or disharmony in the body. Colour has a powerful effect on our emotions. Colours activate the chakra system. Each chakra resonates in harmony with one of the spectrum colours. The chakras can be stimulated and energised with their particular colour vibration to restore balance and harmony.

Colour therapy and aromatherapy work together in synergy. Essential oils and colour can recharge the aura and cleanse negative vibrations from the subtle bodies. Each essential oil has its own colour vibration or signature, so you can blend a harmonious mix of essential oils that resonate at the same frequency as the colours you wish to treat. You can complement the treatment with the use of a colour lamp, coloured towels and the colour of the room.

Red

Red is the element of fire. It is the colour of the base chakra. Red governs the genitals and reproductive organs, blood and circulation. It is drive and willpower.

The colour red is associated with energy, procreation, zest for life, dangers, construction and destruction, being alive and sexuality. It produces restlessness, anger, might and aggression and the will to win, sometimes at all costs.[17]

Red rays produce heat that is vitalising and energising, excellent for contracted muscles.[18] Red activates blood circulation, raises the pulse and heart beat. It tends to motivation, stimulation and power. Red light can be used when one is feeling tired and rundown. It rids the body of toxins and of any psyche negativity.

Essential oils which reflect the red ray are black pepper, cedarwood, jasmine, benzoin, sage, myrrh, rose and thyme.[18]

Orange

Orange is a combination of red and yellow rays, and its healing power is greater than the two individual rays. Orange is the colour of the sacral chakra. Orange governs the area of the lower back and lower intestines, the abdomen and kidneys. It has an antispasmodic effect and it stimulates the pulse rate without affecting the blood pressure.

The colour orange is about feeling and sensations, good-naturedness and flamboyance, giving one back their self-esteem, worth and importance, emotional force, and pleasurable experiences. It is related to being sociable, ambitious, enthusiastic and leads to a concern for others. It helps in cases of identity crises by promoting self-assurance.[17]

Orange is the colour for dealing with grief, bereavement and loss. Essential oils which reflect the orange ray are benzoin, cardamom, marjoram, neroli, bergamot, carrot seed, nutmeg, orange, neroli, patchouli, pine, mandarin, aniseed, caraway, ginger, cedarwood, sandalwood and cypress.[18]

Yellow

This is the colour of the solar plexus chakra. The solar plexus is the part of us that absorbs emotions. Yellow governs the pancreas, spleen, middle stomach, liver, gall bladder, digestive system and the nervous system.

Yellow is associated with the colour of intellect and the use of the mind in concrete, scholarly ways.[5] Because many individuals with stress-related disorders, such as ulcers, tend to be mentally focused and sometimes emotionally repressed, the yellow ray can be helpful in treating various types of stomach problems and indigestion.[5]

Yellow is associated with the search for self-knowledge. It is the re-energiser of the mind, promoter of mental activity, ingestion and assimilation, study and thought.[17] Yellow is associated with those who can be stubborn and opinionated, have a good business head and are the protectors of innate wisdom. It relates to higher emotions like joy and happiness, emotional sensitivity, reactivity and reaction.

Yellow is the colour of the mind and the ego. It is an excellent colour for the nerves and brain. It is a good eliminator, ridding the body of toxins. It can help to relieve constipation. Psychologically, yellow is uplifting, bringing hope and light, giving a feeling that everything will be alright.[18]

Essential oils that reflect the yellow ray are bergamot, cardamom, cajeput, citronella, lemon, lemongrass, grapefruit, basil, fennel, carrot seed, dill, sandalwood, tea tree, vetiver, aniseed, petitgrain and ginger.[18]

Green

Green is the colour of peace and healing and the colour of the heart chakra. Green governs the thymus gland, heart, shoulders, chest and lower lungs. Green is made up of yellow and blue.

Green exercises some control over distribution of blood supply though its effects are on the heart.[5]

Green helps prevent stagnation and represents a new place and pace, affections of the heart, freedom, adaptability, harmony and brings good judgements, balance and understanding, maturity and self-control, love for humanity, generosity, nature, regeneration, karma or opportunities for new beginnings, breathing space, compassion, and co-operation, understanding, caring, stability, giving, growth, willingness and a positive expression of the inner self.[17]

Green is cooling, soothing and calming on all levels. It is emotionally stabilising and balancing and is also regulating on the metabolism. It is a muscle builder and tissue builder. It helps to dispel negativity. It soothes headaches.[18]

Essential oils that reflect the colour green are melissa, rosewood, palmarosa, geranium, eucalyptus, peppermint, lemon, bergamot, petitgrain and aniseed.[18]

Blue

Blue is the colour of the throat chakra, it rules the throat area and is linked to upper lungs and arms, base of skull and weight. Blue is peaceful and cool.

Blue is associated with nurturing, communicating, peace, faith, idealism, sincerity, expression of thoughts, languages and images, the mother, cool and calm, a natural antiseptic, stability, gentleness and meditation.[17]

The blue vibration is very helpful for throat problems, helping to dispel the fear of 'speaking out' or 'speaking the truth'. Blue increases vitality. The coolness of blue makes it an excellent colour for treating inflammatory diseases. Blue can reduce stress and anxiety and can help to reduce blood pressure.[18]

Essential oils that reflect the blue ray are German chamomile, Roman chamomile, marjoram, myrtle, pine, hyssop, rosemary, cypress, mandarin and eucalyptus.[18]

Indigo

Indigo is made up of dark blue and dark violet, it is the colour of the third eye chakra. Indigo rules the endocrine system, the spine, lower brain, eyes and sinuses.

Indigo is pacifying and calming, pure spiritual thoughts, devotion to an ideal, psychic matters, the eye of the soul, contact with the higher self, spiritual communications, a higher level of intellect, insight, imagination and self-realisation.[17]

Indigo provides the greatest analgesic benefits in the spectrum. It is useful for treating sciatica, migraine, bruising and inflammations. It promotes skin repair. It is a balancer for high blood pressure and is said to be great for insomnia.[18]

Essential oils that reflect the indigo ray include tea tree, bay laurel, clove, yarrow, myrtle and cinnamon.[18]

Violet

Violet is a light shade of purple. Violet is the colour of the crown chakra. It governs the pineal gland. Violet is considered a very spiritual colour and has a spiritual dedication. Violet is intuition, it calms emotional upsets and it aids psychic ability and is a great colour for meditation.

Violet is associated with creativity, inspiration, mental strength, inspired leadership, evolution of the soul, religion, spirituality, the gateway to attainment, aspiration, humanitarian and devotion.[17]

Violet is good for bone growth. It is a blood purifier and helps to build up white blood cells. It is used as a treatment for varicose veins, inflammation and pain. Because violet vibrates at such a high frequency, it has the ability to break down fears associated with the mind. Newton says that it is a cleanser of impure thoughts and emotions in the mind as well as the room.[18]

Essential oils that reflect the violet ray include juniper, lavender, frankincense, hyssop, grapefruit, basil, patchouli, sandalwood and sage.[18]

Utilising Colour Therapy in Healing

There are intricate systems and approaches to colour healing that are utilised by various practitioners. Colours may be applied alone or in special therapeutic combinations that tend to enhance the potential of colour therapy through synergistic effects. The methods by which the frequencies of colour may be transmitted to patients are numerous. The methods include:

- direct light from electric lamps (or natural sunlight) which has passed through various colour screens and filters
- coloured tinctures or flower essences
- colour breathing.[5]

Gerber outlines a procedure for colour breathing and the benefits of visualisation and affirmations. This could be utilised with the appropriate essential oils that reflect the colour you are visualising.[5]

> *Color breathing involves visualising oneself breathing in a particular color during the inspiratory phase of respiration. Following inspiration, the visualised color is mentally directed to areas of illness, blockage and dysfunction, or those bodily systems which are in need of visualisation. There are many variations on this particular technique of colour breathing which allow visualised color to be used for altering the level of one's consciousness and for cleansing the chakras, as well as achieving particular types of healing. Color breathing at the mental level involves directing energies that work with the mental and astral bodies and chakras.*
>
> *In general, visualisation of the color, gem, or flower being vibrationally applied can powerfully augment the effectiveness of the treatment. Mental affirmations — inwardly spoken statements that reaffirm the desired physical or emotional change — can also be helpful in amplifying the efficacy of the various vibrational therapies. … The more the individual becomes actively involved with the therapy, as in the use of visualisation and affirmations, the greater the chances are for a successful healing outcome to occur.*[5]

Chakras and Aromatherapy

The chakras are said to resemble whirling vortexes of subtle energy. They are involved in taking in higher energies and transforming them to a form that can be utilised by the human body.[5]

Chakras exist on the outside of the etheric body, and are points of connection through which energy flows from one being to another. Gerber describes chakras as energy transformers, stepping down energy of one form and frequency to a lower level energy. This energy is then translated into hormonal, physiological and cellular changes throughout the body.[5]

There are seven major chakras associated with the physical body. Anatomically, each of the chakras is associated with a major nerve plexus and a major endocrine gland. The chakras are situated in a vertical line ascending from the base of the spine to the head.

Gerber says that each of the major chakras is associated with a particular type of psychic perceptual functioning.[5]

The Base Chakra

The journey through the chakras begins with the base chakra. It is also known as the root or coccygeal chakra. Its Sanskrit name, *Muladhara*, means 'root' or 'support'. The root chakra is concerned with physical needs and basic human survival. It has the lowest vibrational rate of all the chakras, resonating to the colour red. The root chakra is located at the base of the spine, between the anus and genitals.[19]

The root chakra reflects the degree to which we feel connected to the earth or are grounded in our activities. The amount of energy flow through the root chakra is a reflection of one's ability to link with the earth and to function effectively upon the earth plane from day to day. On a practical level this refers to the ability to keep one's feet firmly upon the ground.[5] The base chakra provides us with the ability to provide for life's necessities, the ability to stand up for oneself and a sense of security.[20]

Mastering the root chakra helps you grasp the importance of a fit, healthy body as you travel upward through higher and higher levels of consciousness.[19]

Essential Oils for the Base Chakra

Essential oils that resonate at the base chakra are generally grounding, strengthening and centring. Essential oils such as myrrh, patchouli and vetiver have the greatest benefit when the base chakra energy is depleted.[6]

The Sacral Chakra

The sacral chakra is also known as the navel chakra, gonadal chakra or splenic chakra. It represents our creative energy and is associated with the functions of our reproductive organs. This chakra vibrates from the pubic bone, between the navel and genitals.[6]

The Sanskrit name for the sacral chakra is *Svadhisthana*, meaning 'sweetness' and its associations are indeed what makes life sweet — pleasure, sexuality, nurture, movement and change.[19]

Gerber describes the sacral chakra as the subtle-energy seat of sexuality. The sacral chakra is associated with the gonads and reproductive organs, in addition to the urinary bladder, large and small intestines, the appendix and the lumbar vertebrae. He says that from a psychoenergetic standpoint, the sacral chakra is associated with the expression of sensual emotion and sexuality.[5]

The sacral chakra leads us from basic existence to help us embrace what makes life worth living.[19] Physical dysfunctions associated with the sacral chakra include chronic lower back pain, sciatica, gynaecological problems, sexual potency and urinary problems.[20]

Essential Oils for the Sacral Chakra

Essential oils that have the greatest affinity with the sacral chakra include sandalwood, jasmine and rose absolute. They are deeply sensual and warming in nature. These oils connect with sexual and reproductive energy and with the great love of beauty.[6]

The Solar Plexus Chakra

The Sanskrit name for the solar plexus chakra is *Manipura* — 'lustrous gem'. It resonates to the colour yellow.[19]

The solar plexus chakra relates to our connection with others, but without the root chakra's reliance on the 'tribe' or the sacral chakra's emphasis on partnerships. It is about the power of being an individual, to be unique, while celebrating our continuing connection with all humanity.[5]

The solar plexus chakra supplies nutritive subtle energy to most of the major organs of digestion and purification. These include the stomach, pancreas, liver, gall bladder, spleen, adrenal glands, lumbar vertebrae and the general digestive system.[5]

Gerber says that from an emotional and spiritual standpoint, the solar plexus chakra is linked to the issue of personal power. Personal power can be described as a feeling of control over one's life. Personal power also relates to how people view themselves in relation to others in their lives. Individuals with a so-called 'victim consciousness', who have no sense of control over their lives, will often manifest an imbalance in the solar plexus chakra. Domination, anger and abuse of others can also be associated with abnormal function of the solar plexus.[5]

Imbalances of the solar plexus chakra can affect any one of the digestive organs of the body that receive energy from this centre. The adrenal glands are linked to the solar plexus chakra. The adrenal glands play an important role in hormonal activation of the body systems during times of stress.[5,20]

By strengthening and stimulating the solar plexus chakra you will attain a state in which you can shake off the fears of rejection, criticism, and standing apart from the group and create your own, unique identity.[19,20]

Essential Oils for the Solar Plexus Chakra

Two very important essential oils include juniper berry and vetiver. Vetiver is a protector and a balancer and juniper is a purifier. Davis recommends using vetiver if you are going to a crowded public place. For any situation that makes you feel uncomfortable it is good to anoint the solar plexus chakra with a drop or two of vetiver. It should be applied in an anti-clockwise direction.[6]

The Heart Chakra

The Sanskrit *Anahata* means 'sound made by two things striking' or 'unstuck', describing the coexistence of body and spirit.

This chakra is concerned with forgiveness and compassion — unconditional love through which we accept others for doing their best. We thus begin to develop true self-acceptance.

Gerber says that the heart chakra is integral to an individual's ability to express love. He says that love may manifest as brotherly love towards neighbours and friends, as emotional love in a love relationship between lovers and also as spiritual love. The highest form of spiritual love is unconditional love towards others.[5]

Mastering the heart chakra helps us to enhance our emotional development and recognise the potency of that powerful energy we call 'love'.[19]

Physical dysfunctions associated with the heart chakra include heart diseases, asthma, lung cancer, bronchial pneumonia and breast cancer.[20]

Essential Oils for the Heart Chakra

Rose absolute and otto intensify the loving energy of the heart chakra. They are deeply healing when the chakra is closed through grief. Bergamot, melissa, ylang ylang and neroli all help open the heart chakra and help the love energy to radiate out.[6]

The Throat Chakra

The throat chakra is the first of the higher centres — associated with communication, self-expression, and creativity through sound. The Sanskrit *Vishuddha* means 'purification'. Developing the throat chakra means choosing words that bring value to communication.

The throat chakra has influence over the major glands and structures in the neck region. These include the thyroid and parathyroid glands, the mouth, vocal cords and trachea. There is also an association between the throat chakra and the parasympathetic nervous system. Gerber says that at a physical/emotional level, dysfunctions of the throat chakra may reflect difficulties in communication.[5]

The throat chakra is the centre of higher creativity such as the creation of word and song. Speech and sound are means by which we can vibrationally communicate with one another and verbally express new ideas.[5]

The throat chakra is also known as the centre of the will. Difficulties in self-expression may be seen here as a problem in exerting will to communicate one's true inner feelings.[5]

Mastering the throat chakra helps us grasp the importance of purifying ourselves by honestly recognising how we feel, following one's dream, using personal power to create and having the confidence to communicate our emotions to others.[19,20]

Physical dysfunctions associated with the throat chakra include chronic sore throat, mouth ulcers, gum problems, scoliosis, laryngitis, swollen glands and thyroid problems.[20]

Essential Oils for the Throat Chakra

German chamomile and Roman chamomile both impart calm strength and enable the truth to be spoken without anger. These oils resonate with the throat chakra and encourage the expression of spiritual truth.[6]

The Third Eye Chakra

Also known as the 'brow chakra'. The third eye chakra, known as *Ajna* in Sanskrit, means, 'to perceive' or 'to know'. Our physical eyes are the tools with which we perceive tangibles, while the 'third eye', above and between the eyebrows, offers us the ability to see and understand all things. It is the connection with the higher functions of consciousness. The third eye chakra is a psychic tool reminding us that everything we see, smell, touch, or taste started as an inner vision or 'in-sight'.[19]

Gerber says that the third eye chakra is one of the psychic centres that gradually develops with meditation. An individual who has a highly developed brow chakra has the ability to 'see within', an aspect of consciousness also related to introspection.[5]

Physically, the brow chakra is associated with the pineal gland, the pituitary gland, and the spinal cord, as well as the eyes, ears, nose and sinuses. Diseases caused by dysfunction of the brow chakra may be caused by an individual's not wanting to see something that is important to his or her soul growth.[5]

Mastering the third eye chakra will help you to keep your mind focused on related issues, including the awareness of the benefits to be gained from transcending the purely physical world and opening yourself up to intuitive sight and wisdom: the ability to learn from experience and emotional intelligence.[19,20]

Essential Oils for the Third Eye Chakra

Used with appropriate visualisation, essential oils such as juniper berry, everlasting, rosemary, thyme and basil help us to connect with the higher levels of the mind and bring clarity to our understanding of spiritual truths.[6]

Davis says that everlasting activates the right side of the brain, deepening intuition and facilitating access to the unconsciousness while thyme stimulates the left brain and all conscious and intellectual thoughts.[6]

The Crown Chakra

The crown chakra, known in Sanskrit as *Sahasrara*, meaning 'thousandfold'. Developing the other chakras was like walking on stepping stones taking us toward this ultimate goal — enlightenment, self-realisation, fulfilment and divine self.[19]

Gerber says that the crown chakra is considered one of the highest vibrational centres in the subtle body and it is associated with deep inner searching: the so-called spiritual quest. This chakra is most active when individuals are involved in religious and spiritual quest for the meaning of life and in the inner search of their origins as conscious evolving beings.[5]

On a physical level the crown chakra is associated with the activity of the cerebral cortex and general nervous system functioning. In addition, the proper activation of the crown chakra influences the synchronisation between the left and right hemispheres of the brain. The crown chakra is also closely linked with the pineal gland. For the crown chakra to be fully awakened there must occur a balance of the body, mind and spirit.[5]

Physical dysfunctions associated with the crown chakra include energetic disorders, mystical depression, extreme sensitivities to light, sound and other environmental factors.[20]

When we awaken the crown chakra we open to the possibilities of infinity of space and time and have divine wisdom and understanding of humanity, selflessness, spirituality and devotion.[19,20]

Essential Oils for the Crown Chakra

Essential oils for the crown chakra include French alpine lavender, rosewood, sandalwood, frankincense and myrrh. Davis says that rosewood facilitates the opening of the crown chakra and frankincense has the ability to connect us with the divine within and without.[6]

Crystals and Aromatherapy

Gerber says that the use of crystal technologies for the development of electronic systems has resulted in great advances in the ways that we are able to perceive the universe around us. Because of the important role of silicon technology in integrated circuitry and the development of computer systems, we have been provided with new tools that can amplify our powers of memory and information storage.[5]

Humankind is now using crystals for communication, information storage, solar power, time keeping and in laser technology!

According to Gerber, the reason that quartz crystals are so good at keeping the time is that when they are stimulated with electricity (a form of energy), their oscillations are so regular and precise that they form a handy reference by which bits of time may be measured and displayed. This property of quartz crystals is a reflection of what is known as the 'piezoelectric effect'. When quartz crystals are subjected to mechanical pressure they produce a measurable electric voltage. Conversely when an electric current is applied to a crystal, it will induce mechanical movement. Most electronic devices utilise a slice or plate of quartz. Each plate of quartz has a particular natural resonant frequency that is dependent upon its thickness and size.[5]

This is the basis for crystal oscillators components used in many electronic systems to generate and maintain very precise energy frequencies. Of particular interest is the way in which crystals affect the subtle energetics of the body. Gerber quotes crystal researcher Marcel Vogel, a senior scientist with IBM for 27 years:

> *The crystal is a neutral object whose inner structure exhibits a state of perfection and balance. When it is cut to proper form and when the human mind enters into relationship with its structural perfection, the crystal emits a vibration which extends and amplifies the powers of the user's mind. Like a laser, it radiates energy in a coherent, highly concentrated form, and this energy may be transmitted into objects or people at will.*
>
> *Although the crystal may be used for 'mind to mind' communication, its higher purpose … is in the service of humanity for the removal of pain and suffering. With proper training, a healer can release negative thought forms which have taken shape as disease patterns in a patient's physical body.*
>
> *As psychics have often pointed out, when a person becomes emotionally distressed, a weakness forms in his subtle energy body and disease may soon follow. With a properly cut crystal, however, a healer can, like a surgeon cutting away a tumor, release negative patterns in the energy body, allowing the physical body to return to a state of wholeness.*[5]

Dr Vogel is saying that the quartz crystal is capable of amplifying and directing the natural energies of the healer.

Gerber suggests that the healing energies transmitted by crystals work at the subtle level of our subtle energetic bodies. When healing energy is focused through the quartz crystal, it is sent into the body of the patient and distributed to the areas most in need of an energy balancing.[5]

The quartz crystal may be held in the hand while touching the patient, and the healing energies sent through the palm chakra. As the energies pass through the crystal, they are amplified and directed to those parts of the subtle anatomy which require energetic healing.

Quartz crystals may also be used for rebalancing and cleansing abnormally functioning or 'blocked' chakras. When cleansing a chakra, the crystal is placed over the particular chakra region and energy is sent through the crystal. The cleansing action may be induced by the energy of the therapist or the individual in need of chakra balancing.

If the therapist is the active energy source, subtle energy is transmitted from the healer's palm chakra, through the crystal, and into the individual's unbalanced chakra, while the healer focuses his/her mind on the task at hand. Conversely, an individual can use the crystal to cleanse his/her own chakras by placing a single terminated crystal over the chakra with the point facing away from the body. In this technique, the individual directs energy from inside the body out through the chakra and the overlying crystal.

Another method of utilising the energies of crystals is through the application of gem elixirs (similar to flower essences but made by using crystals). The energy imprint of the crystal is transferred to the water.

In the realm of personal healing, the quartz crystal is an excellent tool to assist in meditation. Gerber says that in meditation, the crystal should be held in the left hand. He says that the reason for this practice is that the left hand is neurologically connected to the right cerebral hemisphere, which is attuned to the higher dimensional fields of consciousness of the higher self because the right brain has unique crystalline connections to the pineal gland.[5]

The Subtle Energy of Crystals

The quartz crystal is but one of many stones and gems that can be used for the purpose of healing, energising and gaining access to higher dimensions of consciousness. The quartz crystal that we have been discussing up to now is the rock crystal of the quartz family. All crystals in the quartz family are composed of silicon dioxide.

There are many different colours and variations of quartz, because within the mixture of silicon dioxide there are also traces of other elements. For instance, amethyst is a violet type of quartz. There is also a smoky quartz, rose quartz, green quartz, blue quartz, etc. Each variety of quartz has its own special subtle energy and healing properties.

It appears that each coloured crystal has an affinity or subtle-energy resonance with a particular subplane of energy.

Crystals will enhance the action of the essential oils that you are using. Many of the coloured crystals correspond to various essential oils.[6] For example, Davis says that rose quartz harmonises exquisitely with rose absolute and both relate to the heart chakra. German chamomile has a strong affinity with blue stones such as lapis lazuli and blue agate which share the ability to calm and soothe, while the clear quartz crystal can be used with any essential oil.[6]

Therapists use crystals in many different ways. One of the simplest ways of using crystals with aromatherapy is to place a small crystal in the bowl of massage oil to potentise it. Davis says you should use only 1% or less dilution when using crystals in this way.[6]

Another way of using crystals is to place a crystal at each corner of the massage table while you are massaging the client. Davis says that it is important to use two evenly matched crystals for this purpose.[6]

Essential Oils and Meditation

Meditation has been described by Wright and Sayre-Adams as a method by which a person empties the mind of all thoughts, stimuli and expectations while, paradoxically, becoming more alert.[1] They cite Longaker who says:

> *Instead of looking outward toward the world, in meditation we shift our attention inward, to help us connect with our innermost essence — a pure, boundless awareness and natural simplicity. Training in meditation, we can experience breaks in our endless mental suffering — moments of freedom, spaciousness and deep peace. By committing ourselves to study, contemplation and meditation, we can learn to sustain and integrate into our entire way of being the openness, clarity and boundless compassion of our true nature, until we transcend suffering entirely.*[1]

People who have been ill have reported a wide range of benefits from meditation. Meditation tends to focus on personal and experiential rather than intellectual knowledge — a deepening of understanding of ourselves and our relationship with the beyond. It shifts our attention from active, outward consciousness and events to what is taking place inside us.[1]

Much of the teaching of meditation in the West has been greatly influenced by eastern philosophy. Carl Jung is said to have believed that the greatest impact upon Western thinking will come from the integration of Buddhist psychology.[1]

Whatever the source, all meditation techniques appear to have a number of common benefits such as:

- producing a state of physical and mental relaxation
- promoting a sense of wellbeing
- reducing stress and anxiety
- improving the autoimmune response and helping with the healing of damaged tissue
- helping us to be 'fully human' to expand our consciousness and go beyond insight into life's daily difficulties and the need to relax into a deeper awareness of who we are, how to be in the world and our relationship with our inner self, and perhaps our God.[1]

How to Meditate

Meditation can be developed around everyday activities such as eating. Indeed, may people can experience a meditative-like state by simply becoming very focused on a particular task, such as a hobby, painting, writing or sporting activities. Many Buddhists teach that being fully present in the moment, with whatever the moment holds, is the purpose of meditation.

Wright and Sayre-Adams describe a simple technique that can be used to achieve a meditative state:

> *Sit quietly with your eyes closed in a quiet room. Begin to count your breathing. Count each time you exhale up to a count of four, then inhale and count again from one to four. Continue to do this so that you become aware only of your breathing and your counting. See how long you can keep this up before you lose count or your mind begins to wander.*[1]

This technique can help us to calm the mind and relax us, and it shows us how tense or anxious we are, how easily the mind wanders, and how difficult it is to stay focused on a task as simple as counting our breath. One of the goals of meditation is, through practice, to develop the skill and attention that help us to master the will and the mind that distracts us and to bring the degree of focused, quiet attention into our daily lives.

A range of activities will assist us in meditation to induce a relaxed state or alter our consciousness so that we become more open, aware and focused in our meditation. These include:[1]

- Particular postures or movements, such as the classic 'lotus' position (sitting cross-legged, with feet over both thighs) or the many yoga positions, or movements associated with Tai Chi and Chi Gung.
- Smell: such as the use of incense or use of essential oils in vaporisers.
- Sound: adding suitable background music, or the use of chants and mantras (words or phrases repeated verbally or silently in the mind to induce a state of quietness and attention. These may be well-established words such as 'aum' or 'om'.
- Focusing on bodily rhythms, such as breathing.
- Visual techniques, for example the use of an inspiring picture, icon, view, flowers and so on, or the use of special lighting such as a candle.

However, Wright and Sayre-Adams warn us not to get caught up in the materialism of spirituality; 'I can not meditate because I don't have my favourite crystal with me.' They stress that it is important to see these aids as tools to help towards a meditative state rather than a end in themselves. Further guidance includes:[1]

- If using a sitting meditation, choose a posture that is most comfortable for you. Particular schools use different methods, but a comfortable chair offering an upright position may be all that you need. Avoid lying down if you want to avoid falling asleep.
- Prepare your environment, especially prepare a sacred place and time if this is possible. Experienced meditators will be able to meditate anywhere, but for the novice it is usually necessary to have:
  - a quiet, undisturbed room
  - lighting adjusted to a comfortable level
  - even, comfortable temperature
  - a cushion or suitable chair for comfort
  - music, incense, candles or other aids according to your choice or method.
- Remove any possible interruptions such as the telephone.
- Read and study widely about the options for meditation, find a technique that suits you and pursue it in depth.
- Find a good teacher or course or group of like-minded people who can give you expert tuition, guidance and support, but be very wary of 'gurus' who ask you to surrender yourself, your body or your money to them in return for their 'unique' knowledge! Meditation is an empowering process, it does not require you to surrender yourself to others.
- Relax in your meditation technique — whatever is happening is meant to happen. Avoid getting caught up in the outcome and do not judge your meditations as good or bad. If you fall asleep that's cool, you probably needed it. If it seemed confused, that's okay. What did it teach you about your state of mind? You can always come back to it later.
- Develop a routine. Part of your sacred space might be to allocate a specific time each day when you meditate, and then commit yourself to it as much as possible, whether it be an hour or five minutes.
- Keep a reflective diary or journal of your experiences which you can share with a trusted person and use this as a reference point to observe how your practice is developing.

Wright and Sayre-Adams summarise the benefits of meditation:

> *Meditation can help us find meaning and purpose in a world which is often confusing and perplexing. Many teachers of meditation believe that the benefits reach out beyond the individual. If we are more relaxed and attentive in our lives, then that impacts upon others around us. They too can feel more calm in the presence of someone who seems so centered and unruffled. With practice it can deepen our understanding of ourselves and our place in the grander scheme of things. We become easier in the world and better able to relax into the 'all that is'. In doing so, we receive revelation and inspiration that to some is divine in origin. We may find ourselves relaxing into the possibility that not just ourselves, but the whole universe, is in a state of meditation.*[1]

The Role of Essential Oils in Meditation

Essential oils and aromatic substances have long been used to facilitate meditation and prayer. Essential oils can be used in meditation for the following reasons:

- They purify and prepare the place where we intend to meditate.
- They assist in deepening and slowing the breath, increasing awareness of the breath and helping to focus on breathing.

- They balance chakra energy, opening the higher chakra centres.
- They heighten awareness, raising consciousness to a higher level.
- They ground and earth energy.
- They harmonise the energies of individuals in a group.
- The most useful way to use essential oils as an aid to meditation is in a vaporiser.[6]

Some of the essential oils that are beneficial for meditation include:[6]

Frankincense: Deepens and slows the rate of respiration. Helps to bring about a calm and meditative state.

Juniper: A psychic cleanser, very good for clearing rooms before meditation.

Rose: Opens the heart chakra, allows love to be given and received. Stimulates creativity, especially useful in meditation that involves visualisation.

Rosewood: Ability to open crown chakra — creates a feeling a calm without inducing drowsiness.

Sandalwood: Balancing, calming and grounding — traditionally used in incense.

Vetiver: Has a balancing action, very good for bringing the energy of all the major chakras into alignment and for harmonising group energies.

References

1. Wright S, Sayre-Adams J. *Sacred space*. Churchill Livingstone, UK, 2000.
2. Jones J. *In the middle of the road we call life*. Harper Collins, London, 1996.
3. Oschman J. *Energy medicine*. Churchill Livingstone, UK, 2000.
4. Gerber R. *Vibrational medicine for the 21st century*. Piatkus, England, 2000.
5. Gerber R. *Vibrational medicine*. Bear & Company, USA, 1988.
6. Davis P. *Subtle aromatherapy*. The C.W. Daniel Company Limited, Great Britain, 1991.
7. Tisserand R. *The art of aromatherapy*. The C.W. Daniel Company Limited, Great Britain, 1977.
8. Price S. *Practical aromatherapy*. Thorsons Publishers Limited, Great Britain, 1983.
9. Price S, Price L. *Aromatherapy for health professionals*. Churchill Livingstone, UK, 1995.
10. Rose J. *The aromatherapy book*. Herbal Studies Course, California, 1992.
11. Holmes P. *Energy medicine*. The International Journal of Aromatherapy, 1998/1999; 9(2): 53–56.
12. Worwood V. *The fragrant heavens*. Doubleday. London, 1999.
13. Classens C. *Aroma: The cultural history of smell*. Routledge, London, 1994.
14. Stoddart M. *The scented ape: The biology and culture of human odour*. Cambridge University Press, Great Britain, 1990.
15. Frank R. *Aromatic signatures: the doctrine of signatures in the practice of aromatherapy*. Aromatherapy Today, 2000; 13: 34–39.
16. Lavabre M. *Aromatherapy workbook*. Healing Art Press, USA, 1997.
17. Cooper A. *Colour the cosmic code*. Unicorn 2000/Aura Light, England, 1999.
18. Newton J. *Aromatherapy and colour*. Aromatherapy Today, 2000; 13: 42–45.
19. Simpson L. *The book of chakra healing*. Simon & Schuster, Australia, 1999.
20. Myss C. *Anatomy of the spirit*. Bantam Books, Australia, 1996.

Recommended Reading

Davis P. *Subtle aromatherapy*. The C.W. Daniel Company Limited, Great Britain, 1991.

Gerber R. *Vibrational medicine*. Bear & Company, USA, 1988.

Gerber R. *Vibrational medicine for the 21st century*. Piatkus, England, 2000.

Myss C. *Anatomy of the spirit*. Bantam Books, Australia, 1996.

Worwood V. *The fragrant heavens*. Doubleday. London, 1999.

Wright S, Sayre-Adams J. *Sacred space*. Churchill Livingstone, UK, 2000.

Essential Oil Safety

Objectives

After careful study of this chapter, you should be able to:

- identify the factors contributing to the safe use of essential oils in aromatherapy
- outline correct handling, storage and labelling requirements for essential oils
- identify the potential hazards of using essential oils in aromatherapy
- identify hazardous constituents found in essential oils
- outline corrective procedures for undesirable reactions to essential oils.

Introduction

The recent interest in holistic therapies such as aromatherapy and the realisation that one's well-being is a personal responsibility has led to a growth in the over-the-counter sales of essential oils.

This has raised a number of important issues regarding the efficacy and safety of essential oils. The safety of essential oils is a concern to all aromatherapists and individuals who use them. Safety is of fundamental importance to the practice of aromatherapy. The factors that need to be considered to ensure the safe use of essential oils include:

- quality of the essential oils being used
- packaging and labelling
- compliance with relevant legislative and regulatory bodies
- chemical composition of essential oils
- identifying essential oil hazards.

Quality

The use of the highest quality essential oils is of the utmost importance in ensuring that aromatherapy is practised safely. Most of the essential oils produced are by the fragrance or flavouring industries. The aromatherapy sector accounts for approximately 5% of the world's consumption of essential oils. It is therefore important that essential oils that are used in aromatherapy meet the standards set by the aromatherapy industry and not by other industries using essential oils.

To ensure that the highest quality essential oils are used in aromatherapy it is necessary to:

- clearly identify the essential oil
- avoid using essential oils that are subject to contamination and adulteration.
- avoid using essential oils that have undergone degradation.

If these criteria are not satisfied, not only is the efficacy of the essential oil undermined, there is a higher risk that the essential oil may be hazardous or not safe to use.

Identifying the Essential Oil

To identify an essential oil the following information should be readily available:

- botanical name
- part of the plant used
- country of origin
- extraction method
- chemical specificity (when applicable)

For example, *Thymus vulgaris* ct. *thymol* has potent antimicrobial activity. However, as it is high in phenols it needs to be used with care in topical preparations as it may be aggressive on the skin.[1]

On the other hand, *Thymus vulgaris* ct. *linalool* has less thymol and carvacrol. It is considered to be much more immunostimulant and less anti-infectious and, having less phenols, it is a safer choice for children.[1]

Contamination and Adulteration

Contamination of an essential oil may include pesticide or herbicide residues while adulteration means that a substance has been added to modify the composition of the essential oil. Typically the substance is a synthetic aroma chemical or an aroma chemical extracted from a less-expensive essential oil.

For example, lavender oil is subjected to extensive adulteration. The most common additives or 'cutting' materials are acetylised lavandin oil, synthetic linalool and linalyl acetate, fractions from the production of linalyl acetate from ho wood or rosewood.[2]

Contaminants and adulterants may potentiate the toxicity of an otherwise safe essential oil. It is believed that some of the allergic reactions to essential oils have been due to the pesticide or herbicide residue and not the essential oil.[3]

Pesticides and herbicides are used in large-scale essential oil crop cultivation to control pests, diseases, parasites, weeds and to raise harvest yields. It is known that biocides used in the cultivation of aromatic plants can be carried over during steam distillation. Solvent-extracted essential oils and expressed oils are even more likely to retain biocides.[3]

Some of the pesticides are considered extremely persistent and there is a chance that, following extraction, pesticide residues will be found in the essential oil.[3]

According to Wabner many biocide molecules contain chlorine or another halogen, which are readily soluble in oils and fats. If contaminated oils are applied to the skin during an aromatherapy treatment, these substances are likely to be transported into the nerve and fatty tissue of the body. While acute toxicity can be prevented by restricting the level of pesticide residue, there is very little research on the long-term accumulative effect of pesticides.[3]

It has been argued that the level of pesticide found in essential oils is usually not higher than levels found in food. Therefore since essential oils are used in much smaller quantities and much less frequently than food products, this leads to the conclusion that aromatherapy is much safer than eating.[3]

However, by definition, biocides are toxic, therefore they should not be welcome in either food or essential oils, even in trace amounts. While limiting values of residues have been established, the regulations state that only 0.1 to 0.5 ppb (parts per billion) of pesticide residue is allowable in drinking water, while the pesticide residue allowable in food is 0.5 to 1.0 ppm (parts per million).[3]

It is of concern that such levels of biocides are allowable in our food, certainly a tempting reason to grow your own vegetables or buy organic cultivated products.

Degradation

Degradation of essential oils is a process by which the quality of the essential oil is reduced over time. This usually occurs with essential oils because of prolonged storage or poor storage conditions. The main factors responsible for essential oil degradation are:

- oxygen
- heat
- light.

The effect of oxygen on essential oils is called oxidation and tends to occur in essential oils rich in monoterpene hydrocarbons such as citrus and pine oils. Oxidation is accelerated by heat and light.

Not only do many essential oils lose their therapeutic properties with age, but the chemical changes that occur may make the essential oil more hazardous.[4]

Wabner cites research which found that oxidised tea tree oil was found to be the cause of severe dermatitis, whereas fresh tea tree oil on the same patients did not elicit the same negative reaction.[4] Oxidised lemongrass oil was found to lose much of its antibacterial activity, when compared to fresh unoxidised lemongrass.[5]

To avoid degradation of essential oils ensure:

- The oils are stored in dark glass bottles.
- Small amounts of essential oils in large bottles should be transferred to smaller bottles to reduce the risk of oxidation.

Packaging and Labelling

The use of the integral dropper-dispenser is very important in limiting the quantity of essential oil that a child could accidentally ingest. Essential oils in open neck bottles probably represent the greatest risk of accidental ingestion in aromatherapy today.

As many essential oils are sold undiluted, it is important to consider the following:

- Do the essential oil bottles carry the appropriate warning and safety instructions?
- Are the essential oils packaged according to the current legislation of the country in which they are being sold or of any industry standard?
- What information should be on the label?

In Australia, these issues have been addressed by the Therapeutic Goods Administration (TGA). This means that essential oil labels should contain the following information:

- Proper identification of the essential oil such as botanical name and the part of the plant.
- The amount of the essential oil in the bottle.
- The concentration of the essential oil — normally expressed in ml/ml.
- Indication of useful shelf life of the essential oil.
- Storage conditions and precautions.
- A unique batch number to ensure traceability to the original source of the essential oil.
- An AUSTL or AUSTR registration number, which indicates that the essential oil has been packaged to strict code of Good Manufacturing Practice (GMP).
- Clear instructions for the use of the essential oil.
- First aid procedure if the essential oil is scheduled as a poison.
- Only therapeutic claims which can be validated according to the Therapeutic Goods Administration code of advertising.

Some essential oils are scheduled as poisons or may require specific cautions and safety instructions. In Australia the National Poisons Scheduling Committee is responsible for maintaining these standards. Some essential oils are classified in Schedule 5 or Schedule 6:

> *Schedule 5: Caution — Substance with a low potential to cause harm, the extent of which can be reduced through the use of distinctive packaging with simple warnings and safety directions on the label.*
>
> *Schedule 6: Poison — Substances with a moderate potential for causing harm, the extent of which can be reduced through the use of distinctive packaging with strong warnings and safety directions on the label.*[6]

It must be emphasised that an essential oil is not necessarily scheduled on the basis of toxicity. While toxicity is one of the factors considered, there are other factors such as purpose of use, potential for abuse and the safety in use.[6]

Any essential oil scheduled as a poison is required by Australian law to carry a label giving the appropriate first aid advice if poisoning occurs. This advice is as follows:

> *For advice, contact a Poisons Information Centre (Phone e.g., Australia 131 126; New Zealand 03 4747 000) or a doctor (at once). If swallowed, do not induce vomiting.*[6]

At the time of writing the following essential oils require specific cautions, first aid instructions or are classified as poisons:

Schedule 5 Essential Oils

Aniseed oil except when it is packaged in containers having a nominal capacity of 50 mL or less fitted with a restrictive flow insert; is labelled with the following warning: KEEP OUT OF REACH OF CHILDREN and in preparations containing 50% or less of anise oil.[6]

Basil oil except when it is packaged in containers having a nominal capacity of 25 mL or less fitted with a restrictive flow insert; is labelled with the following warning: KEEP OUT OF REACH OF CHILDREN and in preparations containing 5% or less of methyl chavicol.[6]

Bergamot oil except when it is steam-distilled or rectified, in preparations for internal use; in preparations containing 0.4% or less of bergamot oil; in soaps or bath and shower gels that are washed off the skin; or when packed in containers with labels that state that application to the skin may increase sensitivity to sunlight.[6]

Camphor as a natural component in essential oils containing 10% or less camphor except when it is in containers having a nominal capacity of 25 mL or less fitted with a restrictive flow insert; is labelled with the following warning: KEEP OUT OF REACH OF CHILDREN and NOT TO BE TAKEN; in rosemary oil, sage oil (Spanish), or lavandin oils; or in preparations containing 2.5% or less of camphor.[6]

Cassia oil and **cinnamon bark oil** except in food additives or in preparations containing 2% or less of these essential oils.[6]

Clove oil and **eugenol** for topical use in the mouth in a pack containing 5% or less of clove or eugenol, except in preparations containing 25% or less of clove oil or eugenol.[6]

Lemon oil except when it is steam-distilled or rectified, in preparations for internal use, in preparations containing 0.05% or less of lemon oil, in soaps or bath and shower gels that are washed off the skin, or when packed in containers with labels that state that application to the skin may increase sensitivity to sunlight.[6]

Lime oil except when it is steam-distilled or rectified, in preparations for internal use, in preparations containing 0.5% or less of lemon oil, in soaps or bath and shower gels that are washed off the skin, or when packed in containers with labels that state that application to the skin may increase sensitivity to sunlight.[6]

Marjoram oil except when it is packaged in containers having a nominal capacity of 50 mL or less fitted with a restrictive flow insert; is labelled with the following warning: KEEP OUT OF REACH OF CHILDREN or in preparations containing 50% or less of marjoram oil.[6]

Methyl salicylate in liquid preparations containing 25% or more of methyl salicylate except when included in Schedule 6.[6]

Nutmeg oil except when it is packaged in containers having a nominal capacity of 25 mL or less fitted with a restrictive flow insert; is labelled with the following warning: KEEP OUT OF REACH OF CHILDREN or in preparations containing 50% or less of nutmeg oil.[6]

Bitter orange oil except when it is steam-distilled or rectified, in preparations for internal use, in preparations containing 1.4% or less of lemon oil, in soaps or bath and shower gels that are washed off the skin, or when packed in containers with labels that state that application to the skin may increase sensitivity to sunlight.[6]

Thyme oil except when it is packaged in containers having a nominal capacity of 25 mL or less fitted with a restrictive flow insert; is labelled with the following warning: KEEP OUT OF REACH OF CHILDREN or in preparations containing 50% or less of nutmeg oil.[6]

Schedule 6 Essential Oils

Bay oil except when it is packaged in containers having a nominal capacity of 15 mL or less fitted with a restrictive flow insert; is labelled with the following warning: KEEP OUT OF REACH OF CHILDREN and NOT TO BE TAKEN; or in preparations containing 25% or less of bay oil.[6]

Cajeput oil except when it is packaged in containers having a nominal capacity of 15 mL or less fitted with a restrictive flow insert; is labelled with the following warning: KEEP OUT OF REACH OF CHILDREN and NOT TO BE TAKEN; or in preparations containing 25% or less of cajeput oil.[6]

Cineole except when it is packaged in containers having a nominal capacity of 15 mL or less fitted with a restrictive flow insert; is labelled with the following warning: KEEP OUT OF REACH OF CHILDREN and NOT TO BE TAKEN; or in preparations containing 25% or less of cineole; or in rosemary oil or white camphor oil.[6]

Cinnamon leaf oil except when it is packaged in containers having a nominal capacity of 15 mL or less fitted with a restrictive flow insert; is labelled with the following warning: KEEP OUT OF REACH OF CHILDREN and NOT TO BE TAKEN; or in preparations containing 25% or less of cinnamon leaf oil.[6]

Clove oil and **eugenol** except when it is packaged in containers having a nominal capacity of 15 mL or less fitted with a restrictive flow insert; is labelled with the following warning: KEEP OUT OF REACH OF CHILDREN and NOT TO BE TAKEN; or in preparations containing 25% or less of clove oil or eugenol.[6]

Eucalyptus oil except when it is packaged in containers having a nominal capacity of 15 mL or less fitted with a restrictive flow insert; is labelled with the following warning: KEEP OUT OF REACH OF CHILDREN and NOT TO BE TAKEN; or in preparations containing 25% or less of eucalyptus oil.[6]

Melaleuca oil (Tea tree oil) except when it is packaged in containers having a nominal capacity of 15 mL or less fitted with a restrictive flow insert; is labelled with the following warning: KEEP OUT OF REACH OF CHILDREN and NOT TO BE TAKEN; or is in preparations containing 25% or less of melaleuca oil.[6]

Pennyroyal oil except when it is packaged in containers having a nominal capacity of 15 mL or less fitted with a restrictive flow insert; is labelled with the following warning: KEEP OUT OF REACH OF CHILDREN and NOT TO BE TAKEN; or in preparations containing 4% or less of d-pulegone.[6]

Sassafras oil or **safrole** except for internal use; or in preparations containing 1% or less of safrole.

Sage oil except when it is packaged in containers having a nominal capacity of 15 mL or less fitted with a restrictive flow insert and child-resistant closure; is labelled with the following warning: KEEP OUT OF REACH OF CHILDREN and NOT TO BE TAKEN; or in preparations containing 4% or less of thujone.[6]

Materials Safety Data Sheets (MSDS)

Also known as safety data sheets. Legislation requires suppliers and manufacturers of essential oils to provide material safety data sheets. Material safety data sheets are required when the user intends to use that essential oil at work or if the substance is classified as dangerous. In most circumstances the information on the label should suffice.

The National Occupational Health and Safety Commission (NOHSC) has published a National Code of Practice for the preparation of MSDSs. The MSDS includes information on the composition of the essential oil, analytical data, health hazards, first aid procedures, fire and explosive hazards, environmental implications, handling procedures and transportation and labelling information.[8]

A typical MSDS for an essential oil can be found in Appendix 5.

Chemical Composition

An essential oil may have 100 or more different constituents, which in combination give the essential oil its unique odour, therapeutic properties and in some cases, its toxicity or potential hazards.

Aldehydes

Some aldehydes can cause skin irritation and allergic reactions.[7,9,12] Cinnamic aldehyde found in *Cinnamomum zeylanicum* (Cinnamon bark) is reported to be a powerful dermal sensitiser.[7] The International Fragrance Research Association (IFRA) recommends that cinnamon bark oil can be used at 1% maximum on the skin.[7]

Citral, an aldehyde, has been found to have an irritating effect on the skin. When essential oils such as may chang or lemongrass, which are high in citral, are blended in a 50/50 mix with essential oils such as lemon or sweet orange (both high in limonene, a monoterpene hydrocarbon), a quenching effect was observed. It has been suggested that the d-limonene is responsible for neutralising the irritancy effects of citral.[9]

Esters

Like alcohols, esters are considered non-hazardous with the exception of sabinyl acetate found in savin and methyl salicylate found in wintergreen.

Ketones

Ketones are considered the most common toxic constituents of all essential oil constituents. However, it is incorrect to assume all ketones are toxic.

Ketones such as fenchone found in fennel, jasmone found in jasmine, italidone found in everlasting and carvone found in essential oils such as dill, caraway and spearmint essential oils are classified as non-toxic.[7,10]

Ketones are known to be toxic and neurotoxic. The most common toxic and neurotoxic ketones are camphor, thujone and pinocamphone. Thujone is found in essential oils such as mugwort, sage, tansy, thuja and wormwood. While essential oils such as mugwort, tansy, thuja and wormwood should not be used in aromatherapy, sage essential oil needs to considered more carefully.

The thujone content of *Salvia officinalis* is anywhere from 35–60%. This alone would certainly render sage quite toxic. However, this contradicts most research on and experience with this oil that clearly does not indicate the toxicity one would expect from such a thujone content.[10]

As a result it may be concluded that the traditional use of sage in aromatherapy should not be considered hazardous. However, it would be wise to exercise extra care when using sage and it should not be used by children or pregnant or nursing mothers.[10]

Another toxic ketone is pulegone. It is found (up to 85%) in pennyroyal essential oil.[7,10]

Essential Oil	Toxic Ketone	Oral LD_{50} (gm/kg)
Pennyroyal	pulegone	0.40
Sage	thujone	2.60
Tansy	thujone	1.15
Thuja	thujone	0.83
Wormwood	thujone	0.96
Hyssop	pinocamphone	1.40

Toxicity of essential oils with ketone constituents[7]

Pinocamphone is the primary constituent found in hyssop. Hyssop, according to the LD_{50}, is distinctly more toxic than sage. Hyssop should always be used carefully in low doses and should not be used by individuals with epilepsy, fever, during pregnancy or by children under 2 years of age.[7]

It is preferable to use *Hyssop officinalis* subspecies *decumbens*, as this oil is free of the potentially toxic ketones.[7,11]

Phenols

While many essential oils that contain phenols are considered valuable in aromatherapy, they warrant a certain amount of caution. Essential oils such as thyme, oregano and savory are very useful essential oils in aromatherapy because of their antimicrobial activity. However, they also have an irritant effect on the skin and on the mucous membrane.

The toxic and carcinogenic phenols are actually classified as phenyl propane derivatives. Some of the more hazardous essential oil constituents are methyl chavicol, found in basil oil; safrole, found in sassafras and yellow or brown camphor essential oils; apiole, found in parsley seed, and asorone, found in calamus.

Monoterpene Hydrocarbons

Monoterpene hydrocarbons are the most commonly occurring essential oil constituents and are generally considered to have very little risk associated with them. However, they are considered to be reactive (they tend to oxidise easily) and may cause skin irritations.[12]

Essential Oil Hazards

The undesirable side-effects or hazards of essential oils are:

- toxicity
- skin reactions
- carcinogenesis
- neurotoxicity
- hepatotoxicity
- hazards during pregnancy.

Toxicity

Toxicity is what is commonly called 'poisoning' and, at a certain level, may become fatal. In aromatherapy, the degree of toxicity depends to a certain extent on the method of application. The toxicity of essential oils used in aromatherapy is usually classified as:

- oral toxicity
- dermal toxicity.

Oral toxicity is the degree of toxicity of a substance when it is ingested by swallowing. Dermal toxicity is the degree of toxicity of a substance when it is absorbed through the skin. Both types of toxicity are determined by lethal dose, which is the amount necessary to kill the organism.

The greatest hazard is associated with oral toxicity. In fact the majority of incidents involving toxicity are from oral dosing. Toxicity is usually classified as acute or chronic.[7]

Acute toxicity is the result of the short-term use of an essential oil, usually involving a single dose and may result in death. When the amount administered is less than a lethal dose, damage may occur to the liver and/or the kidneys.

Balacs cites a case in which a child who ingested clove oil almost died:

> *A two year old boy had drunk between 5–10ml of clove oil from an open neck bottle. One hour after ingestion the boy was conscious but drowsy and distressed. Within three hours, the boy had fallen into a deep coma, had a very low blood glucose level and had a marked acidosis. Twenty four hours after ingestion the boy was still in a coma and was showing signs of disseminated intravascular coagulopathy with concurrent liver failure.*
>
> *After three days of treatment with heparin, plasma, fibrinogen, antithrombin III, protein C and*

factor VII, the child began to recover. By the fifth day the boy's neurological state improved and he was fully conscious by the sixth. He made full recovery. It was suggested by the author that all essential oils should not be sold in open neck bottles (I fully concur) and that labelling should be more explicit.[13]

Chronic toxicity is the result of long-term use of small doses of essential oil. An example of chronic toxicity is cited by Lassak.

It appears that he had been in the habit, for about the past five years, of swallowing five to ten drops of eucalyptus oil to keep colds at bay and 'make him feel good'. Later during those five years he started to feel discomfort and even pain in the region of his liver. On entering hospital for a check-up the matron apparently informed him that he suffered with cirrhosis of the liver and that, unless he stopped drinking immediately, his condition would further deteriorate. Now it so happened he was a tee-totaller and never so much as touched alcohol. The cause of his condition, as it turned out, was most likely the cineo1e he so regularly took to improve his health.[14]

The result of chronic toxicity is usually organ tissue damage, most commonly degenerative changes in the liver and kidneys. Death may eventually result, but the problem here is one of slow tissue damage, rather than fatality. Chronic toxicity usually involves oral administration and it would be reasonable to assume the same applies to dermal administration.

Determining the Level of Toxicity

A common method of establishing a measure of toxicity is the LD_{50} experiment. LD_{50} is the dose of a specific substance that has been lethal for 50% in a group of test animals.[7] This is usually not given as an absolute value but in grams of toxin per kilogram body weight. For example:

LD_{50} = 1 [gm/kg]

Means that 1 gram of essential oil per kilogram of body weight induces death in 50% of test animals. Using this value as a guide to toxicity in humans, it would mean, assuming the body weight to be 70kg, that

1 [g/kg] x 70 [kg] = 70 [g]

Therefore 70 g of essential oil would be a lethal dose in humans. LD_{50} values generally refer to oral toxicity. LD_{50} values are commonly accepted in establishing toxicity of a given substance in humans.

The LD_{50} value is not absolute. The LD_{50} value for the same substances frequently varies between the types of animals being used for testing, different laboratories, and method of administration (e.g., oral, dermal or by injection).[7]

Clearly the toxicity of the same substance in animals and humans can be quite different. The following table indicates the gross error that is often assumed in using animal toxicity data to determine lethal doses in humans.

Essential oil	LD_{50} (gm/kg)	Actual lethal dose for 70kg person	Comment
Boldo	0.13	9.1 gm	Toxic
Hyssop	1.40	98.0 gm	Caution
Sage	2.52	176.0 gm	Safe
Chamomile	8.56	600.0 gm	Safe

LD_{50} values and corresponding lethal dose.[7]

Nor does the LD_{50} value tell us anything about the risks during pregnancy or carcinogenesis.

Cases of Poisoning

There are many recorded cases of poisoning from essential oils. All the cases of severe poisoning from essential oils arose from oral ingestion and in every case the amount taken was much higher than normal therapeutic amounts.

The following oils have frequently appeared in cases of poisoning:

camphor, cinnamon, citronella, eucalyptus, hyssop, nutmeg, parsley, pennyroyal, sage, thuja, sassafras, wintergreen, wormwood, wormseed.[7]

This does not mean that oils not appearing here are necessarily safe. It is very likely that any essential oil, ingested in sufficient quantities, may cause serious problems.

The Validity of Animal Testing

The RIFM (The Research Institute of Fragrance Materials) often conducts acute dermal toxicity studies on rabbits. It has, however, been clearly identified that human skin and rabbit skin do not absorb the same essential oils at the same rate. Hotchkiss says that absorption is usually higher through animal skin therefore existing information regarding dermal toxicity probably gives no useful indication of the toxicity of dermally applied essential oils.[15]

Tisserand says that it is a mistake to extrapolate LD_{50} values obtained from animal testing to determine oral toxicity in human beings.[16]

Apart from the ethical issues involving testing to determine the LD_{50} value, clearly the toxicity of the same substance in animals and humans can be quite different.

The following table gives you an indication of the gross errors that may be assumed in using animal toxicity data to determine lethal doses for humans.[16]

Essential oil	Type of toxicity	Animal toxicity [gm/kg]	Human toxicity [gm/kg]
Eucalyptus	Acute oral	2.5	0.4–0.8
Wintergreen	Acute oral	1.2	0.23–0.37
Camphor	Acute oral	0.5–0.15	0.005–0.5
Pennyroyal	Acute oral	0.4	0.4

Skin Reactions

Skin reactions that often occur when using essential oils are:

- skin irritations
- sensitisation
- phototoxicity
- idiosyncratic reactions.

Compared with toxicity, skin reactions may vary considerably from one individual to another, and are therefore very difficult to predict.

Patch Test

If there is any reason to believe that an individual is likely to encounter a skin reaction, then a patch test should be conducted. Tisserand and Balacs outline a procedure for performing a patch test:[7]

1. Apply the oil at twice the concentration you plan to use it, to the inside of the forearm for 48 hrs.
2. Apply two drops of the oil to the inside of a plaster.
3. Repeat a second time in order to test for sensitisation.

Procedure for Dealing with an Adverse Skin Reaction

If a reaction from a patch test, an accident or from an aromatherapy treatment does occur, immediately wash the skin with a mild unperfumed soap to remove the oil from the surface of the skin. If necessary apply an aloe vera gel to soothe the skin.

Irritation

An irritation is produced on the skin when the skin is exposed to a 'primary irritant', such as a corrosive chemical. Typically the reaction occurs rapidly; the severity is dependent upon the concentration of the irritant.[7]

Essential oils that are known to be potential irritants are those that generally provoke dermal irritation at certain concentrations, although there is no guarantee that this will happen on a particular individual. At the same time, essential oils that are not considered to be irritants may occasionally cause irritation in someone with sensitive skin.[7]

Essential oils such as horseradish and mustard are considered severe dermal irritants while oils such as rectified cade, massoia, onion and garlic and oxidised pine oils are considered strong dermal irritants.[7]

Oils such as ajowan, betel leaf, birch, cassia, cinnamon bark and leaf, clove bud, leaf and stem, sweet fennel, fig leaf, oregano, parsley leaf, parsley seed, pimento berry, rue, Dalmatian sage, sassafras, summer and winter savory, tagetes, tarragon, thyme, verbena and wintergreen are reported to be moderate dermal irritants.[7]

Sensitisation

A dermal sensitisation reaction is sometimes referred to as an allergic urticaria. The skin normally reacts in the form of a rash, blotchy redness, often accompanied by irritation or slight blistering.

Sensitisation refers to an allergic reaction to a substance by an organism that involves the interaction of its immune system with a substance. Substances that are capable of inducing an immune response from an organism are called antigens. The antigens interact with the lymphocytes, causing the formation of antibodies that will in turn react with the antigen, rendering it harmless. When an antigen induces an immune response at first exposure, the organism will experience altered body reactivity to subsequent exposure to the same or similar antigens. This may cause exaggerated reactions like sneezing and itching. This is defined as the allergic reaction.

Sensitisation is considered to be unpredictable as some individuals will be sensitive to a potential allergen and some will not.[7] Essential oil constituents such as cinnamic aldehyde, found in cinnamon oil and cassia oil, and the lactones such as those found in costus and elecampane are known to be dermal sensitisers.

If an essential oil caused an allergic reaction, its use should be discontinued immediately. What we do know about sensitisation is that once an individual has become sensitised to an essential oil, a severe inflammatory response may be evoked even with a small quantity of the sensitising essential oil.

Essential oils such as costus, elecampane, tea absolute and verbena are considered severe skin sensitisers and must not be used on the skin or mucous membrane.[7]

Essentials oils which should be avoided on the skin and mucous membrane because they are considered strong dermal sensitisers include cassia, cinnamon bark, bitter fennel, fig leaf, garlic, oakmoss, tree moss and verbena.[7]

Essential oils which may be considered a slight risk of causing dermal sensitisation include aniseed, catnip, citronella, khella, laurel leaf, lavender absolute, lemongrass, may chang, melissa, myrrh absolute, onion, Perilla, dwarf pine, Scotch pine, Star anise and ylang ylang.[7]

Photosensitisation

Photosensitisation is a skin reaction that occurs in the presence of ultra violet light. Certain constituents of essential oils are capable of absorbing energy from ultraviolet light much more effectively than the skin. Essential oils listed as photosensitisers are hazardous only in this context. To simply apply these oils to the skin diluted or undiluted will not in itself produce a photosensitisation, which can only be achieved if the skin is covered in a photosensitising oil, and then exposed to the sun or any other source of ultraviolet light.

The most common phototoxic agents are psoralens, otherwise known as furocoumarins.

> *These polycyclic molecules whose structure gives them the ability to absorb ultraviolet photons, store them for a while, and then release them in a burst on to the skin.*[7]

Citrus oils extracted by direct expression without distillation are the major group of phototoxic essential oils containing furocoumarins. Bergamot and other expressed citrus oils contain small quantities of a furocoumarin known as bergaptene or 5 methoxypsoralen or 5-MOP.[7]

As can be seen from the table below, the phototoxic potential of citrus oils is minimised when the furocoumarin content is reduced to 0.0075%. According to these results we can make the following conclusions:

Phototoxic essential oils — bergamot, cold-pressed lime, cold-pressed bitter orange, angelica root, cumin, rue, opoponax.

Mildly phototoxic essential oils — cold-pressed grapefruit, cold-pressed lemon, cold-pressed sweet orange, cold-pressed tangerine.

Essential Oil	Furocoumarin average content	Photo-toxicity at 100%	Level when not phototoxic
Bergamot	0.44%	strong	1.0–2.0%
Lime	0.25%	strong	2.0–3.5%
Bitter orange	0.072%	moderate	3.5–7.0%
Lemon	0.0032%	weak	5.0–10.0%
Grapefruit	0.0012%	weak	10.0–20.0%
Sweet orange	0.00005%	mild	No limit
Tangerine	0.00005%	mild	No limit
Mandarin	trace	mild	No limit

Phototoxic potential of citrus oils[17]

Other oils known to be phototoxic because they contain psoralens are fig leaf absolute, verbena oil, tagetes, angelica root, rue.

Tisserand and Balacs suggest that the risk of phototoxicity will remain for up to 12 hours, following the topical application of any phototoxic essential oil.[7]

The best advice regarding the use of an essential oil that may cause a phototoxic reaction is to use less than 1% in a blend. Also, advise your client to wear protective clothing and a sunscreen that will block out the UV light and not to go into the sun for at least 12 hours after a treatment.

Idiosyncratic Sensitisation

An idiosyncratic sensitisation is an allergic reaction to a substance that is generally not known to be an allergen. Like a food allergy, it is a phenomenon which can appear and disappear again with no apparent logic. The allergic reaction may be induced by dermal application, inhalation or by any other means. As with other types of sensitisation, the substances responsible can produce a severe reaction even in quite low dilutions, especially if the subject is already sensitised.

There is not much we can do in situations like this except to ensure that when a person does have a history of allergic reactions to do a patch test first and to avoid the use of that oil in future.

Carcinogenesis

This is defined as the stimulation of the formation and growth of cancerous cells in the body. Carcinogenesis involves at least three stages — *initiation, promotion,* and *progression*, before the formation of a malignant neoplasm.[18]

Initiation involves the rapid, irreversible alteration in the cell's genetic material that primes the cell for the subsequent neoplastic development. The initiated cell may remain dormant until exposed to a tumour-promoting agent that then allows the growth of clones from initiated cells which will eventually produce a tumour.[18]

Promoting agents are chemicals that are not in themselves carcinogens, but when they are given repetitively, after a low dose of an initiating agent, they will increase the incidence of cancer.[18] Progression is the development of a malignant tumour from a benign tumour.[18]

It has been suggested that at least 70 to 90% of all cancers are attributed to environmental chemical causes. Many substances such as benzene and asbestos have been identified as carcinogens. However, there may be many unidentified carcinogens.[7]

Studies have shown that carcinogens require repeated application, usually several weeks or months, before any cancerous growth can be detected.[7]

Essential Oils that are Carcinogenesis

The following essential oil constituents have been identified as potentially carcinogenic.

Safrole

Tisserand cites research that indicates safrole as a carcinogenic essential oil constituent. It is a major component of sassafras essential oil and of the yellow and brown fractions of camphor.[7] Studies have shown that safrole is a hepatocarcinogenic.[7,18]

Estragole

Estragole is also known as methyl chavicol. It is found in tarragon oil (70–87%) and in basil oil (5–87%). Methyl chavicol is a procarcinogen, becoming a carcinogen following metabolic activation. Studies on the toxicity of estragole conclude that estragole-containing essential oils should present no risk when used periodically at low doses.[19] This conclusion is supported by the fact that rapid detoxification reactions occur immediately after estragole is metabolised into its carcinogenic form. It has also been determined that the level of estragole used in animal carcinogenicity studies is several hundred times higher than the estimated human daily intake.[19]

However, it is recommended that tarragon and the Comoros Islands basil chemotype should not be used in aromatherapy. The linalool basil chemotype is much safer to use.[7]

β-asarone

β-asarone is a potential hepatocarcinogenic constituent found in calamus oil.[19] Calamus essential oil should not be used in aromatherapy.[7]

β-asarone must first undergo metabolic l'hydroxylation in the liver before becoming toxic. Cytochrome P_{450} in the hepatocytes is responsible for secreting the hydrolysing enzymes that convert β-asarone into its genotoxic epoxide structure.[19]

Benzo[a]pyrene

Benzo[a]pyrene is a chemical constituent present in unrectified cade oil. It is considered a potential polynuclear hydrocarbon, which is well known as a carcinogen. Cade oil is from the destructive distillation of the wood of *Juniperus oxycedrus*. Unrectified cade oil should not be used in aromatherapy.[7]

Massage and Cancer

There is a common belief that massage will spread cancer cells from one part of the body to another, by stimulating lymph flow. However, there is no clinical evidence that massage can spread cancer.

It would be reasonable to assume that gentle massage would stimulate the lymph flow no more than gentle exercise or body movement. However, the following precautions should be observed before massaging a client with cancer:

- Avoid deep massage of any kind, over or near the lymph glands
- Avoid areas of the body that have been treated with radiation therapy, as the skin is usually very fragile.
- Massage should also be avoided over areas of skin cancer.

There are numerous clinical trials that report on the positive effects on the wellbeing of patients with cancer.

Any health professionals who decide to use massage should have a comprehensive understanding of massage and cancer.

Neurotoxicity

Neurotoxicity is defined as an adverse effect in either the structure or function of the nervous system following exposure to a chemical agent. At a molecular level, a substance might interfere with protein synthesis, leading to reduced production of neurotransmitters and brain dysfunction.[18]

The potential adverse effects that essential oils can have on the central nervous system are:

- convulsant effects
- psychotropic effects.

Convulsant Effects

A convulsant is an agent that produces convulsions. Fenchone, pinocamphone, camphor and thujone have all been found to have convulsant activity.[7] However, Tisserand and Balacs say that the doses used in the studies were extremely high and have no relevance to the dosage used in aromatherapy.[7]

It has been suggested that essential oils that contain the above ketones may trigger seizures in individuals with epilepsy.

Hyssop, camphor, mugwort, sage, wormwood and thuja essential oils have all been identified as having a convulsant effect.[7,20,21]

It has been recommended that rosemary not be used by individuals with epilepsy.[22,23] Valnet states that the essence of rosemary in excessive quantities has a strong tendency to induce epilepsy. However, he also suggests using rosemary oil in small internal doses to prevent seizures.[24]

A clinical study with animal experiments, in vivo, found that rosemary induced tonicoclonic convulsions. It was found that the oil inhibited oxygen consumption and the electrolyte gradients of sodium and potassium. It has been postulated that there may be a relationship between the metabolic effects of rosemary essential oil in vitro and convulsant activity in vivo.[25]

Tisserand and Balacs state that epileptics should exercise caution with rosemary, especially orally.[7] The assumption being made here that it is okay to use rosemary oil as long as you do not take it orally, even if you are prone to epileptic seizures.

However, it is known that individuals who are prone to epilepsy may have idiosyncratic reactions to essential oils and odours in general.[7] It becomes almost impossible to predict the adverse effects. It is apparent that whether rosemary oil is taken orally, applied topically or inhaled, the potential exists to trigger a seizure. Therefore, since the effect of rosemary on seizures is unpredictable, I recommend that individuals with epilepsy use rosemary with caution.

Fennel is also listed as being contraindicated for individuals with epilepsy,[22,23] presumably for its fenchone content. The fenchone content is usually higher in bitter fennel than sweet fennel.[26]

However, I was not able to find any herbal references which supported the claim that fennel oil is contraindicated for persons with epilepsy.

The essential oil constituents believed to be responsible for the convulsant effects are ketones. Some consider that all ketones are highly stimulating to the CNS, and therefore are a risk to those prone to epilepsy. I believe there is no reason to assume that all other ketones found in essential oils present any danger to people prone to epilepsy.

Psychotropic Effects

A psychotropic substance affects the brain in a way which causes changes in the mood and behaviour. Reports of essential oils having psychotropic effects include:

- nutmeg
- thujone rich oils
- anethole.

Some of the psychotropic effects reported after having used the above include hallucinogenic effects. These substances may also be classified as hallucinogens that are described as:

> *Chemicals which, in non-toxic doses, produce changes in perception, in thought, and in mood, but which seldom produce mental confusion, memory loss, or disorientation for person, place and time.*[18]

Nutmeg

Most of the speculation regarding the psychotropic qualities of nutmeg oil focuses on two of its major constituents, myristicin and elimicin. Reports have shown that these two constituents are the principal psychotropic components. It has been suggested that a metabolic pathway converts the elimicin and myristicin to TMA (3,4,5-trimethoxyamphetamine) or MMDA (3-methoxy-4,5-methylenedioxyamphetamine), both known as hallucinogens.[7]

Myristicin has been shown to be an inhibitor of an enzyme important in eliminating monoamine oxidase. This may be the reason for nutmeg's euphoric properties. In animal tests, myristicin was found to increase levels of serotonin in rat brain. If this were also the case for humans, this would explain the psychotropic effect.[7] However, closer investigation has revealed the following:[7]

Component	Psychotropic
Whole nutmeg	Highly active
Whole nutmeg less essential oil	Non activity
Nutmeg oil	Weakly active
myristicin	No activity

It appears that the psychotropic properties are due not only to the myristicin and elimicin, but to other constituents found in the whole nutmeg.

While ground nutmeg is moderately to strongly psychotropic when taken in high doses, the effect of the essential oil is very weak, and it appears that non-oral doses will not have any effect at all.

Thujone-rich oils

It has been suggested that thujone and delta-9-tetrahydrocannabinol, the most active ingredient in cannabis, interact with a common receptor in the CNS and so have similar psychotropic effects.[7]

Anethole

Tisserand cites a study in which trans-anethole had psychotropic activity in mice at levels over 0.3 gm/kg. However, he states that this is a very high dose and has no relevance to aromatherapy.[7]

It should also be mentioned that no reference to anethole's potential psychotropic effects could be found in any of the major herbal reference texts.

Hepatotoxicity

The liver has a wider variety of functions than any other organ in the body. Apart from its major roles of carbohydrate and lipid metabolism, protein synthesis and secretion of bile, it is responsible for the detoxification of the blood. A substance is defined as a hepatotoxin if it causes damage to the liver cells.

It is unlikely that any essential oil is a hepatotoxic through dermal application. However, studies have shown that substances such as eugenol (clove and cinnamon leaf), cinnamaldehyde (cinnamon bark and cassia) and trans-anethole (aniseed) have caused depletion of glutathione in oral doses in laboratory experiments on rodents.[7]

Pulegone, found in pennyroyal, has also shown to be hepatotoxic similar to that of paracetamol toxicity. A toxic metabolite of pulegone, menthofuran, is produced in the liver's enzyme system and was found to produce acute liver and lung damage in rats.[7,19] The following table lists the essential oils and their corresponding constituents which are potentially hepatotoxic.

Constituent	Essential oil
Trans-anethole	Aniseed, fennel
Cinnamaldehyde	Cassia, cinnamon bark
Methyl chavicol	Basil (methyl chavicol), tarragon
Eugenol	West Indian bay, cinnamon, clove
Pulegone	Buchu, pennyroyal
Safrole	Camphor, Spanish marjoram

Hazards during Pregnancy

There is often a concern that some essential oils may not be safe to use during pregnancy. Some aromatherapists suggest that essential oils should not be used during pregnancy. This is being overcautious, as aromatherapy can be immensely beneficial in maintaining the general health of the expectant mother and in minimising the various discomforts of pregnancy. The main concerns during pregnancy in using some essential oils are that they:

- may have a hormone-like activity, disturbing the normal, finely tuned balance of hormones
- may cause injury or malformation in the development of the foetus
- may cause abortion.[7]

Essential Oils with Oestrogenic Properties

Circulating levels of oestrogen and progesterone are much higher during pregnancy than at other times. The two most important female hormones are oestradiol, which is an oestrogen, and progesterone. Oestradiol controls the development and maintenance of the female sexual organs and gives a person her essentially feminine shape and physiology. Progesterone prepares the uterine lining for pregnancy each month.

Some essential oil constituents have hormone-like behaviour because their structure is similar to the hormones, so they interact with the same receptors that identify hormones. Oestrogenic activity has been found in essential oils of aniseed and fennel.[27]

Anethole, the main constituent in both these essential oils, is a methyl ether of oestradiol and is believed to be responsible for the oestrogenic activity of these oils. Essential oils with oestrogenic activity are known to influence menstrual cycle, lactation and secondary sexual characteristics.[27]

Balacs suggests that until the absolute safety of anethole-rich oils such as aniseed and fennel is established it would be prudent to avoid their use in pregnancy.[27]

Teratogenic Effect of Essential Oils

Studying the effect of essential oils and drugs during pregnancy is highly problematic. Results of animal studies often correlate even more poorly with the human situation than in other fields of research. Interpreting the results obtained in animal toxicity studies to the human is very difficult indeed, if not totally inaccurate.

There are very few studies on the distribution and fate of drugs within the human embryo, because it is almost impossible to design safe clinical experiments. It is often assumed that drug or essential oil concentrations in the embryo would reach similar levels to that in the mother's serum. This may be inaccurate and the truth is that we simply do not know whether foreign substances such as essential oils circulating in the mother's bloodstream reach the developing child. As a rule of thumb, molecules which can cross the blood–brain barrier into the CNS are likely to reach the fetus. Essential oils would therefore be in this category.

So can we safely use essential oils during pregnancy without harming the foetus? Tisserand and Balacs cite several studies involving rats, which showed that cineole does cross the placenta in sufficient quantities when given by subcutaneous injection to pregnant rats at a dose of 0.5 gm/kg for 4 days.[7]

Tisserand and Balacs cite another study that involved a mother who ingested 2 ounces of camphorated oil and had the first of three seizures 20 minutes later. She was admitted to hospital and gastric lavage was performed. The next morning she had a spontaneous labour and the baby was born without complications, but smelling distinctly of camphor. The baby was closely monitored for several days and found to be okay. Another baby unfortunately died when the mother ingested the same amount of camphorated oil.[7]

In these cases the amount of camphor ingested is approximately 12 mL. According to Tisserand and Balacs this amount of camphor was more than the LD_{50} values given for camphor.[7] Tisserand and Balacs suggests that if the maximum concentration of essential oil for application by aromatherapy massage is 2%, then there is very little risk to the embryo and foetus.[7] They are of the opinion:

> *...that the external use of camphor-rich oils such as rosemary are safe in pregnancy.*[7]

However, they state that;

> *...oral administration of camphor-rich essential oils should be avoided during pregnancy.*[7]

Other toxic oils discussed include safrole-rich oils such as sassafras and thujone-rich oils such as wormwood and sage. These oils are obviously toxic and should be avoided altogether in aromatherapy.

Abortifacient Effect of Essential Oils

An abortifacient is an agent used to induce an abortion.[19] There is no clear evidence that essential oils are abortifacients. Most essential oils that have been labelled as abortifacients are potentially toxic and are not recommended for use in aromatherapy.

All the 'abortifacient' oils are known to have a strong emmenagogue action. However, not all emmenagogues will induce abortion, and not all emmenagogue oils are toxic.

Many essential oils such as clary sage, cedarwood, cypress, sweet marjoram, peppermint, rosemary and rose are classified as contraindicated during pregnancy. However, they are not abortifacients. It has been suggested that these essential oils present no danger in pregnancy as long as they are not used orally.[7,19]

However, it would be prudent to avoid using these essential oils as there is anecdotal evidence that indicates that they may be unsafe to use during pregnancy.

The following essential oils are known to have an abortifacient effect: mugwort, parsley seed, pennyroyal, rue, sassafras, savin, thuja, tansy and wormwood.[7] These oils are toxic and appear to be abortifacients in lethal dosages.

Miscarriages are common, and women who use essential oils and then miscarry often suspect that the essential oils contributed or caused the miscarriage. However, in most cases there is no definite conclusion that the essential oils were actually responsible.

General Safety Guidelines

Safety Guidelines for the Aromatherapist's Wellbeing

When using essential oils please ensure that:

- the treatment room has good ventilation
- regular breaks are taken between clients
- hands are washed between appointments.

Safety Guidelines for the General Public

When recommending essential oils to the general public ensure that they:

- keep essential oils out of reach of children
- use less rather than more
- do not take essential oils internally
- do not purchase undiluted essential oils unless the bottles have a restrictive flow insert
- do not use undiluted essential oils on the skin
- do not use essential oils directly on the eyes to treat eye conditions
- avoid essential oils that are poorly identified.

If someone accidentally gets an essential oil in their eye, wash thoroughly with cold, clean water for 5 minutes. If the stinging has not subsided after 15 minutes seek medical attention.

Safety Guidelines for Applications

Baths

It is preferable to add essential oils to a bath with a dispersing agent. There is a higher risk of irritation, since the essential oil clumps together on the surface of the water and creates a higher risk of irritation to sensitive areas of the skin. It is recommended to use a dispersant, which will ensure that the essential oil will be dispersed in the bath water. Follow the manufacturer's instructions when using a dispersant.

Use of Undiluted Oils

As a general rule undiluted essential oils are not used in massage, applied to broken skin (cuts, wounds, surgery, sores etc.) or diseased skin. There may be some instances where the benefits of direct topical application may outweigh the risks. This might include instances such as insect bites and stings, burns, tinea and warts.

Inhalations

While asthma often responds well to the inhalation of essential oils, please be careful when recommending a steam inhalation, as it can be contraindicated for someone with asthma. Never leave a child unsupervised when using a steam inhalation.

Safety Guidelines for the Care of Essential Oils

To ensure the integrity of essential oils and the safe practice of aromatherapy, ensure the following:

- essential oils have a use-by date
- essential oils are stored in a dark glass bottle only (e.g., amber)
- store essential oils below 30° C
- keep the essential oils in a cool place away from the sun
- small amounts of essential oil remaining in large bottles should be transferred to smaller bottles, to reduce the risk of oxidation.

Procedure in Case of Essential Oil Poisoning

If a child ingests an essential oil, do the following:

- Telephone a general practitioner.
- Take the child to a hospital accident or emergency department and take the bottle with you.
- If the ingestion took place some time ago and the child shows severe signs of poisoning, such as loss of consciousness, telephone the ambulance emergency service.
- Do not induce vomiting, unless advised to do so by a general practitioner.

References

1. Soulier J. *Properties and indications: Thymus vulgaris*. Aromatherapy Record, 1995; 1: 50–53.
2. Arctander S. *Perfume and flavour materials of natural origin*. Allured Publishing, USA, 1994.
3. Wabner D. *Purity and pesticides*. The International Journal of Aromatherapy 1993; 5(2): 27–29.
4. Wabner D. *The peroxide value — A new tool for the quality control of essential oils*. The International Journal of Aromatherapy 2002; 12(3): 142–144.
5. Orafidiya LO. *The effect of autoxidation of lemongrass oil on its antibacterial activity*. Phytotherapy Research 1993; 7: 269–271.
6. *Standard for the uniform scheduling of drugs and poisons*. No. 17 Effective Date 2 June 2002, Australian Health Ministers' Advisory Council.
7. Tisserand R, Balacs T. *Essential oil safety*. Churchill Livingstone, UK, 1995.
8. *Planning occupational health & safety*. 5th edn, CCH Australia Limited, 2000.
9. Price S, Price L. *Aromatherapy for health professionals*. 2nd edn, Churchill Livingstone, England, 1999.
10. Schnaubelt K. *Medical aromatherapy*. Frog Ltd, USA, 1999.
11. Schnaubelt K. *Advanced aromatherapy*. Healing Art Press, Canada, 1995.
12. Bowles J. T*he basic chemistry of aromatherapeutic essential oils*. Australia, 1991.
13. Balacs T. cites Hartnoll G, et al. *Near fatal ingestion of oil of cloves*. Arch. Diseases in Childhood, 1993; 69: 392–393. in Research Reports, The International Journal of Aromatherapy 1994; 6(2): 33.
14. Lassak E. Australian medicinal plants. Methuen Australia, 1983.
15. Hotchkiss S. *How thin is your skin*. New Scientist, 29th January 1994:24–27.
16. Tisserand R. *New perspectives on essential oil safety*. Aroma' 95 Conference Proceedings, Aromatherapy Publications, England, 1995.
17. *The IFRA's guidelines and recommendations on citrus oils*. Perfumer and Flavorist 1980; 5(1): 1–17.
18. Hodgson E, Levi P. A textbook of modern toxicology. 2nd edn, McGraw-Hill Higher Education, USA, 2000.
19. McGuffin M, et al. Botanical safety handbook. CRC Press, USA, 1997.
20. Bruneton J. *Pharmacognosy*. 2nd edn, Lavoisier Publishing Inc, France, 1999.
21. Blumenthal M, et al. *The complete German commission E monographs: Therapeutic guide to herbal medicine*. American Botanical Council USA, 1998.
22. Davis P. *Aromatherapy: An A–Z*. 2nd edn, The C.W. Daniel Company Limited, Great Britain, 1999.
23. Lawless J. *The encyclopaedia of essential oils*. Element Books Limited, Great Britain, 1992.
24. Valnet J. *The practice of aromatherapy*. The C.W. Daniel Company Limited, Great Britain, 1980.
25. Steinmetz MD, et al. *Actions of essential oils of rosemary and certain of its constituents (eucalyptol and camphor) on the cerebral cortex of the rat in vitro*. J. Toxicology Clin Exp 1987; 7(4): 259–271.
26. Leung A, Foster S. *Encyclopedia of common natural ingredients used in food, drugs and cosmetics*. John Wiley & Sons Inc, USA, 1996.
27. Balacs T. *Hormones and Health*. The International Journal of Aromatherapy 1993; 5(1): 18–20.

Unit III

The Remedies

Unit III provides you with an extensive and systemic survey of a range of essential oils and carrier oils. It contains monographs of over 60 essential oils including:

- Botanical names
- Country of origin, traditional uses
- Chemical constituents
- Properties
- Indications for use, energetics
- Subtle effects
- Personality profile and safety.

Unit III includes the following chapters:

CHAPTER 13

The Essential Oils

Objectives

After careful study of this chapter, you should be able to:

- state the botanical origins
- identify the organoleptic characteristics
- outline the historical and traditional uses
- state the method of extraction
- identify the principal chemical constituents
- review clinical trials conducted
- examine the therapeutic properties
- describe the personality profile and emotional effects
- discuss the subtle effects
- outline the energetics
- state the mode of administration and the safety requirements

for a range of essential oils commonly used in aromatherapy.

Introduction

The criticism of aromatherapy has been that much of the data on essential oils has not been evaluated. In this second edition, every effort has been made to evaluate the original publications available to assure that the information presented is reputable.

It is with this in mind that these monographs have been prepared. The monographs are headed and ordered according to the English common name of each essential oil. This is followed by the current accepted botanical name of the plant from which the essential oil is derived and the following.

Synonyms

Other English names, alternative botanical names and common names in other languages are listed.

Family

The name of the plant family is listed. The modern botanical nomenclature has been adopted. This requires all the plant family names to end in '-aceae.'

Botany and Origins

A brief description of the plant is provided along with the origins of the plant and the essential oil.

Method of Extraction

The typical method of extracting the essential oil is identified.

Essential Oil Characteristics

A detailed organoleptic description of the essential oil is described.

Historical and Traditional Uses

The historical and background information about the plant and the essential oil is outlined. The traditional uses of the essential oil are documented. This can provide a valuable insight into the therapeutic uses of the essential oil.

Chemical Composition

A typical chemical profile of the essential oil is outlined. The main chemical constituents and the typical percentage of the constituents are provided.

Pharmacology and Clinical Studies

This section summarises a range of clinical studies and research which scientifically validates much of what we now know about essential oils.

Therapeutic Actions

The actions of the essential oils which are supported by reliable scientific and/or anecdotal evidence are listed.

Indications

Where applicable the indications are divided into categories such as analgesic, cardiovascular system, children's remedy, detoxification, digestive system, integumentary system, lymphatic system, musculoskeletal system, nervous system, reproductive system, respiratory system, urinary system, skin care.

Energetics

The energetics of the essential oils described in these monographs draw essentially on the principles of Traditional Chinese Medicine (TCM).

Personality Profile

Also referred to as the character profile or the characterologies of an essential oil. It is known that individuals are often drawn towards the scent of a particular essential oil. Often the scent corresponds to the physical, emotional and mental characteristics of a person. This section investigates this phenomenon.

Subtle Aromatherapy

This section investigates the subtle or spiritual influences of essential oils.

Mode of Administration

The mode of administration refers to the method of application of the essential oils. The modes of administration include topical application — massage, ointments, compress, bath, sitz bath, douche, skin care; Inhalation — direct inhalation, diffusers, oil vaporiser.

For instructions on each of the modes of administration refer to *Chapter 21 — Methods of Administration*.

Safety

This section lists contra-indications for the use of the essential oils in aromatherapy. In some cases the safety information presented may be contradictory. In such circumstances the source of the contradictory information which relates to the misunderstanding of the botanical name or the use of herbal texts as a reference has been provided.

Angelica Root

Angelica archangelica

Synonyms

Angelica officinalis

Family

Umbelliferae or Apiaceae

Botany and Origins

Angelica is a stout biennial or perennial herb which grows up to 2 m high with a large rhizome. It is cultivated in Belgium, Holland, France, Germany, Hungary and northern India.[1]

It is preferable that the oil be distilled from roots that are not more than two years old. The oil from older roots is different from that of young roots, but not inferior. The monoterpene hydrocarbons have resinified and in oil from older roots has little or no peppery top note.[1]

Method of Extraction

Angelica root oil is steam-distilled from the dried roots of *A. archangelica.*

Essential Oil Characteristics

Angelica root oil is a pale-yellow to orange-brown-coloured liquid. Its viscosity varies according to the root material used for distillation and the age of the essential oil. Beneath the peppery top note is a rich, somewhat herbaceous-earthy, woody base note of unique tenacity and great diffusive power. The base note is also slightly musky-animal-like with a spicy undertone.[1]

Historical and Traditional Uses

The virtues of angelica have been known for centuries. Folk lore testifies to its merits as a protection against contagion, for purifying the blood and for curing every conceivable malady. It was held a sovereign remedy for poisons and all infectious maladies.[2]

Culpeper describes the properties of angelica root:

> *The stalks and roots are candied and eaten fasting are good preservatives in time of infection, and will warm and comfort a cold stomach ... A water distilled from the root, as steeped in wine and distilled, and drank two or three spoonfuls at a time easeth all pains and torments coming of cold and wind, and taken with some of the root in powder, helpeth the pleurisy, as also all other diseases of the lungs and breast, as coughs, phthisic and shortness of breath.*[3]

Angelica was closely linked with Christianity beliefs. According to one legend, angelica was revealed in a dream by an angel to cure the plague. Another explanation for the name of this plant is that it blooms on the day of Michael the Archangel, and on that account is used as a preservative against evil spirits and witchcraft.

Most old herbals refer to angelica as a purifying agent, easing rheumatism and gout, warming, comforting and sudorific and it is particularly effective in drying out the body and expelling toxins.

The powdered root is extensively used in herbal preparations to treat bronchitis, pleurisy and other diseases of the lungs. It is also recommended for menstrual regulation.[6]

Chemical Composition

The chemistry of angelica essential oil is complex. The oil contains up to 70% monoterpene hydrocarbons, small quantities of esters, alcohols, coumarins and lactones.

The furocoumarins found in angelica oil are omelliferone, archangelicine, angelicine and bergaptene. These constituents are responsible for angelica's phototoxicity. Coumarins have a strong affinity with the nervous system and can raise the threshold from which one registers nervous stress.[4]

A typical chemical composition of angelica root is reported as follows:

α-pinene (21.12–25.24%), camphene (1.42–1.43%), α-pinene (1.28–1.48%), sabinene, δ-3-carene (7.94–10.38%), α-phellandrene (2.38–9.58%), myrcene (4.00–4.62%), limonene (8.54–11.53%) β-phellandrene (14.04–16.03%), cis-ocimene (0.24–0.28%), trans-ocimene (0.9–2.12%), p-cymene (6.25–11.3%), terpinolene (0.28–0.38%), copaene (0.93–1.29%), bornyl cryptone (0.44–0.99%), α-bisabolene (0.09–0.19%), rho-cymen-8-ol (0.14–0.35%), humulene monoxide (0.18–0.21%), tridecanolide (0.58–0.81%), pentadecanolide (0.87%).[5]

Pharmacology and Clinical Studies

Angelica root oil has been reported to exhibit antibacterial and antifungal properties.[6]

Therapeutic Actions

Antiseptic, antispasmodic, carminative, cholagogue, depurative, diaphoretic, digestive, diuretic, emmenagogue, expectorant, nervine, stomachic and tonic.

Indications

Digestive System

The oil is an excellent tonic for the digestive system.[12] It is recommended for flatulence and indigestion.[16]

Lymphatic System

Angelica root oil is reputed to have excellent detoxifying and diuretic properties.[7,12] Used in a massage oil it improves lymph drainage, relieves rheumatism and arthritis, fluid retention and cellulite.

Nervous System

Angelica root oil is well known for its tonic effect on the nervous system.[12] It is recommended for weakness and nervousness and for convalescents and old people.[7]

It is ideal for fatigue and stress-related disorders:

> *Angelica aids people with an upset nervous system who urgently need to rebuild body and soul. The oil helps soothe all kinds of weakness. It's like super-growth fertiliser you might feed a sickly plant. The essential oil of*

angelica root will help you rediscover your own inner strength and stamina.[8]

Respiratory System

It is an expectorant and may be used for chronic bronchial asthma, sinus infections, chronic respiratory problems and coughs.[9,12,13]

Skin Care

Angelica root essential oil is not commonly used in skin care. The oil is used as a fragrance ingredient in soaps, detergents, creams, lotions and perfumes.[1,6]

Energetics

Angelica root is *warming* and *drying*. It has been described as follows:

> *Draining the yin, warming and restoring, warming and invigorating the stomach/spleen and intestines, awakens the appetite, abates distension and dispels mucous damp.*[9]

It is beneficial in all *yin excess* conditions such as cold, damp and phlegm congestion in the lungs, intestines and uterus.[9]

Personality Profile

Fischer-Rizzi suggests that angelica root will assist people who are afraid, weak or who lack perseverance and have a tough time making decisions.

> *Don't give up! Stick with it — nothing has been lost. Don't be afraid — begin to rebuild. You are strong — nothing will knock you down.*[8]

Subtle Aromatherapy

It has been suggested that the oil helps the user to be more open to angelic powers.[10] The oil is recommended for strengthening the mind and spirit.

> *The source of angelica's strength is the earth, since the plant itself has been strongly influenced by the elements of the soil. As an essential oil, angelica has a fiery temperament and lends us more physical vitality or earthly strength than cosmic or spiritual energy. Angelica is particularly suited to people who need solid grounding or who search for reality.*[8]

Mode of Administration

Topical application — massage; Inhalation — direct inhalation, diffuser, oil vaporiser.

Safety

The oil is non-toxic and non-irritant. The furanocoumarins present in angelica root essential oil sensitise the skin to UV light. It is considered phototoxic. [6,11,15]

Herbal preparations of angelica root are contra-indicated in pregnancy as it is a uterine stimulant and an emmenagogue.[14] Davis and Tisserand do not state that the oil is contra-indicated during pregnancy. However, Lawless says that it should not be used during pregnancy. [12,15,16]

References

1. Arctander S. *Perfume and flavour materials of natural origin.* Allured Publishing, USA, 1994.
2. Grieve M. *A modern herbal.* Penguin Publishing, England, 1931.
3. Potterton. W. ed., *Culpeper's colour herbal.* Foulsham, Great Britain, 1983.
4. Whitton S. *Herb of angels.* Aromatherapy Quarterly, Issue No. 39, Winter 1993.
5. Lawrence B. *Angelica root oil.* Perfumer and Flavorist, 1977:1(6): 31.
6. Leung A, Foster S. *Encyclopedia of common natural ingredients used in food, drugs and cosmetics.* 2nd edn, John Wiley and Sons Inc, USA, 1996.
7. Lavabre M. *Aromatherapy workbook.* Healing Art Press, USA, 1990.
8. Fischer-Rizzi S. *Complete aromatherapy handbook.* Sterling Publishing Company, USA, 1990.
9. Holmes P. *The energetics of western herbs Vol I.* Artemis Press, USA, 1989.
10. Davis P. *Subtle aromatherapy.* The C.W. Daniel Company Limited, Great Britain, 1991.
11. Blumenthal M. *The complete German commission E monographs: Therapeutic guide to herbal medicines.* American Botanical Council, USA, 1998.
12. Davis P. *Aromatherapy: An A–Z.* 2nd edn, The C.W. Daniel Company Limited, Great Britain, 1999.
13. Evans WC. *Trease and Evans pharmacognosy.* 15th edn, WB Saunders, UK, 2002.
14. McGuffin M et al. *American herbal products association botanical safety handbook.* CRC Press, USA, 1997.
15. Tisserand R, Balacs T. *Essential oil safety.* Churchill Livingstone, UK, 1995.
16. Lawless J. *The encyclopaedia of essential oils.* Element Books Limited, Great Britain, 1992.

Aniseed (and Star Anise)

Pimpinella anisum, Illicium verum Hook

Synonyms

Aniseed *Anisum vulgare*; *A. officinarum.* Aniseed oil is also known as anise oil, sweet cumin. **Star Anise** is also known as Chinese anise, Chinese star anise.

Family

Aniseed: Umbelliferae or Apiaceae; **Star anise**: Illiciaceae

Botany and Origins

Aniseed is an annual herb, usually less than 0.6 m high. The seeds are reddish-brown, ribbed and aromatic, with a distinctive liquorice-like smell and taste. It is a native to Greece and Egypt, now widely cultivated in Spain.

Star anise is an evergreen tree usually 4–6 m high, but may grow up to 12 m. It is indigenous to south-eastern Asia, is extensively cultivated in southern China, Vietnam, India and Japan. The part of the plant used is the dried, ripe fruit that consists of 5 to 13 (usually 8), seed-bearing woody follicles attached to a central axis in the shape of a star, hence the name star anise. China is the major producer of star anise.[1]

Japanese star anise should not be confused with true star anise. It is obtained from a related species, *I. lanceolatum*, which grows in southern China, Taiwan and Japan. It is described as a smaller, deformed version of the Chinese star anise.[1]

Method of Extraction

Aniseed oil is distilled from the dried ripe fruit (seeds) of *P. anisum*. Star anise is steam-distilled from the fresh or partly dried whole or comminuted fruits of *I. verum.*

Essential Oil Characteristics

Aniseed oil is a clear to very pale-yellow-coloured oil with an intensely sweet clean odour, truly reminiscent of the crushed seeds. A very common description used is that of a 'licorice-like odour'.[2]

Historical and Traditional Uses

It was cultivated by the ancient Egyptians as a medicine and culinary spice, and was thought to 'refresh the heart'. It was well known to the Greeks and Romans as a 'pick-me-up'. Combined with orris root it was used by Edward IV for scenting linen and clothes.[3]

Ancient Chinese physicians used star anise as a digestive aid, the treatment of flatulence and as a breath freshener.[1] Aniseed has been extensively used for the treatment of hard, dry coughs where expectoration is difficult. It is used in lozenges and the seeds have been used for smoking, to promote expectoration.[4] The oil was mixed with spirits of wine to create a liqueur, Anisette, which was recommended for bronchitis and spasmodic asthma.[4]

Aniseed oil is used in flavours for candy, liqueurs, alcoholic beverages, tobacco, baked goods, spice blends, canned foods and pickles.[3]

Chemical Composition

The main chemical constituent is anethole, a phenyl propane derivative. It also contains methyl chavicol or estragole which is a phenolic ether. These constituents account for aniseed's excellent antispasmodic properties.[14]

Most pharmacopoeias allow the use of both essential oils indiscriminately as the anethole content is up to 90–95% in both oils.[1]

A typical chemical composition of *P. anisum* oil is reported as follows: α-pinene (0.17%), camphene (0.07%), β-pinene (0.01%), linalool (0.18%), cis-anethole (2.29%), trans-anethole (85.0%), safrole (0.58%), anisaldehyde (0.91%), acetoanisole (0.94%).[5]

A typical chemical composition of *I. verum* oil is reported as follows: trans-anethole (71.19%), feniculin (14.56%), estragole (5.04%), limonene (1.68%), linalool (0.69%), β-caryophyllene (0.63%), trans-α-farnesene (0.68%), anisaldehyde (0.41%), nerolidol (0.3%), cinnamyl acetate (0.25%), cis-ocimene (0.32%).[6]

Pharmacology and Clinical Studies

The oestrogenic activity of anethole is well documented.[1] Anethole is a methyl ether of oestrone, and seems to have potent oestrogenic activity. Research suggests that the active oestrogenic compounds are polymers of anethole such as dianethole and photoanethole.[1,7] Anethole has been reported to exhibit spasmolytic properties, to stimulate respiratory secretions and expectoration.[17]

Therapeutic Actions

Antiseptic, antispasmodic, carminative, expectorant, galactagogue, stimulant, stomachic.

Indications

Digestive System

Aniseed is well known for its effect on the digestive system as a carminative, digestive and an antispasmodic. It may be used to relieve dyspepsia, colic and flatulence.[1,11,12,15,16]

Reproductive System

Aniseed may be used to increase the milk flow of nursing mothers.[1,10,15] However, for this purpose, a herbal infusion of the crushed anise seeds is preferred. Aniseed can also be used for the treatment of amenorrhoea.[8]

Respiratory System

As it is an expectorant and antispasmodic it is excellent for any asthmatic or respiratory condition associated with copious white phlegm, coughing, wheezing or chronic bronchial asthma.[1,10,11,16] The expectorant action of *P. anisum* is better than caraway or fennel; on the other hand, the carminative effect is much less than that of fennel or caraway.[9]

Skin Care

Aniseed is generally not used in skin care.

Energetics

Aniseed is described as warming and drying. It increases the *Qi* and replenishes deficiency so it is ideally suited as a tonic for those suffering from overwork, chronic illness and weak constitution.[10]

Personality Profile

The warm spicy scent of aniseed has an uplifting and comforting effect on the mind. It is good for introverted, melancholic or fearful people who tend to be withdrawn or frigid.[2]

Mode of Administration

Topical application — massage; Inhalation — direct inhalation, diffuser, oil vaporiser.

Many herbalists suggest taking aniseed essential oil internally. Holmes suggests two to four drops in a little warm water.[10] The German Commission E Monographs suggest 0.3 g essential oil as a bronchial expectorant for upper respiratory tract congestion and for dyspeptic complaints.[11]

Schnaubelt suggests that the preferred mode of use is internal and that:

> *a drop of anise oil on a teaspoon of sugar will restore equilibrium to an acutely out-of-whack autonomic nervous system.*[8]

Safety

Information regarding the safe use of aniseed is conflicting. Some sources suggest that aniseed is highly toxic:

> *... very toxic and dangerous, causing a muscular numbness followed by paralysis. It can be more dangerous than pure alcohol, and should never be left where children might find it.*[13]

It is difficult to believe that aniseed is so toxic, knowing that herbalists are recommending its use internally and the only contra-indications identified are the occasional allergic reactions of the skin.

The oestrogenic effects of aniseed are relatively weak, but suggest that it would be safe not to use orally during pregnancy and breast feeding.[7]

References

1. Leung A, Foster S. *Encyclopedia of common natural ingredients used in food, drugs and cosmetics.* 2nd edn, John Wiley and Sons Inc. USA. 1996.
2. Arctander S. *Perfume and flavour materials of natural origin.* Allured Publishing, USA, 1994.
3. Lawless J. *Aromatherapy and the mind.* Thornsons, Great Britain, 1994.
4. Grieve M. *A modern herbal.* Penguin, England, 1931.
5. Lawrence B. *Anise oil. Perfumer and Flavorist.* 1983; 8(3): 65.
6. Jian-Qin Cu et al. *GC/MS analysis of star anise oil.* Journal of Essential Oil Research, March/April 1990; 91–92.
7. Balacs T. *Hormones and health.* The International Journal of Aromatherapy 1993; 5(1): 18–20.
8. Schnaubelt K. *Medical aromatherapy.* Frog Ltd, USA, 1999.
9. Weiss RF. *Herbal medicine.* Beaconsfield Publishers Ltd, England, 1988.
10. Holmes P. *The energetics of western herbs Vol II.* Artemis Press, USA, 1989.
11. Blumenthal M. et al. *The complete German commission E monographs: Therapeutic guide to herbal medicine.* American Botanical Council USA, 1998.
12. Davis P. *Aromatherapy: An A–Z.* 2nd edn, The C.W. Daniel Company Limited, Great Britain, 1999.
13. Ryman D. *Aromatherapy.* Piatkus Press, Great Britain, 1991.
14. Schnaubelt K. *Advanced aromatherapy.* Healing Art Press, USA, 1995.
15. Lavabre M. *Aromatherapy workbook.* Healing Art Press, USA, 1990.
16. Lawless J. *The encyclopaedia of essential oils.* Element Books Limited, Great Britain, 1992.
17. Bruneton J. *Pharmacognosy*, 2nd edn, Lavoisier Publishing, France, 1999.

Basil

Ocimum basilicum

Synonyms

Sweet basil and common basil

Family

Labiatae or Lamiaceae

Botany and Origins

Basil is an annual herb, which grows to about 0.5 m in height. It is a native of tropical Asia and Africa. There are many varieties of basil cultivated all over the world. Each variety produces a unique essential oil which is dependent on environmental factors such as temperature, geographic location, soil and the amount of water.[1]

The two most commonly available basil oils are:[2]

- The true Sweet basil oil, also known as European or Sweet basil. This oil has a higher percentage of linalool. This oil is generally regarded as safe to use in aromatherapy.
- Exotic or Reunion basil, which is distilled in the Comoro Islands, Malagasy Republic, Thailand and occasionally in the Seychelles. This oil has a higher percentage of methyl chavicol.

According to an extensive analysis of over 200 individual basil plants, five chemotypes of basil oil have been identified:[3]

- linalool
- methyl chavicol
- methyl eugenol
- (E)-methyl cinnamate
- eugenol.

Method of Extraction

Basil oil is steam-distilled from the leaves and flowering tops of *O. basilicum*.

Essential Oil Characteristics

Sweet basil oil is a pale-yellow or almost colourless mobile liquid with a sweet-spicy, slightly green, fresh top note and a balsamic-woody undertone.

Exotic basil oil is a pale-yellow to pale-green mobile liquid with a slightly coarse-herbaceous, camphoraceous top note and it displays an intense aniseed-like sweetness associated with the methyl chavicol content.[1]

Historical and Traditional Uses

Basil takes its name from Latin for a royal 'basileum', possibly because the plant was so highly prized that it was considered a king among plants.

In India, basil is dedicated to Vishnu and is regarded as the incarnation of his wife, Lakshmi, goddess of fortune and beauty. The basil species that we are referring to in India is *O. sanctum*, also called Tulsi. Tulsi is called upon for life and death, for various acts of life and above all for giving children to those who want them. According to tradition, basil protects from unfortunate destinies and evil spirits.[4]

Basil was recommended by Pliny against jaundice and epilepsy, and as a diuretic. It was also known as an aphrodisiac. In the Middle Ages it was prescribed for melancholy and depression.

The 16th century herbalist John Gerard wrote:

> *The smell of basil ... taketh away sorrowfulness and maketh a man merry and glad.*[5]

Chemical Composition

Estragole is also known as methyl chavicol. There are some safety concerns with the estragole content of basil, therefore in aromatherapy, it is preferable to use the linalool chemotype. The methyl chavicol chemotype is preferred in the manufacture of expensive perfumes whereas the linalool chemotype is preferred in food flavouring and less expensive perfumes.[9]

The phenolic ethers found in basil confirm basil's antispasmodic properties which make it ideal for the treatment of spasmodic abdominal pain and for asthmatic conditions.[11]

The typical chemical composition of basil oil is as follows.[15]

Compound	Origin		
	Comoro Is.	France	Egypt
α-pinene	0.18%	0.11%	0.25%
camphene	0.06%	0.02%	0.07%
β-pinene	0.25%	0.07%	0.43%
myrcene	0.12%	0.13%	0.35%
limonene	2.64%	2.04%	4.73%
cis-ocimene	2.52%	0.03%	0.63%
camphor	0.37%	1.43%	0.57%
linalool	1.16%	40.72%	45.55%
methyl chavicol	85.76%	23.79%	26.56%
α-terpineol	0.84%	1.90%	1.09%
citronellol	0.65%	3.57%	1.76%
geraniol	0.03%	0.38%	0.20%
methyl cinnamate	0.05%	0.34%	0.25%
eugenol	0.74%	5.90%	5.90%

Pharmacology and Clinical Studies

Methyl cinnamate and methyl chavicol have insecticidal activities.[3,6] Basil ct methyl chavicol essential oil was found to have potent antimicrobial and antifungal properties.[7]

Therapeutic Actions

Analgesic, antidepressant, antiseptic, antispasmodic, carminative, cephalic, digestive, emmenagogue, expectorant, febrifuge, nervine, sudorific.

Indications

Digestive System

Basil is also useful in digestive disorders such as vomiting, gastric spasms, nausea, dyspepsia and hiccups.[8,9]

Nervous System

It is considered to be one of the 'finest remedies' for the brain and a cephalic.[10,11,12] It is reputed to clear the head, relieve intellectual fatigue, and give the mind strength and clarity. It may be used in all types of nervous disorders, especially those associated with weakness, indecision or hysteria.

Basil oil is recommended for those in need of protection, due either to debilitating illness and low resistance levels, nervous exhaustion, a constitutional weakness or a change in life resulting in feelings of vulnerability.[5]

Mailhebiau says that *O. basilicum* is remarkably relaxing, due to its high methyl ether content.

> *We recommend it for people with schizoid tendencies as it soothes, calms and relaxes; it is the antistress essence par exellence.*[4]

It is recommended as a carminative and sedative for digestive insomnia — people who 'digest' their worries during the night.[4]

Immune System
Basil's sudorific and febrifuge properties mean it may be used for all types of fever. In Ayurvedic medicine it is combined with black pepper for malarial fever.[8,12]

Respiratory System
Basil's antispasmodic property has a beneficial action on the respiratory system and is used for the relief of sinus congestion, asthma, bronchitis, influenza and whooping cough.[8,12]

Reproductive System
Basil is recommended for delayed menstruation, scanty periods and abdominal cramps.[10]

Skin Care
Basil oil has been used in low dilutions to improve the tone and appearance of the skin.[12]

Energetics

Basil is a warming oil which tonifies yang and lifts the spirit. It is recommended for people who are physically or mentally exhausted, suffer from nervous depression and have become complacent and melancholic.[10]

Personality Profile

The scent of basil is uplifting, awakening, clarifying and stimulating.[13]

Mode of Administration

Topical application — massage, ointment; Inhalation — direct inhalation, diffuser, oil vaporiser.

Safety

Avoid using basil oil with a high content of methyl cinnamate and methyl chavicol as it will be an irritant to people with sensitive skin. Basil oil is contra-indicated during pregnancy.[8,12]

Methyl chavicol administered to experimental mice is partially metabolised to 1'-hydroxy-estragole, a carcinogen.[9]

It must be noted that international authorities have not set any limits to the use of basil as it is unlikely that the amount of methyl chavicol absorbed in normal usage would be minimal.[9] Only basil with a methyl chavicol content of 5% or less should be used in aromatherapy.[14]

References

1. Arctander S. *Perfume and flavour materials of natural origin.* Allured Publishing, USA, 1994.
2. Leung A, Foster S. *Encyclopedia of common natural ingredients used in food, drugs and cosmetics.* 2nd edn, John Wiley and Sons, USA, 1996.
3. Lawrence B. *Essential oils: From agriculture to chemistry.* The World of Aromatherapy III Conference Proceedings, NAHA, 2000: 8–26.
4. Mailhebiau P. *Portraits in oils.* The C.W. Daniel Company Limited, Great Britain, 1995.
5. Tisserand R. *The art of aromatherapy.* 2nd edn, The C.W. Daniel Company Limited, Great Britain, 1979.
6. Chokechaijaroenporn O. et al. *Mosquito repellent activities of ocimum volatile oils.* Phytomed, 1994; 1:135–139. Cited in the Aromatherapy Database, Bob Harris, Essential Oil Resource Consultants, UK, 2000.
7. Ndounga M, Ouamba J. *Antibacterial and antifungal activities of essential oils of Ocimum gratissimum and O. basilicum from Congo.* Fitoterapia 1997; 68(2): 190–191. Cited in the Aromatherapy Database, Bob Harris, Essential Oil Resource Consultants, UK, 2000.
8. Lawless J. *The encyclopaedia of essential oils.* Element Books Limited, Great Britain, 1992.
9. Bruneton J. *Pharmacognosy.* 2nd edn, Lavoisier Publishing, France, 1999.
10. Holmes P. *The energetics of western herbs Vol II.* Artemis Press, USA, 1989.
11. Schnaubelt K. *Advanced aromatherapy.* Healing Art Press, USA, 1995.
12. Davis P. *Aromatherapy: An A–Z.* 2nd edn, The C.W. Daniel Company Limited, Great Britain, 1999.
13. Worwood V. *The fragrant mind.* Doubleday, Great Britain, 1995.
14. Tisserand R, Balacs T. *Essential oil safety.* Churchill Livingstone, UK, 1995.
15. Lawrence B. *Basil.* Perfumer and Flavorist, 1980; 4(6): 31.

Bay, Laurel

Laurus nobilis

Synonyms

Bay, laurel, bay sweet, true bay and Mediterranean bay

Family

Lauraceae

Botany and Origins

L. nobilis is an evergreen tree, up to 20 m high; however, it is usually pruned to below 3 m. The bark on mature trees is greyish and on younger stems it is smooth and shiny, often with a reddish tint.[1]

It is believed to have originated in Asia Minor, but is now considered a native to the Mediterranean region. There are several botanical species known under the name bay. These include *Pimenta racemosa,* commonly known as West Indian bay, and *Umbellularia california,* commonly known as Californian bay.[1]

It is commonly planted in gardens as a hedge and in tubs to produce fresh leaves for culinary purposes.

Method of Extraction

Bay laurel oil is produced by steam distillation of the leaves and branchlets.

Characteristics

The oil is a pale-yellow to very pale-olive-green or almost colourless liquid of a fresh, strong but sweet, camphoraceous and spicy odour.

Historical and Traditional Uses

L. nobilis was sacred to the god Apollo in classical Greece. According to legend, when Daphne, the nymph daughter of the earth goddess Gaia, was pursued by Apollo, slayer of her bridegroom, she entreated the gods for assistance, who changed her into a laurel tree. Apollo then crowned himself with a circle of laurel leaves, and declared the tree sacred to his divinity.[1]

A garland of woven laurel leaves was awarded as a symbol of honour or victory in Rome. In the Middle Ages, distinguished men were crowned with a wreath of berried laurel, hence the term Poet Laureate. University graduates were known as bachelors from the Latin *baccalaureus* (*bacco,* a berry, and *laureus,* of laurel). They were forbidden to marry as it was believed that this would distract them from their studies.[1]

Bay laurel was said to confer the gift of prophecy. A withering laurel tree in the garden predicted a disaster.[1]

Bay laurel has long been used in herbal medicine. An infusion of the berries was supposed to suppress profuse menstruation and hasten childbirth. Infusions of the bark and leaves were frequently prescribed to alleviate kidney disorders and respiratory problems.[1]

Chemical Composition

The composition of bay laurel is fascinating. It contains constituents from almost all the functional groups (oxides, esters, alcohols and phenols), which explains its spectrum of uses.[2]

A typical chemical composition of *L. nobilis* is as follows:

1,8-cineole (40%), α-terpinyl acetate (9%), sabinene (7%), α-pinene (7%), β-pinene (4%), terpinene-4-ol (4%), α-terpineol (3%), linalool (10%), p-cymene (1%), γ-terpinene (1%), methyl eugenol (5%).[3]

Pharmacology and Clinical Studies

Bay laurel oil has been reported to have bactericidal and fungicidal properties. It depresses the heart rate and lowers blood pressure in animals.[3]

Therapeutic Actions

Antiseptic, bactericidal, carminative, expectorant, diaphoretic, digestive, tonic.

Indications

Digestive System

It has a pronounced effect on the digestive system and may be useful as an appetite stimulant. Expels wind, settles the stomach pain and has a tonic effect on the liver and kidneys.[5,6]

Nervous System

It has been described as an excellent cerebral stimulator and nerve tonic for those who doubt themselves.[4,5]

Respiratory System

Bay laurel oil is a good antiseptic for the respiratory system. It is an expectorant with mucolytic properties. It is recommended for the treatment of chronic bronchitis.[4]

Skin Care

Bay laurel is recommended for conditions such as ulcers, boils, acne and abscesses.[4]

Energetics

Energetically, bay laurel's principal actions are to circulate and regulate *Qi energy* and to clear *cold phlegm.*[5]

Personality Profile

It is particularly beneficial for individuals who lack energy and confidence. It is well suited to people who lack self-esteem and doubt their abilities and intellect.[5]

Subtle Aromatherapy

The oil is best suited to writers, poets, painters, musicians and creative artists — those with psychic tendencies who depend on intuition and inspiration for their work. It promotes confidence, insight and courage.[7]

Mode of Administration

Topical application — massage, compress, bath, skin care; Inhalation — direct inhalation, diffuser, oil vaporiser.

Safety

Bay laurel oil is generally regarded as safe. Frequent use of bay laurel oil on the skin over a longer period of time (approximately 3 weeks) can result in sensitisation and irritations.[2,6]

References

1. Weiss EA. *Essential oil crops*. CAB International, UK, 1997.
2. Schnaubelt K. *Advanced aromatherapy*. Healing Art Press, USA, 1995.
3. Leung A, Foster S. *Encyclopedia of common natural ingredients used in food, drugs and cosmetics*. 2nd edn., John Wiley and Sons, USA, 1996.
4. Mailhebiau P. *Portraits in oils*. The C.W. Daniel Company Limited, Great Britain, 1995.
5. Mojay G. *Aromatherapy for healing the spirit*. Healing Arts Press, USA, 1999.
6. Lawless J. *The encyclopaedia of essential oils*. Element Books Limited, Great Britain, 1992.
7. Lawless J. *Aromatherapy and the mind*. Harper Collins Publishers, England, 1994.

Bay, West Indian

Pimenta racemosa

Synonyms

P. racemosa is commonly known as bay rum tree or bay. In the Caribbean, it is known as wild cinnamon and bay-berry.[1]

Family

Myrtaceae

Botany and Origins

West Indian bay is a small to medium-size forest tree which grows up to 15 m. It is a native of the West Indies and is cultivated in Venezuela, Puerto Rico and the Caribbean Islands.

Method of Extraction

West Indian bay essential oil is steam- or water-distilled from the leaves.

Essential Oil Characteristics

The oil is a pale straw to brownish orange in colour, with an intensely fresh-spicy, somewhat camphor-aceous, with a lasting sweet-balsamic undertone.[2]

Historical and Traditional Uses

The major use of West Indian bay leaf oil is in hair lotions, such as *Bay Rum* which was originally produced by distilling rum over the leaves but it is now formulated by blending the essential oil with alcohol and rum.

Chemical Composition

The main components of West Indian bay essential oil are eugenol (up to 56%), chavicol (up to 22%), and myrcene (up to 21%).[1] A typical chemical composition of West Indian bay is reported as follows:

Myrcene (31.6%), limonene (1.4%), 1,8-cineole (2.0%), trans-ocimene (2.1%), 3-octanone (1.0%), p-cymene (0.5%), 3-octanol (0.5%), 1-octen-3-ol (1.3), linalool (3.0%), terpinen-4-ol (0.3%), caryophyllene (0.9%), methyl chavicol (0.3%), neral (0.8%), α-terpineol (0.8%), geranyl acetate (0.8%), eugenol (38.6%), chavicol (11.0%).[1]

Pharmacology and Clinical Studies

West Indian bay oil has antiseptic and astringent properties.[3]

Therapeutic Actions

Analgesic, antiseptic, astringent, general stimulant, expectorant.

Indications

Musculoskeletal System

The essential oil may be used in massage for muscular aches and pain, strains and sprains.[4]

Respiratory System

Because of the high amount of phenols, the essential oil is a good antiseptic for the respiratory system and is recommended for the treatment of colds, flu, tonsillitis and viral infections.[4]

Skin Care

The oil is recommended in hair care as a scalp stimulant, a hair rinse for dandruff and for greasy, lifeless hair. West Indian bay is extensively used as a fragrance ingredient in *Bay Rum*, in creams, lotions, soaps, detergents and perfumes.[3]

Mode of Administration

Topical application — massage, compress, bath, skin care; Inhalation — direct inhalation, diffuser, oil vaporiser.

Safety

The high eugenol content in West Indian bay oil suggests that the oil should be used with caution. It is a mucous membrane irritant. Tisserand and Balacs suggest avoiding oral dosages of essential oils rich in eugenol because eugenol is an inhibitor of platelet activity and impairs liver activity.[5]

It does not appear to be a dermal sensitiser like bay laurel.[4,5]

References

1. Weiss EA. *Essential oil crops*. CAB International, UK, 1997.

2. Arctander S. *Perfume and flavour materials of natural origin.* Allured Publishing, USA, 1994.
3. Leung A, Foster S. *Encyclopedia of common natural ingredients used in food, drugs and cosmetics.* 2nd edn, John Wiley and Sons, USA, 1996.
4. Lawless J. *The encyclopaedia of essential oils.* Element Books Limited, Great Britain, 1992.
5. Tisserand R, Balacs T. *Essential oil safety.* Churchill Livingstone, UK, 1995.

Bergamot

Citrus bergamia

Synonyms

Citrus aurantium subsp. *bergamia*

Family

Rutaceae

Botany and Origins

The botany and origin of bergamot is somewhat obscure.[1] It is an upright tree up to 12 m with a single trunk and numerous branches. Under cultivation, the trees are pruned to 4–5 m and the branches are cut back to maintain a tree diameter of 5 m. The fruit is generally globoid to 7.5 cm, the peel is thin, tough, smooth and green, becoming yellow when ripe.[1]

The bergamot fruit is not edible because the pulp is too sour. As a result, the bergamot tree is primarily cultivated for its essential oil. The tree cannot be propagated by seed; bergamot buds are grafted onto other citrus rootstocks. Bitter orange is commonly used. Other citrus species have proven to be more disease-resistant. Some growers believe that lemon and citron rootstock gives an oil of finer quality, but there are no technical data that support this claim.[1]

The tree grew almost exclusively in a narrow coastal strip in the southern part of Calabria, Italy. Bergamot is now cultivated and produced in the Ivory Coast, Guinea, Morocco and Corsica.

Method of Extraction

Bergamot oil is produced by cold expression from the peel of the nearly ripe fruit from the small bergamot tree, *C. bergamia*.

Essential Oil Characteristics

Bergamot oil is a green or olive-green, mobile liquid of an extremely rich, sweet-fruity top note followed by a oily-herbaceous and somewhat balsamic body and dry-out. The colour of the oil fades on aging, particularly when the oil is exposed to light. The oil turns yellow or pale olive-brown.[2]

Historical and Traditional Uses

The origins of the word bergamot are shrouded in mystery. Guenther says that it might have been derived from the shape of a fruit which resembles the bergamot pear.[3]

Another account is that bergamot was brought by Columbus from the Canary Islands to the city of Berga, in the Province of Barcelona, Spain, and it was introduced from there to Calabria in southern Italy, the principal growing region.[3]

Davis says that it is named after the Italian city of Bergamo in northern Italy, where the oil was first sold.[4]

The development of the toilet water known as *eau-de-cologne*, originally made in Italy by the Feminis family in the sixteenth century, stimulated bergamot oil production, as the oil is an essential ingredient.[1]

The oil has been used in Italian folk medicine for the treatment of fever and worms.[5]

Bergamot imparts a pleasant flavour to Earl Grey tea and is considered one of the most popular essential oils for use in perfumery.

Chemical Composition

Bergamot essential oil is primarily composed of monoterpene hydrocarbons, monoterpene alcohols and esters. A typical chemical composition of bergamot is reported as follows:

α-pinene (1.0%), β-pinene (5.7%), myrcene (0.9%), limonene (33.0%), α-bergamotene [bergaptene] (0.23%), β-bisabolene (0.57%), linalool (13.45%), linalyl acetate (31.3%), nerol (0.1%), neryl acetate (0.42%), geraniol (0.05%), geraniol acetate (0.46%), α-terpineol (0.13%).[6]

Pharmacology and Clinical Studies

Bergaptene, known as 5-methoxypsoralen, which is present in bergamot oil, has been shown to be phototoxic when tested on human skin.[7]

Therapeutic Actions

Analgesic, antidepressant, antiseptic, antiviral, carminative, cicatrisant, deodorant, digestive, febrifuge, sedative, stomachic, tonic, vermifuge, vulnerary.

Indications

Digestive System

Its action on the digestive system is carminative and digestive, and it is useful in relieving colic, flatulence and indigestion.[9,10]

Bergamot oil is particularly indicated for nervous indigestion and loss of appetite due to emotional stress.

Immune System

Bergamot has been found to inhibit the *herpes simplex* I virus which causes cold sores.[4] It is particularly effective in combination with tea tree and lavender for the treatment of cold sores, chicken pox and shingles.

Nervous System

The fruity and lively but gentle, floral scent of bergamot gives the oil a sedative and yet uplifting quality.[8]

Bergamot oil is recommended for people who are tense, anxious or depressed. Bergamot's antidepressant property combined with its regulatory effect on appetite would seem to indicate its use in treating eating disorders such as anorexia nervosa.[4]

Urinary System

Bergamot oil is recommended for the treatment of cystitis and urinary tract infections. It can be used in the very early stages of cystitis to prevent the infection spreading. This can be done by adding no more than three drops of bergamot essential oil to a bath and using it as a local wash.[4,5,9]

Skin Care

Bergamot's antiseptic action makes it beneficial for treating wounds, herpes and acne. It is recommended for oily skin types and is used as an effective deodorising agent.[4] It is recommended for treating eczema and psoriasis. For this purpose, Fischer-Rizzi suggests blending bergamot with rock rose and everlasting.[8]

Energetics

The energetics of bergamot are neutral with cooling and warming potential. It is described as relaxing, restoring and calming.[9] Bergamot's energetic qualities enhance the circulation and free flowing of *Qi*.[10]

Mojay describes bergamot's antidepressant properties according to the principles of TCM:

> *Depression due to stagnant Qi energy is the result of accumulated stress or repressed emotion. The emotion most often involved is that of unexpressed anger... Like lavender, bergamot encourages the release of pent up feelings — feelings that can lead not only to depression but to insomnia, anxiety and sudden mood swings... Bergamot oil helps us to relax and 'let go'.*[8]

Whenever the flow of *Qi* is disrupted or constrained nervous behaviour develops such as irritability, neuralgic pain, palpitations, sleep disturbances and anxiety.

Personality Profile

Bergamot personalities are young, fresh, caring, considerate and full of energy. They are not necessarily young in years, but they are always young at heart and have a joyful approach to life.[11]

Fischer-Rizzi ideally describes bergamot:

> *Thanks to bergamot's sunny and warming disposition, the oil helps people regain self-confidence, and it uplifts and refreshes the spirit. The gentle fragrance, like a bouquet of flowers, evokes joy and warms the heart.*[8]

Subtle Aromatherapy

The green colour of bergamot has an affinity with the heart chakra, and is useful when the heart chakra is affected by grief.[12]

Mode of Administration

Topical application — massage, compress, bath, sitz bath, douche, skin care; Inhalation — direct inhalation, diffuser, oil vaporiser.

Safety

Bergaptene has been found to be phototoxic on the skin. Avoid exposure to the sun after having used bergamot in massage or bath.[7,13]

The International Fragrance Research Association (IFRA) says that the amount of bergamot used in topical preparations should be limited to a maximum of 0.4%, except in bath preparations such as soaps and other bath preparations which are washed off the skin.[14]

References

1. Weiss EA. *Essential oil crops*. CAB International, UK, 1997.
2. Arctander S. *Perfume and flavour materials of natural origin.* Allured Publishing, USA, 1994.
3. Guenther E. *The essential oils. Volume III.* Robert Krieger Publishing Company, USA, first published 1949.
4. Davis P. *Aromatherapy: An A–Z.* 2nd edn, The C.W. Daniel Company Limited, Great Britain, 1999.
5. Tisserand R. *The art of aromatherapy*. The C.W. Daniel Company Limited, Great Britain, 1979.
6. Lawrence B. *Bergamot oil.* Perfumer and Flavorist. 1982; 7(5): 43.
7. Leung A, Foster S. *Encyclopedia of common natural ingredients used in food, drugs and cosmetics*. 2nd edn, John Wiley and Sons, USA, 1996.
8. Fischer-Rizzi S. *Complete aromatherapy handbook.* Sterling Publishing Company, USA, 1990.
9. Holmes P. *The energetics of western herbs Vol II.* Artemis Press, USA, 1989.
10. Mojay G. *Aromatherapy for healing the spirit.* Hodder and Stoughton, UK, 1996
11. Worwood V. *The fragrant mind.* Doubleday, Great Britain, 1995.
12. Davis P. *Subtle aromatherapy.* The C.W. Daniel Company Limited, Great Britain, 1991.
13. Lawless J. *The encyclopaedia of essential oils.* Element Books Limited, Great Britain, 1992.

14. Tisserand R, Balacs T. *Essential oil safety.* Churchill Livingstone, UK, 1993.

Black Pepper

Piper nigrum

Synonyms

pepper

Family

Piperaceae

Botany and Origins

P. nigrum is a native of southern India and Indonesia. It has been cultivated in the same areas for over 2,000 years.

It is a perennial vine climbing to about 5 m. The inflorescence is a spike of about 20–30 sessile flowers, which develop into sessile fruits. The fruits on a spike do not mature together and when a few fruits are ripe the spike is harvested. Ripe fruits are removed and allowed to ferment or are soaked in running water to remove the pericarps. The seeds are dried and powdered to give us the white pepper of commerce.[1]

Black peppers are more pungent and are produced from the unripe fruits on the harvested spikes. These are sun-dried usually after soaking in hot water. The pungency is due to the presence of various resins and a yellow crystalline alkaloid called piperine.[1]

Method of Extraction

The essential oil of black pepper is produced by the steam distillation of the dried, crushed but not quite ripe fruits of the pepper vine, *P. nigrum*.

Essential Oil Characteristics

The essential oil of black pepper is a clear to pale-greenish-coloured mobile liquid. It has a fresh, dry-woody, warm-spicy odour reminiscent of dried black pepper.[2]

It was believed that black pepper oil, which is green, was of a higher quality; however, Arctander and Weiss say this is not so.[1,2] They claim that the green colour is simply due to the presence of azulenes. If this is so, I would suggest that the green-coloured black pepper oil would be of higher quality for use in aromatherapy.

Historical and Traditional Uses

Pepper has been esteemed as a spice in India since time immemorial and dispersed in trade throughout the world. Pepper was so important that the search for the source of the spice and the control of the trade was a significant factor influencing world exploration and history.

The word originates from the Latin 'piper', which in turn comes from the Sanskrit *pippali*. Black pepper is one of the oldest known spices, being described by Theophrastus in the 4th century BC.[1]

By the Middle Ages pepper was of great importance in Europe to season and preserve meats, and to overcome odours of rancid food. Peppercorns were very expensive and accepted as currency.[1]

The warming and stimulating properties of pepper were well known to early European herbalists such as Joseph Miller:

> *Pepper is heating and drying, expelling wind, and of great use against coldness and windiness of the stomach, and the colic; it strengthens nerves and head, and helps the sight; outwardly it is good for toothache and for cold affections of the nerves, and pains in the limbs.*[4]

Black and white pepper are used extensively as domestic spices. They are widely used as flavour ingredients in most food products.[3]

Pepper is used in TCM and Ayurvedic medicine for its carminative, warming and eliminative properties.[3]

Chemical Composition

The oil of black pepper is rich in monoterpene hydrocarbons and sesquiterpene hydrocarbons. Monoterpene hydrocarbons are known for their analgesic, antiseptic and tonic properties while sesquiterpene hydrocarbons may account for black pepper's antiviral properties.

The composition of black pepper oil can vary considerably according to origin and method of preparation. The greatest variation is within the monoterpene hydrocarbon group as follows:

limonene (0–40%), β-pinene (5–35%), α-phellandrene (1–27%), β-phellandrene (0–19%), sabinene (0–20%), d-3-carene (trace to 15%), myrcene (trace to 10%).[1]

A typical chemical composition of black pepper is as follows:

α-pinene (5.8%), camphene (0.1%), β-pinene (10.4%), d-3-carene (20.2%), limonene (17.1%), g-terpinene (0.2%), p-cymene (0.8%), terpinolene (1.0%), d-elemene (2.5%), α-copaene (2.3%), β-elemene (0.4%), β-caryophyllene (27.8%), α-humulene (1.4%), d-cadinene (0.8%), caryophyllene oxide (0.6%).[1]

Therapeutic Actions

Analgesic, antiseptic, antispasmodic, carminative, diaphoretic, diuretic, febrifuge, laxative, rubefacient, stomachic, tonic.

Pharmacology and Clinical Studies

Black pepper oil was spasmogenic on isolated jejunum at concentrations exceeding 70 μg/mL.[5] The essential oil of *P. nigrum* was found to have antibacterial properties.[6]

Indications

Circulatory System

Black pepper oil is recommended for the treatment of anaemia, as a stimulant of the spleen, which is involved in the production of new blood cells, and for the treatment of bruises.[7] It is also recommended for the treatment of chilblains.[9]

Digestive System

Black pepper's stomachic, antispasmodic and carminative properties make it an excellent choice for treating disorders of the digestive system.[7] It is recommended for atonic dyspepsia, constipation, flatulence and loss of appetite.[4]

Musculoskeletal System

Black pepper oil is recommended in a massage blend for the relief of rheumatism and arthritis, muscular aches and pains, tired and aching limbs and muscular stiffness. It can be used before training or a performance to prevent pain and stiffness and possibly improve performance.[7]

Skin Care

Black pepper essential oil is generally not used in skin care.

Energetics

The warming qualities of black pepper indicate that it is the ideal essential oil to use to dispel any cold pathology.

In TCM, cold is associated with poor digestive function, the onset of an infection with headaches, chills and fatigue, fluid congestion and general aches and pains.[8]

Personality Profile

The personality of black pepper is associated with that of a stern older person. Black pepper personalities are often extremely dictatorial, self-righteous and tend to take responsibility for everyone in their family circle. While black pepper is a warming oil, a black pepper personality is not easily able to express feelings of love.[10]

Subtle Aromatherapy

Black pepper oil will help us 'get a move on' at times when our lives feel 'stuck'.[11]

Mode of Administration

Topical application — massage, compress, ointment; Inhalation — direct inhalation, diffuser, oil vaporiser.

Safety

Black pepper oil is non-irritating and non-sensitising and there are no contra-indications. It has been said that excessive use can overstimulate the kidneys.[4,7] I could not find any clinical evidence to confirm this.

References

1. Weiss EA. *Essential oil crops*. CAB International, UK, 1997.
2. Arctander S. *Perfume and flavour materials of natural origin*. Allured Publishing, USA, 1994.
3. Leung A, Foster S. *Encyclopedia of common natural ingredients used in food, drugs and cosmetics*. 2nd edn, John Wiley and Sons, USA, 1996.
4. Tisserand R. *The art of aromatherapy*. The C.W. Daniel Company Limited, Great Britain, 1979.
5. Ramadan A et al, *Some pharmacodynamic effects and antimicrobial activity of essential oils of certain plants used in Egyptian folk medicine*. Vet Med J Giza, 42(1): 263–270. Cited in the Aromatherapy Database, Bob Harris, Essential Oil Resource Consultants, UK, 2000.
6. Jain SR, Kar A. *The antibacterial activity of some essential oils and their combinations*. Planta Medica, 20(2): 118–123. Cited in the Aromatherapy Database, Bob Harris, Essential Oil Resource Consultants, UK, 2000.
7. Davis P. *Aromatherapy: An A–Z*. 2nd edn, The C.W. Daniel Company Limited, Great Britain, 1999.
8. Holmes P. *The energetics of western herbs Vol II*. Artemis Press, USA 1989.
9. Lawless J. *The encyclopaedia of essential oils*. Element Books Limited, Great Britain, 1992.
10. Worwood V. *The fragrant mind*. Doubleday, Great Britain, 1995.
11. Davis P. *Subtle aromatherapy*. The C.W. Daniel Company Limited, Great Britain, 1991.

Cajeput

Melaleuca cajeputi

Synonyms

M. leucadendron var. *cajeputi*, also known in Malaysia and Indonesia as *kayaputi* and *cajeputi*, and in the USA as punk tree.[1]

Family

Myrtaceae

Botany and Origins

M. cajeputi is a medium-sized tree to 30 m, with a single trunk to 1.5 m, but several stems may grow from the original root stock. The trees often have small crowns, especially in pure stands, with smaller branches and often slender twigs. The bark is whitish, papery, thin and flaking.[1]

Method of Extraction

Cajeput oil is steam-distilled from the fresh leaves and twigs of *M. cajeputi*.

Essential Oil Characteristics

The essential oil is a colourless to pale-yellow or greenish-coloured liquid with a powerful fresh, eucalyptus-like and camphoraceous odour.

Historical and Traditional Uses

Cajeput has been traditionally used for its antiseptic, carminative and local analgesic properties by Australian aborigines.

> *Cajeput has been used by local aborigines on Groote Eylandt for the treatment of aches and pains. The leaves are crushed in the hand and rubbed on. Sometimes young leaves and twigs are crushed and steeped in hot water; the liquid is used to bathe the affected area and the rest is poured over the head. Crushed leaves are sniffed to cure headache.*[2]

Cajeput has long been used in Malaysia and Indonesia for its therapeutic values. It was considered particularly valuable for colds, flus and chronic rheumatism and was prescribed for cholera. It was first introduced to Europe in the 17th century. Until the Dutch gained territory in the Moluccas, it remained a very rare and expensive oil in France.[3]

Ryman says that cajeput was first mentioned in *The Natural History of Simple Drugs* by Dr G Guibourt in 1876. He described its properties as antiseptic for intestinal problems, dysentery, enteritis, urinary complaints, cystitis and infections of the urethra.[3]

Chemical Composition

A typical chemical composition of cajeput is reported as follows:

α-pinene (38.9%), β-pinene (1.5%), myrcene (0.5%), α-terpinene (0.2%), limonene (2.9%), 1,8-cineole (21.1%), γ-terpinene (1.0%), p-cymene (3.1%), terpinolene (0.8%), linalool (0.3%), terpinen-4-ol (1.9%), α-terpineol (3.3%).[4]

Therapeutic Actions

Analgesic, antiseptic, antispasmodic, expectorant, febrifuge, stimulant, sudorific, vermifuge.

Pharmacology and Clinical Studies

Cajeput oil is reported to have carminative, stimulant, diaphoretic and antimicrobial properties.[5]

Indications

Digestive System

Soothes colic and inflammation of the intestines such as enteritis, dysentery, gastric spasm and intestinal parasites.[6]

Integumentary System

It is used to alleviate itching due to insect bites, and the relief of eczema and psoriasis.[6]

Musculoskeletal System

Cajeput oil is used in a massage oil or an ointment for all painful conditions, especially arthritis and rheumatism. Its pain-relieving properties make it useful in massage for neuralgia, gout, sciatica, lumbago, sports injuries, muscle stiffness and general aches and pain.[5,6,9]

Nervous System

Cajeput oil is a tonic to the nervous system and may be used to alleviate fatigue, drowsiness and restlessness.[5]

Respiratory System

Cajeput oil is recommended for catarrhal conditions such as asthma, sinusitis, sore throats, coughs, colds and flus. A steam inhalation with cajeput is recommended for cleansing the congested nasal passages. It has analgesic properties that will help to reduce the discomfort of sore throats.[5,6,7,8,10]

Skin Care

It is recommended for the treatment of oily skin.[7]

Energetics

Cajeput is described as having a hot, stimulating nature and it is recommended for *cold* and *deficient* conditions.[9]

Mode of Administration

Topical application — massage, compress, bath, ointment, skin care; Inhalation — direct inhalation, diffuser, oil vaporiser, steam inhalation.

Safety

Cajeput is non-toxic and non-sensitising. However, Davis says that it can irritate the skin, therefore it needs to be well diluted and never allowed to come into contact with mucous membranes.[10]

References

1. Weiss EA. *Essential oil crops*. CAB International, UK, 1997.
2. Lassak EV, McCarthy T. *Australian medicinal plants*. Methuen Australia, Australia, 1983.
3. Ryman D. *Aromatherapy*. Piatkus Publishers, Great Britain, 1991.

4. Williams L. *The composition and bactericidal activity of the oil of melaleuca alternifolia. The International Journal of Aromatherapy.* 1989; 1(3): 15.
5. Leung A, Foster S. *Encyclopedia of common natural ingredients used in food, drugs and cosmetics.* 2nd edn, John Wiley and Sons, USA, 1996.
6. Blumenthal M et al. *The complete German commission E monographs: Therapeutic guide to herbal medicine.* American Botanical Council USA, 1998.
7. Lawless J. *The encyclopaedia of essential oils.* Element Books Limited, Great Britain, 1992.
8. Schnaubelt K. *Medical aromatherapy.* Frog Ltd, USA, 1999.
9. Holmes P. *The energetics of western herbs Vol II.* Artemis Press, USA 1989.
10. Davis P. *Aromatherapy: An A–Z.* 2nd edn, The C.W. Daniel Company Limited, Great Britain, 1999.

Cardamom

Elettaria cardamomum

Synonyms

Cardamom seed and cardamon

Family

Zingiberaceae

Botany and Origins

Cardamom is a perennial herb with lance-shaped leaves borne on long sheathing stems, up to 4 m high. It is a native of tropical Asia and is now cultivated in Sri Lanka, India, Guatemala and El Salvador.

Method of Extraction

Cardamom oil is produced by the steam distillation of the seeds of *E. cardamomum.* The seeds are enclosed in husks and should not be removed from the almost odourless hulls until prior to distillation.

Characteristics

Cardamom oil is an almost colourless or pale-yellow liquid which darkens when exposed to sunlight. The odour of cardamom is warm-spicy with a slightly penetrating camphoraceous-cineole-like odour. The odour becomes balsamic-woody with a sweet and almost floral dry-out.[1]

Essential oil produced from the 'green' types of cardamom smells more of cineole than the oil produced from the bleached or pale-yellow-coloured cardamom seeds.[1]

Historical and Traditional Uses

Cardamom is reputed to be one of the oldest spices known. It has been used for thousands of years in Chinese and Ayurvedic medicine. It was bought to Europe by the Greeks in the 4th century BC.[2]

The name *cardamom* is thought to have originated from the Arab word *hehmama*, a derivation of the Sanskrit term for something hot and pungent. The seeds have remained an important culinary spice not only in India but all over the world.[2]

Chemical Composition

A typical chemical composition of cardamom is reported as follows:

α-pinene (1.5%), β-pinene (0.2%), sabinene (2.8%), myrcene (1.6%), α-phellandrene (0.2%), limonene (11.6%), 1,8-cineole (36.3%), γ-terpinolene (0.5%), linalool (3.0%), linalyl acetate (2.5%), terpinen-4-ol (0.9%), α-terpineol (2.6%), α-terpinyl acetate (31.3%), citronellol (0.3%), nerol (0.5%), geraniol (0.5%), methyl eugenol (0.2%), trans-nerolidol (2.7%).[3]

Therapeutic Actions

Antiseptic, antispasmodic, carminative, cephalic, digestive, diuretic, expectorant, stimulant, stomachic, tonic.

Pharmacology and Clinical Studies

Cardamom oil has been reported to have antispasmodic activity on excised mouse intestine.[4] The oil has anti-inflammatory, analgesic and antispasmodic properties.[5] Cardamom oil was found to have significant analgesic activity, and had a suppressive action of carrageenan-induced oedema, exerting its effect by reducing the synthesis of eicosanoid mediators of inflammation.[5]

Indications

Digestive System

Cardamom is reputed to be a general tonic of the body. It is also recommended for the treatment of digestive complaints such as colic, cramps, dyspepsia and flatulence.[6,7,9]

Nervous System

Cardamom oil has been described as a cephalic and a gentle tonic of the nervous system.[2] It is also recommended for nervous exhaustion and depression.[6]

Respiratory System

Cardamom oil is recommended for catarrhal conditions of the respiratory system such as chronic bronchitis.[6]

Skin Care

Cardamom is generally not used in skin care.

Energetics

Cardamom oil is a *Qi* tonic. It has warming qualities which make it an excellent choice as a digestive stimulant and as a remedy for mucolytic damp catarrhal conditions of the respiratory and digestive system.[6]

It is indicated for problems associated with the earth element. It is ideal for persons burdened by worries and by responsibilities that test our endurance.[2]

Personality Profile

Cardamom personalities are strong, forthright, motivating and enthusiastic; they instil inspiration in others and tend to make good leaders.[8]

Mode of Administration

Topical application — massage, compress, bath; Inhalation — direct inhalation, diffuser, oil vaporiser.

Safety

Cardamom oil is non-toxic, non-irritant and non-sensitising.

References

1. Arctander S. *Perfume and flavour materials of natural origin.* Allured Publishing, USA, 1994.
2. Mojay G. *Aromatherapy for healing the spirit.* Hodder and Stoughton, UK, 1996.
3. Lawrence B. *Major tropical spices — cardamom.* Essential Oils 1976–1978. Allured Publishing, USA.
4. Leung A, Foster S. *Encyclopedia of common natural ingredients used in food, drugs and cosmetics.* 2nd edn, John Wiley and Sons, USA, 1996.
5. Al-Zuhair H, El-Sayeh B, Ammen HA, Al Shoora H. *Pharmacological studies of cardamom in animals.* Pharmacological Research, 34(1/2): 79–82. Cited in the Aromatherapy Database, Bob Harris, Essential Oil Resource Consultants, UK, 2000.
6. Holmes P. *The energetics of western herbs Vol I.* Artemis Press, USA, 1989.
7. Lawless J. *The encyclopaedia of essential oils.* Element Books Limited, Great Britain, 1992.
8. Worwood V. *The fragrant mind.* Doubleday, Great Britain, 1995.
9. Lavabre M. *Aromatherapy workbook.* Healing Art Press, USA, 1997.

Carrot Seed

Daucus carota

Synonyms

Oil of carrot, wild carrot

Family

Umbelliferae or Apiaceae

Botany and Origins

Carrot is an annual or biennial herb with erect multi-branched stems up to 1.5 m high. The common cultivated carrot, *D. carota* L. subsp. *sativus*, has an edible fleshy orange-red tap root, while the wild carrot, *D. carota* L. subsp. *carota*, has an inedible, tough whitish root. Wild carrot is a native to Europe, Asia and North America.[1]

Method of Extraction

Carrot seed oil is steam-distilled from the dried seed of the wild carrot. The essential oil is produced in France, Holland and Hungary.

A carrot root oil is obtained by solvent extraction of the red fleshy root of the common edible carrot root. It has a high concentration of carotenes.

Essential Oil Characteristics

Carrot seed oil is a yellow or amber-coloured to pale-orange-brown liquid with a peculiar dry-woody somewhat earthy odour. The top note is sweet and fresh, but the tenacious undertone and dry-out is very heavy, earthy and slightly spicy.[2]

Historical and Traditional Uses

Carrot is better known for its edible root than its essential oil. Most of the historical references refer to the carrot root and not the essential oil from the seed.

Carrot seed oil is used as a fragrance component in soaps, detergents, creams, lotions and perfumes. Carrot root oil is used in some sun-screen preparations and as a source of β-carotene and vitamin A.[1]

Chemical Composition

Carrot seed oil contains α-pinene (up to 13.3%), β-pinene (up to 18.29%), carotol (up to 18.29%), ducol, limonene, β-bisabolene, β-elemene, *cis*-β-bergamotene, γ-decalactone, β-farnesene, geraniol, geranyl acetate (up to 10.39%), caryophyllene, caryophyllene oxide, methyl eugenol, nerolidol, eugenol, *trans*-asarone, vanillin, asorone, α-terpineol, terpinen-4-ol, γ-decanolactone, coumarin and β-selinene.[1]

Therapeutic Actions

Carminative, cytophylactic, depurative, diuretic, emmenagogue, hepatic.

Pharmacology and Clinical Studies

Carrot seed oil has been reported to exhibit vasodilatory and smooth-muscle relaxant effects on isolated animal organs. It also depressed cardiac action in frog and dog hearts, among other activities.[1]

Indications

Detoxification

It is highly regarded for its hepatic, depurative and diuretic properties. Carrot seed oil is an excellent regenerator of liver cells and should be prescribed after the acute phase of hepatitis, a violent bilious attack, drug poisoning, but not at the critical moment of the pathology.[3]

Integumentary System
The excellent depurative property of carrot seed oil means that it can be used to treat eczema, psoriasis and ulcerative conditions of the skin.[3,5,7]

Carrot seed is excellent as a cellular regenerator for the skin. It vitalises the hypodermis and is recommended for the treatment of aged skin, dermatitis, skin irritations, skin rashes and wrinkles.[3,4,5] For this purpose, Mailhebiau recommends blending it with lavender and wheatgerm oil.[3]

Skin Care
It can be used to improve the complexion of the skin and has been described as one of the strongest revitalising essential oils. It is recommended for dull, pallid, lifeless and tired skin which is tired from environmental stress.[4]

Personality Profile

Mailhebiau refers to *D. carota* as the symbol of life or death, the gift of self or egoism in the middle of the crowd, for those who seem to use both these tendencies according to the opportunity of the moment and the advantage that one hopes to get out of it.[3]

Mode of Administration

Topical application — massage, compress, bath, skin care; Inhalation — direct inhalation, diffuser, oil vaporiser.

Safety

Carrot seed essential oil is non-toxic, non-irritant and non-sensitising.

References

1. Leung A, Foster S. *Encyclopedia of common natural ingredients used in food, drugs and cosmetics*. 2nd edn, John Wiley and Sons, USA, 1996.
2. Arctander S. *Perfume and flavour materials of natural origin*. Allured Publishing, USA, 1994.
3. Mailhebiau P. *Portraits in oils*. The C.W. Daniel Company Limited, Great Britain, 1995.
4. Lavabre M. *Aromatherapy workbook*. Healing Art Press, USA, 1997.
5. Schnaubelt K. *Advanced aromatherapy*. Healing Art Press, USA, 1995.
6. Lawless J. *The encyclopaedia of essential oils*. Element Books Limited, Great Britain, 1992.
7. Davis P. *Aromatherapy: An A–Z*. 2nd edn, The C.W. Daniel Company Limited, Great Britain, 1999.

Cedarwood, Atlas

Cedrus atlantica

Synonyms

Moroccan Cedarwood

Family

Pinaceae

Botany and Origins

Atlas cedarwood is believed to have originated from the famous Lebanon cedars which grow wild in Lebanon and on the island of Cyprus. These trees are now protected from being felled for essential oil distillation or lumber.[1]

Atlas cedarwood is entirely different from Virginian cedarwood oil — both chemically and olfactorily. The tree *C. atlantica* is a pine, not a cypress such as the Virginian cedarwood.

Atlas cedarwood is related to *C. deodara* and *C. libani*. *C. deodara* is known as Himalayan Cedarwood, which grows at high altitude in the Himalaya mountains. *C. libani* is known as Lebanon cedarwood and grows wild in the mountains of Lebanon and on the island of Cyprus. The tree is protected by law against felling or any kind of exploitation. Any oil offered as Lebanon cedarwood oil is most likely to be oil distilled from *C. atlantica*.

Method of Extraction

Atlas cedarwood is steam-distilled from the wood, stumps or from the sawdust. Most of the distillation takes place in Morocco and the north-western regions of Algeria.[1]

The best quality essential oil is obtained from distilling wood chips from trees that are 20 to 30 years old. The essential oil distilled from the heartwood is considered warmer, more balsamic and aromatic.[2]

Essential Oil Characteristics

Atlas cedarwood is a yellowish to orange-yellow or deep amber-coloured, viscous oil that is occasionally turbid. Its odour is described as interesting to say the least — it is not exactly pleasant with a slightly camphoraceous-cresylic top note with a sweet, tenacious woody undertone.[1]

Historical and Traditional Uses

Atlas cedarwood was believed to used by the ancient Egyptians for embalming purposes, cosmetics and perfumery. The Lebanon cedar was prized as a building wood.[3] The cedar trees were mentioned in the bible, symbolising everything that was fertile and abundant. Later, Dioscorides and Galen referred to cedar's resin being used to preserve the body from putrefaction. In 1698, Nicholas Lemery mentioned the therapeutic nature of the oil as a urinary and pulmonary antiseptic. Doctors Michel and Gilbert in France recorded in 1925 the good results obtained in cases of chronic bronchitis.[4]

According to the Song of Solomon, cedarwood was used to build Solomon's temple. Cedarwood symbolised abundance, fertility and spiritual strength. The name *Cedrus* originates from the Arabic word *kedron*, meaning 'power'.[6]

Chemical Composition

The presence of 7 to 10% sesquiterpene ketones gives Atlas cedarwood oil an anti-inflammatory action which acts in the first phase of inflammation (reduction of globulins), associated with a mucolytic effect; this also gives an effective action in certain afflictions such as hay fever.[2]

The sesquiterpene alcohols (approximately 7%) take part in decongestive action on the mucosa. The richness in sesquiterpenes helps the anti-inflammatory action, most particularly in arteriocapillary pathologies and in the case of cellulite.[2]

A typical chemical profile of *C. atlantica* is as follows:

Sesquiterpenes (himachalenes 14.5%, α-himachalene 10%, β-himachalene 42%, cis-bisabolene 1.2%); sesquiterpene alcohols (himachalol 4%, allo-himachalol 2.3%); ketones (α-atlantone 2.65%, γ-atlantone 5%); oxides (himachalene oxide 1%).[2]

Pharmacology and Clinical Studies

A clinical study was conducted, in which *C. atlantica* essential oil was used in an aromatherapy massage blend for the treatment of *alopecia areata* — a disorder in which the hair falls out in patches, producing baldness. Although the results were variable, the group using the massage blend containing Atlas cedarwood showed a significant improvement of 44%.[5]

Therapeutic Actions

Antiseptic, astringent, antiseborrheic, diuretic, expectorant, insecticide, sedative.

Indications

Lymphatic System

Atlas cedarwood is reputed to encourage lymphatic drainage and stimulate the breakdown of accumulated fats. It is mildly diuretic and may be used for the treatment of cellulite and oedema.[6]

Nervous System

Atlas cedarwood may be used for reducing stress, anxiety and tension.[3,6,7,11]

Respiratory System

The presence of sesquiterpene ketones gives Atlas cedarwood oil its excellent mucolytic effect and may be used for treating catarrhal conditions, coughs and chronic bronchitis.[3,7,11]

Urinary System

The oil is recommended for the treatment of cystitis and urinary tract infections.[3,6,7]

Skin Care

Because of its astringent and antiseptic properties Atlas cedarwood is recommended in hair and skin care for improving oily skin, acne, dandruff and seborrhoea of the scalp.[3,6,11] It is also reputed to strengthen hair growth and alleviate dandruff.[3,7]

Energetics

Atlas cedarwood is fortifying and strengthening and it is considered a powerful tonic of the body's *Qi*.[6] The oil is tonifying to the kidneys and spleen-pancreas and may be used for general lethargy, nervous debility, lower backache and poor concentration.[6]

The oil is effective in treating conditions classified as cold damp. It has decongesting qualities and combined with its antiseptic properties it is useful for genitourinary and respiratory infections.[6]

Personality Profile

The qualities of Atlas cedarwood are grounding, strengthening and dignity.[8] Worwood describes the cedarwood personality as someone gliding through life as if they had a royal charter. They may actually appear haughty and just too grand to be approached about anything mundane, but this assumption is usually incorrect as they are a tower of strength in almost all situations. Cedarwood personalities instil confidence and security in people less able to cope with life's stresses and strains.[8]

Subtle Aromatherapy

Atlas cedarwood has a strengthening and comforting effect:

> *The essential oil of cedarwood is warming, harmonising and thought to be life giving. It calms during times of fear and nervous tension. In difficult situations the oil may provide comfort and warmth, and help stabilise energies thrown out of balance.*[7]

Cedarwood oil can give us immovable strength in times of crisis. Steadying the conscious mind, it will help us to resist the sudden events and powerful emotions that threaten to undermine our confidence and morale.[6]

Mode of Administration

Topical application — massage, compress, bath, sitz bath, douche, skin care; Inhalation — direct inhalation, diffuser, oil vaporiser.

Safety

Atlas cedarwood is non-toxic, non-irritant and non-sensitising.

Price, Lawless and Fischer-Rizzi say that *C. atlantica* should not be used during pregnancy.[3,7,9] It is said to have neurotoxic and abortive effects; toxic doses are cumulative.[9] Tisserand and Balacs state that Atlas cedarwood is safe to use and do not suggest that it should be contra-indicated during pregnancy.[10]

References

1. Arctander S. *Perfume and flavour materials of natural origin.* Allured Publishing, USA, 1994.
2. Collins P. *Cedarwood.* The Aromatherapist, 1996; 3(2): 30–33.
3. Lawless J. *The encyclopaedia of essential oils.* Element Books Limited, Great Britain, 1992.
4. Ryman D. *Aromatherapy.* Piatkus Ltd, Great Britain, 1991.
5. Hay, IC, Jamieson. M, Ormerod, AD, *Randomized trial of aromatherapy: Successful treatment of alopecia areata.* Arch Dermatol 1998; 134: 1349–1352. Cited in the Aromatherapy Database, Bob Harris, Essential Oil Resource Consultants, UK, 2000.
6. Mojay G. *Aromatherapy for healing the spirit.* Hodder and Stoughton, UK, 1996.
7. Fischer-Rizzi S. *Complete aromatherapy handbook.* Sterling Publishing Company, USA, 1990.
8. Worwood V. *The fragrant mind.* Doubleday, Great Britain, 1995.
9. Price S, Price L. *Aromatherapy for health professionals.* Churchill Livingstone, UK, 1995.
10. Tisserand R, Balacs T. *Essential oil safety.* Churchill Livingstone, UK, 1993.
11. Davis P. *Aromatherapy: An A–Z.* 2nd edn, The C.W. Daniel Company Limited, Great Britain, 1999.

Cedarwood, Virginian

Juniperus virginiana

Synonyms

Cedar oil, red cedarwood

Family

Cupressaceae

Botany and Origins

J. virginiana is a slow-growing evergreen tree with a narrow, dense and pyramidal crown. It grows in a fairly continuous belt running approximately from the central part of Virginia, through North Carolina and the northern edge of South Carolina, into Tennessee, central Kentucky and northern Alabama.[1]

Other species include the *J. Sabina,* known as savin, *J. mexicana,* known as Texas cedarwood, and *J. procera,* known as East Africa cedarwood.

Texas cedarwood is a small alpine evergreen tree up to 7 m tall. It is a small and poor-looking relative of the cypress. The oil is steam-distilled from the heartwood of this tree which is felled exclusively for the purpose of producing the essential oil which is extensively used in perfumery.[2]

East African cedarwood is steam-distilled from the waste wood in the sawmills of Kenya, where the wood is extensively used for the manufacture of pencils, boxes and wood carvings.

Method of Extraction

Virginian cedarwood oil is obtained by steam distillation of the wood, sawdust, shavings and other lumber wastes of *J. virginiana.*

Essential Oil Characteristics

Virginian cedarwood oil is a pale-yellow to slightly orange-yellow-coloured oil that is slightly less viscous than Atlas cedarwood. The odour is at first oily and woody with a sweet balsamic scent typical of cedarwood lumber. The odour becomes drier and more woody, less balsamic as the oil dries out.[2]

Historical and Traditional Uses

The wood from *J. virginiana* is highly prized for furniture making. Older trees are preferred since they contain more of the reddish heartwood which not only gives a beautiful surface when polished, but also yields more essential oil than wood from young trees.[2]

Virginian cedarwood oil has been used as an insect repellent. Decoctions of the leaves, barks, twigs and fruit were used to treat conditions such as coughs, bronchitis, rheumatism, venereal warts and skin rashes.[3]

Chemical Composition

According to Guenther, trees less than 25 years old should not be felled. Older trees will yield about 3.5% of the volatile oil while younger trees will yield less than 1%. He states that the oil distilled from the older trees and younger trees differs considerably in regard to the odour and chemical composition. Oil produced from older trees is higher in high boiling point constituents while oil from younger trees is richer in cedrol.[1]
A comparion of the chemical compositions of *J. virginiana* and *J. mexicana* is as follows:[4]

Constituent	Virginiana	Texas
α-cedrene	20.0%	21.2%
β-cedrene	6.6%	4.9%
thujopsene	18.9%	29.0%
other sesquiterpenes	13.3%	15.5%
cedrol	31.6%	25.0%
widdrol	4.8%	4.2%

Pharmacology and Clinical Studies

No pharmacological or clinical studies could be found for *J. virginiana*.

Therapeutic Actions

Antiseptic, astringent, antiseborrhoeic, diuretic, emmenagogue, expectorant, insecticide, sedative.

Indications

While the odour profiles of Atlas and Virginian cedarwood are very different the two oils seem to share similar properties.

Nervous System

Virginian cedarwood oil has a sedative effect, and may be used in conditions associated with anxiety and nervous tension.[6] It is generally more useful for chronic conditions than acute ones.[5]

Respiratory System

Virginian cedarwood oil is recommended for treating catarrhal conditions, coughs and chronic bronchitis.[3,7,11]

Urinary System

The oil is recommended for the treatment of cystitis and urinary tract infections.[3,6,7]

Skin Care

Because of its astringent and antiseptic properties Virginian cedarwood is recommended in hair and skin care for improving oily skin, acne, dandruff and seborrhoea of the scalp.[5,6,8] It is regarded as an excellent insect repellent.[5]

Energetics

Virginian cedarwood is fortifying and strengthening and is considered a powerful tonic of the body's *Qi*. The oil is tonifying to the kidneys and spleen-pancreas and may be used for general lethargy, nervous debility, lower backache and poor concentration.[8]

Subtle Aromatherapy

Virginian cedarwood can assist an individual to take a negative or threatening situation and transform it into an experience from which strength and wisdom can be derived.[8]

Mode of Administration

Topical application — massage, compress, bath, sitz bath, douche, skin care; Inhalation — direct inhalation, diffuser, oil vaporiser.

Safety

Virginian cedarwood is non-toxic, non-irritant and non-sensitising. However, Lawless says that Virginian cedarwood should not be used during pregnancy.[6]

Tisserand and Balacs state that Virginian cedarwood is safe to use and they do not suggest that it should be contra-indicated during pregnancy.[9]

I believe that Virginian cedarwood is one of those oils whose botanical name may have been confused with savin — *J. sabina,* a highly toxic oil which is contra-indicated during pregnancy.

References

1. Guenther E. *The essential oils — volume VI.* Robert E. Krieger Publishing Company, USA, 1982.
2. Arctander S. *Perfume and flavour materials of natural origin.* Allured Publishing, USA, 1994.
3. Leung A, Foster S. *Encyclopedia of common natural ingredients used in food, drugs and cosmetics.* 2nd edn, John Wiley and Sons Inc. USA, 1996.
4. Lawrence B. *Virginian and Texan cedarwood oil.* Perfumer and Flavorist 1980; 5(3): 63.
5. Tisserand R. *The art of aromatherapy.* The C.W. Daniel Company Limited, Great Britain, 1977.
6. Lawless J. *The encyclopaedia of essential oils.* Element Books Limited, Great Britain, 1992.
7. Fischer-Rizzi S. *Complete aromatherapy handbook.* Sterling Publishing Company, USA, 1990.
8. Mojay G. *Aromatherapy for healing the spirit.* Hodder and Stoughton, UK, 1996.
9. Tisserand R, Balacs T. *Essential oil safety.* Churchill Livingstone, UK, 1993.

Chamomile, German

Matricaria recutita

Synonyms

Blue chamomile, Hungarian chamomile, *M. chamomilla*

Family

Compositae or Asteraceae

Botany and Origins

German chamomile is a fragrant, low annual herb, up to 0.6 m tall with delicate feather leaves and simple daisy-like white flowers on single stem.

It is native to Europe, particularly to central and northern Europe. It is cultivated in Hungary, Yugoslavia, Bulgaria, Russia, Germany, Belgium and Spain. Hungary is one of the main producers of the oil.[1]

Frequent changes in the interpretation of the scientific name of German chamomile have led to confusion over the past two decades. The current accepted scientific name is *M. recutita*, though *C. recutita* and, to a lesser extent, *M. chamomilla* are commonly seen in literature.[2]

Method of Extraction

German chamomile oil is steam-distilled from the dried flower heads of *M. recutita*. The essential oil content is highest at the beginning of flowering. Drying the flowers at 40–45°C is reported to preserve the matricarin and the essential oil is reputed to be the best.[3]

Essential Oil Characteristics

German chamomile oil is a deep, inky-blue somewhat viscous oil with an intensely sweet, herbaceous odour with a fresh fruity undertone.[1] The pure undiluted oil has an intense odour which many find overwhelming and unpleasant.

Historical and Traditional Uses

Since antiquity chamomile flowers have been used internally for digestive disorders and externally for skin and mucous membrane irritations. It has been difficult to ascertain which species were used historically, as many plants within the *Compositae* family or, in the most recent botanical nomenclature, *Asteraceae* family, were referred to by the common name of Chamomile.[4]

German chamomile flowers are extensively used as a herbal tea. The oil is extensively used in cosmetics.[2]

Chemical Composition

A typical chemical composition of German chamomile is reported as follows:

Chamazulene (2.16–35.59%), α-bisabolol (1.72–67.25%), bisabolol oxide A (55.08%), bisabolol oxide B (4.35–18.93%) and bisabolone oxide A (63.85%).[5]

German chamomile essential oil varies in composition according to the source. Four main chemotypes have been identified as follows.[5]

Type A
α-bisabolol oxide B > α-bisabolol oxide A > α-bisabolol

Type B
α-bisabolol oxide A > α-bisabolol oxide B > α-bisabolol

Type C
α-bisabolol > α-bisabolol oxide B > α-bisabolol oxide A

Type D
α-bisabolol oxide B = α-bisabolol oxide A = α-bisabolol

The content and composition of the essential oil are dependent on the development stage of the plant. For example, the quantity of α-bisabolol, α-bisabolol oxide A and B and bisabolone oxide A reached a maximum in full bloom, whereas the farnesene content decreased rapidly with the growth and development of the flower.[4]

Pharmacology and Clinical Studies

The anti-inflammatory properties of German chamomile oil are well documented when used topically.[6,9]

The accepted wisdom is that the anti-inflammatory activity of chamomile is mainly due to chamazulene. This blue compound is formed from matricarin by steam distillation. In other words the compound found naturally in chamomile is matricarin, and this is converted into chamazulene by the action of the steam.[3]

The antiphlogistic effects of (-)-α-bisabolol found in German chamomile have been proven in experiments on adjuvant arthritis in rats.[8]

Experiments showed that (-)-α-bisabolol had a greater effect than bisabolol oxides A and B. It was suggested that standardising the content of (-)-α-bisabolol was important to the antiphlogistic effectiveness of chamomile.[7]

When sourcing German chamomile oil for its antispasmodic and anti-inflammatory properties, attention should be paid to the presence of (-)-α-bisabolol, as it contributes greatly to its effects.

German chamomile oil is rich in monoterpenes and sesquiterpenes which exhibit cholagogue and choleretic activity.[10] The herbal extract and essential oil have a dose-dependent spasmolytic effect on the smooth muscle of the intestine and also demonstrated liver-regenerating properties.[11,12]

The above research confirms the traditional uses of German chamomile. In many instances it is preferred to use the whole extract rather than just the essential oil alone; in this way the lipophilic and hydrophilic constituents can be utilised.

Therapeutic Actions

Analgesic, anti-allergenic, anti-inflammatory, antiphlogistic, antispasmodic, bactericidal, carminative, cicatrisant, cholagogue, emmenagogue, hepatic, sedative, stomachic, vulnerary.

Indications

Children's Remedy

German chamomile is considered one of the gentlest of essential oils and is particularly beneficial for treating children. It may be used to alleviate the pain associated with teething infants.[13,17]

Digestive System
German chamomile oil can be used in treating colic, dyspepsia and indigestion.[13,18] The oil stimulates the liver and gall bladder and is recommended for poor appetite and slow painful digestion.[16,19]

Immune System
Schnaubelt says that an overlooked quality of German chamomile is its ability to neutralise toxic bacterial metabolic wastes, which are often the cause of fever during acute illness.[14] German chamomile is reputed to stimulate leukocyte production. However, for this purpose, Valnet recommends the internal use of German chamomile.[15]

Integumentary System
German chamomile can be used for wounds that are slow to heal such as open leg sores, abscesses and infected ingrown nails.[18] It is important for the treatment of eczema, urticaria and dry, itchy conditions.[13,17]

Musculoskeletal System
German chamomile oil can be used in a massage for muscular aches and pain, and for inflamed joints associated with rheumatoid arthritis. It is beneficial in treating sprains, inflamed tendons and swollen painful joints in bursitis.[2,13,17]

Reproductive System
German chamomile oil is recommended for promoting and harmonising the menses, for spasmodic dysmenorrhoea and PMS.[18,19]

Urinary System
German chamomile oil is especially beneficial for urinary tract infections such as cystitis.[17] Davis recommends drinking chamomile tea and having compresses and massages over the lower abdomen with the oil. The oil should also be used in a bath.[17]

Skin Care
German chamomile oil is beneficial for sensitive skin problems. It is a local vasoconstrictor and can reduce the redness of cheeks due to enlarged capillaries.[17]

Energetics
According to the principles of TCM, German chamomile promotes the free flow of *Qi* which is important for relaxing the nerves, relieving spasms and easing pain. This makes it beneficial for nervous tension, insomnia, indigestion and headaches.[19,20]

Personality Profile
The German chamomile personalities are very strong, emotional people. They have emotional depth and the ability to draw out the best in other people, but keep their own feelings to themselves. They are usually down-to-earth and up-front. They are always good to have around in an emotional storm, or when grieving, as they provide a strong, solid shoulder to cry on if needed.[21]

Subtle Aromatherapy
German chamomile can be used to counteract agitation or over-activity in any chakra. It should be used to heal the aura wherever heat, redness or anger are present.[22]

Mode of Administration
Topical application — massage, compress, ointment, bath, sitz bath, douche, skin care; Inhalation — direct inhalation, diffuser, oil vaporiser, steam inhalation.

Safety
German chamomile oil has been reported to be non-toxic, non-irritant and non-sensitising.

References

1. Arctander S. *Perfume and flavour materials of natural origin.* Allured Publishing, USA, 1994.
2. Leung A, Foster S. *Encyclopedia of common natural ingredients used in food, drugs and cosmetics.* 2nd edn, John Wiley and Sons, USA, 1996.
3. Balacs T, Tisserand R. *German chamomile.* The International Journal of Aromatherapy, 1998; 9(1): 15–21.
4. Evans WC. *Trease and Evans pharmacognosy.* WB Saunders, 15th edn, UK, 2002.
5. Lawrence B. *Chamomile oil.* Perfumer and Flavorist, 1987; (12)1: 35.
6. Fleischer AM. *Plant extracts: To accelerate healing and reduce inflammation.* Cosmetic Toilet, 1985; 100: 147–153.
7. Isaac O. *Pharmacological investigations with compounds of chamomile.* Planta Med 1979; 35: 188–194. Cited in the Aromatherapy Database, Bob Harris, Essential Oil Resource Consultants, UK, 2000.
8. Jakovlev V, Isaac O, Thiemer K, Kunde R. *Pharmacolgocal investigations with compounds of chamomile. New investigations on the antiphlogistic effects of (-)-a-bisabolol and bisabolol oxides.* Planta Medica, 1979; 35: 125-140. Cited in the Aromatherapy Database, by Bob Harris, Essential Oil Resource Consultants, UK, 2000.
9. Maiche AG et al. *Effect of chamomile cream and almond ointment on acute radiation skin reaction.* Acta Oncol, 1991; 30(3): 395–396. Cited in the Aromatherapy Database, Bob Harris, Essential Oil Resource Consultants, UK, 2000.
10. Rangelov A. *An experimental characterisation of cholagogic and choleretic activity of a group of essential oils.*

Folia Medica, 1989; 31(1): 46–53. Cited in the Aromatherapy Database, Bob Harris, Essential Oil Resource Consultants, UK, 2000.

11. Acterrath-Tuckermann U et al. *Pharmacological investigations with the compounds of chamomile.* Planta Medica, 1980; 39: 38–50. Cited in the Aromatherapy Database, Bob Harris, Essential Oil Resource Consultants, UK, 2000.
12. Gershbein L. *Regeneration of rat liver in the presence of essential oils and their components.* Food Cosmet Toxicol, 1977; 15(3): 173–182.
13. Lawless J. *The encyclopaedia of essential oils.* Element Books Limited, Great Britain, 1992.
14. Schnaubelt K. *Medical aromatherapy.* Frog Ltd, USA, 1999.
15. Valnet J. *The practice of aromatherapy.* The C.W. Daniel Company Limited, Great Britain, 1980.
16. Lavabre M. *Aromatherapy workbook.* Healing Art Press, USA, 1997.
17. Davis P. *Aromatherapy: An A–Z.* 2nd edn, The C.W. Daniel Company Limited, Great Britain, 1999.
18. Fischer-Rizzi S. *Complete aromatherapy handbook.* Sterling Publishing Company, USA, 1990.
19. Holmes P. *The energetics of western herbs Vol. II,* Artemis Press, USA, 1986.
20. Mojay G. *Aromatherapy for healing the spirit.* Hodder and Stoughton, UK, 1996
21. Worwood V. *The fragrant mind.* Doubleday, Great Britain, 1995.
22. Davis P. *Subtle Aromatherapy.* The C.W. Daniel Company Limited, Great Britain, 1991.

Chamomile, Roman

Anthemis nobilis

Synonyms

Chamaemelum nobile, Garden chamomile

Family

Compositae or Asteraceae

Botany and Origins

Roman chamomile is a pleasant-smelling perennial with feathery fern-like leaves and branched stems of a creeping habit with daisy-like flowers.[1] It is a native of Western Europe and is now cultivated in England, Belgium, France and Hungary.[2]

Roman chamomile's common name is derived from the Greek word *chamaimelon* — *chamai* meaning on the ground, and *melon* an apple, referring to its distinctive smell when fresh.[1]

The botanical name of *Anthemis* is derived from the Greek word *anthos* which means a flower. The plant's specific name of *nobilis* means noble or noted — referring to its healing virtues.[1]

Method of Extraction

Roman chamomile is distilled from the flowering tops of *A. nobilis.*

Essential Oil Characteristics

Roman chamomile is a pale-yellow-coloured, mobile liquid of a sweet herbaceous, somewhat fruity-warm and tealeaf-like odour. The odour is extremely diffusive but it has little tenacity.[2]

Historical and Traditional Uses

Since antiquity, chamomile flowers have been used internally for digestive disorders and externally for skin and mucous membrane irritations. It has been difficult to ascertain which species were used historically, as many plants within the *Compositae* family or, in the most recent botanical nomenclature, *Asteraceae* family, were referred to by the common name of chamomile.[3]

Chamomile has long been known for its therapeutic properties. Decoctions of the whole herb have been taken or applied throughout Europe for the relief of complaints such as:

> *... the wind and pains and torments of the belly, the pain of colic and stone, as a mollifyer of swellings and sinews, inflammation of the bowels, cramps and aches all over, pains and stiches in the side, for weak or irritable stomachs.*[1]

Culpeper was familiar with the pronounced effect that chamomile had on the mind and nervous system. He suggested that it comforts the head and the brain.[4]

Mrs Grieve says that chamomile tea is an old-fashioned but extremely effective remedy for hysterical and nervous afflictions in women, and is also used as an emmenagogue.[3]

Chamomile flowers are recommended as a tonic in dropsical complaints for their diuretic and tonic properties. The flowers may be used in a poultice and fomentation for external swelling, inflammatory pain or congested neuralgia.[4]

Valnet recommends chamomile oil as a stimulant of leucocytosis and for anyone with a low resistance and repeated susceptibility to infection.[5]

Tisserand associates chamomile's ability to soothe restlessness, nervous irritability or impatience with its action on the liver — the emotional state of anger is associated with the choleric humour and the liver according to traditional herbalists.[6]

Chemical Composition

While Roman chamomile shares similar properties with German chamomile, its chemical profile is very different. Roman chamomile essential oil contain very little if any chamazulene or α-bisabolol — the major constituents responsible for German chamomile's anti-inflammatory and anti-allergenic properties.[8]

A typical chemical composition of Roman chamomile is:

α-pinene (0.5–10.0%), camphene (0–0.5%), β-pinene (0–10.0%), sabinene (0–10.0%), myrcene (0–0.5%), 1,8 cineole (0.5–25%), γ-terpinene (0–0.5%), caryophyllene (0–10.0%), propyl angelate (0.5–10.0%), butyl angelate (0.5–10.0%).[7]

Pharmacology and Clinical Studies

Roman chamomile has been identified as having sedative and anti-inflammatory properties.[10] It was found that the oil from the white-headed variety was significantly more sedative than the oil from the yellow-headed variety. The white-headed variety contained significantly more angelic esters and this may have contributed to the increased sedative and anti-inflammatory properties.[11]

Therapeutic Actions

Analgesic, antiphlogistic, antiseptic, antispasmodic, bactericidal, carminative, cholagogue, digestive, emmenagogue, febrifuge, hepatic, sedative, stomachic, sudorific, vulnerary.

Indications

Children's Remedy

Roman chamomile is considered one of the gentlest of essential oils and is particularly beneficial for treating children. It may be used to alleviate the pain associated with teething infants.[13,17]

Digestive System

Roman chamomile is used in treating colic, diarrhoea, poor appetite, indigestion.[12,13,14,16]

Nervous System

The sweet scent of Roman chamomile oil is soothing, calming and antidepressant. It is particularly beneficial for alleviating anxiety and stress.[13,17] It is used to alleviate migraines and headaches and for insomnia.[13,16]

Respiratory System

Roman chamomile oil is recommended as an emergency remedy during an asthma attack. Schnaubelt recommends rubbing the oil on the solar plexus, wrists and temples until more specific help becomes available.[15]

Reproductive System

Roman chamomile oil is very helpful for treating amenorrhea, dysmenorrhea and PMS.[16,18]

Skin Care

Roman chamomile oil is beneficial for sensitive, red or dry skin.

Energetics

According to the principles of TCM, Roman chamomile promotes the free flow of *Qi* which is important for relaxing the nerves, relieving spasms and easing pain. This makes it beneficial for nervous tension, insomnia, indigestion and headaches.[12,19]

Personality Profile

Roman chamomile personalities are full of sunshine and joy, with a harmonious disposition and emotional life. While they are serene and gentle, they sometimes appear to be in a dreamlike state.[20]

Fischer-Rizzi describes the type of person who might benefit from Roman chamomile oil:

> *... someone who feels grumpy, discontented or impatient, chamomile is a good remedy. it is beneficial for people who feel short tempered, self-involved, overly sensitive or rarely satisfied.*[18]

Subtle Aromatherapy

Roman chamomile is harmonising, peaceful and soothing to the spirit.[20] It relates to the throat chakra and can be used to help individuals to express their highest spiritual truth.[21]

Mode of Administration

Topical application — massage, compress, ointment, bath, sitz bath, douche, skin care; Inhalation — direct inhalation, diffuser, oil vaporiser.

Safety

Roman chamomile oil has been reported to be non-toxic, non-irritant and non-sensitising.

Not to be used if allergies to Roman chamomile and other Compositaes exist. The sensitisation potency is moderate and frequency rare.[22]

References

1. Le Strange R. *A history of herbal plants*. Angus and Robertson, UK, 1977.
2. Arctander S. *Perfume and flavour materials of natural origin*. Allured Publishing, USA, 1994.
3. Grieve M. *A modern herbal*. Penguin, Great Britain, 1931.
4. Evans WC. *Trease and Evans pharmacognosy*. 15th edn, WB Saunders, UK, 2002.
5. Valnet J. *The practice of aromatherapy*. The C.W. Daniel Company Limited, Great Britain, 1980.

6. Tisserand R. *The art of aromatherapy*. The C.W. Daniel Company Limited, Great Britain, 1977.
7. Lawrence B. *Roman chamomile oil*. Perfumer and Flavorist, 1981; 6(2): 59.
8. Bruneton J. *Pharmacognosy*. 2nd edn, Lavoisier Publishing Inc, France, 1999.
9. Fleischer AM. *Plant extracts: To accelerate healing and reduce inflammation*. Cosmetic Toilet, 1985: 100; 147–153.
10. Rossi T, Melegari M, Bianchi A, Albasini A, Vampa G. *Sedative, anti-inflammatory and anti-diuretic effects induced in rats by essential oils of varieties of anthemis nobilis: A comparative study*. Pharmacological Research Communications 1988; 20 (suppl 5): 71–74. Cited in the Aromatherapy Database, by Bob Harris, Essential Oil Resource Consultants, UK, 2000.
11. Melegari M et al. *Chemical characteristics and pharmacological properties of the essential oils of Anthemis nobilis*. Fitoterapia, 1989; 59(6): 449–455. Cited in the Aromatherapy Database, Bob Harris, Essential Oil Resource Consultants, UK, 2000.
12. Holmes P. *The energetics of western herbs Vol. II*. Artemis Press, USA, 1989.
13. Lawless J. *The encyclopaedia of essential oils*. Element Books Limited, Great Britain, 1992.
14. Leung A, Foster S., *Encyclopedia of common natural ingredients used in food, drugs and cosmetics*. 2nd edn, John Wiley and Sons Inc, USA, 1996.
15. Schnaubelt K. *Medical aromatherapy*. Frog Ltd, USA, 1999.
16. Lavabre M. *Aromatherapy workbook*. Healing Art Press, USA, 1997.
17. Davis P. *Aromatherapy: An A–Z*. 2nd edn, The C.W. Daniel Company Limited, Great Britain, 1999.
18. Fischer-Rizzi S. *Complete aromatherapy handbook*. Sterling Publishing Company, USA, 1990.
19. Mojay G. *Aromatherapy for healing the spirit*. Hodder and Stoughton, UK, 1996.
20. Worwood V. *The fragrant mind*. Doubleday, Great Britain, 1995.
21. Davis P. *Subtle Aromatherapy*. The C.W. Daniel Company Limited, Great Britain, 1991.
22. Blumenthal M et al. *The complete German commission E monographs: Therapeutic guide to herbal medicine*. American Botanical Council USA, 1998.

Cinnamon

Cinnamomum zeylanicum Blume

Synonyms

Cinnamomum verum

Family

Lauraceae

Botany and Origins

Cinnamon is a bushy, evergreen tree up to 15 m. The bark and leaves are strongly aromatic. Three distinct essential oils (bark, leaf and root) are produced from the cinnamon tree.

Cinnamon is often confused with *C. cassia*, which is known as cassia. Cinnamon is native to Sri Lanka, India and South East Asia. It has been introduced to the Seychelles, Zanzibar and Indonesia. Cinnamon produces the finest bark in sunny regions with an average temperature of 27–30°C.[1]

Method of Extraction

Cinnamon bark essential oil is obtained by steam or water distillation with cohobation. Cinnamon bark contains water-soluble volatile aromatic components, which can be recovered by extracting distillation water and adding the extract to water-distilled oil.[1]

Essential Oil Characteristics

Cinnamon bark oil is a pale-yellow to dark-yellow or brownish-yellow liquid with an extremely powerful, diffusive, warm-spicy and tenacious odour.[2]

Cinnamon leaf oil is a yellow to brownish-yellow oil with a warm-spicy, but rather harsh odour which lacks the rich body of the bark oil. It has some resemblance to the odour of clove leaf and clove stem oil.[2]

Historical and Traditional Uses

Both cassia and cinnamon have been used for several thousand years in Eastern and Western cultures in treating chronic diarrhoea, rheumatism, colds, abdominal and heart pains, kidney problems, hypertension and female disorders such as amenorrhoea and cramps.[4]

Cinnamon and cassia are mentioned in the bible. In Exodus, God told Moses to take myrrh, cinnamon, olive oil and bulrushes with him from Egypt. The ancient Egyptians were known to have used cinnamon in mummification. Diodorus described how after cleaning the body with palm wine and spices and anointing it with cedar oil and other unguents it was then rubbed down with myrrh, cinnamon and other aromatics to preserve it.[5]

The Arab traders, who kept its origin a secret, supplied the spice to the Greeks and Romans. The quest for cinnamon was pursued so enthusiastically that it was the principal incentive of the Portuguese in discovering the route around the Cape to India and Ceylon.[6]

Ceylon was occupied by the Portuguese in 1536, the Dutch in 1656 and the English East India Company in 1796. The Dutch started cinnamon cultivation in 1770 and exercised a strict monopoly on the cinnamon trade comparable with their monopoly of nutmegs. This continued until the monopoly of the English East India company was abolished in 1833.[6]

The Dutch introduced cinnamon into their East Indian colonies, particularly Java and Indonesia.

Cinnamon bark oil is used in pharmaceutical preparations as a carminative, stomachic, tonic or counterirritant and it is often included in mouth washes, liniments, nasal sprays and toothpaste.[4]

Cinnamon leaf is used as a fragrance component of soaps, detergents, creams, lotions and perfumes.[4]

Chemical Composition

A typical chemical composition of cinnamon leaf and bark oil is reported as follows:

Leaf: eugenol (80–96%), eugenol acetate (1.0%), cinnamaldehyde (3%), benzyl benzoate (3%).[3]

Bark: cinnamaldehyde (40–50%), eugenol (4–10%), benzyl benzoate (1.0%), α-pinene (0.2%), 1,8-cineole (1.65%), linalool (2.3%), caryophyllene (1.35%).[3]

Therapeutic Actions

Anaesthetic, antiseptic, antispasmodic, aphrodisiac, cardiac, carminative, emmenagogue, haemostatic, insecticide, stimulant, stomachic, vermifuge.

Pharmacology and Clinical Studies

The potential antibacterial and antifungal activity of cinnamon has been extensively demonstrated.[4,7]

A carbon dioxide extract of cinnamon bark at a 0.1% concentration completely suppressed the growth of numerous micro-organisms, including *Escherichia coli, Staphylococcus aureus* and *Candida albicans*.[7] Cinnamon bark oil was also found to have potent antifungal properties against fungi causing respiratory tract mycoses.[8]

Indications

Antimicrobial Properties

Cinnamon bark is regarded as one of the strongest antibacterial agents known.[10,12] It is useful for resisting viral infections and contagious diseases.

Digestive System

Cinnamon bark oil is regarded as an excellent gastrointestinal stimulant. It calms spasms of the digestive tract, relieves conditions such as dyspepsia, colitis, flatulence, diarrhoea, nausea and vomiting. It stimulates secretions of gastric juices and is recommended for loss of appetite.[9,10,12,13,15]

The strong antimicrobial properties of cinnamon bark and leaf oil are quite effective in cleansing the intestinal tract of pathogenic bacteria. The phenylpropanoid compounds such as cinnamic aldehyde and eugenol act against the pathogenic bacteria and at the same time support the intestinal flora.[9]

Nervous System

Cinnamon bark and cinnamon leaf are very warming, therefore they can be used to relieve aches and chills in the early stages of colds and flu, and the feeling of debility that often remains after the initial stage of a fever. The oil is also beneficial during convalescence.[11]

Valnet recommends using cinnamon for general debility and older persons during the winter months as a tonic.[10] It is recommended for persons who are devitalised, emaciated and suffering from nervous depression.[15]

Energetics

Cinnamon bark is classified as a hot and stimulating remedy. It will stimulate circulation, generate warmth, support the immune system, warm and invigorate the digestion and relieve pain.[12]

Personality Profile

Those who have a cinnamon personality are described as strong personality, affable, practical, intelligent and larger than life.[14]

Subtle Aromatherapy

It has been described as a physical essence, which restores a taste and vigour for life to the depressed, and the fire of courage to the belly of those who may have lost it in the maze of melancholia.[15]

Mode of Administration

Topical application — it is often not recommended for topical application[13,16]; Inhalation — diffuser, oil vaporiser.

It is interesting to note that as cinnamon bark is a potential skin irritant and sensitiser, the preferred mode of use is internally.[9,12] Schnaubelt says that the internal application of cinnamon bark is well tolerated and is safe and effective, provided it is used in appropriate small dosages. He recommends one drop of oil into one tablespoon of edible vegetable oil and then ingesting that mixture in a gelatin capsule.[9]

Safety

Cinnamon bark oil has been reported to be a severe dermal irritant and sensitiser.[9,11,13,16] If cinnamon bark is used externally, the dilution should not be more than 0.1%.[16]

The German Commission E Monographs state that internal use of cinnamon bark is contraindicated during pregnancy.[17]

Cinnamon leaf oil is a mild dermal irritant and its eugenol content suggests that it may be hepatotoxic and may inhibit blood clotting.[16]

References

1. Weiss EA. *Essential oil crops*. CAB International, UK, 1997.
2. Arctander S. *Perfume and flavour materials of natural origin*. Allured Publishing, USA, 1994.
3. Lawrence B. *Cinnamon leaf and cinnamon bark oil*. Perfumer and Flavorist, 1978; 3(4): 54.
4. Leung A, Foster S. *Encyclopedia of common natural ingredients used in food, drugs and cosmetics*. 2nd edn, John Wiley and Sons, USA, 1996.
5. Manniche L. *An ancient Egyptian herbal*. British Museum Press, Great Britain, 1993.
6. Evans WC. *Trease and Evans pharmacognosy*. 15th edn, WB Saunders, 2002.
7. Bruneton J. *Pharmacognosy*. 2nd edn, Lavoisier Publishing, France, 1999.
8. Singh, HB et al. *Cinnamon bark oil, a potent fungitoxicant against fungi causing respiratory tract mycoses*. Allergy, 1995; 50(12): 995–999. Cited in the Aromatherapy Database, Bob Harris, Essential Oil Resource Consultants, UK, 2000.
9. Schnaubelt K. *Medical aromatherapy*. Frog Ltd, USA, 1999.
10. Valnet J. *The practice of aromatherapy*. The C.W. Daniel Company Limited, Great Britain, 1980.
11. Davis P. *Aromatherapy: An A–Z*. The C.W. Daniel Company Limited, Great Britain, 1999.
12. Holmes P. *The energetics of western herbs Vol. I*, Artemis Press, USA, 1989.
13. Lawless J. *The encyclopaedia of essential oils*. Element Books Limited, Great Britain, 1992.
14. Worwood V. *The fragrant mind*. Doubleday, Great Britain, 1995.
15. Mailhebiau P. *Portraits in oils*. The C.W. Daniel Company Limited, Great Britain, 1995.
16. Tisserand R, Balacs T. *Essential oil safety*. Churchill Livingstone, UK, 1993.
17. Blumenthal M et al. *The complete German commission E monographs: Therapeutic guide to herbal medicine*. American Botanical Council USA, 1998.

Citronella

Cymbopogon nardus

Synonyms

C. winterianus, Andropogon nardus. C. winterianus is named after Mr Winter, a pioneer of the Sri Lankan essential oil industry and is locally known as Winter's grass.[1]

Family

Poaceae or Gramineae

Botany and Origins

C. nardus and *C. winterianus* are tufted, perennial grasses with long narrow leaves, and numerous stems arising from short rhizomatous roots. *C. nardus* has a more vigorous, extensive and penetrating root system than *C. winterianus*. This allows the species to withstand periods of drought and to grow well in a wider range of soil types.[1]

Commercial cultivation of *C. nardus* is limited to Sri Lanka and *C. winterianus* is commercially cultivated in Indonesia, Guatemala, Honduras, Haiti, China and, more recently, India and Vietnam.[1]

The essential oil industry generally defines the oils as Ceylon and Java types as there are characteristic differences, the most important being the geraniol content.[1]

Method of Extraction

Citronella oil is obtained from the steam distillation of the leaves of *C. nardus* or *C. winterianus*.

Essential Oil Characteristics

C. nardus, commonly known as Ceylon citronella oil is a yellow to brownish-yellow liquid with a distinctive warm-woody and yet fresh, grassy odour.[2]

C. winterianus, commonly known as Java citronella, is a colourless to pale-yellow liquid with a sweet, fresh and lemony odour.[2]

Historical and Traditional Uses

Poultices of the leaves were widely used in India and Sri Lanka to treat minor cuts, abrasions and swellings. Extracts of the leaves were used as a febrifuge, stomachic, diaphoretic, diuretic, emmenagogue and as a vermifuge.[1,3]

The oil is used extensively in detergents, waxes, household soaps and cleaners and to a minor extent in cheap perfumes and toiletries.[1] Java citronella is used as a major source for the isolation of citronellal and geraniol.[3]

The oil is extensively used as an insect repellent.[3]

Chemical Composition

The main constituents found in Java and Ceylon citronella oil are as follows:[1]

Constituent	Java	Ceylon
α-pinene	—	2.6%
camphene	—	8.0%
limonene	1.3%	9.7%
cis-ocimene	—	1.4%
trans-ocimene	—	1.8%
citronellal	32.7%	5.2%
camphor	—	0.5%

β-caryophyllene	2.1%	3.2%
4-terpinenol	trace	0.7%
citronellyl acetate	3.0%	1.9%
geranyl formate	2.5%	4.2%
1-borneol	trace	6.6%
citronellol	15.9%	8.4%
nerol	7.7%	0.9%
geraniol	23.9%	18.0%
geranyl butyrate	trace	1.5%
methyl eugenol	trace	1.7%
elemol	6.0%	1.7%
methyl iso-eugenol	2.3%	7.2%

Therapeutic Actions

Antiseptic, bactericidal, deodorant, diaphoretic, febrifuge, insecticide, tonic.

Pharmacology and Clinical Studies

Citronella oil has been reported to have antibacterial and antifungal activities.[3] *C. nardus* is reputed to be as active as penicillin against certain gram-positive bacteria.[3]

C. nardus essential oil was found to give almost complete protection against *Anopheles cullicifacies* (a principal malaria carrier) for up to eleven hours. The oil was considered comparable with synthetic repellents of dimethyl and dibutyl phthalate.[4]

Indications

Musculoskeletal system

Citronella oil is recommended in a massage oil for the relief of arthritic and rheumatic pain, muscular pain and neuralgia.[5,6]

Nervous System

Citronella oil has a fresh invigorating scent indicating that it may be used to alleviate nervous exhaustion and fatigue.[5,7]

Respiratory System

The aldehyde content suggests that citronella oil has excellent antimicrobial properties. It is recommended as an inhalation against colds, flus and minor infections.[7]

Skin Care

Citronella oil is well known as an insect repellent. For this purpose, it may be used in a spray, diffused into the air or applied to the skin in a massage oil.[3,6,7] It is also recommended for excessive perspiration and oily skin conditions.[7]

Mode of Administration

Topical application — massage, bath, skin care; Inhalation — direct inhalation, diffuser, oil vaporiser.

Safety

Citronella oil has been reported to be non-toxic, non-irritant and non-sensitising. It may cause contact dermatitis in some individuals.[3]

References

1. Weiss EA. *Essential oil crops*. CAB International, UK, 1997.
2. Arctander S. *Perfume and flavour materials of natural origin*. Allured Publishing, USA, 1994.
3. Leung A, Foster S. *Encyclopedia of common natural ingredients used in food, drugs and cosmetics*. 2nd edn, John Wiley and Sons, USA, 1996.
4. Ansari MA, Razdan RK. *Relative Efficacy of Various Oils in Repelling Mosquitoes*. Indian J. Malariol, 32(3): 104–111. Cited in the Aromatherapy Database, Bob Harris, Essential Oil Resource Consultants, UK, 2000.
5. Blumenthal M et al. *The complete German commission E monographs: Therapeutic guide to herbal medicine*. American Botanical Council USA, 1998.
6. Schnaubelt K. *Advanced aromatherapy*. Healing Art Press, Canada, 1995.
7. Lawless J. *The encyclopaedia of essential oils*. Element Books Limited, Great Britain, 1992.

Clary Sage

Salvia sclarea

Synonyms

Clary, muscatel sage

Family

Labiatae or Lamiaceae

Botany and Origins

Clary sage is a biennial herb or perennial herb, growing 30 to 120 cm high, with greyish, velvety, heart-shaped leaves and numerous pale-blue, violet-pink or white flowers.[1] It is cultivated in central Europe, Russia, England, Morocco and the USA.[2]

Method of Extraction

Clary sage oil is steam-distilled from the flowering tops and foliage of *S. sclarea*.

Essential Oil Characteristics

Clary sage oil is a colourless to pale-yellow or pale-olive coloured liquid with a sweet fruity, floral and herbaceous odour.

Historical and Traditional Uses

The English name clary is derived from the Latin word *sclarea*, a word derived from *clarus*, meaning 'clear'. The name clary was gradually modified to

Clear Eye, possibly because the herb was once used for clearing mucus from the eyes.[3]

Culpeper suggested that a compress of the mucilage made from the seeds would reduce tumours or swellings.[1] Originally grown in southern Europe, it was planted in German vineyards. It was also used as a substitute for hops in brewing beer.[3] Clary sage is used as a source of sclereol which is used as a flavouring in tobaccos.[4]

Chemical Composition

A typical chemical composition of clary sage is reported as follows:

Linalool, (10–20%), linalyl acetate (60–70%), caryophyllene (1.5–2.5%), α-terpineol (0.5–2.5%), geraniol (trace–1.5%), neryl acetate (0.3–1.0%), sclareol (0.5–2.0%), germacrene D (3.0–5.0%).[5]

The essential oil of clary sage is rich in esters, which are known for their antispasmodic and sedative properties.

Therapeutic Actions

Antidepressant, antispasmodic, deodorant, emmenagogue, hypotensive, nervine, sedative, tonic.

Pharmacology and Clinical Studies

Clary sage has been reported to show anticonvulsive activity in animals.[4]

Balacs reports a clinical trial by an Italian group who have been researching the anti-inflammatory and peripheral analgesic effects of clary sage. In rats, clary sage oil showed a significant anti-inflammatory effect and mild analgesic action after subcutaneous injection at 259 mg/kg. The anti-inflammatory response was more marked in carrageen-induced oedema than in histamine-induced inflammation. Balacs suggests that clary sage's activity is mediated via modulation of prostaglandin synthesis rather than via histamine.[6]

A clinical trial involving the use of essential oils being used during labour found clary sage was beneficial for its analgesic effects, relaxing effects and its ability to accelerate labour.[7]

Indications

Nervous System

Clary sage is well known for its euphoric action.[9] It is beneficial for treating anxiety, stress, nervous tension and depression.[11,12,13,14]

Clary sage is well known for its ability to balance. It is strengthening yet relaxing — while it is a general tonic indicated for mental and nervous fatigue, the oil is, on the other hand, effective for calming the mind and easing tension.[9]

Reproductive System

Clary sage is one of the most important essential oils as a women's remedy. All three phases of a woman's life stand to benefit from clary sage — the menstrual cycle, childbirth and menopause.[8]

Clary sage is renowned for the relief it brings to menstrual cramps because of its spasmolytic and analgesic action on the womb. Clary sage is also a uterine stimulant and an emmenagogue that promotes menstruation when delayed, scanty or completely absent.[8,11,12,14]

Holmes suggests that clary sage's oestrogenic action on the system results from pituitary-gonadal stimulation. It is very likely that this oil exerts a regulating action on the pituitary gland. Clary sage is recommended for managing menopause. Holmes suggests blending it with geranium oil to use in a bath or foot bath.[8]

In childbirth, clary sage's relaxant effect can help the mother release some tension and anxiety usually present in pre-labour and labour, right up to the transition phase. It is suggested that clary sage takes the edge off the physical and emotional intensity involved in the work of riding the contraction waves.[8]

Respiratory System

Clary sage is recommended for treating asthma as it relaxes spasms in the bronchial tube and helps reduce anxiety and emotional tension often associated with asthma sufferers.[9,11,13]

Skin Care

Clary sage is suggested for preventing excessive sweating. It is recommended for oily skin, greasy hair and dandruff as it regulates sebum production.[9,11]

Energetics

According to TCM, clary sage is reputed to strengthen *Qi* that is depleted and it relaxes and improves circulation of *Qi*. This means that it is a general tonic and an excellent antispasmodic.[13]

Personality Profile

Clary sage personalities have the ability to probe deeply into the psyche of others. They appear pensive at times, are gentle, melancholic and thoughtful.[15]

Clary sage brings long-lasting inner tranquillity, and, thanks to its warmth and liveliness, it helps dispel melancholy. This oil may be compared to a colourful clown or comedian who cheers and entertains with a sort of dance.[10]

Clary sage has been particularly recognised as useful for people involved in creative work. It opens the path to the unknown, unusual, creative and intuitive.[10]

Subtle Aromatherapy

Mojay suggests that clary sage is able to 'uplift' one's spirit without 'disconnecting' one from reality. The earthy quality of its herbaceous, musky sweetness reflects its ability to steady and calm the mind, while its gentle pungency enlivens the senses and restores clarity.[13]

Davis says that clary sage helps to bring us more closely in touch with the dream world. It is reputed to encourage vivid dreams, or it may be that it encourages dream recall.[16]

Mode of Administration

Topical application — massage, compress, bath, skin care; Inhalation — direct inhalation, diffuser, oil vaporiser.

Safety

Clary sage oil has been reported to be non-toxic, non-irritant and non-sensitising.[11] The oil is contra-indicated during pregnancy.[9,11]

However Tisserand and Balacs suggest that just because clary sage is labelled as an emmenagogue does not imply that the oil is an abortifacient in the amounts used in aromatherapy and, as such, it should present no danger in pregnancy.[17]

References

1. Le Strange R. *A history of herbal plants.* Angus and Robertson, Great Britain, 1977.
2. Arctander S. *Perfume and flavour materials of natural origin.* Allured Publishing, USA, 1994.
3. Grieve M. *A modern herbal.* Penguin, Great Britain, 1931.
4. Leung A, Foster S. *Encyclopedia of common natural ingredients used in food, drugs and cosmetics.* 2nd edn, John Wiley and Sons, USA, 1996.
5. Lawrence B. *Clary sage oil.* Perfumer and Flavorist, 1986; (11)5: 111.
6. Balacs T. *Research reports.* The International Journal of Aromatherapy, 1998; (8)4: 41–43.
7. Burns E, Blamey C. *Soothing scents in childbirth.* The International Journal of Aromatherapy, 6(1): 24–28.
8. Holmes P. *Clary sage.* The International Journal of Aromatherapy, 1993; 5(1): 15–17.
9. Davis P. *Aromatherapy: An A–Z.* 2nd edn, The C.W. Daniel Company Limited, Great Britain, 1999.
10. Fischer-Rizzi S. *Complete aromatherapy handbook.* Sterling Publishing Company, USA, 1990.
11. Lawless J. *The encyclopaedia of essential oils.* Element Books Limited, Great Britain, 1992.
12. Lavabre M. *Aromatherapy workbook.* Healing Art Press, USA, 1997.
13. Mojay G. *Aromatherapy for healing the spirit.* Hodder and Stoughton, UK, 1996.
14. Schnaubelt K. *Medical aromatherapy.* Frog Ltd, USA, 1999.
15. Worwood V. *The fragrant mind.* Doubleday, Great Britain, 1995.
16. Davis P. *Subtle aromatherapy.* The C.W. Daniel Company Limited, Great Britain, 1991.
17. Tisserand R, Balacs T. *Essential oil safety.* Churchill Livingstone, UK, 1995.

Clove Bud

Syzygium aromaticum

Synonyms

Eugenia aromatica; *E. caryophyllata*

Family

Myrtaceae

Botany and Origins

The clove is an evergreen tree, up to 15 m high, with glossy green leaves, fragrant red flowers and purple fruits.[1] The buds appear with a rosy-pink corolla at the tip and as the corolla fades the calyx slowly turns deep red. The calyxes are beaten from the tree and, when dried, provide the clove buds of commerce.

It is a long-lived tree and is reported to remain productive for 150 years.[1] The modern English name of clove is from the French *clou,* meaning nail, derived from the Latin *clavus*.[1] The clove is indigenous to the Moluccas, now part of Indonesia. The first recorded use was in the Chinese Han period 220–206 BC where it was used to sweeten the breath.[1]

The origins of cloves became known in Europe following a publication by Marco Polo in AD 1298. Venice was the leading European source of cloves and other spices in the 13th century. Cloves were traded in Europe via the Arabs, who for centuries had a monopoly of the seaborne spice trade until it was broken by the Portuguese in the 16th century. The Portuguese had a monopoly in the trade of cloves for over a century.[1]

The Dutch subsequently broke the Portuguese monopoly, instituting their own, which they maintained with the utmost ruthlessness. In order to prevent other countries from obtaining cloves, the Dutch issued a proclamation in 1621 which ensured that all clove trees be destroyed except on Amboina and adjacent islands. This destruction of wild and cultivated trees resulted in a great loss of genetic diversity.[1]

Cloves were introduced to Zanzibar in the 19th century. Zanzibar, now part of Tanzania, has become the world's largest exporter of cloves.[1]

Method of Extraction

Clove bud oil is water-distilled from the dried flower buds of *S. aromaticum.*

The clove buds are comminuted prior to distillation. If the cloves are steam-distilled, hydrolysis takes place, and most of the natural acetyl eugenol is converted to eugenol. Compared to steam distillation the level of hydrolysis that occurs during water distillation is minimal.[2]

The eugenol content of water distillation is typically 85–89%, while the eugenol content of steam-distilled clove bud oil is typically 91–95%.[1]

Essential Oil Characteristics

Clove bud oil is a clear to yellow mobile liquid, becoming brown with a strong, sweet and spicy odour.[2]

Adulterants of clove bud oil are usually clove stem or leaf oil, or clove terpenes remaining after eugenol extraction.[1]

Clove leaf oil is a dark-brown mobile liquid with a harsh, woody, phenolic, slightly sweet aroma. The leaf oil is often rectified and is usually a pale-yellow colour with a sweeter, less harsh, dry woody odour closer to that of eugenol.[1]

Historical and Traditional Uses

During the Renaissance, pomanders were made with cloves to keep epidemics and the plague at bay. Cloves are used in traditional medicine as a carminative, anti-emetic, and counterirritant. Clove tea is used to relieve nausea and the oil is well known for its ability to alleviate toothache.[3]

In TCM, clove oil is used for diarrhoea, hernia and bad breath.[3] Clove buds are recommended in the German Commission E Monographs as a mouthwash for the treatment of inflammatory changes of the oral and pharyngeal mucosa and for topical analgesia in dentistry.[4]

The main use of cloves, whole and ground, is as a domestic culinary spice and for the production of sauces and pickles.[1]

Indonesia is one of the largest consumers of clove buds. The comminuted clove buds are used to the extent of up to 8% in Indonesian *kretek* cigarettes.[1,2]

Chemical Composition

A typical composition of the bud, stem and leaf oil can be differentiated as follows[5]:

Compound	clove leaf	clove stem	clove bud
eugenol	85–90%	87–92%	80–85%
eugenyl acetate	0–10%	3–3.5%	8–12%
isoeugenol	—	trace	—
caryophyllene	10–15%	6–8%	6–10%
isocaryophyllene			0–2.0%

Therapeutic Actions

Analgesic, antiseptic, antispasmodic, carminative, stomachic.

Pharmacology and Clinical Studies

Clove oil is reported to be antiseptic, exhibiting broad antimicrobial activities, as well as having anthelmintic and larvicidal properties.[3] The oil is also reported to have antihistaminic and spasmolytic properties.[3] It is a potent inhibitor of platelet aggregation.[7]

Clove oil has long been used as a local analgesic for the relief of toothache.[6,7] Eugenol, like other phenols, acts to depress sensory receptors involved in pain perception. The mechanism of action involves a pronounced inhibition of prostaglandin biosynthesis resulting from blockages of the cyclo-oxygenase and lipoxygenase pathways.[6,7]

At high doses (0.5 mL/kg) clove oil is toxic, especially in young children, in whom it causes CNS depression, hepatic necrosis, convulsions and/or major haemostatic abnormalities.[7]

Indications

Analgesic

The dental value of cloves is well known.[8,9,10,12] The oil has a minor anaesthetic effect. A cotton bud dipped in the undiluted oil and applied to the surface of the aching tooth and surrounding tissue or, if possible, inserted directly into the cavity will alleviate the pain for several hours.

Antiseptic Properties

Clove oil has excellent antiseptic properties, because of the high proportion of eugenol. It may be used for the prevention of colds and flus.[10,11,12] A 1% emulsion of clove oil has an antiseptic strength three to four times greater than phenol.[11]

Digestive System

Being a carminative and antispasmodic, it helps stimulate digestion, restores appetite and relieves flatulence.[10,12]

Musculoskeletal System

For rheumatic pains, clove oil will help relieve arthritis, rheumatism and sprains.[10]

Nervous System

Clove oil is a physical and mental tonic and should be used in conjunction with peppermint to ward off drowsiness.[9,12]

Skin Care

While clove bud oil may be used as an insect repellent, it is generally not used in skin care as it is a potential dermal irritant and sensitiser.

Energetics

According to TCM, clove oil is warming and it tonifies *Qi*. It may be used to generate warmth and to eliminate any condition associated with cold.

Personality Profile

The rich spicy aroma of clove oil suggests that the clove personality is dynamic, self-assured and full of energy.

Mode of Administration

Topical application — massage, compress, ointment; Inhalation — direct inhalation, diffuser, oil vaporiser.

Safety

Clove bud oil has been reported to be a potential skin irritant and sensitising agent. A near-fatal ingestion of clove oil was reported involving a 2-year-old boy who had drunk between 5–10 mL of clove oil.[13]

References

1. Weiss EA. *Essential oil crops*. CAB International, UK, 1997.
2. Arctander S. *Perfume and flavour materials of natural origin*. Allured Publishing, USA, 1994.
3. Leung A, Foster S. *Encyclopedia of common natural ingredients used in food, drugs and cosmetics*. 2nd edn, John Wiley and Sons Inc, USA, 1996.
4. Blumenthal M et al. *The complete German commission E monographs: Therapeutic guide to herbal medicine*. American Botanical Council, USA, 1998.
5. Lawrence B. *Major tropical spices — Clove. Essential oils: 1976–1977*. Allured Publishing Corporation, USA, 1979: 84–145.
6. Tyler V. *Herbs of choice: The therapeutic use of phytomedicinals*. Pharmaceutical Products Press, USA, 1994.
7. Bruneton J. *Pharmacognosy*. 2nd edn, Lavoisier Publishing Inc, France, 1999.
8. Davis P. *Aromatherapy: An A–Z*. 2nd edn, The C.W. Daniel Company Limited, Great Britain, 1999.
9. Mailhebiau P. *Portraits in oils*. The C.W. Daniel Company Limited, Great Britain, 1995.
10. Lawless J. *The encyclopaedia of essential oils*. Element Books Limited, Great Britain, 1992.
11. Valnet J. *The practice of aromatherapy*. The C.W. Daniel Company Limited, Great Britain, 1980.
12. Lavabre M. *Aromatherapy workbook*. Healing Art Press, USA, 1997.
13. Hartnoll G et al. *Near fatal ingestion of oil of clove. Arch. Diseases in Childhood*. 1993; 69: 392–393.

Cypress

Cupressus sempervirens

Synonyms

Italian Cypress, Mediterranean cypress

Family

Cupressaceae

Botany and Origins

The tree originates in the eastern Mediterranean countries and can be found along the coast of southern France, Italy, Corsica, Sardinia, Sicily, North Africa, Spain, Portugal and the Balkan countries. Most of the oil is distilled in southern France.

It is an extremely old species of tree dating back to the Pliocene era (5.3 to 1.8 million years). It is exceptionally long-lived. Some cypress trees are believed to be two thousand years old.[1]

Method of Extraction

Cypress oil is steam-distilled from the leaves (needles) and twigs of *C. sempervirens* which are obtained by pruning the trees in autumn.

Essential Oil Characteristics

Cypress is a pale-yellow to almost colourless, mobile liquid with a sweet balsamic, yet refreshing odour, reminiscent of pine needles and juniper berry oil with a unique dry-out of a delicate and tenacious sweetness.[2]

Historical and Traditional Uses

Cypress was well known to the ancient Egyptians. The ancient Greeks dedicated the tree to Pluto, god of the underworld — thus the use of the trees in cemeteries. Hippocrates recommended cypress for severe cases of haemorrhoids with bleeding. Dioscorides and Galen recommended macerating the leaves in wine with a little myrrh for a fortnight. This was recommended for bladder infections and internal bleeding.[3]

Culpeper says of cypress:

> *The cones, or nuts, are mostly used, the leaves but seldom; they are accounted very drying and binding, good to stop fluxes of all kinds, as sitting of blood, diarrhoea, dysentery, the immoderate flux of the menses, involuntary miction; they prevent the bleeding of the gums, and fasten loose teeth: outwardly, they are used in styptic restringent formentations and cataplasms.*[4]

Chemical Composition

A typical chemical composition of cypress is reported as follows:

α-pinene (20.4%), camphene (3.6%), sabinene (2.8%), β-pinene (2.9%), δ-3-carene (21.5%), myrcene and α-terpinene (1.1%), terpinolene (6.3%), linalool (0.07%), bornyl acetate (0.3%), cedrol (5.35%), cadinene (1.7%).[5]

Pharmacology and Clinical Studies

No pharmacological or clinical studies could be found for cypress.

Therapeutic Actions

Antiseptic, antispasmodic, astringent, deodorant, diuretic, haemostatic, hepatic, styptic, sudorific, venous decongestant, tonic.

Indications

Circulatory System

Cypress oil is renowned as an excellent venous decongestant and is used for the treatment of varicose veins, oedema and haemorrhoids.[6,7,8,9,12] Holmes describes the therapeutic properties of cypress:

> *Cypress is the only essential oil which is a true venous blood decongestant as well as an astringent ... it gives a lift to the side of the circulation liable to congestive stasis, relieving resultant menstrual imbalances with heavy periods and intermenstrual bleeding. Part of cypress' blood activating action is a restorative effect on the veins themselves, useful with ailments ranging from haemorrhoids to phlebitis.*[11]

Nervous System

Fischer-Rizzi suggests that cypress oil strengthens an overburdened nervous system and helps to restore calm.[6]

Reproductive System

Cypress oil is known as a menstrual regulator. It may be used to relieve painful periods. It is recommended for dysmenorrhoea, menorrhagia and menopausal problems.[7,8] It is recommended for severe hot flashes during menopause.[6]

Respiratory System

Cypress oil is reputed to be effective as a cough remedy for the management of acute and chronic bronchitis and whooping cough.[7,8,9,12]

Skin Care

Cypress oil is used in skin care preparations for its antiseptic and astringent properties. It used for acne, oily and over-hydrated skins and is recommended for excessive perspiration.[7,8,12] It is also recommended in a foot bath for excessive sweating of the feet.[6,8,12]

Energetics

Mojay says that not only does cypress move blood, but it also circulates *Qi*. Like lavender, it has a wide-ranging antispasmodic effect which is beneficial for treating spasmodic colitis, PMS and asthma.[10]

Personality Profile

> *The cypress tree, standing dark and silent, is like a finger pointing to heaven! It does not indulge in needless movements, like other trees that stretch out limbs, allowing them to sway in the wind.*[6]

This description gives you a clear indication of the cypress personality. Cypress represents the strength within, wisdom and is seen as a symbol of eternity. Cypress personalities tend to be forceful, outspoken and firm in their views and are seen as strong people who are able to resolve most problems.[13]

Mailhebiau describes the cypress personality:

> *The splendour of the cypress, a fine slender tree rising like a flame towards the starry, endless sky, represents the sacred flame of life, the unchangeable, eternal essence, and powerfully evokes the spiritual archetype of cypress, a tall, fine-looking old man with the wisdom granted by a thousand years of intense, disciplined life ...*[1]

He suggests that anyone who has lost touch with a sense of harmony and serenity will benefit from a blend of cypress, atlas cedarwood, rosemary and sandalwood.

Subtle Aromatherapy

Cypress oil is helpful at times of transition such as career changes, moving home and is always helpful with painful transitions such as bereavement or ending of close relationships.[14]

Mode of Administration

Topical application — massage, compress, bath, skin care; Inhalation — direct inhalation, diffuser, oil vaporiser.

Safety

Cypress oil has been reported to be non-toxic, non-irritant and non-sensitising.

References

1. Mailhebiau P. *Portraits in oils*. The C.W. Daniel Company Limited, Great Britain, 1995.
2. Arctander S. *Perfume and flavour materials of natural origin*. Allured Publishing, USA, 1994.
3. Ryman D. *Aromatherapy*. Piatkus Ltd, Great Britain, 1991.
4. Tisserand R. *The art of aromatherapy*. The C.W. Daniel Company Limited, Great Britain, 1977.
5. Lawrence B. *Cypress oil*. Perfumer and Flavorist, 1977; 1(6): 31.
6. Fischer-Rizzi S. *Complete aromatherapy handbook*. Sterling Publishing Company, USA, 1990.
7. Lawless J. *The encyclopaedia of essential oils*. Element Books Limited, Great Britain, 1992.

8. Davis P. *Aromatherapy: An A–Z.* 2nd edn, The C.W. Daniel Company Limited, Great Britain, 1999.

9. Schnaubelt K. *Medical aromatherapy.* Frog Ltd, USA, 1999.

10. Mojay G. *Aromatherapy for healing the spirit.* Hodder and Stoughton, UK, 1996.

11. Holmes P. *The energetics of western herbs Vol. I.* Artemis Press, USA, 1986.

12. Valnet J. *The Practice of aromatherapy.* The C.W. Daniel Company Limited, Great Britain, 1980.

13. Worwood V. *The fragrant mind.* Doubleday, Great Britain, 1995.

14. Davis P. *Subtle aromatherapy.* The C.W. Daniel Company Limited, Great Britain, 1991.

Eucalyptus

This monograph will examine the cineole-rich eucalyptus oils.

Family

Mytaceae

Botany and Origins

Almost all eucalypts are indigenous to Australia where they constitute approximately 75% of all tree flora.[1]

The large eucalyptus plantations in other countries have been established mainly from Australian seed, and are now so extensive that eucalypts form a significant proportion of the forested area in countries such as Ethiopia and South Africa.[1] The ability of some eucalyptus species to grow quickly makes eucalyptus valuable where wood fuel is of great domestic importance.[1]

Eucalypts are known to produce the hardest, heaviest and most durable wood known as 'ironbark'.[1]

The genus *Eucalyptus* was named by French botanist CL Brutelle L'Heritier from the Greek words *eu* (well) and *kalipto* (covered), referring to the cup-like structure which is thrown off as the flower expands.[1]

Of the 600 species of eucalyptus, fewer than 20 have ever been exploited commercially.[2] The species of eucalyptus most commonly used for the production of essential oil are those with a high content of cineole.

Species	Cineole (%)	Oil yield (%) on fresh wt basis
E. globulus	65–85	0.7–2.4
E. polybractea	60–93	0.7–5.0
E. radiata	65–75	2.5–3.5
E. dives (cineole variant)	60–75	3.0–6.0
E. smithii	70–80	1.0–2.2
E. vridis	70–80	1.0–1.5
E. eneorifolia	40–90	approx 2.0
E. camaldulensis	10–90	0.3–2.8
E. dumosa	33–70	1.0–2.0
E. leucoxylon	65–75	0.8–2.5
E. oleosa	54–52	1.0–2.1
E. sideroxylon	60–75	0.5–2.5
E. tereticornis	45	0.9–1.0

Commercial Eucalyptus Oil Species[2]

The species discussed in this monograph will be:

- *E. globulus* — Also known as Tasmanian blue gum or blue gum. It is principally cultivated in Portugal, Spain and China. The timber is strong and durable and is used for construction purposes.[3]
- *E. polybractea* — The name *E. fruticetorum* has been incorrectly but commonly applied to this species.[2] It is the prime source of cineole-rich eucalyptus oils and is currently the major species used in commercial oil production in Australia. It is ideally suited to mechanical harvesting.[3] It appears that E. *polybractea* does not thrive outside of Australia.[1]
- *E. radiata* — This is one of the more important sources of eucalyptus oil. It varies from a small tree with a bushy crown to a large tree of good form. The oil is also known as 'narrow-leafed peppermint gum'.[2]
- *E. smithii* — Commonly known as 'gully gum', 'white ironbark' and Smith's gum after HG Smith, Australia's foremost pioneer of eucalyptus oil.[3] This species is extensively grown in southern Africa.[2]

The active therapeutic and principal constituent of the medicinal oils is 1,8-cineole. The quality of the oil is specified by the minimum standards which are defined in the British Pharmacopoeia (BP). It requires a eucalyptus oil to contain not less than 70% 1,8-cineole and to be free of α- and β-phellandrene.[1]

Although many eucalyptus species contain 1,8-cineole in their oils, only a limited number combine a composition high in 1,8-cineole with consistently high total yields and are suitable for commercial exploitation. Rectification and blending of eucalyptus oils has therefore become common practice.[1]

Rectification is done by redistillation in a vacuum in which the low boiling point fractions of the oil are removed and the high boiling residues remain.[1]

Lassak cites work conducted by Penfold and Grant who noticed that the high boiling residues of eucalyptus oil extracted from the rectified essential oil exhibited a greater germicidal power than the rectified oil.[3]

Many eucalyptus oils sold as BP grade are blended and redistilled. Today the major eucalyptus producing countries are China, Spain, Portugal, South Africa and Chile. China is presently the world's largest producer of eucalyptus oil.[1]

Method of Extraction

Eucalyptus oil is steam-distilled from the fresh or partially dried leaves of the Eucalypt species.

Essential Oil Characteristics

E. globulus is a cineole-rich oil with a refreshing, slightly camphoraceous but typical eucalyptus odour.[1,4]

E. smithii is a colourless or very pale-yellow, mobile liquid with a fresh cineole type odour.[1]

E. australiana, which is also known as *E. radiata,* is a colourless to pale-yellow oil, with a fresh, very powerful, peppery camphoraceous odour.[3,4]

E. polybractea is yellow to brown, becoming almost colourless to pale-yellow on rectification, with a pronounced sweet-camphoraceous odour.[1,4]

Historical and Traditional Uses

It was Baron Ferdinand von Mueller, the first government botanist of Victoria in 1853, who convinced his friend Joseph Bosisto, a Melbourne pharmacist, of the virtues of eucalyptus oils and the potential for developing an indigenous industry.[2]

In 1854, Bosisto built his first distillation plant on the banks of Dandenong Creek near Dandenong on the outskirts of Melbourne. He distilled eucalyptus oil from what was then known as *E. amygdalina,* now known as *E. radiata.*[2]

By the 1880s the eucalyptus oil industry had firmly established itself. Bosisto received financial backing from Melbourne businessmen Alfred Felton and Frederick Grimwade and together they formed the 'Eucalyptus Mallee Company'. Today this company still produces eucalyptus oil which is marketed under the name Bosisto's Brand Eucalyptus oil.[2]

Eucalyptus oil was in huge demand during World War I, as it was used to help control a meningitis outbreak and for the influenza of 1919. However, by 1930, the impact of overseas eucalyptus plantations impacted dramatically on Australian produced oil.[2]

The eucalyptus oil industry in Australia reached its peak in the early post-war years when, in 1947, total production reached almost 1,000 tonnes, of which 70% was exported. Since then the industry has declined. In 1989 the world eucalyptus market was about 2,000 to 3,000 tonnes per annum, of which about 5 to 10% was produced in Australia.[2]

The cineole-rich eucalyptus oils are widely used in medicine for inhalations, soaps, gargles and lozenges.[3]

Chemical Composition

A typical chemical composition of various eucalyptus oils is reported as follows:

E. globulus: α-pinene (10.66%), β-pinene (0.18%), α-phellandrene (0.09%), 1,8-cineole (69.10%), limonene (3.29%), terpinen-4-ol (0.22%), aromadendrene (1.63%), epiglobulol (0.80%), piperitone (0.1%), globulol (5.33%).[2]

E. radiata: α-pinene (15.0–21.0%), 1,8-cineole (57.0–71.0%), limonene (5.0%), p-cymene (0.3–1.0%).[2]

E. polybractea: α-pinene (0.90%), β-pinene (0.23%), 1,8-cineole (91.90%), limonene (1.10%), terpinen-4-ol (0.51%), globulol (0.05%).[2]

E. smithii: α-pinene (4.08%), β-pinene (0.11%), 1,8-cineole (80.54%), limonene (3.29%), terpinen-4-ol (0.11%), globulol (2.36%).[2]

Therapeutic Actions

Analgesic, antibacterial, anti-inflammatory, antineuralgic, antirheumatic, antiseptic, antispasmodic, antiviral, astringent, balsamic, cicatrisant, decongestant, deodorant, diuretic, expectorant, febrifuge, hypoglycaemic, rubefacient, vermifuge, vulnerary.

Pharmacology and Clinical Studies

Eucalyptus oil and 1,8-cineole have been reputed to have antiseptic and expectorant properties and strong antibacterial activity against several strains of *Streptococcus.*[5,6,7]

There is some confusion over eucalyptus oil's antimicrobial properties. For example, Williams cites two clinical trials, one which reported eucalyptus as having a high antimicrobial activity and one which indicated that eucalyptus oil has little to no antimicrobial activity. Williams conducted his own research which revealed little to no antimicrobial activity against *Candida albicans, Staphylococcus aureus* and *E. coli*. He also tested 1,8-cineole and it also failed to show any zone of inhibition against a range of micro-organisms.[9]

Williams concluded that the selection of eucalyptus oil for the use in household disinfectants is because of price rather than efficacy of their disinfectant properties. Lassak also says that the only reason that eucalyptus gained a reputation as an antiseptic is because of the clean crisp smell. He suggests that the clearing effect of cineole vapour on the nasal passage results in easier and deeper breathing. Good deep breathing and fresh air have always been associated with good health.[3]

Another clinical trial suggests that 1,8-cineole is not responsible for the antimicrobial activity of eucalyptus oil. The activity is due to the presence of minor constituents such as the alcohols — borneol, trans-pinocarveol, nerol and citronellol. It was suggested that the presence of these alcohols increased antimicrobial activity provided that no nonfavourable components were present such as myrtenol, geraniol and cedrol.[8]

However, Balacs cites research which indicates that cineole has considerable antimicrobial activity against gram-positive and gram-negative bacteria, as well as some fungi, and was more potent than citronellal and caryophyllene.[10]

Indications

Analgesic Properties

Eucalyptus oil has been used to relieve insect bites and muscular aches and pains. It is indicated for rheumatic pain of a cold nature and may be used to relieve muscular aches and pains and neuralgia.[12,13,16]

Davis recommends using *E. radiata* to alleviate the acute pain of shingles. She recommends blending it with bergamot for the treatment of cold sores and genital herpes.[12]

Nervous System

Eucalyptus oil is recommended for the treatment of headaches, neuralgia and debility.[13]

Respiratory System

Eucalyptus is best known as a decongestant inhalation for colds and catarrh.[12]

Schnaubelt recommends using *E. radiata* as an inhalation and for topical use for rhinitis, flu, otitis, sinusitis and bronchitis.[15] According to Valnet the spraying of a 2% emulsion containing eucalyptus oil kills off 70% of local, airborne staphylococci.[14]

Balacs suggests that during a respiratory tract infection such as a common cold, the nasal and lower respiratory passages become constricted which in turn makes breathing difficult. Research indicates that aromatic inhalations containing eucalyptus oil can significantly improve respiratory function. It has been suggested that the mechanisms of action of such respiratory congestion may be reflex, and related to nerve stimulation by the essential oils.[10]

Balacs says that the reputation of eucalyptus as a decongestant relies on its ability to stimulate cold receptors in the nose. During an infection with a common cold virus, the nasal and lower respiratory passages restrict the passage of air into the lungs because of vasoconstriction. Along with menthol and camphor, eucalyptus oil and cineole have the effect of reducing surface tension between water and air in the lungs, a property which would presumably enhance the effects of the lungs' own surfactant.[10]

Skin Care

Eucalyptus oil is effective as an insect repellent and is used to treat burns, blisters, cuts and wounds.[12,13]

Energetics

According to TCM, eucalyptus is an exceptional remedy for clearing lung-phlegm and wind-heat. This makes it beneficial for the onset of flu or fever, sore throat, the common cold, sinusitis and chronic bronchitis.[16,17]

It is classified as a tonic of the lung *Qi* and is used to enhance the breathing function, promoting the uptake of oxygen by the red blood cells.[16]

Personality Profile

The psychological properties of the eucalyptus oils are closely related to the action of the lungs. Its aroma helps to dispel melancholy, it revives the spirits and restores vitality and a positive outlook.[16]

> *Eucalyptus oil is suited to people who feel emotionally 'hemmed in' or constricted by their surroundings — whether at home, at work or in society. They sense the possibility of achieving greater freedom and a wider life experience, but dare not seek to create this due to excessive caution, habit, fear or responsibility. Eucalyptus oil helps to disperse the negative feelings associated with such situations, and gives us, inwardly, 'room to breathe.*[16]

Subtle Aromatherapy

Eucalyptus may be used at a subtle level to cleanse any place where there has been conflict or where negative energies are felt.[18] Eucalyptus is also described as a fragrance of newness and renewal and is recommended for those seeking new horizons.[19]

Mode of Administration

Topical application — massage, compress, bath, liniment, skin care; Inhalation — direct inhalation, diffuser, oil vaporiser, steam inhalation.

Safety

Eucalyptus oil has been reported to be non-toxic, non-irritant and non-sensitising. However, there is some confusion and controversy regarding its safety.

The leaves of some eucalyptus are a source of food for the koalas. A koala is known to eat 10 g of 1,8-cineole a day with no adverse effects. It appears that the oil is conjugated with glucuronic acid present in the koala's blood and is excreted in a water-soluble form in urine.[3]

Unfortunately humans are not able to metabolise 1,8-cineole in the same way as koalas. Lassak cites an incident, where, for about the past five years, a man had been in the habit of swallowing five to ten drops of eucalyptus oil to keep colds at bay and to make him feel good. He began to feel discomfort and pain in the region of the liver. After entering hospital for a check-up, he was informed that he suffered from cirrhosis of the liver, and that, unless he stopped drinking immediately, his condition would continue to deteriorate. This man had never drunk alcohol and the apparent cause of his condition was the ingested eucalyptus that he had assumed would improve his health.[3]

Eucalyptus oil is scheduled as a poison in Australia. While it is freely available, it must be sold with a child-resistant closure. Balacs suggests that the evidence that eucalyptus oil is dangerous is very thin indeed:

> *... There have been cases of oral poisoning, but these are most notable for the fact that remarkably large doses have been survived, usually with no permanent ill-effect. It should be noted that this author* [Balacs] *is very concerned to highlight potential toxicity wherever it exists: it does seem however, that eucalyptus and cineole are two of the least toxic materials one comes across in essential oils.*[10]

Balacs cites recorded fatalities resulting from the ingestion of eucalyptus. Some of the reports date back to 1893, the amount of eucalyptus oil ingested ranged between 15 mL and 90 mL. As the records are old, it was not clearly recorded as to whether it was pure eucalyptus oil that was ingested or a blend of eucalyptus and other substances.[10]

An Australian study over an 11-year period from 1981 to 1992 recorded that 109 children were admitted to a Melbourne hospital for eucalyptus poisoning. According to the report 31 had some degree of CNS depression, 3 were unconscious, having ingested between 5 and 10 mL, and one child who ingested about 75 mL was unconscious. Vomiting occurred in 37%, ataxia in 15% and pulmonary dysfunction in 11%.[10]

The treatment for 21% of the cases was ipecac, 57% received a nasogastric activated charcoal and 12% required no treatment. It also needs to be noted that not one child died from eucalyptus poisoning. Balacs cites a report from Queensland where 33 out of the 41 children admitted to hospital with suspected eucalyptus poisoning were entirely without symptoms, despite the fact that in some cases they had consumed as much as 30 mL of oil.[10]

On the other hand clinical trials have suggested that cineole has a similar neurotoxic profile to that of camphor in tests.[6,10] The clinical trial studied the effects of 1,8-cineole on cortical sodium and potassium. It was found that 1,8-cineole altered brain sodium and potassium in a similar way to camphor and consistent with increased susceptibility to convulsions.[10]

References

1. Weiss EA. *Essential oil crops*. CAB International, UK, 1997.
2. Boland DJ et al. *Eucalyptus leaf oils*. Inkata Press, Australia, 1991.
3. Lassak E. *Australian medicinal plants*. Methuen Australia, Australia, 1983.
4. Arctander S. *Perfume and flavour materials of natural origin*. Allured Publishing, USA, 1994.
5. Leung A, Foster S. *Encyclopedia of common natural ingredients used in food, drugs and cosmetics*. 2nd edn, John Wiley and Sons Inc, USA, 1996.
6. Bruneton J. *Pharmacognosy*. 2nd edn, Lavoisier Publishing Inc, France 1999.
7. Benouda A et al. *The antiseptic properties of essential oils in vitro, tested against pathogenic germs found in hospitals*. Fitoterapia, 1988; 59(2): 115–119. Cited in the Aromatherapy Database, Bob Harris, Essential Oil Resource Consultants, UK, 2000.
8. Zakarya D et al. *Chemical Composition — Antimicrobial activity relationships of eucalyptus essential oils*. Plantes Medica Phytotherapy, 1993; 26(4): 319–331. Cited in the Aromatherapy Database, Bob Harris, Essential Oil Resource Consultants, UK, 2000.
9. Williams L. *Australian eucalyptus oils*. Simply Essential, 1994; 12: 21–25.
10. Balacs T. *Cineole-rich eucalyptus*. The International Journal of Aromatherapy, 1997; 8(2): 15–21.
11. Peneol D. *Winter shield*. The International Journal of Aromatherapy, 1992; 4(4): 10–12.
12. Davis P. *Aromatherapy: An A–Z*. 2nd edn, The C.W. Daniel Company Limited, Great Britain, 1999.
13. Lawless J. *The encyclopaedia of essential oils*. Element Books Limited, Great Britain, 1992.
14. Valnet J., *The practice of aromatherapy*. The C.W. Daniel Company Limited, Great Britain, 1980.
15. Schnaubelt K. *Medical aromatherapy*. Frog Ltd, USA, 1999.
16. Mojay G. *Aromatherapy for healing the spirit*. Hodder and Stoughton, UK, 1996.
17. Holmes P. *The energetics of western herbs Vol. I*, Artemis Press, USA, 1996.
18. Worwood V. *The fragrant spirit*. Doubleday, Great Britain, 1999.
19. Davis P. *Subtle aromatherapy*. The C.W. Daniel Company Limited, Great Britain, 1991.

Eucalyptus, Broadleaf Peppermint

Eucalyptus dives

Synonyms

Broad-leaf peppermint, Peppermint tree

Family

Myrtaceae

Botany and Origins

It is a small tree with a large crown which prefers open conditions and occurs in south-eastern Australia. The oil is produced on a large scale in Australia and South Africa.[1]

E. dives contains at least three chemotypes. The cineole-rich chemotype is known as *E. dives* var "C" yields an oil similar to the cineole-rich eucalyptus oils.[1]

The piperitone chemotype is known as *E. dives* "type" yields an oil with approximately 40 to 54% piperitone.[1]

The phellandrene chemotype is known as *E. dives* var. "A" yields an oil with approximately 60% a-phellandrene and 2 to 8% piperitone.[1]

Method of Extraction

Broadleaf peppermint eucalyptus oil is steam-distilled from the leaves of *E. dives.*

Essential Oil Characteristics

E. dives "type" is a colourless to pale-yellow, mobile liquid that has a strong and very fresh, camphoraceous, spicy and minty odour.[2]

Historical and Traditional Uses

The Australian aborigines fumigated people by burning leaves of *E. dives* for the relief of fever.[4]

E. dives type "A" oil is used as a solvent, and in industrial perfumery and in insecticides.[3]

The piperitone-rich oil is used as a source of *l*-piperitone which in turn is used for the production of synthetic menthol, a white crystalline solid with a clean, fresh odour of true peppermint. Menthol is used in gargles, mouth washes, liniments as well as flavourings.[1]

Chemical Composition

A typical chemical composition of *E. dives* "type" is reported as follows:

α-pinene (1.10%), α-phellandrene (19.52%), α-terpinene (2.20%), limonene (0.3%), β-phellandrene (1.70%), p-cymene (3.36%), terpinolene (2.02%), terpinen-4-ol (4.0%), piperitone (52.27%), globulol/viridiflorol (6.03%).[1]

Therapeutic Actions

Analgesic, antiseptic, antineuralgic, balsamic, decongestant, expectorant, mucolytic, rubefacient, stimulant, vermifuge.

Pharmacology and Clinical Studies

E. dives oil has been found to have antifungal activity against *C. albicans.*[5]

Indications

Musculoskeletal System

E. dives is recommended for the treatment of arthritis, muscular aches and pains, rheumatism, sports injuries and sprains.[6]

Nervous System

E. dives oil is recommended for the treatment of headaches, neuralgia and debility.[6]

Respiratory System

E. dives is recommended for the treatment of asthma, bronchitis, catarrh, coughs and throat or mouth infections.[6] Schnaubelt says that piperitone, a ketone found in *E. dives,* is a very effective mucolytic and is recommended for bronchitis.[7]

Mode of Administration

Topical application — massage, compress, ointment; Inhalation — direct inhalation, diffuser, oil vaporiser.

Safety

Dr Penoel recommends not using *E. dives* due to its high content of piperitone, which he says is neurotoxic.[8] However, Lawless and Schnaubelt state that the oil is not toxic.[6,7]

References

1. Boland DJ, Brophy JJ, House APN. *Eucalyptus leaf oils: use, chemistry, distillation and marketing.* Inkata Press, Australia, 1991.
2. Arctander S. *Perfume and flavour materials of natural origin.* Allured Publishing, USA, 1994.
3. Weiss EA. *Essential oil crops.* CAB International, UK, 1997.
4. Lassak E. *Australian medicinal plants.* Methuen Australia, Australia, 1983.
5. Beylier MF, Givaudan SA. *Bacteriostatic activity of some Australian essential oils.* Perfumer and Flavorist, 1979; 4: 23–25.
6. Lawless J. *The encyclopaedia of essential oils.* Element Books Limited, Great Britain, 1992.
7. Schnaubelt K. *Medical aromatherapy.* Frog Ltd, USA, 1999.
8. Peneol D. *Winter shield.* The International Journal of Aromatherapy, 1992; 4(4): 10–12.

Eucalyptus, Lemon Scented

Eucalyptus citriodora

Synonyms

Lemon-scented gum, Lemon-scented spotted gum.

Family

Myrtaceae

Botany and Origins

E. citriodoria is distinguished from all the other eucalyptus species by the strong smell of citronellal in the leaves. It is a medium to tall tree with an attractive pink or spotted bark and a rather sparse crown. It is confined to subtropical and tropical zones in Australia. Today it is cultivated and grows wild in Brazil, Zaire, the Seychelles, South Africa, Indonesia, Morocco and Guatemala.[1]

Method of Extraction

Lemon scented eucalyptus oil is steam-distilled from the leaves of *E. citriodoria.*

Essential Oil Characteristics

E. citriodora is a colourless to pale-yellow, mobile liquid that has a strong and very fresh, citronella-like odour and a sweet, balsamic-floral dry-out note.[2]

Historical and Traditional Uses

E. citriodora oil is used in less expensive perfumes, soaps and disinfectants. It is also used for the isolation of citronellal, which is a source of many aromatic chemicals including hydroxycitronellal and menthol.[3] The kino (a red or orange exudate of the tree) contains an antibiotic substance, citriodorol.[4]

Chemical Composition

A typical chemical composition of *E. citriodora* is reported as follows:

α-pinene (0.14%), β-pinene (0.36), citronellal (80.1%), linalool (0.66%), isopulegol (3.41%), iso-isopulegol (8.51%), β-caryophyllene (0.39%), citronellyl acetate (0.02%), citronellol (4.18%).[1]

Therapeutic Actions

Antiseptic, bactericidal, deodorant, fungicidal, insecticidal.

Pharmacology and Clinical Studies

E. citriodora has bacteriostatic activity towards *S. aureus*. This is due to the synergy between citronellol and citronellal present in the oil.[4,5]

Indications

Antimicrobial Properties

Pharmacological studies indicate that *E. citriodora* has bacteriostatic activity towards *S. aureus.*[4,5]

Respiratory System

E. citriodora oil is recommended for the treatment of asthma, laryngitis and sore throat.[6]

Skin Care

E. citriodora oil is recommended for the treatment of athlete's foot, cuts, dandruff, herpes and as an insect repellent.[6] Lavabre recommends using *E. citriodora* in skin care because of its deodorising properties.[7]

Personality Profile

The *E. citriodora* personalities are fresh, alive and love freedom. They are constantly expressing new ideas and are full of vitality and laughter. Citriodora personalities get excited over new ideas and new gadgets. However, they cannot stand being tied down or feeling hemmed in — they need freedom.[8]

Mode of Administration

Topical application — massage, compress, ointment, skin care; Inhalation — direct inhalation, diffuser, oil vaporiser.

Safety

E. citriodora oil has been reported to be non-toxic, non-irritant and non-sensitising.

References

1. Boland DJ, Brophy JJ, House APN. *Eucalyptus leaf oils: use, chemistry, distillation and marketing,* Inkata Press, Australia, 1991.
2. Arctander S. *Perfume and flavour materials of natural origin.* Allured Publishing, USA, 1994.
3. Weiss EA. *Essential oil crops.* CAB International, UK, 1997.
4. Lassak E. *Australian medicinal plants.* Methuen Australia, Australia, 1983.
5. Low, D et al, *Antibacterial action of the essential oils of some Australian myrtaceae with special references to the activity of chromatographic fractions of the oil of eucalyptus citriodora.* Planta Medica, 1974; 26: 184–189. Cited in the Aromatherapy Database, Bob Harris, Essential Oil Resource Consultants, UK, 2000.
6. Lawless J. *The encyclopaedia of essential oils.* Element Books Limited, Great Britain, 1992.
7. Lavabre M. *Aromatherapy workbook.* Healing Art Press, USA, 1997.
8. Worwood V. *The fragrant mind.* Doubleday, Great Britain, 1995.

Everlasting

Helichrysum angustifolium DC.

Synonyms

H. italicum. Commonly known as helichrysum or immortelle.

Family

Compositae or Asteraceae

Botany and Origins

A strongly aromatic shrub with many branched stems that are woody at the base and grows up to 0.6 m high.[1]

When dried the brightly coloured, daisy-like flowers retain their colour and shape — hence the name *everlasting* or *immortelle*.[2,3] The plant grows wild and is cultivated in the south of France, Italy, former Yugoslavia and other Mediterranean countries.[2]

There are about 500 species of helichrysum, but many of these do not produce an essential oil. The main species used for the production of essential oil include:[3]

- *H. italium* or *H. angustifolium* (Corsica and former Yugoslavia)
- *H. stoechas* DC (France)
- *H. gymnocephalum* H. Humb (Madagascar)
- *H. patulum* (South Africa)

Method of Extraction

Everlasting oil is steam-distilled from the flowering tops of *H. angustifolium*.

Essential Oil Characteristics

The oil is a pale-yellow, oily liquid with a powerful and diffusive odour which is unique. It has a sweet-fruity and tea-like odour with an excellent tenacity.[2]

Historical and Traditional Uses

The name *Helichrysum* comes from the Greek word helios (sun) and chrysos (gold) because of the way these plants bloom gives the impression of little golden suns.[3]

In traditional herbal medicine, everlasting is used as an expectorant, antitussive, choleretic, diuretic, anti-inflammatory and antiallergenic agent in Europe. It has been used for bronchitis, asthma, whooping cough, psoriasis, burns, rheumatism, headache, migraines, allergies and liver ailments and it is usually taken in the form of a decoction or infusion.[1]

Chemical Composition

A typical chemical composition of everlasting oil contains 30–50% of nerol and neryl acetate; α-pinene, β-pinene, myrcene, limonene, 1,8-cineole, borneol, linalool, 4,7-dimetyl-6-octen-3-one, several diketones and 3,5-dimethyloctane-4, 6-dione and 2,4-dimethylheptane-3,5-dione reported to be the odour principles.[1]

Therapeutic Actions

Anti-inflammatory, antimicrobial, antitussive, antiseptic, cholagogue, cicatrisant, diuretic, expectorant, hepatic, mucolytic.

Pharmacology and Clinical Studies

Everlasting oil has been reported to exhibit antimicrobial properties *in vitro* against *Staphyloccus aureus*, *Escherichia coli*, a *Mycobacterium* species and *Candida albicans*.[1]

Indications

Circulatory System

Among its chemical constituents is a group of ketone-like compounds called beta-diones. It is this group of constituents that contributes to the oil's anticoagulant properties, making it applicable in the treatment of any severe bruising that results in haematoma.[4,6,8]

Detoxification

Everlasting is well known for its ability to purify the blood. Fischer-Rizzi says that everlasting helps drain the lymph glands. She recommends using the everlasting when performing a lymphatic drainage massage.[7] It is well known as a stimulant to the liver, gall bladder, kidney, spleen and pancreas — the organs responsible for detoxifying the body.[5,7]

Integumentary System

Everlasting is reputed to have anti-inflammatory properties and is recommended for eczema and allergies.[5,6]

Fischer-Rizzi recommends blending everlasting with rock rose and lavender for treating skin allergies, eczema, rashes and psoriasis.[7]

Schnaubelt says that everlasting may be used for the treatment of large injuries until professional care is available. He recommends applying undiluted oil onto the wound, before it is bandaged for the trip to the hospital. It will not cause any irritation and will reduce swelling and inflammation and speed up the wound-healing process.[8]

Musculoskeletal System

Everlasting's analgesic and anti-inflammatory properties make it beneficial for the treatment of rheumatoid arthritis.[5,6]

Respiratory System

Everlasting has mucolytic, antispasmodic and expectorant properties which make it beneficial for treating sinus infections, bronchitis and coughs.[5,6]

Skin Care

Everlasting oil is used in skin care because of its excellent anti-inflammatory activity. It is recommended where there is inflamed tissue which needs to be calmed down and regenerated.[8]

Energetics

Mojay compares the properties of everlasting with Roman chamomile and yarrow. He states that all three oils regulate the flow of *Qi* and clear heat. Therefore they are beneficial for conditions associated with the liver and encourage the flow of bile.[4]

Personality Profile

The everlasting personality profile is one of quietness, introversion and youth, with a quiet knowing that comes from being sure of the spirituality of all things. The everlasting person is described as being spiritually highly evolved and often seems fairy-like, having high consciousness and mental agility.[9]

Mojay describes the type of individual who specifically benefits from everlasting's ability to disperse more deeply embedded repression:

> *Such individuals are emotionally "blocked" in a profound way, unable not only to give expression to their anger and despair but to admit to themselves the fact of their own deep wounding. Instead of seeking ways to release these feelings — feelings which may stem from childhood trauma — they respond instead by developing rigid, self-denying thought patterns, and judging harshly those who are not open and spontaneous.*[4]

Subtle Aromatherapy

Everlasting oil is ideal for people who feel cold or who may have received too little warmth and affection as children. The oil is beneficial for people who have lost contact with the earth, have become too cerebral, or have acquired cold feet.[7]

Lawless recommends using everlasting to increase dream activity and awareness and to stimulate the right side of the brain.[10]

Mode of Administration

Topical application — massage, compress, bath, ointment, skin care; Inhalation — direct inhalation, diffuser, oil vaporiser.

As a liver stimulant, Fischer-Rizzi and Schnaubelt suggest that everlasting oil be taken orally in small doses.[7,8] Fischer-Rizzi recommends taking one drop twice daily.[7]

Safety

Everlasting oil has been reported to be non-toxic, non-irritant and non-sensitising.

References

1. Leung A, Foster S. *Encyclopedia of common natural ingredients used in food, drugs and cosmetics.* 2nd edn, John Wiley and Sons Inc, USA, 1996.
2. Arctander S. *Perfume and flavour materials of natural origin.* Allured Publishing, USA, 1994.
3. Mailhebiau P. *Portraits in oils.* The C.W. Daniel Company Limited, Great Britain, 1995.
4. Mojay G. *Aromatherapy for healing the spirit.* Hodder and Stoughton, UK, 1996.
5. Lawless J. *The encyclopaedia of essential oils.* Element Books Limited, Great Britain, 1992.
6. Davis P. *Aromatherapy: An A–Z.* 2nd edn, The C.W. Daniel Company Limited, Great Britain, 1999.
7. Fischer-Rizzi S. *Complete aromatherapy handbook.* Sterling Publishing Company, USA, 1990.
8. Schnaubelt K. *Medical aromatherapy.* Frog Ltd, USA, 1999.
9. Worwood V. *The fragrant mind.* Doubleday, Great Britain, 1995.
10. Lawless J. *Aromatherapy and the mind.* Harper Collins Publishers, UK, 1994.

Fennel, Sweet

Foeniculum vulgare

Synonyms

F. officinale, Anethum foeniculum; F. vulgare is also known as Roman fennel.

Family

Umbelliferae or Apiaceae

Botany and Origins

Fennel is a biennial or perennial herb that grows up to 2 m high, with fine, feathery leaves and umbels of golden-yellow flowers. It is indigenous to Mediterranean countries such as Italy, Greece and France.[1] The name of fennel comes from Latin *foenum*, meaning hay, and the Romans called it *foeniculum*.[2]

There are two subspecies of fennel:

- *F. vulgare* var. *amara*, known as bitter fennel.
- *F. vulgare* var. *dulce*, known as sweet fennel.

Method of Extraction

Fennel oil is produced from the distillation of the crushed seeds of *F. vulgare*.

Essential Oil Characteristics

Sweet fennel oil is a colourless to pale-yellow liquid with a very sweet, but slightly earthy or peppery-spicy odour and a clean, sweet aromatic dry-out.[1]

Historical and Traditional Uses

Fennel was well known to the ancient Egyptians, the Greeks and the Romans. It was cultivated for its aromatic fruits and succulent edible shoots. Pliny had high regard for its medicinal properties.[2]

The Greeks were the first to recognise its value as a slimming aid. The ancient Greek name of the herb, *Marathron*, from *maraino* (to grow thin), probably refers to this property. It was said to convey longevity, and to give strength and courage. The ancient Greeks ate the seeds for this reason and to help control their weight while training for the Olympics.[2]

The seeds were carried by Roman soldiers on long marches, to chew when they did not have time to stop and cook a meal, and by devout Christians to satisfy the cravings of hunger on fasting days.[3]

During the Middle Ages the use of fennel was entwined with witchcraft and superstition. It was used with St John's Wort as protection against evil forces. It was hung inside houses and churches or above doors to protect those inside against the devil.[4]

William Cole, a 17th century herbalist, affirms the properties of fennel:

> *... fennel is much used in drinks and broths for those that are grown fat, to abate their unwellness and cause them to grow more gaunt and lank.*[2]

Culpeper was well aware of fennel's qualities:

> *... Fennel is good for breaking of wind, ... to provoke urine, ... to break and ease the pain of the stone, ... stay the hiccough, ... allay the heat and loathing of the stomach, and the gripings thereof, ... open obstructions of the liver, gall and spleen, ... and to ease the painful and windy swellings of the spleen ... as also in gout and cramps.*[4]

The dried, aromatic fruits or seeds are widely used in culinary preparations for flavouring bread and pastry, in candies, alcoholic liqueurs as well as in oral and medicinal preparations.[5]

In TCM, fennel has been used for centuries to treat snake bites, for which the powdered herb is used as a poultice.[5]

Chemical Composition

A typical chemical composition of sweet fennel is reported as follows:

α-pinene (1.8–3.3%), myrcene (0.5–0.8%), fenchone (19.0–21.6%), trans-anethole (64.0–69.2%), methyl chavicol (3.9–6.5%), limonene and 1,8-cineole (1.2–1.7%), anisic aldehyde (0.1–0.3%).[6]

The concentration of trans-anethole in fennel oil varies from 50 to 90%, depending on the varieties, sources and the ripeness of the seeds.[5]

Sweet fennel contains less fenchone and more anethole than bitter fennel oil.

Therapeutic Actions

Antiseptic, antispasmodic, carminative, depurative, diuretic, emmenagogue, expectorant, galactagogue, splenic, stomachic.

Pharmacology and Clinical Studies

Fennel oil has been reported to have spasmolytic effects on smooth muscles of experimental animals.[5] It was found to be antispasmodic towards smooth muscle of isolated rat ileum and urinary bladder. It inhibits contractions induced by acetylcholine in a calcium-free medium. It was concluded that fennel oil inhibited calcium release from intracellular stores and/or blocked binding proteins.[7]

Fennel oil exhibited antibacterial activities in vitro.[5] Anethole and fenchone have been found to stimulate secretions of the upper respiratory tract.[5] Fennel oil and anethole were found to have cholagogue and choleretic effect on rats and guinea pigs.[8,9] Research suggests that polymers of anethole are active oestrogenic compounds.[5,10]

Indications

Digestive System

Fennel oil is traditionally used as a stomachic and a carminative in treating flatulence and other digestive problems.[3,5] The oil is recommended in the German Commission E Monographs for peptic discomforts, spastic disorders of the gastrointestinal tract, feelings of fullness and flatulence.[11]

Lymphatic System

Fennel is a diuretic and lymphatic decongestant, assisting the body to eliminate toxins. It is often used for treating fluid retention, cellulite and obesity, as an essential oil and herbal tea.[3,12]

Reproductive System

Fennel is recommended for regulating the menstrual cycle, particularly where periods are scanty and painful.[3,5] It may be used during menopause to reduce symptoms caused by fluctuating hormonal levels.[3]

Respiratory System

Like aniseed, fennel oil is an antispasmodic and expectorant and is recommended for catarrh of the upper respiratory tract.[5,11,12]

Urinary System

Fennel is a diuretic and traditionally used as an urinary tract antiseptic. It may be used for the treatment of urinary tract infections.[3]

Skin Care

Fennel oil is recommended in skin care preparation for the treatment of dull, oily and mature skin types.[12]

Energetics

Fennel is classified as a warming and drying remedy. It removes stagnancy in the stomach, frees spasms, clears flatus, settles the stomach and expels phlegm. It is recommended for bronchial asthma, wheezing and asthmatic breathing in any condition.[13,14]

Personality Profile

Worwood says that the fennel personalities are constantly active and always on the move.

> *They don't walk — they hurry along — leaping up the stairs rather than waiting for a lift. Fennels buy exercise tapes to use at home; they belong to swimming clubs and probably play squash at the weekend. They excel at any type of competition — at work as well as at play.*[15]

Fennel oil is closely related to the *earth* element and the intellect. According to TCM, an important aspect of the *earth* element is the need and capacity to be productive and creative.[14]

Mojay says that fennel is suited to the type of individual who tends to over-think and over-analyse.[14]

> *While they may easily generate concepts and ideas, they rarely communicate them or put them into practice. They may find it difficult to articulate and express themselves, feelings, too, tend to churn within. The more such emotions are locked inside, the more they intensify, building up tension that affects the bowels. The unacceptable, unexpressed thoughts and emotions that are pushed below consciousness accumulate in the intestines as nervous spasm and gas.*[14]

Subtle Aromatherapy

Davis refers to the traditional uses of fennel as a form of protection against witches and evil. She recommends using fennel if you feel threatened at any time by psychic attack. To do this, Davis suggests rub a drop or two on your hands and smooth them over your aura at a little distance from the surface of the body.[16]

Mode of Administration

Topical application — massage, compress, bath, skin care; Inhalation — direct inhalation, diffuser, oil vaporiser.

For digestive complaints the German Commission E Monographs recommend 10 to 20 g of fennel honey syrup which is made with 0.5 g fennel oil/kg.[11]

Safety

Sweet and bitter fennel oil are often contra-indicated for use by persons suffering from epilepsy or during pregnancy.[12,3]

I have a suspicion that some aromatherapists may be concerned about the fenchone content, which is a ketone. As we know, some ketones are reputed to be neurotoxic. There is no pharmacological evidence to suggest that fenchone or trans-anethole are neurotoxic in the doses used in aromatherapy.[17] Bitter fennel may cause sensitisation in some individuals.[11,12,17]

The German Commission E Monographs state that fennel oil should not be used during pregnancy or for infants and toddlers.[11] Due to trans-anethole's oestrogen-like action, Tisserand and Balacs advise to avoid the oral doses of fennel oil, until conclusive data is available, during breast feeding or pregnancy, for oestrogen-dependent cancers or endometriosis.[17]

References

1. Arctander S. *Perfume and flavour materials of natural origin.* Allured Publishing, USA, 1994.
2. Grieve, M, *A modern herbal.* Penguin, England, 1931.
3. Davis P. *Aromatherapy: An A–Z.* 2nd edn. The C.W. Daniel Company Limited, Great Britain, 1999.
4. Le Strange R. *A history of herbal plants.* Angus and Robertson, Great Britain, 1977.
5. Leung A, Foster S. *Encyclopedia of common natural ingredients used in food, drugs and cosmetics.* 2nd edn, John Wiley and Sons Inc, USA, 1996.
6. Lawrence B. *Fennel oil.* Perfumer and Flavorist, 1979; 4(2): 53.
7. Saleh MM et al. *Volatile oil of Egyptian sweet fennel and its effects on isolated smooth muscles.* Pharm Pharmacol Lett, 1996; 6(1): 5–7. Cited in the Aromatherapy Database, Bob Harris, Essential Oil Resource Consultants, UK, 2000.
8. Rangelov A. *An experimental characterisation of cholagogic and cholesteric activity of a group of essential oils.* Folia Med, 1989; 31(1): 46–53. Cited in the Aromatherapy Database, Bob Harris, Essential Oil Resource Consultants, UK, 2000.
9. Rangelov A et al. *Experimental study of the cholagogic and choleretic action of some of the basic ingredients of essential oils on laboratory animals.* Folia Med, 1988; 30(4): 30–38. Cited in the Aromatherapy Database, Bob Harris, Essential Oil Resource Consultants, UK, 2000.
10. Balacs T. *Hormones and health.* The International Journal of Aromatherapy, 1993; (5)1: 18.
11. Blumenthal M et al. *The complete German commission E monographs: Therapeutic guide to herbal medicine.* American Botanical Council, USA, 1998.
12. Lawless J. *The encyclopaedia of essential oils.* Element Books Limited, Great Britain, 1992.
13. Holmes P. *The energetics of western herbs Vol. I.* Artemis Press, USA, 1989.
14. Mojay G. *Aromatherapy for healing the spirit.* Hodder and Stoughton, UK, 1996.
15. Worwood V. *The fragrant mind.* Doubleday, Great Britain, 1995.

16. Davis P. *Subtle aromatherapy.* The C.W. Daniel Company Limited, Great Britain, 1991.

17. Tisserand R, Balacs T. *Essential oil safety.* Churchill Livingstone, UK, 1995.

Fir

Abies alba

Synonyms

A. excelsa, A. pectinata, A. picea, silver fir needle, silver spruce or white spruce.

Family

Pinaceae

Botany and Origins

A. alba is a relatively small tree which grows in Austria, Eastern France, Germany, Poland, Russia and Canada. The tree is planted in many European countries for lumber, wood pulp and for Christmas trees.[1]

Fir oil is produced from the leaves and twigs of various members of the conifer family which are sold under the name fir oil.

Siberian fir needle oil is made from the leaves of *A. siberica*. This is considered one of the most popular fir needle oils in Europe. [1]

Japanese fir needle oil is also called pine needle oil and is made from the leaves and twigs of *A. mayriana*. [1]

Balsam fir needle oil is made from the leaves and twigs of the Canadian and northeast American 'balsam fir'. Scandinavian fir needle oil is known as *Pinus sylvestris*. [1]

Method of Extraction

Fir oil is produced from the steam distillation of the leaves and twigs of various *abies* species.

Essential Oil Characteristics

Fir oil is a colourless to pale-yellow liquid with a rich balsamic-sweet and pleasant coniferous fragrance.[1]

Historical and Traditional Uses

Fir pine tree exudes a resin called fir balsam. This was used by North American Indians for medicinal and religious purposes.[2]

A. alba oil is used in perfumes for bath preparations, air fresheners, disinfectants, fougere colognes, soap perfumes and detergents.[1]

Chemical Composition

A typical chemical composition of fir is reported as follows:

Santene (1.2–4.0%), tricylene (0.4–1.2%), α-pinene (4.7–9.4%), camphene (3.9–10.9%), β-pinene (21.4–44.3%), myrcene (1.0–2.5%), carene (7.3–35.6%), limonene (2.7–19.7%), phellandrene (2.7–5.8%), terpinolene (0.3–0.7%), borneol (0.1–0.6%), terpinen-4-ol (trace to 0.2%), α-terpineol (0.1–0.4%), bornyl acetate (8.7–23%), piperitone (0–0.3%).[3]

Pharmacology and Clinical Studies

The antimicrobial properties of *A. alba* essential oil has been investigated and has been found to have moderate activity to very little activity.[4]

Therapeutic Actions

Analgesic, antiseptic, expectorant, deodorant, rubefacient, stimulant.

Indications

Musculoskeletal System

Fir oil is recommended for the relief of muscular aches and pains due to rheumatism or arthritic conditions.[2,5,6]

Nervous System

Fir oil is recommended for alleviating anxiety and stress.[2]

Respiratory System

Fir oil is recommended for catarrhal illness of the upper and lower respiratory tract.[2,6,7]

Subtle Aromatherapy

Fir oil is said to encourage protection and clarity of mind and spirit. It allows us to achieve strength and inner unity.[7] It is considered elevating and grounding and is recommended for the third eye and crown chakra.[2]

Mode of Administration

Topical application — massage, compress, bath, ointment; Inhalation — direct inhalation, diffuser, oil vaporiser, steam inhalation.

Safety

Fir oil has been reported to be non-toxic, non-irritant and non-sensitising.

The German Commission E Monographs state that fir is contra-indicated for bronchial asthma and whooping cough as it increases bronchial spasms.[5]

References

1. Arctander S. *Perfume and flavour materials of natural origin.* Allured Publishing, USA, 1994.

2. Lavabre M. *Aromatherapy workbook.* Healing Art Press, USA, 1990.

3. Lawrence B. *Fir oil.* Perfumer and Flavorist, 1979; 3(6): 54.

4. Bagci E, Digrak M. *Antimicrobial activity of essential oils of some Abies (fir) species from Turkey.* Flavour and Fragrance Journal, 1996; 11(4): 251–256.
5. Blumenthal M. *The complete German commission E monographs: Therapeutic guide to herbal medicine.* The American Botanical Council, USA, 1998.
6. Lawless J. *The encyclopaedia of essential oils.* Element Books Limited, Great Britain, 1992.
7. Worwood V. *The fragrant heavens.* Transworld Publishing, Great Britain, 1999.

Frankincense

Boswellia ssp.

Synonyms

Olibanum

Family

Burseraceae

Botany and Origins

Frankincense, also known as olibanum, is a natural oleo-gum-resin formed from the physiological exudate from the bark of various *Boswellia* species.[1] The most commonly used species are as follows:[1]

- *B. sacra* — from Oman, Yemen and southern Saudi Arabia.
- *B. carteri* Birdwood — from Somalia.
- *B. frereana* Birdwood — from Somalia.
- *B. papyifera* — from western Ethiopia
- *B. serrata* — from western India.

The trees originate from the mountainous areas of western India, southern Arabia and north-eastern Africa. The trees are not cultivated, and the collection of the resin is made where the trees are most abundant.[1] The major frankincense-producing countries are Somalia and Ethiopia.[2]

The resin is collected by making incisions into the bark. A milky-white liquid appears which then solidifies into amber or orange-brown crystals of resin. The resin is sorted and graded. The age, appearance, moisture level and odour characteristics determine the quality of the oil.[1]

The resin appears as pale-yellow or pale-amber-coloured, tear-shaped or drop-shaped, egg-shaped or almost round lumps, varying from pea size to walnut size. Other grades may be orange-yellow, orange-red or brownish in colour, and the tears may be agglutinated into large lumps. There is no simple rule to determine which colour of frankincense 'tears' or 'lumps' will yield the best oil.[1]

Method of Extraction

Frankincense oil is produced from the steam distillation of the resin of various *boswellia* species. A resinoid absolute of frankincense is also produced for the perfume industry by solvent extraction.[1]

Essential Oil Characteristics

Frankincense oil is a pale-yellow or pale-amber-greenish mobile liquid with a strongly diffusive odour. The odour is fresh and terpene-like with a subtle green-lemon note.[2]

Historical and Traditional Uses

The name olibanum is thought to be derived from Latin, *olium libanum*, meaning oil from Lebanon. The name frankincense is derived from the Old French word *franc,* meaning free, pure or abundant, and Latin *incensum,* meaning to smoke.[8]

Frankincense played a very important role in the religious and domestic lives of Ancient Egypt, Persian, Hebrew, Greek and Roman civilisations. It has always been considered an important ingredient in cosmetics, as an aromatic incense and in religious rituals of these ancient civilisations.

The Egyptians obtained frankincense from the land of Punt, believed to have been a region in Somalia. The famous kyphi, a renowned scent used by them, was made with frankincense. Kyphi was used as an incense and also added to beverages.[3]

Kohl, a black powder used by Egyptian women to paint their eyelids, is made from charred frankincense.[4]

According to Herodotus, the Babylonians used large amounts of frankincense during their religious rites.[4] Roman emperor Nero is said to have burnt more frankincense than Arabia could produce in a year at his wife Poppaea's funeral.[5]

Frankincense is regularly mentioned in the Bible, being used in religious ceremonies. The most famous reference to frankincense was in the bible when it was given as a gift to the infant Jesus. Pliny recommended frankincense as an antidote to hemlock, Avicenna recommended it for tumours, ulcers, vomiting, dysentery and fever.[4]

Frankincense continues to be used in many Christian churches nowadays. It is still used in many parts of the Arab world. For example, the Muslim inhabitants of the United Arab Emirates say that a dirty smelly body is vulnerable to evil, the scented person is surrounded by angels. They believe that the most useful scent for attracting angels and dispelling evil spirits is frankincense. For this reason, children, houses and mosques are censed weekly with frankincense.[5]

Chemical Composition

A typical chemical composition of frankincense is reported as follows.[6]

Constituent	B. carteri	B. frereana	B. serrata
α-pinene	1.0—4.6%	34.4–43%	7.7%
α-thujene	0.0–1.5%	—	61.4%
sabinene	—	0.9–1.3%	5.1%
para-cymene	—	1.7–14.0%	4.3%
octyl acetate	50–60%	<1.5%	—
octanol	3.5–12.7%	—	—
incenysl acetate	3.0–4.1%	—	—
incensol	2.1–2.7%	—	—
limonene	1.7–2.4%	1.1–6.0%	1.6%
linalool	0.2–2.5%	—	—
cembrene	<2.3%	—	—
isocembrene	<1.8%	—	—
1,8-cineole	<1.6	—	—
(E)-β-ocimene	1.5–1.5%	—	—
camphene	<1.1%	<2.0%	—
viridoflorol	—	<15.2%	—
α-phellandrene	—	<14.6%	2.2%
verbenone	—	<6.5%	—
myrcene	—	2.0–6.0%	—
β-pinene	—	1.0–4.1%	—
β-caryophyllene	—	0.1–1.2%	—
estragole	—	—	2.7%
(Z)-β-ocimene	—	Tr–1.0%	—
α-thujone	—	—	1.7%
β-bourbonene	—	—	1.5%
β-thujone	—	—	1.4%
δ-3-carene	—	—	1.2%
zingiberene	—	—	1.0%

Pharmacology and Clinical Studies

A nonphenolic fraction of *B. serrata* has been reported to have strong analgesic effects on rats. It was identified as having anti-inflammatory and anti-arthritic properties.[1]

Therapeutic Actions

Antiseptic, astringent, carminative, cicatrisant, cytophylactic, diuretic, emmenagogue, expectorant, sedative, uterine, vulnerary.

Indications

Nervous System

Frankincense can be used to alleviate anxiety, nervous tension and stress-related conditions.[8]

Respiratory System

Frankincense has traditionally been used to treat respiratory conditions such as asthma, bronchitis, catarrhal conditions and asthma.[8,9]

Davis says that frankincense has the ability to *deepen the breath* — that is, to slow down the rate of breathing and increase the amplitude of breathing. She suggests that it is an ideal choice for someone with an asthmatic condition associated with nervousness.[7]

Skin Care

Frankincense is well known in skin care for its cicatrisant, cytophylactic and vulnerary properties and is recommended for dry and mature skin, scars, wounds and wrinkles.[8,9]

Energetics

Mojay recommends frankincense to smooth the free flow of *Qi*. It is best used whenever there is an accumulation of stress that has led to irritability, restlessness and insomnia.[10]

Personality Profile

Worwood says that frankincense people often display an air of mystery and secretiveness. There is a sense of maturity, confidence and efficiency about these people, who seem to have an understanding of the nature of the universe. While they are not necessarily religious people, they have a profound love of God in their hearts. They are usually good communicators, are friendly, warm and loving.[11]

Frankincense personalities often have parapsychological tendencies — they are sensitive to atmospheres, sensing unhappiness or evil in a room or house.[11]

Subtle Aromatherapy

Mojay recommends frankincense for aiding meditation, contemplation and prayer, helping to cease mental chatter and stilling the mind.[10] Frankincense is recommended as a meditation aid and to cut ties with the past, especially where these may block personal growth.[12]

Mode of Administration

Topical application — massage, compress, bath, liniment, skin care; Inhalation — direct inhalation, diffuser, oil vaporiser, steam inhalation.

Safety

Frankincense oil has been reported to be non-toxic, non-irritant and non-sensitising.

References

1. Leung A, Foster S. *Encyclopedia of common natural ingredients used in food, drugs and cosmetics*. 2nd edn, John Wiley and Sons Inc, USA, 1996.
2. Arctander S. *Perfume and flavour materials of natural origin*. Allured Publishing, USA, 1994.
3. Manniche L. *An ancient Egyptian herbal*. British Museum Press, London, 1993.

4. Grieve M. *A modern herbal.* Penguin, Great Britain, 1931.
5. Classens C et al. *Aroma: The cultural history of smell.* Routledge, England, 1994.
6. Lawrence B. *Essential oils 1992–1994.* Allured Publishing, USA, 1995.
7. Davis P. *Aromatherapy: An A–Z.* 2nd edn., The C.W. Daniel Company Limited, Great Britain, 1999.
8. Lawless J. *The encyclopaedia of essential oils.* Element Books Limited, Great Britain, 1992.
9. Lavabre M. *Aromatherapy workbook.* Healing Art Press, USA, 1997.
10. Mojay G. *Aromatherapy for healing the spirit.* Hodder and Stoughton, UK, 1996.
11. Worwood V. *The fragrant mind.* Doubleday, Great Britain, 1995.
12. Davis P. *Subtle aromatherapy.* The C.W. Daniel Company Limited, Great Britain, 1991.

Geranium

Pelargonium graveolens

Synonyms

There are several types of geranium oil produced from cultivated forms, varieties and hybrids of the *Pelargonium* species. The main species are *P. capitum, P. graveolens, P. radens and P. odoratissimum.*

Bourbon geranium is produced from the cultivar Rose, which is a hybrid of *P. capitum* and *P. radens,* and is commonly known as *P. graveolens.*[1]

Family

Geraniaceae

Botany and Origins

There is actually a great deal of confusion over the origins of geranium. This is not surprising considering that there are over 250 natural species of *Pelargonium*, hundreds of hybrids and thousands of cultivars.[1]

P. graveolens is a perennial, shrubby, hairy plant, up to 1 m high with fragrant leaves.

Geraniums originate from South Africa. They were introduced to Europe in the 17th century and hybridised. Some of these scented-leaf hybrids were distributed around the world and later grown for geranium oil production.[1]

The first geranium plants grown for the French perfume industry were planted in Algeria in 1847 and in the 1880s extensive plantations were established on Reunion. Geranium oil is also produced in other parts of the world such as China and Egypt. The Chinese geranium is very similar to Bourbon, while Egypt geranium is quite different.[1]

Other *Pelargonium* species grown in gardens for their fragrant leaves include *P. citriodorum* (citron-scented), *P. Fragrans* (nutmeg-scented) and *P. tomentosum* (peppermint-scented).[1]

A number of geranium oils are available and they are usually distinguished by a country of origin prefix: Reunion, Chinese, Egyptian or Moroccan.[1]

Bourbon geranium, which is produced on the Reunion Islands, is considered the most important of the geranium oils.

An oil from Bulgaria known as zdravetz oil is distilled from *Geranium macrorrhium*. Zdravetz oil is a pale olive-green or pale-yellowish-green somewhat viscous liquid which at room temperature is normally 30% liquid and 70% crystals. The crystals begin to dissolve at 32°C. The main constituents of zdravetz oil are sesquiterpenes (to 90%) of which about half is germacrone.[1]

Method of Extraction

Geranium oil is steam-distilled from the leaves and branches of *P. graveolens.*

Essential Oil Characteristics

Bourbon geranium is a greenish-olive oil with a pronounced green, leafy-rosy scent.

The odour of freshly distilled bourbon geranium has a peculiar, rather obnoxious top note which is partly due to dimethyl sulphide. It is produced during the rapid decaying of the plant material immediately prior to the distillation. The unpleasant top note will disappear after proper aeration or aging of the oil.[2]

Moroccan geranium is usually darker to medium-yellow colour and the Egyptian geranium is yellow to yellowish-green colour. Both have a sweet, rosy, herbaceous odour somewhat similar to Reunion geranium.[1]

The Chinese geranium is dark green, often with a brownish or brownish-yellow tinge and the odour is harsher than Bourbon geranium and is often more lemony and rosy, with a sweet-herbaceous note.[1]

Historical and Traditional Uses

The first reference to geranium is in Dioscorides' *Materia Medica*, as *geranion* from the Greek *geranos*, a crane, because of the shape of the long beaked fruit. The plant and its fragrant leaves were used by the Romans.[1]

Much confusion exists over the therapeutic activity of geranium oil. This originates from transcribing Culpeper's and other herbal texts which refer only to *G. robertianium*, which has a completely different chemical composition to the geranium oil of today.[3]

Geranium oil is widely used as a fragrance component in all kinds of cosmetic products such as soaps, detergents, creams, lotions and perfumes.[4]

Its main medicinal use in the past was the treatment of diarrhoea and dysentery. This is possibly due to the antispasmodic action on smooth muscle.[4]

Chemical Composition

There can be quite some difference in the chemical composition of geranium essential oil from different places of origins.[1]

Constituent	Bourbon	Chinese	Egypt
linalool	12.90%	3.96%	9.47%
citronellol	21.28%	40.23%	27.40%
nerol	1.24%	0.67%	0.88%
geraniol	17.45%	6.45%	18.00%
citronellyl formate	8.37%	11.35%	6.74%
geranyl formate	7.55%	1.92%	4.75%
geranyl butyrate	1.34%	0.98%	1.48%
geranyl tiglate	1.04%	1.32%	1.06%
iso-menthone	7.20%	5.70%	5.39%
guaia-6,9-diene	3.90%	4.40%	0.27%

Therapeutic Actions

Antidepressant, antiseptic, astringent, cicatrisant, cytophylactic, diuretic, deodorant, haemostatic, styptic, tonic, vermifuge, vulnerary.

Pharmacology and Clinical Studies

Geranium oil has been reported to exhibit antifungal and antibacterial activities *in vitro*.[4,5]

Indications

Detoxification

Geranium oil is a diuretic and has a stimulating effect on the lymphatic system. It is beneficial for treating cellulite, fluid retention and oedema of the ankles.[6,8,9]

Integumentary System

Geranium oil has excellent astringent and haemostatic properties which make it useful for treating wounds and bruises.[6,8,9] It is recommended for its anti-inflammatory properties for conditions such as eczema and psoriasis and is used for treating acne.[8,9] It has cytophylactic properties and is recommended for the treatment of burns and wounds.[8,9]

Nervous System

Geranium oil has an excellent regulating effect on the nervous system and may be used in a bath, massage or vaporiser to relieve stress, nervous tension, depression, headaches and anxiety.[7,8] The action of geranium oil on the nervous system is sedative and uplifting.[7]

Reproductive System

Geranium oil may be a stimulant of the adrenal cortex, whose hormones are essentially regulating and balancing. This is why geranium oil is recommended for conditions where fluctuating hormones are a problem. In particular, geranium oil may be used to relieve premenstrual tension and menopause.[6,8,9]

Skin Care

It is popular in skin care, not only for its delightful aroma, but for its action in balancing the production of sebum. This makes it valuable for skin that is either dry, oily or combination skin.[7,8,9]

Energetics

According to the principles of TCM, geranium oil is cooling and moist. It clears heat and has the ability to strengthen the flow of *Qi*. It is therefore able to calm the mind, relax the body, ease frustration and irritability.[10]

Personality Profile

Geranium is described as one of the mothering personalities — a person who is always ready to take care of someone or something.[11]

The geranium personalities are able to create a sense of security and stability wherever they go. They are friendly and comforting, although not in any way extroverted or over-talkative. They tend to have the ability to wash away your tension and stress.[11]

Subtle Aromatherapy

Geranium is ideal for the workaholic perfectionist — the person who has forgotten imagination, intuition and sensory experience.[10]

Mode of Administration

Topical application — massage, compress, bath, ointment, skin care; Inhalation — direct inhalation, diffuser, oil vaporiser.

Safety

Geranium oil has been reported to be non-toxic, non-irritant and non-sensitising. However, cases of dermatitis in hypersensitive individuals caused by geranium oil have been documented.[4]

References

1. Weiss EA. *Essential oil crops.* CAB International, UK, 1997.
2. Arctander S. *Perfume and flavour materials of natural origin.* Allured Publishing, USA, 1994.
3. Lis-Balchin M. *Geranium oil.* The International Journal of Aromatherapy, 1996; 7(3): 18.

4. Leung A, Foster S. *Encyclopedia of common natural ingredients used in food, drugs and cosmetics.* 2nd edn, John Wiley and Sons Inc, USA, 1996.
5. Lis-Balchin M. *Bioactivity of geranium oils from different sources.* Journal of Essential Oil Research, 1996; 8(3): 281–290.
6. Davis P. *Aromatherapy: An A–Z.* 2nd edn. The C.W. Daniel Company Limited, Great Britain, 1999.
7. Tisserand R. *The art of aromatherapy.* The C.W. Daniel Company Limited, Great Britain, 1977.
8. Lawless J. *The encyclopaedia of essential oils.* Element Books Limited, Great Britain, 1992.
9. Lavabre M. *Aromatherapy workbook.* Healing Art Press, USA, 1997.
10. Mojay G. *Aromatherapy for healing the spirit.* Hodder and Stoughton, UK, 1996.
11. Worwood V. *The fragrant mind.* Doubleday, Great Britain, 1995.

Ginger

Zingiber officinale

Synonyms

Another member of the same family is *Languas officinarum,* known as ginger root or Chinese ginger.

Family

Zingiberaceae

Botany and Origins

Ginger is a tropical perennial herb growing 0.6 to 1.2 m high, with reed-like stems, lanceolate leaves and yellow flowers with purple markings. The stem grows directly from the thick tuberous rhizome, from which the spice and essential oil are produced.

Originally from India, ginger is now cultivated in India, China, most of South East Asia, Australia and the tropical regions of Africa.

Method of Extraction

Ginger oil is produced by steam distillation, occasionally by water and steam distillation of the dried, unpeeled, ground rhizomes of *Z. officinale.*

An oleoresin is produced by solvent extraction of the dried and unpeeled rhizome of *Z. officinale.*

Characteristics

Ginger oil is a pale-yellow to light-amber-coloured mobile liquid. Its odour is warm, but fresh-woody, spicy with a slight fresh top note. The sweet and heavy undertone is tenacious, sweet and rich, almost balsamic-floral.[1]

Ginger oleoresin is a dark-brown or very dark amber-coloured, viscous liquid, with a warm-spicy, sweet aroma.[1]

Historical and Traditional Uses

Ginger was originally used as a spice. In India, it is mentioned in the earliest Sanskrit literature, but not in the oldest Vedic works. In China, the first known recorded use of ginger is from Confucius (*c.* 500 BC), who claimed never to be without ginger when he ate. It was used to treat rheumatism, toothache and malaria.[2]

In TCM, ginger is used for colds and chills, to promote sweating, expel mucous and stimulate the appetite. The dried ginger has been used to treat stomach ache, diarrhoea, nausea, cholera and bleeding.[3]

Ginger was one of the first spices to find its way to Europe along the spice route, where both the Greeks and Romans made extensive use of it. The Greek physician Dioscorides recommended using ginger as a digestive stimulant.[3]

Chemical Composition

Some 100 constituents have been identified in distilled ginger oil. The main components are sesquiterpene hydrocarbons (50–66%), oxygenated sesquiterpenes (up to 17%), and the rest is made up of monoterpene hydrocarbons and oxygenated monoterpenes.

A typical chemical composition of a range of distilled ginger oils are reported as follows:[2]

Constituent	Australia	Sri Lanka	India
α-pinene	Trace	0.2–3.3%	0.4%
camphene	Trace	0.9–14.1%	1.1%
geranial	3–20%	1.0–7.7%	1.4%
nerol	1–10%	2.5–10.1%	0.2%
1,8-cineole	Trace	2.1–12.23%	Trace
ar-curumeme	6–10%	5.7–17.7%	17.7%
zingiberene	20–28%	0.3–1.2%	35.6%
(z)-β-farnesene	–	0.5–1.2%	–
β-sesquiphellandrene	7–11%	0–0.3%	–
β-bisabolene	5–9%	20.1–60.4%	0.2%
β-eudesmol	Trace	1.0–5.4%	Trace

Australian ginger oil typically has a higher citral content (geranial) compared with most other ginger oils. This gives the oil a distinctly fresh, lemon-like aroma. This is probably due to more careful drying of the rhizomes.[2]

Ginger oleoresin contains the pungent principles gingerols and shogaols as well as zingerone.[3]

Pharmacology and Clinical Studies

As a medicinal herb, ginger may be prepared by either decocting the fresh root or by preparing an alcoholic tincture or fluid extract with it. A tincture is considered the most complete preparation as it contains the essential oil constituents as well as the pungent alcohols; shogaol and gingerol.[4]

While it may be tempting to suggest that the essential oil and herbal extract have similar properties, Holmes points out that because the distilled essential oil contains no pungent components, the essential oil can not have diaphoretic properties. He therefore says that it is a waste of time using ginger essential oil as a diaphoretic at the onset of a cold.[4]

The oleoresin may be of interest to aromatherapists as it contains more of the pungent and warming components found in the herb. Gingerol and shogoal may have a local irritant effect on mucous membranes and it is possible that vascular stimulation that follows from taking ginger comes either from direct action on metarterioles or by reflex from sensory receptors at other sites.[5]

A considerable number of pharmacological studies involving the digestive, central nervous and cardiovascular systems have been reported for gingerol and shogoal. It has been identified that these constituents have potent inhibitory action against prostaglandin synthetase which corresponds with anti-inflammatory and anti-platelet aggregation.[6]

Clinical trials have shown that the oleoresin is a cholesterol-lowering agent. Gingerol has been found to be a cholagogue and is a hepatoprotective agent.[6,7]

Clinical trials have identified that ginger has antiemetic properties. Most of the trials revealed an activity superior to that of a placebo for motion sickness, postoperative nausea or morning sickness (at the usual dose of 1 g per day). The antiemetic action may be a consequence of the direct stimulating effect on the gastrointestinal tract.[7]

The German Commission E Monographs recommend using the rhizome powder for gastrointestinal distress and to prevent motion sickness (2 g/day). It is described as having antiemetic, positive inotropic and stimulant effects on intestinal peristalsis, salivary and gastric secretions.[8]

The antipyretic (reducing fever) activity of ginger has been attributed to shogaol and gingerol. The antipyretic activity of ginger can be attributed to ginger's diaphoretic activity in febrile states.[9]

Bone and Mills cite several studies which have investigated the possible thermogenic (warming) effects of ginger. Zingerone, found in the oleoresin, increased the secretion of catecholamines, especially adrenaline, from the adrenal medulla ater intravenous injection in rats.[9]

Therapeutic Actions

Analgesic, antiseptic, carminative, expectorant, febrifuge, laxative, rubefacient, stimulant, stomachic, sudorific, tonic.

Indications

Circulatory System

Mojay describes ginger as a circulatory stimulant and tonic of the heart. It is recommended for poor circulation, cold hands and feet, cardiac fatigue and angina pectoris.[11]

Digestive System

Ginger stimulates and warms the digestive system, therefore it is indicated for poor digestion, abdominal distenstion and flatulence. Mojay says that it should be blended with Roman chamomile and sweet orange to relieve travel and morning sickness.[11]

Musculoskeletal System

Ginger oil may be used in a compress or massage for rheumatism, arthritis and muscular pain of a cold contracting type.[10,11]

Respiratory System

Ginger oil is recommended for catarrhal conditions, coughs, sinusitis and sore throats.[10]

Energetics

The properties of ginger oil are described as warming. Not only is this warming quality beneficial for stimulating arterial circulation, but it also helps dispel cold conditions associated with the digestive system, respiratory system and reproductive system.[4,11]

It has a warming and stimulating effect on the lungs and is ideally suited to treat chronic bronchitis. Ginger's ability to tonify the yang energy of the kidneys makes it a useful oil for relieving lower back pain associated with muscular fatigue.[11]

Personality Profile

Ginger is ideal for people who have clear plans and good intentions, but who lack the personal drive and optimism to manifest initiative and take real or immediate action.[11]

A ginger personality is a strong, silent type. The character of ginger is warming, strengthening and encouraging.[12]

Subtle Aromatherapy

The scent of ginger will increase determination and clarity. It is recommended for conditions associated with loss of motivation, will or inner strength, especially when these present apathy, listlessness, indecision, confusion and disconnection.[4]

Mode of Administration

Topical application — massage, compress, bath, ointment; Inhalation — direct inhalation, diffuser, oil vaporiser.

Safety

Ginger oil is non-toxic and non-irritant. It may cause sensitisation in some individuals.

References

1. Arctander S. *Perfume and flavour materials of natural origin.* Allured Publishing, USA, 1994.
2. Weiss EA. *Essential oil crops.* CAB International, UK, 1997.
3. Leung A, Foster S. *Encyclopedia of common natural ingredients used in food, drugs and cosmetics.* 2nd edn, John Wiley and Sons Inc, USA, 1996.
4. Holmes P. *Ginger oil.* The International Journal of Aromatherapy, 1996; 7(4): 16.
5. Mills S. *The essential book of herbal medicine.* Arkana Penguin Books, England, 1991.
6. Evans WC. *Trease and Evans pharmacognosy.* WB Saunders, 15th edn, England, 2002.
7. Bruneton J. *Pharmacognosy.* 2nd edn, Lavoisier Publishing Inc, France, 1999.
8. Blumenthal M et al. *The complete German commission E monographs: Therapeutic guide to herbal medicine.* American Botanical Council, USA, 1998.
9. Bone K, Mills S. *Principles and Practice of Phytotherapy.* Churchill Livingstone, UK, 2000.
10. Lawless J. *The encyclopaedia of essential oils.* Element Books Limited, Great Britain, 1992.
11. Mojay G. *Aromatherapy for healing the spirit.* Hodder and Stoughton, UK, 1996.
12. Worwood V. *The fragrant mind.* Doubleday, Great Britain, 1995.

Grapefruit

Citrus paradisi Macf.

Synonyms

C. racemosa, C. decumana var. *racemosa, C. mazima* var. *racemosa,* Shaddock fruit.

Family

Rutaceae

Botany and Origins

C. paradisi is considered to be a hybrid between *C. maxima* and *C. sinensis.*[1]

Grapefruit is the only citrus species native to the New World and probably originated in the West Indies from a natural cross between introduced parents some time in the 17th century.[1]

The oil is produced in USA, the West Indies, Brazil, Israel and Nigeria.

Grapefruit is a large, vigorous tree that grows up to 30 m, with a single trunk, many branches, and has a round to blunt conical shape if left unpruned. The fruit is large, up to 15 cm diameter, generally spherical but often compressed laterally, light yellow to orange. The shape and colour of the fruit are dependent on the cultivar.[1]

The difference between the essential oil from the white- and red-fleshed cultivars is that the former generally has a higher aldehyde content and lower evaporative residue than the latter, which also contains a small percentage of linalool.[1]

Method of Extraction

Grapefruit oil is expressed from the peels of the grapefruit.

Essential Oil Characteristics

The oil is a mobile, yellowish to greenish-yellow or pale-orange-yellow oil with a fresh-citrus and sweet odour.[2] The characteristic grapefruit aroma and flavour is reported to be due to nootkatone.[3]

Historical and Traditional Uses

Apart from its recent use in aromatherapy, grapefruit is extensively used as a flavour in soft drinks and as a fragrance component in soaps, detergents and personal care products.[3]

Chemical Composition

Cold-pressed grapefruit oil contains mostly limonene, a monoterpene hydrocarbon. A typical chemical composition of grapefruit oil is reported as follows:

α-pinene (0.38%), β-pinene (0.02%), sabinene (0.42%), myrcene (1.37%), d-limonene (84.0%), citronellal (0.1%), decanol (0.4%), linalool (0.1%), nootkatone (0.1%).[1]

Pharmacology and Clinical Studies

Studies indicate that grapefruit oil has considerable antimicrobial activity when tested against *Candida albicans, Aspergillus niger* and the generally difficult to inhibit *Pseudomonas aeruginosa.*[1]

Therapeutic Actions

Antidepressant, antiseptic, depurative, diuretic, disinfectant, stimulant.

Indications

Grapefruit's properties have been described as being similar to that of lemon oil.[4,5]

Lymphatic System

Grapefruit oil is a lymphatic stimulant and is indicated for cellulitis, obesity and water retention.[4,6,7]

Nervous System
Grapefruit oil has an uplifting and reviving effect which makes it valuable for treating stress, depression and nervous exhaustion. It is recommended for people who are depressed and lethargic, particularly in winter.[7]

Skin Care
It is beneficial for treating oily skin and acne, and has a tonic effect on the skin and scalp.[7]

Energetics

It is cooling, cleansing and decongesting and is beneficial for an overheated liver and sluggish lymphatic system.[4] According to TCM, symptoms associated with an overheated liver includes abdominal distension, constipation, nausea and a feeling of general irritability.[4]

Personality Profile

The oil is most suited to people who are tense. Under pressure they tend to resort to 'comfort eating' as a means of dealing with difficult situations.[4]

The grapefruit personality is described as a warm, happy person who is bursting with energy, loves life and people.[8] Grapefruit oil has been described as stimulating self-esteem, creating euphoria and self-worth.[9]

Mode of Administration

Topical application — massage, compress, bath, skin care; Inhalation — direct inhalation, diffuser, oil vaporiser.

Safety

Grapefruit oil is reported to be non-toxic, non-irritating, non-sensitising and is not phototoxic to humans.[3]

References

1. Weiss EA. *Essential oil crops*. CAB International, UK, 1997.
2. Arctander S. *Perfume and flavor materials of natural origin*. Allured Publishing Corporation, USA, 1994.
3. Leung A, Foster S. *Encyclopedia of common natural ingredients used in food, drugs and cosmetics*. 2nd edn, John Wiley and Sons Inc, USA, 1996.
4. Mojay G. *Aromatherapy for healing the spirit*. Hodder and Stoughton, UK, 1996.
5. Lawless J. *Aromatherapy and the mind*. Harper Collins Publishers, England, 1994.
6. Lavabre M. *Aromatherapy workbook*. Healing Art Press, USA, 1997.
7. Davis P. *Aromatherapy: An A–Z*. 2nd edn, The C.W. Daniel Company Limited, Great Britain, 1999.
8. Worwood V. *The fragrant mind*. Doubleday, Great Britain, 1995.
9. Miller L and B. *Ayurveda and aromatherapy*. Lotus Press, USA, 1995.

Hyssop

Hyssopus officinalis var. *decumbens*

Synonyms

H. officinalis, creeping hyssop

Family

Labiatae or Lamiaceae

Botany and Origins

A perennial aromatic small sub-shrub which grows up to 0.5 m high, with slender herbaceous stems arising from a woody base, bearing whorls of small purplish-blue flowers.

It is native to southern Europe and has been cultivated as a culinary herb and for medicinal uses for hundreds of years. The major producing countries include France, Hungary and Holland.[1]

Method of Extraction

Hyssop oil is steam-distilled from the leaves and flowering tops of *H. officinalis*.

Essential Oil Characteristics

Hyssop oil is a pale-yellow or faintly greenish-yellow colour to almost colourless oil with a powerful, sharp, sweet-camphoraceous odour with a warm, spicy undertone.[1]

Historical and Traditional Uses

The name comes from the Greek word *hyssopus*, itself derived from the Hebrew word *ezob*, meaning good scented herb. The flowers and leaves have been highly valued since antiquity for their therapeutic properties, and it was one of the bitter herbs mentioned in the Old Testament. Hippocrates prescribed it for pleurisy and bronchitis.[2]

It was commonly used in the Middle Ages for its therapeutic properties. Culpeper recommended:

> *It is good to wash inflammations, and takes away the blue and black marks that come by strokes, bruises or falls … it is an excellent medicine for the quinsy, or swelling in the throat, to wash and gargle it … The hot vapours of the decoction taken by a funnel in the ears, eases the inflammation and singing noise of them … It is good for falling sickness (epilepsy), expectorates tough phlegm, and is effectual in all cold griefs, or diseases of the chest and lung.*[3]

The herb is used for sore throats, coughs, colds, digestive disorders, intestinal ailments, menstrual complaints. It is a diaphoretic and may be used externally for treating skin irritations, burns, bruises and frostbite.[9]

Chemical Composition

A typical chemical composition of hyssop is reported as follows:

α-pinene (0.74%), camphene (0.14%), β-pinene, sabinene (1.72%), myrcene (0.72%), limonene (0.68%), pinocamphone (42.66%), isopinocamphene (30.88%), α-terpineol (1.00%), 1,8-cineole (0.64%), β thujone (0.33%).[4]

It is important to distinguish between the oil of *H. officinalis* and *H. officinalis* var. *decumbens*. The latter is free of the potentially toxic ketones, whereas the oil of *H. officinalis* contains a high percentage of pinocamphone.[5]

Therapeutic Actions

Antiseptic, antispasmodic, cicatrisant, digestive, emmenagogue, expectorant, febrifuge, hypertensive, nervine, sudorific, vulnerary.

Pharmacology and Clinical Studies

Herbal extracts of hyssop have been reported to exhibit antiviral activities.[9]

Indications

Circulatory System

As a hypertensive it has a regulatory effect on the circulation and helps raise low blood pressure.[7,8] It is recommended in a cold compress for the treatment of bruises.[7]

Digestive System

It is a tonic to the digestive system and acts as an appetite stimulant, mild laxative, relieves stomach cramps and expels wind.[9,10]

Immune System

H. officinalis var. *decumbens* is reputed to have potent antiviral effects and is suitable for treating herpes.[6]

Nervous System

It has an invigorating effect on the mind and is recommended for poor concentration, mental fatigue and nervous debility.[10,11]

Respiratory System

Hyssop has a special affinity with the respiratory system. It liquefies mucus and relieves bronchial spasms. It is effective for treating colds, sore throats, influenza, bronchitis and asthma.[6,7,8,11]

Reproductive System

Hyssop relieves menstrual problems associated with water retention during periods and is effective for treating amenorrhoea and leucorrhoea.[9,11]

Energetics

Hyssop is described as hot and stimulating and is a tonic of yang *Qi*. It is reputed to strengthen and warm the lungs and is recommended for chronic bronchitis, poor vitality, breathlessness and immune deficiency.[10,11]

Personality Profile

It is reputed to strengthen one's sense of personal 'boundary'. It therefore benefits the type of person who is easily influenced by others' moods and emotions, and who, as a result, absorbs any negativity and tension in the environment.[10]

Subtle Aromatherapy

Hyssop is reputed to be a cleansing herb and is recommended to cleanse any area in which you are planning to meditate or use for healing purposes.[13]

Mode of Administration

Topical application — massage, compress, bath, liniment; Inhalation — direct inhalation, diffuser, oil vaporiser, steam inhalation.

Safety

Hyssop oil should not be used during pregnancy or on individuals with epilepsy.[7,10,12]

H. officinalis var. *decumbens* contains very little of the hazardous ketones and is considered relatively safe to use.[5,14]

References

1. Arctander S. *Perfume and flavour materials of natural origin.* Allured Publishing, USA, 1994.
2. Le Strange R. *A history of herbal plants.* Angus and Robertson, Publishers, Great Britain, 1977.
3. Grieve M. *A modern herbal.* Penguin, England, 1931.
4. Lawrence B. *Hyssop oil.* Perfumer and Flavorist, 1984; 9(3): 35.
5. Schnaubelt K. *Medical aromatherapy.* Frog Ltd, USA, 1999.
6. Schnaubelt K. *Advanced aromatherapy.* Healing Art Press, USA, 1995.
7. Davis P. *Aromatherapy: An A–Z.* 2nd edn, The C.W. Daniel Company Limited, UK, 1999.
8. Lavabre M. *Aromatherapy workbook.* Healing Art Press, USA, 1997.
9. Leung A, Foster S. *Encyclopedia of common natural ingredients used in food, drugs and cosmetics.* 2nd edn, John Wiley and Sons Inc, USA, 1996.
10. Mojay G. *Aromatherapy for healing the spirit.* Hodder and Stoughton, UK, 1996.
11. Holmes P. *The energetics of western herbs Vol. I.* Artemis Press, USA, 1989.
12. Lawless J. *The encyclopaedia of essential oils.* Element Books Limited, Great Britain, 1992.
13. Davis P. *Subtle aromatherapy.* The C.W. Daniel Company Limited, Great Britain, 1991.
14. Tisserand R, Balacs T. *Essential oil safety.* Churchill Livingstone, UK, 1995.

Jasmine

Jasminum grandiflorum

Synonyms

J. officinale

Family

Oleaceae

Botany and Origins

The *Jasminum* species are evergreen deciduous shrubs or shrubby climbers with white, pink or yellow very fragrant flowers.

Jasmine is native to the Indian and South East Asian region. The three commercially cultivated species used for essential oil production are:[1]

- *J. auriculatum*
- *J. grandiflorum*
- *J. sambac*

J. auriculatum is native to southern India and has adapted to regions with high temperature and above average rainfall.[1]

J. grandiflorum is native to northern Iran, Afghanistan and Kashmir, and has been introduced and is commercially cultivated in many countries, principally around the Mediterranean. It has adapted to a milder climate.[1]

Grasse, a town in the south of France, became the principal supplier of jasmine absolute. However, due to the high costs of production, most jasmine cultivation is now in countries such as Algeria, Morocco, Egypt and India.[1]

J. sambac is native to southern India and has a long history of cultivation in India. It is commonly referred to as Mogra.[1]

Method of Extraction

Jasmine absolute is produced by alcohol extraction of jasmine concrète, which is prepared by extraction with hydrocarbon solvents or by enfleurage. The enfleurage process has been described as follows:

> *Jasmine season began at the end of July, the perfume of this flower was both so exquisite and so fragile that not only did the blossoms have to be picked before sunrise, but they also demanded the most gentle and special handling. Warmth diminished their scent; suddenly to plunge them into hot macerating oil would have completely destroyed it.*
>
> *The souls of these noblest of blossoms could not be simply ripped from them, they had to be methodically coaxed away. In a special impregnated room, the flowers were strewn on glass plates smeared with cool oil or wrapped in oil soaked clothes, there they would die slowly in their sleep. It took three or four days for them to wither and exhale their scent into the adhering oil. then they were carefully plucked off and new blossoms spread out.*
>
> *This procedure was repeated a good, ten, twenty times, and it was September before the pomade had drunk its fill and the fragrant oil could be pressed from the clothes. The yield was considerably less than with maceration.*
>
> *But in purity, it was unequalled, the jasmine oil radiated the sticky sweet, erotic scent of the blossoms with lifelike fidelity.*[2]

This well-known method of extraction which has been employed for over 200 years is today becoming increasingly impractical and uneconomical due to the high costs of labour.[3]

Today, most jasmine absolute is commonly obtained by solvent extraction, via the concrète from the flowers of *J. grandiflorum*, cultivated in Egypt, Italy, Morocco and India, and of *J. sambac* from China and India.

The flowers open in the early morning and there is a rapid and significant loss of essential oil once the buds have opened. For example, one of the constituents, indole, dropped by 0.6–0.8 mg/100 g of flowers in the first hours after the buds open.[1]

Flowers are usually picked by hand as a suitable method for mechanical harvesting has not been commercially developed. Flowers must be processed without delay. Approximately 1,000 kg of jasmine flowers will yield 2.5–3.5 kg of concrete, and half this amount as an absolute.[1]

Essential Oil Characteristics

Jasmine absolute is a dark-orange (on aging reddish-brown), somewhat viscous liquid and it possesses an intensely floral, warm, rich and highly diffusive odour with a peculiar waxy-herbaceous, oily-fruity and tea-like undertone.[3]

Historical and Traditional Uses

Jasmine's fragrant flowers have been used since antiquity for personal adornment and in religious ceremonies.[1]

In India, jasmine is known as 'Queen of the Night', because the scent is stronger during the hours of darkness. The importance of the jasmine flower has been symbolically used throughout the centuries.

In China, the jasmine flower symbolises the sweetness of women while in India it symbolises divine hope. In the 15th century, jasmine was cultivated for its fragrant flowers in the gardens of the emperors of China, Afghanistan, Iran and Nepal. It was not until around 1600 when jasmine was bought to Spain by the Moors that it first made its appearance in Europe.

In China, the flowers of *J. officinalis* var. *grandiflorum* are mainly used to treat hepatitis, pain due to liver cirrhosis, and abdominal pain due to dysentery, while the flowers of *J. sambac* are used to treat conjunctivitis, skin ulcers and tumours, as well as abdominal pain due to dysentery.[3]

Jasmine has long been used for its effect on the reproductive system. It can be used as an aphrodisiac and to assist in childbirth.[1]

Dried jasmine flowers from *J. sambac* are used as an ingredient of Chinese jasmine tea.[3]

Chemical Composition

A typical chemical composition of jasmine absolute is reported as follows:

Benzyl acetate (22.09%), linalool (6.44%), benzyl alcohol (0.92%), farnesene (1.86%), indole (2.5%), benzyl benzoate +phytol (24.55%), *cis*-jasmone (2.6%), methyl anthranilate (2.04%), methyl jasmonate (2.99%), phytol acetate (10.25%), eugenol (1.66%), isophytol+jasmone lactone (9.77%).[1]

While the main volatile component of jasmine is benzyl acetate, minor constituents such as indole and *cis*-jasmone significantly contribute to the typical jasmine fragrance.

There is a significant difference between the main volatiles emitted by living and picked flowers. For instance, indole and benzyl acetate, which occurred in relatively high concentration in the headspaces of living jasmine flowers, decreased significantly in the headspace of picked flowers. The linalool content also rose from 3% to 30% of the total volatiles.[1]

Jasmine absolute produced from a pomade varies in odour from jasmine absolute produced from concrète. Generally, the indole note is more pronounced in the pomade-absolute than in the absolute from concrète.[3]

Therapeutic Actions

Antidepressant, antiseptic, antispasmodic, aphrodisiac, galactagogue, parturient, sedative, uterine.

Pharmacology and Clinical Trials

A clinical trial found that jasmine flowers from *J. sambac* were effective for the suppression of puerperal lactation. It was suggested that tactile and olfactory stimuli from the flowers were responsible for the suppression of lactation.[4]

Indications

Nervous System

The therapeutic value of jasmine oil is inseparable from the exquisite, comforting sweetness of its aroma and the effect it has on the mind and emotions. Jasmine is considered one of the most effective essential oils for nervous anxiety, restlessness and depression.[5]

Jasmine absolute has been described as a powerful antidepressant of a stimulating nature. It is recommended when depression has given rise to lethargy.[6]

The effects of jasmine have been described by Fischer-Rizzi as capable of changing our mood so intensely that it offers little choice other than optimism. She says that jasmine is especially helpful for emotional dilemmas, particularly when they involve relationships and sex.[7]

Reproductive System

Jasmine oil is one of the most useful oils to use during childbirth. If it is used as a massage oil on the abdomen and lower back in the early stages of labour it will relieve the pain and strengthen the contractions. It helps with the expulsion of the placenta after delivery and aids post-natal recovery.[6,9] It can be used to relieve spasms of the uterus and delayed and painful menstruation.[7,9]

Skin Care

Jasmine is particularly useful in skin care and is used to treat dry and irritated skin.[6,9,10]

Energetics

Holmes and Mojay describes jasmine as having yang qualities.[5,8] In terms of TCM, this means that it is used to dispel cold and generate warmth.

Holmes describe jasmine as a depression fighter equal to melissa, basil and ylang ylang. However, jasmine acts best on depression of the yang deficiency. This includes symptoms such as apathy, chilliness, fatigue, weakness and restlessness.[8]

Personality Profile

Jasmine is predominantly indicated for problems associated with the emotions. The fragrance of jasmine diminishes fear, it is helpful in enhancing self-confidence and defeating pessimism.

Worwood describes the jasmine personality as the passionate seductress, gentle and charismatic, bewitching all those who come into her presence.[12]

While Worwood is describing the female jasmine personality, she says that the male jasmine is equally charming, charismatic and at ease with his femininity. Jasmine personalities are joyful, happy people, comfortable with themselves. They can be unnerving if you are not used to them, particularly at work.[12]

Subtle Aromatherapy

Lavabre best summarises the subtle qualities of jasmine when he says that it releases inhibition, liberates imagination, develops exhilarating playfulness and has the power to transcend physical love, fully releasing male and female sexual energy.[11]

Mojay recommends jasmine for depression which results from unconscious restraint and repression — an approach to life based on values discordant with the individual soul and its true desires.[5]

Mode of Administration

Topical application — massage, compress, bath, skin care; Inhalation — direct inhalation, diffuser, oil vaporiser, steam inhalation.

Safety

Jasmine absolute is non-irritating, non-sensitising and non-phototoxic. However, Leung has cited coniferyl acetate and coniferyl benzoate as allergenic components of the jasmine absolute.[3]

References

1. Weiss EA. *Essential oil crops*. CAB International, UK, 1997.
2. Suskind P. *Perfume: The story of a murderer.* Penguin Books, England, 1986.
3. Arctander S. *Perfume and flavour materials of natural origin.* Allured Publishing, USA, 1994.
3. Leung A, Foster S. *Encyclopedia of common natural ingredients used in food, drugs and cosmetics.* 2nd edn, John Wiley and Sons Inc, USA, 1996.
4. Shrivastav P et al. *Suppression of puerperal lactation using jasmine flowers.* Aust. NZ J. Obstet Gynaecol, (1988), No. 28, pp. 68–71. Cited in the Aromatherapy Database, Bob Harris, Essential Oil Resource Consultants, UK, 2000.
5. Mojay G. *Aromatherapy for healing the spirit.* Hodder and Stoughton, UK, 1996
6. Davis P. *Aromatherapy: An A–Z.* 2nd edn, The C.W. Daniel Company Limited, Great Britain, 1999.
7. Fischer-Rizzi S. *Complete aromatherapy handbook.* Sterling Publishing Company, USA, 1990.
8. Holmes P. *The energetics of western herbs Vol. I.* Artemis Press, USA, 1986.
9. Lawless J. *The encyclopaedia of essential oils.* Element Books Limited, Great Britain, 1992.
10. Holmes P. *Jasmine*. The International Journal of Aromatherapy, 1998; 8(4): 8–12.
11. Lavabre M. *Aromatherapy workbook.* Healing Arts Press, USA, 1990.
12. Worwood V. *The fragrant mind.* Doubleday, Great Britain, 1995.

Juniper Berry

Juniperus communis

Synonyms

Common juniper

Family

Cupressaceae

Botany and Origins

The shrub *J. communis* grows wild throughout central Europe. It is a small tree reaching the height of 12 m with blue-green needle-like leaves, greenish-yellow flowers and small round berries. The berries take about three years to mature.[1]

The best juniper berries are collected in northern Italy, Austria, Czech Republic, Hungary, Croatia, Serbia and France.[1]

Method of Extraction

The best juniper berry oil is steam-distilled from the crushed, dried or partly dried ripe berries.[1]

Essential Oil Characteristics

Juniper berry oil is a clear or very pale-yellow, mobile oil having a fresh, yet warm, rich-balsamic, woody-sweet and pine-needle like odour.[1]

Historical and Traditional Uses

Juniper was commonly burnt as a fumigant and ritual incense by ancient Greeks to combat epidemics, and by Tibetans and native Americans for ceremonial purposes. The English name *juniper* is derived from the Latin *juniores*, meaning young berries.[12]

Culpeper was well aware of juniper's diuretic and detoxifying properties:

> *It is a remedy for dropsy, brings down the terms, helps fits of the mother, expels wind and strengthens the stomach. It provokes the urine and is good for gout and sciatica, and strengthens the limbs.*[4]

The berries and extract are used as ingredients in diuretic and laxative preparations. The oil is used as a fragrance component in soaps, detergents, creams, lotions and perfumes.[2] Juniper berries are used for making gin.

The berries are used as a carminative and diuretic, to treat flatulence, colic, intestinal worms and gastrointestinal infections.[2]

The German Commission E Monographs recommend a daily dosage of 2–10 g of the dried berries for dyspepsia. However, they warn that prolonged use may cause kidney damage and that it is contra-indicated during pregnancy.[3]

Juniper berries are recommended for acute and chronic cystitis and topical application for rheumatic pain in the joints or muscles.[5]

Chemical Composition

A typical chemical composition of juniper berry is reported as follows:

α-pinene (33.7%), camphene (0.5%), β-pinene (1.1%), sabinene (27.6%), myrcene (5.5%), α-phellandrene (1.3%), α-terpinene (1.9%), γ-terpinene (3.0%), 1,4-cineole (4%), β-phellandrene (1.3%), p-cymene (5.5%), terpinen-4-ol (4.0%), bornyl acetate (0.4%), cayophyllene (0.6%), and trace amounts of limonene, camphor, linalool, linalyl acetate, borneol and nerol.[6]

Therapeutic Actions

Antiseptic, antirheumatic, antispasmodic, astringent, carminative, depurative, detoxicant, rubefacient, stimulating, stomachic, sudorific, tonic, vulnerary.

Pharmacology and Clinical Studies

The oil has an antispasmodic effect on smooth muscles.[2] Juniper berries and juniper oil stimulate the excretion the glomerular filtration rate of the kidney. However, they are known to irritate the renal epithelium and could cause hematuria.[7]

It is believed that the toxicity depends on the hydrocarbon content of the essential oil. Juniper berry oil containing high levels of α– and β-pinene which are known irritants to the urinary tract. Higher levels of pinenes would result from co-distillation of the needles, branches and unripe berries with ripe berries. It has been concluded that oil distilled from the ripe berries can be safely used in diuretic therapy.[8]

Indications

Detoxification

Juniper berry oil is well known for its diuretic and lymphatic decongestant properties. It is recommended for clearing toxins and resolving toxaemia and to reduce levels of uric acid in the body, thus being beneficial for cellulite and rheumatic conditions.[9,10,11,12,13]

Integumentary System

Juniper berry oil is recommended for skin conditions which result as an accumulation of toxins in the body such as weeping type eczema, acne and psoriasis.[9,10,11]

Nervous System

Juniper berry oil is recommended for nervous and intellectual fatigue.[11]

Urinary System

Juniper berry oil is considered one of the best oils to choose for treating cystitis, pyelitis and urinary stones. However, if there is blood or pus in the urine or a fever, do not delay in getting medical assistance.[10]

Energetics

The energetic qualities of juniper are warming and stimulating yang energy.[12,13] Juniper berry oil is considered a powerful tonic of the body. Its warming and invigorating effect benefits tiredness, poor circulation, cold hands and feet and lower backache.[12]

Juniper berry oil is ideal for conditions associated with cold and damp. Cold and damp conditions are likely to be characterised by poor circulation, urinary-genital tract infections, digestive problems such as diarrhoea and poor appetite, and accumulation of toxins.

Personality Profile

Juniper personalities are described as having a profound spiritual ease; they have no concern for human authority, preferring to be directed by their intuition or religious beliefs. They are not afraid to enjoy themselves, therefore they often appear immature because they take delight in new experiences and knowledge.[14]

Subtle Aromatherapy

The fresh clean scent of juniper is associated with purification. It is no wonder that it has been used since ancient times for spiritual purification. It may be used for driving out negative influences. It is recommended for the individuals who, feeling burdened and aloof, are deeply absorbed in their own thoughts — thoughts that revolve around worries, pressures and unpleasant memories.[12]

Mode of Administration

Topical application — massage, compress, bath, sitz bath, douche, skin care; Inhalation — direct inhalation, diffuser, oil vaporiser.

Safety

Juniper berry oil has been reported to be non-toxic, non-irritant and non-sensitising. Juniper oil is contra-indicated during pregnancy or those with kidney disease.[9,10] It must be remembered that this refers to the internal use of herbal extracts of juniper berries.[5,7]

I agree with Tisserand and Balacs, who state that there is a good chance that juniper oil may have been confused with savin, whose botanical name is *J. sabina*.[15]

References

1. Arctander S. *Perfume and flavour materials of natural origin.* Allured Publishing, USA, 1994.
2. Leung A, Foster S. *Encyclopedia of common natural ingredients used in food, drugs and cosmetics.* 2nd edn, John Wiley and Sons Inc, USA, 1996.
3. Blumenthal M. et al. *The complete German commission E monographs: Therapeutic guide to herbal medicine.* American Botanical Council, USA, 1998.
4. Grieve M. *A modern herbal.* Penguin, England, 1931.
5. *British herbal pharmacopoeia.* British Herbal Medicine Association, England, 1987.

6. Lawrence B. *Juniper berry oil*. Perfumer and Flavorist, 1987/1988; 12(6): 59.
7. Bruneton J. *Pharmacognosy*. 2nd edn, Lavoisier Publishing Inc, France, 1999.
8. Cited from *Mediherb Monitor*. No. 7, December 1993.
9. Lawless J. *The encyclopaedia of essential oils*. Element Books Limited, Great Britain, 1992.
10. Davis P. *Aromatherapy: An A–Z*. 2nd edn, The C.W. Daniel Company Limited, Great Britain, 1999.
11. Lavabre, M. *Aromatherapy workbook*. Healing Art Press, USA, 1997.
12. Mojay G. *Aromatherapy for healing the spirit*. Hodder and Stoughton, UK, 1996.
13. Holmes P. *The energetics of western herbs Vol. I*, Artemis Press, USA, 1989.
14. Worwood V. *The fragrant mind*. Doubleday, Great Britain, 1995.
15. Tisserand R, Balacs T. *Essential oil safety*. Churchill Livingstone, UK, 1995.

Lavender

Lavandula angustifolia

Synonyms

L. officinalis Chaix; *L. vera*, True lavender

Family

Labiatae or Lamiaceae

Botany and Origins

Lavender is an aromatic evergreen sub-shrub with linear or lance-shaped leaves. It grows up to 0.9 m high and is native to the Mediterranean region.

The *lavandula* genus has approximately 30 species that grow around the world.[1] The four main species of lavender are: [1]

- *L. angustifolia* — true lavender
- *L. latifolia* — spike lavender
- *L. x intermedia* — lavandin
- *L. stoechas* — maritime lavender.

Lavender essential oil distilled from *L. angustifolia* P.Miller, *L. officinalis* Chaix or *L. vera* de Candolle is referred to as true lavender.

Approximately half of the true lavender produced now comes from cultivated clones such as *Maillette*. This gives a 40 to 50% higher yield than population lavender (raised from seed). Harris says that population lavender from France has a superior fragrance and commands a higher price than cloned lavender and lavender from other countries. Lavendulol and its ester lavendulyl acetate are said to contribute to the aroma of this oil.[1]

The main producers of true lavender are Bulgaria and France. Smaller producers include Australia, Argentina, England, Hungary, Japan, Morocco, Italy, Algeria, India and Russia.[2]

Lavender grown and distilled at a higher altitude (from 600 to 1500 m) has a reputation of being the best quality lavender. This is because distilleries located at higher altitudes distil the oil at 92 to 93 °C instead of 100°C. This produces an oil with a higher ester content. Even at this small decrease of temperature, hydrolysis of the natural linalyl esters takes place at a much slower rate. A rapid distillation at a slightly reduced pressure will also produce an oil with a higher linalyl ester content.[2]

Mrs Grieve goes to great lengths to discuss the ideal method of cultivating lavender and the best time to harvest the plant. She recommends that the blooms be fully developed, because this will produce an essential oil with a high ester content. She suggests that very cold weather prevents the esters from developing. The most refined lavender oil is distilled from the flowers that have been stripped from the stalk. This, however, leads to a very expensive lavender oil.[3]

Lavandin is a hybrid of true lavender and spike lavender. The lavandin plant is larger and much hardier than that of true lavender. It is ideally suited to large-scale cultivation and harvesting methods. It is very popular with the fragrance industry as it yields twice the amount of oil as true lavender and is commonly used in soaps, detergents and cosmetics.[1]

There are three main clones of lavandin in France:[1]

- Abrial
- Super
- Grosso.

Maritime lavender is sometimes known as cotton lavender. The essential oil is predominantly harvested and distilled from the wild in Portugal. It is rich in ketones and while it is used in France for its mucolytic and antimicrobial properties, it should be used with caution as there are concerns about the oil's toxicity.[1]

Lavender is one of the most commonly adulterated essential oils. Adulteration of true lavender in the essential oil trade is common. This is achieved by:[1]

- addition of lavandin oil
- substitution by lavandin oil
- addition of synthetic linalool and linalyl acetate
- addition of linalool and linalyl acetate from other natural sources.

Method of Extraction

Lavender oil is steam-distilled from the freshly cut flowering tops and stalks of *L. angustifolia*.

Essential Oil Characteristics

L. angustifolia oil is a colourless or pale-yellow liquid of a sweet, floral herbaceous refreshing odour with a pleasant, balsamic-woody undertone.[2]

Historical and Traditional Uses

Lavendula comes from *lavare*, meaning 'to wash' in Latin.[3] Lavender essential oil has been widely used as a toilet water and is one of the most common ingredients in pot-pourris and sachets.

Culpeper recommended a decoction of lavender flowers to help prevent falling sickness (epilepsy) and giddiness or turning of the brain.[4]

Mrs Grieve describes lavender as an admirable restorative tonic against fainting, palpitations of a nervous nature, giddiness, spasms and colic. She recommends a few drops of lavender oil in a hot foot bath to relieve fatigue and outwardly applied she recommends it for the relief of toothache, neuralgia, sprains and rheumatism.[4]

Lavender's antiseptic properties were well known by the French Academy of Medicine, where it was used in the swabbing of wounds, treatment of sores, varicose ulcers, burns and scalds.[4]

Chemical Composition

A typical chemical composition of lavender is reported as follows:

α-pinene (0.02–0.67%), limonene (0.02–0.68%), 1,8-cineole (0.01–0.21%), cis-ocimene (1.35–2.87%), trans-ocimene (0.86–1.36%), 3-octanone (1.75–3.04%), camphor (0.54–0.89%), linalool (29.35–41.62%), linalyl acetate (46.71–53.80%), caryophyllene (2.64–5.05%), terpinen-4-ol (0.03–4.16%), lavendulyl acetate (0.27–4.24%).[5]

Therapeutic Actions

Analgesic, anticonvulsive, antidepressant, antiphlogistic, antirheumatic, antiseptic, antispasmodic, antiviral, bactericide, carminative, cholagogue, cicatrisant, cordial, cytophylactic, decongestant, deodorant, diuretic, emmenagogue, fungicide, hypotensive, nervine, restorative, sedative, sudorific, vulnerary.

Pharmacology and Clinical Studies

Lavender oil has been demonstrated to have CNS-depressive activities on mice. It is also reported as having excellent antimicrobial activities.[6] It has been found to be spasmolytic, in vitro on the smooth muscle of guinea pig ileum.[7] The oil has been demonstrated to have a dose-dependent anaesthetic activity.[8]

Lavender oil has been the focus of several clinical trials and has successfully been used in some hospitals as a massage oil, being vaporised to help dispel anxiety, and as an alternative to using orthodox drugs to help patients sleep.[9,10]

Indications

Lavender oil enjoys the status as being the most popular and versatile essential oil in aromatherapy.

Integumentary System

It was Rene-Maurice Gattefosse who observed the healing effects of lavender oil when he burnt his hand in a laboratory accident. Lavender oil is commonly associated with burns and healing of the skin. It has antiseptic, analgesic and cytophylactic properties which will ease the pain of a burn, prevent infection and promote rapid healing.

Lavender is beneficial for conditions involving inflammation such as acne, dermatitis, eczema, psoriasis, boils and wounds.[11,12,13,14]

Lavender is useful for the treatment of sunburn and sunstroke. It can be combined with peppermint in a 1% dilution and used as a massage oil.

Musculoskeletal System

Lavender is very beneficial for the relief of muscular aches and pains. It can also be used for the relief of rheumatism, sciatica and arthritis.[12,13]

Nervous System

Lavender has a harmonising effect on the nervous system. Holmes explains this in terms of lavender's ability to deal with stress. Stress can become counterproductive on the physiological level involves either the sympathetic or parasympathetic nervous system. Sympathetic hyperfunctioning is triggered by emotional stress whereas sympathetic hyperfunctioning is triggered more by physical stress. Both types of stress reactions will produce symptoms such as spasms, cramps, pains, nervous tension, irritability and mental distraction.[17]

Holmes says that lavender oil can inhibit sympathetic or parasympathetic nervous system functions. Therefore lavender can assist our responses to unproductive stress of any kind. Likewise, lavender will tend not to interfere with productive stress — a normal part of life.[17]

Lavender can exert a sedative or a stimulant action depending on one's actual needs. It will act as a sedative in conditions of mental and emotional agitation and unrest, calming the mind, comforting feelings and alleviating fears, while it is uplifting and revives the spirits for someone feeling emotionally depleted and depressed.

Lavender is regarded as the first choice in the treatment of insomnia, especially when the insomnia is due to mental stress and anxiety.[13] It is recommended for the treatment of migraines and headaches.[14]

Reproductive System
Lavender oil is valuable for relieving premenstrual tension and menstrual pain. Davis recommends gently massaging a massage oil with lavender into the lower abdomen or using it in a hot compress.[13]

A clinical trial identified lavender as the most popular essential oil during childbirth and it was found to reduce maternal anxiety, for pain relief and to lighten the mood.[18]

Respiratory System
Lavender is recommended for the treatment of colds and flu, bronchitis, throat infections and catarrhal conditions.[11,12,14] Lavender is particularly beneficial for asthma of a nervous origin or a result of uncontrolled anxiety. Mailhebiau says it relaxes the person and enables easier breathing.[3]

Skin Care
The antiseptic, antiphlogistic and cicatrisant properties of lavender make it beneficial in many skin care preparations. It can be used for all skin types. It can be used as an insect repellent and may also be used to treat insect bites — preventing the itching and scratching.[13,14]

Energetics

According to TCM, lavender oil is cooling. Holmes says that lavender may be used to clear heat, resolve fever, cool an overheated liver, support and stabilise the heart, calm the spirit and relieve irritability.[15]

Mojay says that lavender soothes and supports the *Qi* of the heart. Lavender is recommended for the treatment of nervous tension, insomnia, palpitations and high blood pressure.[16]

Personality Profile

Holmes best summarises the qualities of lavender:

> *The very feminine experience of being surrounded by fields of purple blooming lavender in a French Haute Provence possibly discloses a hint to the nature of this plant: a compassionate herb of the highest order. Pain, infection, inflammation, distress, agitation and acute injuries of everyday life are the main symptoms relieved through its compassionate effects — regardless of the illness or underlying condition.*[17]

Lavender is often referred to as the 'mother' of essential oils. Worwood says that the lavender personality is able to care for a multitude of physical and psychological problems and like a mother can accomplish several jobs at the same time.[19]

Worwood says that lavender is the perfect balance between masculine and feminine traits within us all.[19] Mailhebiau compares lavender to Mother Teresa:

> *Tireless, always even-tempered, with unfailing gentleness and devotion, Lavandula cares for and calms, listens to and remedies a thousand ills. She takes care of children, adults and elderly, animals, plants, the earth and sky. She looks after everyone with equal love and if there is anyone in the world whom she neglects, it is herself.*[3]

Subtle Aromatherapy

Davis says that the calming and relaxing qualities of lavender can help in reaching deeper states of meditation. She recommends using lavender to integrate our spirituality into everyday life. She suggests that it helps to bring together the higher and lower chakra centres into harmony with each other.[20]

Method of Administration

Topical application — massage, compress, bath, sitz bath, douche, ointment, skin care; Inhalation — direct inhalation, diffuser, oil vaporiser, steam inhalation.

Safety

Lavender oil is non-toxic, non-irritating and non-sensitising.

References

1. Harris R. *Lavenders of Provence*. The World of Aromatherapy III Conference Proceedings. NAHA, USA, 1999; 75–81.
2. Arctander S. *Perfume and flavour materials of natural origin.* Allured Publishing, USA, 1994.
3. Mailhebiau P. *Portraits in oils*. The C.W. Daniel Company Limited, Great Britain, 1995.
4. Grieve M. *A modern herbal.* Penguin, Great Britain, 1931.
5. Lawrence B. *Lavender oil.* Perfumer and Flavorist, Dec/Jan 1987/1988; 12(6): 59.
6. Leung A, Foster S. *Encyclopedia of common natural ingredients used in food, drugs and cosmetics.* 2nd edn., John Wiley and Sons Inc, USA, 1996.
7. Lis-Balchin L et al. *Studies on the mode of action of the essential oil of lavender.* Phytotherapy Research, 1999; 3: 540–542. Cited in the Aromatherapy Database, Bob Harris, Essential Oil Resource Consultants, UK, 2000.
8. Ghelardini C et al. *Local anaesthetic activity of the essential oil of lavandula angustifolia.* Planta Medica, 1999; 65: 700–703. Cited in the Aromatherapy Database, Bob Harris, Essential Oil Resource Consultants, UK, 2000.
9. Husdon R. *The value of lavender for rest and activity in the elderly patient.* Complimentary Therapy Medicine, 1996; 4: 52–57. Cited in the Aromatherapy Database, Bob Harris, Essential Oil Resource Consultants, UK, 2000.
10. Henry, J., et al., *Lavender oil for night sedation of people with dementia.* The International Journal of Aromatherapy, 6(2): 28–30.

11. Fischer-Rizzi S. *Complete aromatherapy handbook.* Sterling Publishing Company, USA, 1990.
12. Lawless J. *The encyclopaedia of essential oils.* Element Books Limited, Great Britain, 1992.
13. Davis P. *Aromatherapy: An A–Z.* 2nd edn, The C.W. Daniel Company Limited, Great Britain, 1999.
14. Lavabre M. *Aromatherapy workbook.* Healing Art Press, USA. 1997.
15. Holmes P. *The energetics of western herbs Vol. I.* Artemis Press, USA, 1989.
16. Mojay G. *Aromatherapy for healing the spirit.* Hodder and Stoughton, UK, 1996.
17. Holmes P. *Lavender.* The International Journal of Aromatherapy 1992; 4(2): 20–22.
18. Burn E, Blamey C. *Soothing scents in childbirth.* The International Journal of Aromatherapy 1994; 6(1): 24–28.
19. Worwood V. *The fragrant mind.* Doubleday, Great Britain, 1995.
20. Davis P. *Subtle aromatherapy.* The C.W. Daniel Company Limited, Great Britain, 1991.

Lavender — Spike

Lavandula spica

Synonyms

L. latifolia, aspic

Family

Labiatae or Lamiaceae

Botany and Origins

Spike lavender is an aromatic evergreen sub-shrub with linear or lance-shaped leaves. It grows up to 1 m high and is native to the Mediterranean region. It is easy to distinguish from other lavender species as it has long spatula-shaped leaves and long flowering spikes with greyish-blue flowers.[1]

Spike lavender grows wild around the Mediterranean countries, particularly Spain, France and Italy. Spain is the major producer of the oil.[2]

Method of Extraction

Spike lavender is steam-distilled from the flowering tops of *L. spica.* Most spike lavender is distilled from wild plants.[1]

Essential Oil Characteristics

Spike lavender oil is a pale-yellow to almost clear-coloured mobile liquid with a fresh camphoraceous and herbaceous odour with a somewhat dry-woody undertone.[2]

Historical and Traditional Uses

Commonly called aspic, it is considered as the 'male lavender' in contrast to *L. angustifolia* which is referred to as the 'female lavender'. The term *aspic* comes from the Greek term meaning 'Egyptian cobra' and owes this name to its historical use against the venom of the asp.[3]

Culpeper recommended spike lavender for a variety of ailments such as pains of the head and brain, falling sickness, dropsy, cramps, and convulsions. He described the oil of spike lavender as having a fierce and piercing quality, and recommended using the oil cautiously, a few drops being sufficient for inward or outward griefs.[4]

Spike lavender was an ingredient in the famous *Oleum Spicae* which was used for the treatment of old sprains and stiff joints.[4]

Chemical Composition

The main difference between spike lavender and true lavender is the high camphor and 1,8-cineole content of spike lavender. A typical chemical composition of spike lavender is reported as follows:

α-pinene (1.7%), camphene (0.5%), β-pinene (1.5%), myrcene (1.4%), 1,8-cineole (23.5%), p-cymene (0.6%), camphor (20.0%), linalool (32.4%), terpinen-4-ol (1.5%), borneol (4.6%), geraniol (1.8%).[5]

Therapeutic Actions

Analgesic, antidepressant, antiseptic, cholagogue, cicatrisant, decongestant, emmenagogue, insecticide, rubefacient, vulnerary.

Pharmacology and Clinical Studies

Spike lavender oil has been reported as having spasmolytic effects on the smooth muscles of laboratory animals.[6]

Indications

Analgesic Properties

Mailhebiau suggests blending spike lavender with peppermint for treating headaches, blending it with sage oil for treating late or painful periods and blended with rosemary oil it becomes an excellent anti-inflammatory and efficient painkiller in cases of rheumatism.[3]

Respiratory System

Spike lavender is valued for its expectorant and mucolytic properties.[3,7,8]

Skin Care

Spike lavender may be used as an insect repellent.[9]

Personality Profile

Mailhebiau compares a spike lavender personality with that of Jean-Jacques Rousseau.[3] This comparison is easy to appreciate when one reads the following statement made by Rousseau:

> *I used to rise with the sun and was happy; I used to go for walks and was happy ... I walked in the woods and over the hillsides, wandered through the valleys, read and was idle; I worked in the garden, picked fruit, helped with the cleaning, and happiness followed me everywhere.*[3]

Rousseau was an anti-establishmentarian who loved to challenge the false values of his time. According to Mailhebiau,

> *... a spike lavender person looks like an old student from May 1968 who has come down from his barricades to go and climb hills — long haired, bearded, who away from pollution, is off to shear his sheep, he carries on his self-sufficient lifestyle as a likeable fringe-person and questions — not without reason — social values and the advanced technologies which, he does not shirk from using if the need arises.*[3]

Mailhebiau suggests that this is a very good essence for bringing people back to a more natural lifestyle.[3]

Mode of Administration

Topical application — massage, compress, bath, ointment, skin care; Inhalation — direct inhalation, diffuser, oil vaporiser, steam inhalation.

Safety

The camphor content varies between 10% and 20% and the 1,8-cineole content varies between 25% and 35%. As camphor is considered a neurotoxic, it has been suggested that spike lavender may be neurotoxic as well. Tisserand suggests that it would only be contra-indicated if the oil were taken orally.[9]

Spike lavender oil is non-toxic, non-irritating and non-sensitising.

References

1. Harris R. *Lavenders of Provence*. The World of Aromatherapy III Conference Proceedings. NAHA, USA, 1999; 75-81.
2. Arctander S. *Perfume and flavour materials of natural origin*. Allured Publishing, USA, 1994.
3. Mailhebiau P. *Portraits in oils*. The C.W. Daniel Company Limited, Great Britain, 1995.
4. Grieve M. *A modern herbal*. Penguin, Great Britain, 1931.
5. Lawrence B. *Spike lavender oil*. Perfumer and Flavorist, 1987/1988; 12(3): 58.
6. Leung A, Foster S. *Encyclopedia of common natural ingredients used in food, drugs and cosmetics*. 2nd edn, John Wiley and Sons Inc, USA, 1996.
7. Davis P. *Aromatherapy: An A–Z*. 2nd edn. The C.W. Daniel Company Limited, Great Britain, 1999.
8. Lavabre, M. *Aromatherapy workbook*. Healing Art Press, USA. 1997.
9. Tisserand R, Balacs T. *Essential oil safety*. Churchill Livingstone, UK, 1995.

Lemon

Citrus limon

Synonyms

Expressed lemon oil

Family

Rutaceae

Botany and Origins

The lemon tree is believed to be a native of south-eastern China. It is believed to arrived in Europe via Persia and the Middle East with the returning crusaders in the 12th century.[1]

Columbus brought lemon and orange seeds on his second voyage to the West Indies in 1493. Little did he know he would be founding the world's largest lemon industry by the 20th century.[2]

The lemon tree fruits all year round, the fruits appearing with a deep green colour and ripening to a bright yellow. Lemon oil is mostly cultivated in California and Florida and in southern Europe.[3]

C. limon is divided into two groups with either smooth or rough skinned fruit. Some taxonomists regard the two as distinct species; the smooth as *C. limon* and the rough, commonly known as citronelle as *C. jambhiri*.[1]

Method of Extraction

Lemon oil is obtained from the peel of lemons by cold expression.

Essential Oil Characteristics

Lemon oil is a yellow to greenish-yellow or pale-yellow mobile liquid of a very light, fresh and sweet odour, truly reminiscent of the ripe peel.

Historical and Traditional Uses

Lemon juice was considered the best of all anti-scorbutics (a remedy for scurvy). English ships were required by law to carry sufficient lemon or lime juice for every seaman to have once daily after being at sea for ten days or more.[4]

The juice was used as a diaphoretic and diuretic. Lemon juice is highly recommended in acute rheumatism and sometimes given to counteract narcotic poisons. The juice is a good astringent and is said to be the best cure for severe, obstinate hiccoughs, and is helpful in jaundice and hysterical palpitation of the heart.[4]

Lemon oil is extensively used in pharmaceuticals as a flavouring agent, and as a fragrance ingredient in soaps, detergents and perfumes.[5]

Chemical Composition

The oil is comprised mostly (up to 70%) of limonene, a monoterpene hydrocarbon. A typical chemical composition of lemon is reported as follows:

α-pinene (1.8–3.6%), camphene (0–0.1%), β-pinene (6.1–15.0%), sabinene (1.5–4.6%), myrcene (1.0–2.1%), α-terpinene (0–0.5%), linalool (0–0.9%) β-bisabolene (0.56%), limonene (62.1–74.5%), trans-α-bergamotene (0.37%), nerol (0.04%), neral (0.76%).[6]

Therapeutic Actions

Antimicrobial, antirheumatic, antiseptic, antispasmodic, astringent, bactericidal, carminative, cicatrisant, depurative, diaphoretic, diuretic, febrifuge, haemostatic, hypotensive, insecticidal, rubefacient, tonic, vermifuge.

Pharmacology and Clinical Studies

Lemon oil has exhibited antimicrobial properties.[5] Studies in Japan found that when dispersed through the room, lemon oil reduced typing errors by 54%.[7]

Indications

Circulatory System

Lemon oil is an excellent tonic for the circulatory system, reducing blood viscosity and helping to break up plaque deposits in the arteries, reducing cholesterol.[9,10,12] It is an excellent remedy for tonifying the blood vessels and it may be used for varicose veins, broken capillaries, haemorrhoids and nosebleeds.[10,12]

Immune System

The antimicrobial qualities of lemon oil are very useful for treating the symptoms of colds, flu, bronchitis and asthma.[8] Lemon oil kills *Diphtheria bacilli* in 20 minutes at a dilution of only 0.2%.[9] Lemon oil is often referred to as having immune-stimulating properties, meaning that it stimulates the production of white blood cells to fight off invading bacteria.[10,11]

Lymphatic System

Lemon oil can be used as a mild detoxifier and is very useful for the treatment of toxaemia or for cellulite.[8]

Nervous System

Lemon oil is reputed to have 'high vibrations' which can lift the spirits and overcome mental fatigue.[13] Lemon oil clears the mind very effectively and is said to aid in the decision-making process without over-stimulating the mind. In fact, it can be very calming for those who are emotionally overwrought.

Skin Care

Lemon oil acts as an astringent, counteracting over-production of sebum, and is especially useful for teenage problem skins. It tones aging skin and has antibacterial properties that are beneficial for the treatment of acne and boils.[8,10] It is recommended for treating warts and verrucae. For this purpose it is best to apply the undiluted oil.[10]

Energetics

Lemon oil is cooling and drying and it is recommended to clear heat, dampness and phlegm. For this reason, it is considered an excellent detoxifying essential oil.[12]

Personality Profile

Lemon personalities sparkle and are full of life, with a very positive approach, in the form of an unshakeable confidence in everything that they do.[14] Lemon is like a breath of fresh air, positively wonderful to have around, not too bothered by the struggles and strains of living, able to take everything quite calmly. Lemon personalities radiate with energy, are very active and have a very positive approach to everything that they do.[14]

Subtle Aromatherapy

At a subtle level, Mojay compares lemon oil to rose oil. He says that the oil can help to *open the heart* — by alleviating fears of emotional involvement and of losing oneself in another person.[12] Worwood says that the fragrance of lemon enables our meditations to be deeper and describes the oil as spiritually cleansing.[15]

Method of Administration

Topical application — massage, compress, bath, ointment, skin care; Inhalation — direct inhalation, diffuser, oil vaporiser.

Safety

Lemon oil is non-toxic, non-irritant. Sensitisation can occur in some people. It should not be used on the skin prior to exposure to the sun as it is phototoxic.[8,12]

References

1. Weiss EA. *Essential oil crops*. CAB International, UK, 1997.
2. Guenther E. *The essential oils volume III*. Robert E. Krieger Publishing Company, USA, 1949.
3. Arctander S. *Perfume and flavour materials of natural origin*. Allured Publishing, USA, 1994.
4. Grieve M. *A modern herbal*. Penguin, England, 1931.
5. Leung A, Foster S. *Encyclopedia of common natural ingredients used in food, drugs and cosmetics*. 2nd edn, John Wiley and Sons Inc, USA, 1996.
6. Lawrence B. *Lemon oil*. Perfumer and Flavorist, 1984; 9(4): 37.

7. Tisserand R. *Lemon fragrance increases office efficiency*. The International Journal of Aromatherapy 1988; 1(2): 2.
8. Lawless J. *The encyclopaedia of essential oils*. Element Books Limited, Great Britain, 1992.
9. Valnet J. *The practice of aromatherapy*. The C.W. Daniel Company Limited, Great Britain, 1980.
10. Davis P. *Aromatherapy: An A–Z*. 2nd edn. The C.W. Daniel Company Limited, Great Britain, 1999.
11. Lavabre, M. *Aromatherapy workbook*. Healing Art Press, USA. 1997.
12. Mojay G. *Aromatherapy for healing the spirit*. Hodder and Stoughton, UK, 1996.
13. Fischer-Rizzi S. *Complete aromatherapy handbook*. Sterling Publishing Company, USA, 1990.
14. Worwood V. *The fragrant mind*. Doubleday, Great Britain, 1995.
15. Worwood V. *The fragrant spirit*. Doubleday, Great Britain, 1999.

Lemongrass

Cymbopogon citratus and C. flexuosus

Synonyms

C. citratus is commonly known as West Indian lemongrass or Guatemala lemongrass and *C. flexuosus* is known as East Indian lemongrass, Cochin lemongrass or native lemongrass.

Family

Gramineae or Poaceae

Botany and Origins

Lemongrass oil is produced from two distinctly different species of *Cymbopogon*. *C. citratus* and *C. flexuosus* are tufted perennial grasses with numerous stiff stems arising from a short rhizomatous rootstock.[1]

C. flexuosus is a native of India and *C. citratus* is possibly a native of Sri Lanka. *C. Citratus* is widely cultivated all over the world and has been named West Indian lemongrass.

India is the major producer of East Indian lemongrass and the major producers of West Indian lemongrass are Guatemala, Madagascar, the Comoros Islands, Brazil, Malaysia and Vietnam.[2]

Method of Extraction

Lemongrass oil is steam-distilled from fresh or partly dried leaves of *C. citratus* or *C. flexuosus*.[2]

Essential Oil Characteristics

Lemongrass oil is a yellow or amber-coloured somewhat viscous liquid with a very strong, fresh grassy, herbaceous and citrus odour.

C. citratus usually has an earthy undertone reminiscent of citronella oil, while *C. flexuosus* smells sweeter, distinctly more lemony, fresh and light.[2]

Historical and Traditional Uses

Lemongrass was originally used as a food flavouring in Asia. The fresh leaves are crushed in water and used as a hair wash and toilet water in India.[1]

The leaves can also be used as a source of cellulose and paper production.[1] A majority of the essential oil is used for citral production which is used either for perfumery or flavour use and for pharmaceutical use in the synthesis of vitamin A.[1]

West Indian lemongrass is used in TCM to treat colds, headache, stomach ache, abdominal pain and rheumatic pain.[3]

Chemical Composition

A typical chemical composition of lemongrass is reported as follows:[1]

Constituent	C. flexuosus	C. citratus
myrcene	0.46%	8.2–19.2%
limonene	2.42%	trace
linalool	1.34%	0.8–1.1%
citronellal	0.37%	0.1%
geranyl acetate	1.95%	1.00%
nerol	0.39%	0.3–0.4%
geraniol	3.80%	0.5–0.4%
neral	30.06%	25–28%
geranial	51.19%	45.2–55.9%
citronellol	0.44%	0.1%

C. citratus usually has a slightly lower citral content and a significantly higher amount of myrcene.

Therapeutic Actions

Analgesic, antidepressant, antimicrobial, antiseptic, astringent, bactericidal, carminative, deodorant, febrifuge, fungicidal, galactagogue, insecticidal, nervine, sedative (nervous system), tonic.

Pharmacology and Clinical Studies

C. citratus has been reported to exhibit excellent antifungal and antibacterial properties. Tests identified citral and citronellal as the most active components while dipentene and myrcene had no activity.[4,5,6]

C. citratus essential oil was found to give almost complete protection against *Anopheles cullicifacies* (a principal malaria carrier) for up to eleven hours. The oil was considered comparable with synthetic repellents of dimethyl and dibutyl phthalate.[7]

Indications

Antiseptic

The antiseptic properties of lemongrass indicate that it would be excellent in a vaporiser to disinfect the air.[9]

Digestive System

It is considered a stimulant of the digestive system and is recommended for colitis, indigestion and gastroenteritis.[9,10,11]

Musculoskeletal System

Lemongrass oil is referred to as the *connective tissue oil.* Lemongrass tightens the elastin fibres in the epidermis and in the subcutis. The oil is recommended in the after-care of sports injuries, sprains, bruises and dislocations.[8]

Nervous System

The refreshing scent of lemongrass is uplifting and energising. It aids our logical thinking and is ideal to use at home or work or wherever clear, fresh are thinking and good concentration is needed.[9]

Skin Care

Lemongrass is often recommended as a skin tonic and it is used in cleansing lotions and creams for its astringent properties.[19,10] I caution its use in skin care as it may cause dermal irritation or sensitisation. It is considered a very effective as an insect repellent.[10,11]

Personality Profile

Fisher-Rizzi says that Lemongrass is considered a secret aid for people who have trouble starting in the morning. She describes the effect of the scent of lemongrass as taking a refreshing, cool morning shower.[9]

Method of Administration

Topical application — massage, compress, skin care; Inhalation — direct inhalation, diffuser, oil vaporiser.

Safety

Lemongrass oil is non-toxic. However, it may be irritating and sensitising in some individuals.[10]

References

1. Weiss EA. *Essential oil crops.* CAB International, UK, 1997.
2. Arctander S. *Perfume and flavour materials of natural origin.* Allured Publishing, USA, 1994.
3. Leung A, Foster S. *Encyclopedia of common natural ingredients used in food, drugs and cosmetics.* 2nd edn, John Wiley and Sons Inc, USA, 1996.
4. Onawunmi GO. *Evaluation of the antifungal activity of lemongrass oil.* Int Journal Crude Drug Research, 1989; 27(2): 121–126. Cited in the Aromatherapy Database, Bob Harris, Essential Oil Resource Consultants, UK, 2000.
5. Onawunmi GO, Ogunlana EO. *Antibacterial constituents in the essential oil of Cymbopogon citratus.* J. Ethnopharmacology, 1984; 12(3): 279–286. Cited in the Aromatherapy Database, Bob Harris, Essential Oil Resource Consultants, UK, 2000.
6. Onawunmi GO, Ogunlana, EO. *A study of the antibacterial activity of the essential oil of lemongrass.* Int Journal Crude Drug Research, 1986; 24(2): 64–68. Cited in the Aromatherapy Database, Bob Harris, Essential Oil Resource Consultants, UK, 2000.
7. Ansari MA, Razdan RK. *Relative efficacy of various oils in repelling mosquitoes.* Indian J. Malariol, 32(3): 104–111. Cited in the Aromatherapy Database, Bob Harris, Essential Oil Resource Consultants, UK, 2000.
8. Gumbel D. *Principles of holistic skin therapy with herbal essences.* Karl F. Haug Publishers, Germany, 1986.
9. Fischer-Rizzi S. *Complete aromatherapy handbook.* Sterling Publishing Company, USA, 1990.
10. Lawless J. *The encyclopaedia of essential oils.* Element Books Limited, Great Britain, 1992.
11. Lavabre M. *Aromatherapy workbook.* Healing Art Press, USA. 1997.

Lime

Citrus aurantifolia

Synonyms

C. medica var. acida, West Indian lime, Key lime, Mexican lime, cold-pressed lime, distilled lime, sour lime.

Family

Rutaceae

Botany and Origins

There are two main types of limes. One contains Key, West Indian and Mexican cultivars whose fruit is small, round, moderately seedy with thin peel, smooth and a greenish flesh. The other contains Persian types whose fruit is larger, seedless and mainly sold as fresh limes or lime juice.[1]

Lime is a small spreading evergreen tree usually to 4–6 m, canopy diameter to 7 m, with many irregular spaced often drooping branches which usually have many short, stiff, very sharp spines, although some cultivars are spineless.[2]

Lime is believed to have originated from northern India and adjacent areas of Burma. Guenther suggests that lime reached the west coast of Central and South America via the Pacific islands, carried by the Polynesians. This accounts for the great abundance of wild limes in the jungles and little-known areas of tropical Central and northern South America.[2]

Limes were brought from India to Persia, Palestine, Egypt and Europe by the Arabs at about the same time as the sour orange and the lemon.[2] Key limes are cultivated in Mexico, Peru and West Indies, while the Persian limes are grown mainly in Florida and Brazil.[2]

There are two types of lime oil:

- expressed lime oil
- distilled lime oil

Method of Extraction

Distilled lime oil is produced by steam distillation of the whole fruits or distilled from the juice of the fruit. Expressed lime oil is cold-pressed from the fruit rind of green limes.

Essential Oil Characteristics

Distilled lime oil is a pale-yellow to almost clear mobile liquid with a fresh, sharp, fruity citrus-type odour. Prolonged storage affects the pleasant fresh aroma of distilled lime oil. With age the oil has a rather harsh-terpeney odour.[2]

Cold-pressed lime is a yellowish-green to olive-green mobile liquid with an intensely fresh citrus, rich and sweet odour.[1]

Historical and Traditional Uses

Limes were introduced into Europe by the Moors and subsequently brought to America by the Spanish and Portuguese explorers around the 16th century.[2]

Distilled lime oil is extensively used in flavouring food and beverages, especially soft drinks. Cold-pressed lime is used in high-grade men's toiletries and perfumery.[2]

Chemical Composition

A typical chemical composition of cold-pressed lime is reported as follows:

α-pinene (3%), β-pinene (18.2%), sabinene (3.2%), myrcene (1,2%), limonene (42.7%), γ-terpinene (7.4%), terpinolene (0.5%), 1.0% saturated aldehydes such as octanal, nonanal, decanal, undecanal, dodecanal, tridecanal, tetradecanal, pentadecanal; trans-α-bergaptene (0.6%), caryophyllene (0.5%), β-bisabolene (1.0%), 6.2% citral — neral and geranial, neryl acetate and geranyl acetate (0.5%), α-terpineol (0.3%) and traces of linalool.[3]

A typical chemical composition of distilled pressed lime is reported as follows:

α-pinene (0.5–1.6%), β-pinene (0.4–9.0%), myrcene (0.5–1.4%), limonene (42.5–50.3%), terpinolene (3.6–9.3%), 1,8-cineole (0.25–3.0%), linalool (0.05–1.0%), borneol (0.3–0.5%) and traces of neryl acetate and geranyl acetate.[3]

Therapeutic Actions

Antiseptic, antiviral, astringent, bactericide, disinfectant, febrifuge, haemostatic, insecticide, tonic.

Pharmacology and Clinical Studies

The phototoxicity of bergaptene is well documented. Expressed lime oil contains more of this compound than other citrus oils and has been reported to be phototoxic to humans.[4]

Indications

The indications for cold-pressed lime are considered to be similar to those of lemon oil.[5]

Antimicrobial

It has antimicrobial properties and is recommended for treating throat infections and influenza.

Digestive System

As with most citrus oils, lime oil is considered a digestive tonic and it is recommended for digestive problems.[6]

Lymphatic System

Cold-pressed lime oil is a lymphatic stimulant and may be used for the treatment of fluid retention and cellulite.[6]

Nervous System

Cold-pressed and distilled lime are refreshing and uplifting. They are ideal for fatigue and a tired mind, especially where there is apathy, anxiety and depression.[6]

Skin Care

Cold-pressed lime oil acts as an astringent, counteracting overproduction of sebum, and is especially useful for oily skin. Its antibacterial property is useful for the treatment of acne.

Method of Administration

Topical application — massage, compress, bath, skin care; Inhalation — direct inhalation, diffuser, oil vaporiser.

Safety

Distilled lime oil is non-toxic, non-irritating and non-sensitising. However, cold-pressed lime is phototoxic.

References

1. Arctander S. *Perfume and flavour materials of natural origin.* Allured Publishing, USA, 1994.

2. Weiss EA. *Essential oil crops*. CAB International, UK, 1997.
3. Lawrence B. *Lime oil*. Perfumer and Flavorist, 1976; 1(4): 31.
4. Leung A, Foster S. *Encyclopedia of common natural ingredients used in food, drugs and cosmetics*. 2nd edn, John Wiley and Sons Inc, USA, 1996.
5. Lawless J. *The encyclopaedia of essential oils*. Element Books Limited, Great Britain, 1992.
6. Lavabre M. *Aromatherapy workbook*. Healing Art Press, USA, 1997.

Mandarin

Citrus reticulata

Synonyms

C. nobilis var. *deliciosa*

Family

Rutaceae

Botany and Origins

Mandarin is a small evergreen tree to 4 m, with a single trunk, and many rather thin drooping branches which may be either spined or spineless. The fruit is a flattened globoid, approximately 5–10 cm in diameter. The peel colour varies from yellow to deep orange-red when ripe.[1]

Mandarin is normally divided into four groups, each suited to certain climatic and environmental conditions. The four groups are — Common, King, Willowleaf and Satsuma.

Mandarin is native to China and Indo-China and spread to other countries of the Far East where it is extensively grown for domestic purposes. It was first introduced to Europe in the eighteenth century. It rapidly became popular and was commercially cultivated in southern Europe and North Africa. It was then introduced to the Americas, southern Africa and Australia.[1]

Mandarin and tangerine fruits have been given the same species status. The name tangerine is used in English-speaking countries, but mandarin elsewhere.[1]

Essential Oil Characteristics

Mandarin oil is an orange-brown to dark-yellowish-brown or olive-brown mobile coloured oil with an intensely sweet, not necessarily fresh odour, with an amine-like, 'fishy' top note. This odour is due to the presence of methyl-N-methyl-anthranilate.[2]

Method of Extraction

Mandarin oil is expressed from the fruit rind of *C. reticulata*.

Historical and Traditional Uses

Apart from its use in aromatherapy, mandarin oil is extensively used in flavours, where it gives interesting modifications with sweet and bitter orange oils, grapefruit and lime oil in flavour compositions for soft drinks, candy and liqueurs.[2]

Chemical Composition

A typical chemical composition of mandarin is reported as follows:

α-thujone (0.76–0.96%), α-pinene (2.12–2.54%), camphene (0.02%), sabinene (0.24–0.29%), β-pinene (0.25–1.82%), myrcene (1.69–1.77%), limonene (67.92–74.00%), γ-terpinolene (16.78–21.02%), linalool (0.05–0.16%), citronellal (0.02–0.04%) terpinen-4-ol (0.02–0.06%), nerol (0.01–0.02%), geranial (0.03–0.06%).[3]

Therapeutic Actions

Antispasmodic, carminative, cholagogue, depurative, digestive, diuretic, sedative.

Pharmacology and Clinical Studies

No pharmacological or clinical studies could be found for mandarin oil.

Indications

Mandarin oil has similar properties to tangerine and orange oil.

Children's Remedy

In France, mandarin oil is considered the children's remedy, and is used to relieve tummy upsets of babies and children.[5] Mandarin oil is recommended for soothing restlessness, especially in hyperactive children.[6]

Digestive System

Mandarin has a tonic effect on the digestive system, helping to regulate metabolic processes and it aids the secretion of bile and breaking down of fats. It is beneficial for calming the intestines and relieving flatulence.[4]

Pregnancy

Mandarin oil is recommended in a massage blend to prevent stretch marks during pregnancy.[5] For this purpose it should be blended with essential oils such as lavender, neroli and wheatgerm, and apricot kernel cold-pressed vegetable oil should be used as the carrier. To be effective the massage oil should be used daily from about the fifth month of pregnancy.[5]

Skin Care

Mandarin oil is often used in combination with lavender, neroli and wheatgerm oil to help prevent stretch marks during pregnancy.[4,5]

Mandarin oil is recommended for acne, congested and oily skin.[4]

Personality Profile

The mandarin personalities are described as among the softer personalities. They are sweet, gentle, kind and loving. They are very uplifting people and may be childlike in that they need love and protection and they tend to attract protectiveness in others.[7]

Subtle Aromatherapy

Davis says that the delicate aroma of mandarin breathes a message of happiness, especially to children and the child within each of us. It helps us to get in touch with that inner child. [8]

Mode of Administration

Topical application — massage, compress, bath, skin care; Inhalation — direct inhalation, diffuser, oil vaporiser.

Safety

Mandarin oil is non-toxic, non-irritating and non-sensitising.

References

1. Weiss EA. *Essential oil crops*. CAB International, UK, 1997.
2. Arctander S. *Perfume and flavour materials of natural origin*. Allured Publishing, USA, 1994.
3. Lawrence B. *Mandarin oil*. Perfumer and Flavorist, 1987; 12(4): 69.
4. Lawless J. *The encyclopaedia of essential oils*. Element Books Limited, Great Britain, 1992.
5. Davis P. *Aromatherapy: An A–Z*. 2nd edn. The C.W. Daniel Company Limited, Great Britain, 1999.
6. Schnaubelt K. *Medical aromatherapy*. Frog Ltd, USA, 1999.
7. Worwood V. *The fragrant mind*. Doubleday, Great Britain, 1995.
8. Davis P. *Subtle aromatherapy*. The C.W. Daniel Company Limited, Great Britain, 1991.

Manuka

Leptospermum scoparium

Family

Myrtaceae

Synonyms

New Zealand Tea Tree

Botany and Origins

Manuka is a small tree which is a native of New Zealand. Most manuka is harvested from wild plants as very little commercial cultivation is yet carried out.

There are several different manuka chemotypes. The 'coast' type contains low levels of monoterpenes and relatively high levels of sesquiterpenes and triketones. It has been suggested that this accounts for its higher antimicrobial activity.[1,2,3]

Method of Extraction

Manuka oil is steam-distilled from the leaves and twigs of *L. scoparium.*

Essential Oil Characteristics

Manuka oil is a clear yellow liquid with a distinctive spicy, herbaceous and fresh aroma.

Historical and Traditional Uses

The leaves of manuka were used by the early Maoris as topical applications for wounds, cuts, sores and skin diseases. Topical use of the various parts of manuka was common among early Maoris and settlers.[1]

Manuka oil has been extensively used for generations in New Zealand for its antimicrobial properties.[1,2,3,4]

The therapeutic properties of manuka honey are well established. It is used for slow-healing ulcers and wound healing.[7]

Chemical Composition

Manuka oil contains low levels of monoterpenes and relatively high levels of sesquiterpenes and triketones. A typical chemical composition of Manuka oil obtained from a distinct chemotype found in the East Cape area of the North Island of New Zealand is as follows:

α-thujene (0.03%), α-pinene (1.31%), β-pinene (0.12%), myrcene (0.24%), p-cymene (0.16%), 1,8-cineole (0.22%), limonene (0.1%), terpinene-4-ol (0.04%), α-terpineol (0.09%), α-cubebene (3.955), α-copaene (5.86%), β-elemene (0.55%), α-gurjunene (1.02%), β-caryophyllene (2.63%), aromadendrene (2.09%), cadina-3,5-diene (4.88%), δ-amorphene (3.81%), β-selinene (3.67%), α-selinene + viridflorene (4.35%), calamenene (14.42%, δ-cadinene (6.02%), flavesone (4.91%), cadina-1,4-diene (5.94%), iso leptospermone (4.62%), leptospermone (15.54%).[3]

Therapeutic Actions

Analgesic, antibacterial, antifungal, anti-inflammatory, deodorant, expectorant, immune stimulant, insecticide, sedative.

Pharmacology and Clinical Studies

Manuka oil was found to possess some antimicrobial properties.[2,3,4,5] However, Lis-Balchin reports that the antimicrobial activity of different samples of manuka was variable and mostly lower than that of tea tree.[5]

The antimicrobial activity of standard tea tree compared with manuka obtained from the East Cape region of New Zealand is reported in the table below.

Comparative antimicrobial activity for some essential oils[4]

Oil Sample	Zone of inhibition (mm)	
	Candida albicans	*Staphylococcus aureus*
Tea Tree	9.0	8.5
Aust. Lavender	8.0	7.0
NZ Manuka	2.0	8.0
Lemongrass	30.0	38.0
Eucalyptus	2.0	2.5

Indications

Integumentary System

Manuka is recommended for treating ringworm, insect bites, athlete's foot, acne, skin eruptions, stubborn ulcers and wounds, cuts and abrasions.[6]

It is an excellent insecticidal.[6] It has been suggested that the sesquiterpenes found in manuka are responsible for manuka's ability to reduce skin irritation and promote wound healing.[7]

Musculoskeletal System

Manuka oil has a good analgesic effect and is recommended for the relief of muscular aches and pain.

Respiratory System

Manuka oil is beneficial for all types of respiratory tract infections and can be used to relieve coughs, cold and flu.[6]

Subtle Aromatherapy

Von Braunschweig says that manuka is a protective oil similar to myrrh and cedarwood. She says that old psychic scars get smoothed and that the sesquiterpenes stabilise and protect the nervous - system and balance the sympathetic and parasympathetic nerves. Manuka's vitalising scent is well suited to gentle souls who express themselves through sensitive skin or frequent digestive upsets.[7]

Mode of Administration

Topical application — massage, compress, bath, sitz bath, douche, ointment, skin care; Inhalation — direct inhalation, diffuser, oil vaporiser, steam inhalation.

Safety

Manuka oil is non-toxic, non-irritating and non-sensitising.

References

1. Anthony C. *Aromatherapy in New Zealand: Indigenous use of essential oils from native plants, mauka and kanuka essential oils.* Proceedings of the Australasian Aromatherapy Conference, Sydney, 1996.
2. Cooke A, Cooke MD. *An investigation into the antimicrobial properties of manuka and kanuka oil.* Cawthron Institute Report No. 263, New Zealand, 1994.
3. Porter NG, Wilkens AL. *Chemical, physical and antimicrobial properties of essential oils of Leptospermum scoparium and Kunzea ericoides.* Phytochemistry, 1998; 50(3): 407–415. Cited in the Aromatherapy Database, Bob Harris, Essential Oil Resource Consultants, UK, 2000.
4. Williams LR, Stockley JK, Yan W, Home VN. *Essential oils with high antimicrobial activity for therapeutic use.* The International Journal of Aromatherapy 1998; 8(4): 30–39.
5. Balchin M, Dean SG, Hart S. Bioactivity of New Zealand medicinal plant essential oils. Acta Horticulturae, 1996; 426: 13–29. Cited in the Aromatherapy Database, Bob Harris, Essential Oil Resource Consultants, UK, 2000.
6. Davis P. *Aromatherapy: An A–Z.* 2nd edn. The C.W. Daniel Company Limited, Great Britain, 1999.
7. Von Braunschweig R. *Manuka, kanuka and tea tree oil — 3 essential oils with interesting effects on the psyche.* Proceedings of the Australasian Aromatherapy Conference, Sydney, 1998.

Marjoram, Sweet

Origanum majorana

Synonyms

Marjorana hortensis, Knotted marjoram

Family

Labiatae or Lamiaceae

Botany and Origins

There is much confusion regarding the various species of marjoram. Sweet marjoram should not be confused with Spanish marjoram *(Thymus mastichina),* which belongs to the thyme species, oregano *(Origanum vulgare),* which is used to produce oregano oil, or with pot marjoram *(O. onites).*[1]

Sweet marjoram is a tender, bushy perennial herb with woolly hairy leaves, growing up to 0.6 m high. It is a native of the Mediterranean region and is cultivated in France, Tunisia, Morocco, Italy, Hungary, Bulgaria, Poland, Germany and Turkey.[1]

The name *origanum* is derived from the Greek word *oros* and *ganos* meaning splendid or joy, thus 'joy of the mountains' referring to the colour and scent of their flowers and leaves, and the hills they originally came from.

Method of Extraction

Sweet marjoram oil is steam-distilled from the dried leaves and flowering tops of the well-known culinary herb *O. marjorana*.

Essential Oil Characteristics

Sweet marjoram oil is a pale-yellow or pale-amber-coloured, mobile liquid with a warm-spicy, aromatic-camphoraceous and woody odour.[2]

Historical and Traditional Uses

The herb has been used since antiquity for its medicinal and culinary purposes. The Greeks referred to marjoram as the funeral herb. It was planted on graves to bring spiritual peace to the dead.[3]

Culpeper writes of marjoram's therapeutic properties:

> *Our common sweet marjoram is warming and comforting in cold diseases of the head, stomach sinews and other parts, taken inwardly or outwardly applied.*[3]

Culpeper recommended marjoram for diseases of the chest, obstructions of the liver and spleen, old griefs of the womb and the windiness thereof.[3]

Sweet marjoram oil is used as a flavouring ingredient in many food products. It is used in European herbal medicine for the treatment of respiratory ailments, bronchitis, antispasmodic and an expectorant.[1]

Chemical Composition

A typical chemical composition of sweet marjoram is reported as follows:

Sabinene (3.0%), α-terpinene (3.0%), γ-terpinene (7.3%), p-cymene (5.3%), terpinolene (2.0%), linalool (3.3%), *cis*-sabinene hydrate (7.1%), linalyl acetate (7.4%), terpinen-4-ol (31.6%), α-terpineol (8.3%).[4]

Therapeutic Actions

Analgesic, anaphrodisiac, antiseptic, antispasmodic, antiviral, bactericidal, carminative, cordial, diaphoretic, digestive, diuretic, emmenagogue, expectorant, fungicidal, hypotensive, nervine, sedative, stomachic, vasodilator, vulnerary.

Pharmacology and Clinical Studies

An aqueous extract of sweet marjoram has been reported to have antiviral activities against *Herpes simplex* in vitro.[1]

Indications

Anaphrodisiac

Sweet marjoram is considered an anaphrodisiac. It is reputed to diminish the desire for sexual contact. This property may be associated with the fact that marjoram has a long association with celibacy, such as members of the priesthood or monastic orders.[5,6]

Davis even goes to the point of warning against excessive use of marjoram unless you are committed to lifelong celibacy as it will diminish normal sexual response.[7]

Circulatory System

Its warming properties make it useful for treating chilblains and it helps disperse bruises.[5] Sweet marjoram oil is recommended for alleviating high blood pressure.[5,6,8,9]

Digestive System

Marjoram stimulates and strengthens intestinal peristalsis, therefore it is a good digestive and carminative, relieving constipation, colic, flatulence and spasmodic indigestion.[5]

Musculoskeletal System

Marjoram is warming and analgesic, making it useful for muscular spasm, rheumatic pains, sprains and strains.[5,6,8,9,10]

Nervous System

It has the ability to strengthen and relax the nerves. It is recommended for conditions in which tiredness alternates with nervous tension, stress-related conditions or characterised by anxiety or insomnia.[5] Davis recommends not abusing the sedative properties of marjoram as it can dull the senses and cause drowsiness, and in large amounts it is stupefying.[5]

According to Tisserand most of its functions centre around the autonomic nervous systems. It stimulates the parasympathetic nervous system and lowers the sympathetic function.[9] Marjoram oil may be rubbed into the temple area for relief of headaches and migraines.[8,9]

Marjoram oil is comforting for people who are lonely or suffering grief. However, it should be used only for a short period as extended use may have a deadening effect on the emotions.[6]

Respiratory System

It can be used as an inhalation or a chest rub for the treatment of colds and flus. The oil has antibacterial and antispasmodic properties which means that it is effective for treating whooping cough.[11]

Reproductive System

Sweet marjoram's antispasmodic and emmenagogue properties are valued for their action on the uterine muscles, used as a massage or hot compress over the lower abdomen it will ease menstrual cramps. Mailhebiau recommends using sweet marjoram in conjunction with clary sage for females who experience uterine and nerve spasms during their period.[10]

Energetics

Sweet marjoram oil circulates *Qi*. This means that the oil has excellent antispasmodic properties.[12,13] It may be used for conditions such as muscular stiffness and pain, nervous spasm, intestinal colic and osteoarthritis.

Its ability to loosen constraint indicates that it can be used to calm and regulate the heart, making it useful for palpitations, tachycardia and hypertension. Its antispasmodic action indicates that it is an excellent oil of choice for nervous cough and asthma.[12,13]

Personality Profile

Mojay suggests that marjoram helps to calm obsessive thinking, ease emotional craving and promote the capacity for inner self-nurturing.[13]

The marjoram personality is described as a warm and friendly person who is always ready to offer comfort and solace to those in need.[14]

Mode of Administration

Topical application — massage, compress, bath, ointment, skin care; Inhalation — direct inhalation, diffuser, oil vaporiser, steam inhalation.

Safety

Sweet marjoram oil is non-toxic, non-irritating and non-sensitising. Sweet marjoram is contra-indicated during pregnancy.[5,6,9] While marjoram herb has been classified as an emmenagogue, none of the herbal texts that I reviewed indicated that marjoram was contra-indicated during pregnancy.

References

1. Leung A, Foster S. *Encyclopedia of common natural ingredients used in food, drugs and cosmetics*. 2nd edn, John Wiley and Sons Inc, USA, 1996.
2. Arctander S. *Perfume and flavour materials of natural origin*. Allured Publishing, USA, 1994.
3. Le Strange R. *A history of herbal plants*. Angus and Robertson, Great Britain, 1977.
4. Lawrence B. *Sweet marjoram*. Perfumer and Flavorist, 1984; 9(1): 49.
5. Lawless J. *The encyclopaedia of essential oils*. Element Books Limited, Great Britain, 1992.
6. Davis P. *Aromatherapy: An A–Z*. 2nd edn. The C.W. Daniel Company Limited, Great Britain, 1999.
7. Davis P. *Subtle aromatherapy*. The C.W. Daniel Company Limited, Great Britain, 1991.
8. Lavabre M. *Aromatherapy workbook*. Healing Art Press, USA, 1997.
9. Tisserand R. *The art of aromatherapy*. The C.W. Daniel Company Limited, Great Britain, 1977.
10. Mailhebiau P. *Portraits in oils*. The C.W. Daniel Company Limited, Great Britain, 1995
11. Schnaubelt K. *Medical aromatherapy*. Frog Ltd, USA, 1999.
12. Holmes P. *The energetics of western herbs Vol. I*. Artemis Press, USA, 1989.
13. Mojay G. *Aromatherapy for healing the spirit*. Hodder and Stoughton, UK, 1996.
14. Worwood V. *The fragrant mind*. Doubleday, Great Britain, 1995.

May Chang

Litsea cubeba

Synonyms

The essential oil is often referred to by its botanical name, *Litsea cubeba*.

Family

Lauraceae

Botany and Origins

Most essential oil suppliers refer to may chang by its botanical name, *Litsea cubeba*, It has been known for its fragrant flowers, fruit and leaves for a long time. The small fruit resemble cubeb pepper, hence its name. It was not until the 1950s that the may chang essential oil became commonly known.[1]

May chang is a small fragrant tropical tree which grows in eastern Asia. China is the largest producer of may chang oil.

An oil, the main constituent of which is citronellal, can be distilled from the bark and another, whose main constituent is cineole, can aslo be distilled from the leaves, but both are of no commercial importance.[2]

Method of Extraction

May chang essential oil is steam-distilled from the small, pepper-like fruits of *L. cubeba*.

Essential Oil Characteristics

While it is often compared with lemongrass, its odour is considered to be finer, more lemon-like and less fatty. May chang is a pale-yellow, mobile oil with an intensely lemon-like, fresh and sweet aroma and a soft and sweet-fruity dry-out.[1]

Historical and Traditional Uses

In TCM, may chang is used to treat dysmenorrhoea that improves with heat or pressure, stomach aches, lower back pain, chills, headaches and muscular aches from external conditions.[3] May chang fruits are reputed to alleviate chronic asthma, as well as being a treatment for coronary heart disease and high blood pressure.[3]

The oil serves as a source of citral in China.[1]

Chemical Composition

May chang is chemically similar to lemongrass, melissa and other essential oils rich in citral. Citral, which comprises around 75% of may chang oil, has two isomers, neral and geranial.

A typical chemical composition of may chang is reported as follows:

α-pinene (0.87%), β-pinene (0.39%), myrcene (3.04%), limonene (8.38%), neral (33.80%), geranial (40.61%), nerol (1.09%), geraniol (1.58%), linalool (1.7%), linalyl acetate (1.65%), caryophyllene (0.51%).[4]

Therapeutic Actions

Antidepressant, antiseptic, astringent, carminative, galactagogue, insecticide, stimulant, tonic.

Pharmacological and Clinical Studies

Tisserand and Balacs cite clinical trials using may chang for the treatment of experimentally induced cardiac arrhythmias. It was compared with propranolol (a beta-blocker, antihypertensive and anti-angina drug). The test results confirmed may chang's ability to reduce arrhythmias from 15 minutes to 6.5 minutes, while propranolol reduced the arrhythmia time from 15 minutes to 0.6 minutes.[3]

It is believed that citral is the main constituent responsible for the beneficial effects seen on the experiments involving experimentally induced cardiac arrhythmia. Experiments have found that citral increases blood flow in the rabbit heart, improved the ECG profile in rabbits with experimentally induced cardiac arrhythmia and in rats with isoprenaline-induced cardiac ischaemia.[3]

Indications

Cardiovascular System

May chang oil may be used as a treatment for coronary heart disease and high blood pressure.[3]

Nervous System

The pleasant refreshing citrus aroma of may chang can be used to alleviate stress and anxiety which may lead to depression.

Skin Care

May chang is recommended for the treatment of oily skin and acne. It is also reputed to reduce excess perspiration and is a deodorant.[5,6]

Mode of Administration

Topical application — massage, compress, bath, skin care; Inhalation — direct inhalation, diffuser, oil vaporiser.

Safety

May chang oil is non-toxic, non-irritating and possibly sensitising in some individuals.

References

1. Arctander S. *Perfume and flavour materials of natural origin.* Allured Publishing, USA, 1994.
2. Weiss EA. *Essential oil crops.* CAB International, UK, 1997.
3. Tisserand R, Balacs T. *May chang.* The International Journal of Aromatherapy 1992; 4(3): 25–27.
4. Lawrence B. *May chang.* Perfumer and Flavorist. 1981; 6(3): 46.
5. Lawless J. *The encyclopaedia of essential oils.* Element Books Limited, Great Britain, 1992.
6. Davis P. *Aromatherapy: An A–Z.* 2nd edn. The C.W. Daniel Company Limited, Great Britain, 1999.

Melissa

Melissa officinalis

Family

Lamiaceae or Labiatae

Synonyms

Lemon balm, balm, common balm, bee balm.

Botany and Origins

Melissa is a sweet-scented perennial herb which grows up to 0.9 m high with serrated leaves and tiny white or pink flowers.

Melissa is distilled in the south of France, Germany and in Italy and Spain. However, the total production of genuine melissa oil is only a fraction of the quantity commercially offered. Melissa oil enjoys the reputation of being one of the most frequently adulterated essential oils.[1]

The name is from the Greek word signifying *bee*, indicative of the attraction the plant has for bees, and the word *Balm* is an abbreviation of the term *Balsam*.[2]

Method of Extraction

Melissa oil is steam-distilled from the leaves and flowering tops of *M. officinalis.*

Essential Oil Characteristics

Melissa oil is a pale-yellow or pale-amber-coloured, mobile liquid with an intensely fresh and sweet citrus and herbaceous odour.

Historical and Traditional Uses

The herb was highly esteemed by Paracelsus, who believed it could completely revivify a man.[2] Herbalist John Evelyn wrote of melissa:

> *Balm is sovereign for the brain, strengthens the memory and powerfully chasing away melancholy.*[2]

A Spirit of Balm, made by combining lemon peel, nutmeg, angelica root and other herbs and spices, enjoyed a great reputation under the name of Carmelite water. This was considered beneficial for the treatment of nervous headaches, digestive problems and neuralgic affections.[2]

Chemical Composition

A typical chemical composition of melissa oil is reported as follows:

trans-ocimene (0.2%), *cis*-ocimene (0.1%), 3-octanone (0.6%), methyl hepenone (0.6%), cis-3-hexanol (0.1%), 3-octanol (0.1%), 1-octen-3-ol (1.3%), copaene (4.0%), citronellal (0.7%), linalool (0.4%), β-bourbonene (0.3%), caryophyllene (9.5%), α-humulene (0.2%), neral (24.1%), germacrene D (4.2%), geranial (37.2%), geranyl acetate (0.5%), d-cadinene (1.1%), γ-cadinene (1.0%), nerol (0.1%), geraniol (0.1%).[3]

Therapeutic Actions

Antidepressant, antispasmodic, antiviral, bactericidal, carminative, cordial, diaphoretic, febrifuge, hypotensive, nervine, sedative, sudorific, tonic.

Pharmacology and Clinical Studies

Melissa oil has antibacterial, antifungal and antispasmodic properties.[4,5]

Hot water extracts of melissa have strong antiviral properties against mumps, *Herpes simplex*, and other viruses. Polyphenols and the tannin present have been identified to be responsible for these antiviral properties.[5]

The hydroalcoholic extract of melissa is a CNS sedative (in mouse), however recent studies indicate that the essential oil does not appear to play a role in this activity.[4]

Indications

Cardiovascular System

Melissa oil is reputed to lower high blood pressure and it has a calming effect on over-rapid breathing and heartbeat.[6] Tisserand suggests that melissa is a tonic of the heart. He recommends it for all heart conditions where there is overstimulation, or heat, leading to weakness of the heart.[7]

Digestive System

Melissa oil is reputed to regulate the digestive system, relieve cramps, reduce flatulence and stimulate the gallbladder and liver.[8] The action of melissa oil has been compared with that of peppermint and fennel. It is a tonic and is recommended for nausea, vomiting and indigestion, especially of nervous origins.[7]

Immune System

Studies in Germany have found melissa oil to possess antiviral properties against *Herpes simplex* and *Herpes zoster*. Dr. Wabner suggests using an undiluted blend of rose and melissa oil directly onto the herpes lesions. He states that the herpes often disappear within 24 hours. Care should be taken to apply the oil to the blisters only and not the surrounding skin, to minimise irritation.[9]

Nervous System

Fischer-Rizzi describes melissa as a gift from heaven, and recommends using the oil for overstimulation of the nervous system that causes stress, anxiety, insomnia, depression and lost inner direction.[8]

Melissa as considered a sedative and is recommended for reducing anger in times of crisis or trauma.[10] The oil is well known for its uplifting and antidepressant qualities.[11]

Reproductive System

Melissa's relaxing and antispasmodic properties make it beneficial for treating painful periods.[7]

Skin Care

Melissa oil is often recommended for the treatment of oily skin and acne.[8,12] However, there is a high risk of skin irritation or skin sensitisation and, for this reason, I prefer using essential oils that are less likely to cause an irritation.

Personality Profile

Melissa oil promotes sensitivity and intuition and helps us find inner contentment and strengthens the 'wisdom of the heart'.[8]

Energetics

Energetically, melissa is cooling and drying. It is indicated for stagnation of *Qi* and for reducing heat in the liver and heart.[13] Melissa's cooling, soothing influence on the heart and nervous system makes it effective for alleviating restlessness, insomnia and nervous tension.[13]

Subtle Aromatherapy

Davis has found melissa oil to be of great comfort during bereavement. She says that the sweet fresh fragrance seems to dispel fear and regret and bring acceptance and understanding as the time of death approaches.[14]

Melissa oil is recommended for the heart chakra and suggests using it to expand feelings of love from the individual towards the total acceptance of unconditional love.[14]

Mode of Administration

Topical application — massage, ointment, skin care; Inhalation — direct inhalation, diffuser, oil vaporiser.

Safety

Melissa oil is non-toxic. However, care must be taken as the oil is a possible sensitiser and dermal irritant. Care must also be taken as this is one of the most frequently adulterated essential oils.

References

1. Arctander S. *Perfume and flavour materials of natural origin.* Allured Publishing, USA, 1994.
2. Grieve M. *A modern herbal.* Penguin, England, 1931.
3. Lawrence B. *Lemon balm.* Perfumer and Flavorist, 1978; 3(4): 58.
4. Bruneton J. *Pharmacognosy.* 2nd edn. Lavoisier Publishing Inc, France, 1999.
5. Leung A, Foster S. *Encyclopedia of common natural ingredients used in food, drugs and cosmetics.* 2nd edn, John Wiley and Sons Inc, USA, 1996.
6. Davis P. *Aromatherapy: An A–Z.* 2nd edn. The C.W. Daniel Company Limited, Great Britain, 1999.
7. Tisserand R. *The art of aromatherapy.* The C.W. Daniel Company Limited, Great Britain, 1977.
8. Fischer-Rizzi S. *Complete aromatherapy handbook.* Sterling Publishing Company, USA, 1990.
9. Tisserand R. *In praise of melissa.* The International Journal of Aromatherapy 1989; 1(4): 10–11.
10. Schnaubelt K. *Medical aromatherapy.* Frog Ltd, USA, 1999.
11. Lavabre, M. *Aromatherapy workbook.* Healing Art Press, USA, 1997.
12. Lawless J. *The encyclopaedia of essential oils.* Element Books Limited, Great Britain, 1992.
13. Mojay G. *Aromatherapy for healing the spirit.* Hodder and Stoughton, UK, 1996.
14. Davis P. *Subtle aromatherapy.* The C.W. Daniel Company Limited, Great Britain, 1991.

Myrrh

Commiphora myrrha

Synonyms

Commiphora molmol, C. myrrha, C. madagascariensis, gum myrrh, myrrha, Somali myrrh

Family

Burseraceae

Botany and Origins

The name myrrh is derived from the Arabic and Hebrew word *mur*, which means bitter.[1]

Myrrh is the resinous exudation, or gum, collected from the myrrh bush, botanically known as *C. molmol*, either when it is wounded or from natural fissures. There are several *commiphora* species from which the myrrh resin is produced.

The resin flows out as a thick pale-yellow liquid, and turns reddish-brown as it dries and hardens. The bush, which is a native of north-east Africa and southern Arabia, has sturdy knotted branches, trifoliate leaves and small white flowers.[2]

To increase the yield and production, incisions are made into the bark. Lumps of the gum often fall to the ground and become contaminated with sand, other lumps are peeled off the trunk, and these usually make a better grade of myrrh. However, myrrh cannot be evaluated just by its appearance. Lumps of high odour value may have poor appearance because they have fallen to the ground.[2]

Myrrh resin consists of rounded or irregular tears, or agglutinated masses of smaller and larger tears of a moderate yellow to dark or reddish-brown colour. The lumps are usually covered with a lighter-coloured or yellowish dust.[2]

Method of Extraction

Myrrh essential oil is steam-distilled from the myrrh resin.

Essential Oil Characteristics

Myrrh oil is a pale-yellow to pale-orange-coloured liquid. It has a warm-spicy odour with a sharp-balsamic, slightly medicinal topnote.

Historical and Traditional Uses

Myrrh is one of the oldest known aromatic substances which is mentioned as far back as 4000 years. It was an ingredient of incense used for religious ceremonies and fumigations by the ancient Egyptians. It was an ingredient of the famous Egyptian perfume 'kyphi', and was an important ingredient in embalming.[3]

It was reputed to reduce wrinkles and preserve a youthful complexion. Egyptian women used myrrh in their facial preparations. It has a slightly cooling effect on the skin, and so would be especially useful in a hot dry climate.[4]

Myrrh's therapeutic properties are frequently mentioned in the old and new testaments, the Koran, and in Greek and Roman texts. Myrrh was one of the gifts presented to the infant Jesus.

> *And when they came into the house, they saw the young child with Mary his mother, and falling to their knees they did give him homage. Then, opening their treasures, they offered him gifts of gold and frankincense and myrrh.* (Matthew 2:11)[5]

It was presented at the death of Christ:

> *... brought a mixture of myrrh and aloes, then took the body of Jesus, and wound it in linen clothes with the spices, as the manner of the Jews is to bury.* (The Gospel according to St John)[5]

In the Song of Solomon, a love poem, the constant reference to myrrh suggests that it was for the incomparable financial value of myrrh that the writer used them to compare with the beauty of the maiden.

> *A bundle of myrrh is my beloved to me Your two breasts like two fawns twins of a gazelle, that feed among the lilies. Until the day breaths and the shadows flee I will lie me to the mountain of myrrh and the hill of incense.* (Song of Songs 1.13)[6]

English herbalist Joseph Miller certainly gives us a detailed account of myrrh:

> *Myrrh is of an opening, heating, drying nature, resists putrefaction, and is of great service in uterine disorders, opens the obstruction of the womb, procuring the menses, expediting the birth, and expelling the secundines. It is good likewise for old coughs and hoarseness, and the loss of voice, and is very useful against pestilential and infectious distempers, both taken inwardly, and flung upon burning coals and the fume received. Outwardly applied it cures wounds and ulcers, and prevents gangreens and mortifications.*[4]

Myrrh was introduced in Chinese medicine in the 7th century and was used for treating conditions involving bleeding, pain and wounds.[1]

Myrrh is primarily used as a tincture containing 20% of myrrh in 85% alcohol. The tincture is astringent and is used for inflammation of the mucous membranes of the throat and mouth, indigestion, bronchial congestion and as an emmenagogoue.[3,8]

Chemical Composition

The typical chemical composition of myrrh essential oil is as follows:

Heerabolene, limonene, dipentene, pinene, eugenol, cinnamaldehyde, cuminaldehyde, cumic alcohol, m-cresol, cadinene, curzerene (11.9%), curzerenone (11.7%), dihydropyrocurzerenone (1.1%), furanoeudesma-1,3-diene (12.5%), 1,10(15)-furanodiene-6-one (1.2%), lindestrene and others.[1]

Therapeutic Actions

Anticatarrhal, anti-inflammatory, antimicrobial, antiphlogistic, antiseptic, astringent, balsamic, carminative, cicatrisant, emmenagogue, expectorant, fungicidal, sedative, digestive and pulmonary stimulant, stomachic, tonic, uterine, vulnerary.

Pharmacology and Clinical Studies

Myrrh is reported to have astringent properties on mucous membranes as well as antimicrobial properties.[1]

Indications

Antimicrobial Properties

Myrrh is well known for its antibacterial, antifungal and anti-inflammatory actions. The tincture can be used in the treatment of mouth, gum and throat infections.[8] The oil can be incorporated into an ointment which is applied externally for the treatment of haemorrhoids, bed sores and wounds.[11]

Digestive System

Myrrh oil is reputed to stimulate the stomach and digestive system and is a useful remedy for treating diarrhoea, dyspepsia and loss of appetite.[8,9]

The German Commission E Monographs recommend using 5–10 drops of myrrh tincture in a glass of water as a gargle for oral and pharyngeal mucosa.[7]

Integumentary System

Myrrh oil is used for the treatment of chronic wounds and ulcers. This is due to its antiseptic, astringent, anti-inflammatory and antiphlogistic properties. It is beneficial for mature skin, wounds that are slow to heal, and for weepy eczema and athlete's foot.[8,9,10] It heals cracked and chapped skin and can be added to skin care creams.[8,9]

Nervous System

Myrrh oil instills a deep sense of calm and tranquility on the mind.[11]

Respiratory System

Myrrh oil is an excellent expectorant and as such is beneficial in the treatment of coughs, bronchitis and colds.[8,9,10]

Reproductive System

Myrrh is a uterine stimulant and promotes menstruation thus relieving painful periods.[10] Holmes says that it stimulates the uterus and promotes the menses and childbirth.[12]

Energetics

According to TCM, myrrh is warming and drying.[11,12] It is recommended for conditions associated with dampness such as chronic ulcers and wounds, respiratory tract infections with phlegm and mucus and diarrhoea.[12]

Personality Profile

Myrrh oil should be considered for someone who is prone to over-thinking, worry and mental distraction.[11]

Subtle Aromatherapy

Myrrh's effect on the spirit is like that of frankincense — one of inner stillness and peace, of an awareness free from restlessness and the mundane. Myrrh unites the spiritual with the physical.[11]

Myrrh is thought to enhance spirituality. It should be used as a meditation aid or before any healing session.[13] It can be used to strengthen the base chakra and is particularly valuable for people who feel emotionally or spiritually stuck and want to move forward in their lives.[13]

Mode of Administration

Topical application — massage, compress, bath, douche, ointment, skin care; Inhalation — direct inhalation, diffuser, oil vaporiser.

Safety

Myrrh oil is non-toxic, non-irritating and non-sensitising. Many ancient physicians classified myrrh as an abortifacient. Myrrh oil is contra-indicated during pregnancy.[8,9,12] However, there has been no scientific evidence to confirm this.[14]

References

1. Leung A, Foster S. *Encyclopedia of common natural ingredients used in food, drugs and cosmetics*. 2nd edn, John Wiley and Sons Inc, USA. 1996.
2. Arctander S. *Perfume and flavour materials of natural origin*. Allured Publishing, USA, 1994.
3. Grieve M. *A modern herbal*. Penguin, England, 1931.
4. Tisserand R. *The art of aromatherapy*. The C.W. Daniel Company Limited, Great Britain, 1977.
5. *The Jerusalem bible*. Darton, Longman and Todd Ltd, Great Britain, 1994.
6. Stoddart M. *The scented ape*. Cambridge University Press, UK, 1990.
7. Blumenthal M. *The complete German commission E monographs: Therapeutic guide to herbal medicines*. American Botanical Council, USA, 1998.
8. Davis P. *Aromatherapy: An A–Z*. 2nd edn. The C.W. Daniel Company Limited, Great Britain, 1999.
9. Lawless J. *The encyclopaedia of essential oils*. Element Books Limited, Great Britain, 1992.
10. Lavabre M. *Aromatherapy workbook*. Healing Art Press, USA, 1997.
11. Mojay G. *Aromatherapy for healing the spirit*. Hodder and Stoughton, UK, 1996.
12. Holmes P. *The energetics of western herbs Vol. II*. Artemis Press, USA, 1989.
13. Davis P. *Subtle aromatherapy*. The C.W. Daniel Company Limited, Great Britain, 1991.
14. Riddle J. *Eve's herbs*. Harvard University Press, England, 1997.

Myrtle

Myrtus communis

Family

Myrtaceae

Botany and Origins

Myrtle is an evergreen shrub or small tree, between 3–7 m, with many branches, a brownish-red bark and small sharp pointed leaves. It has fragrant white or pinkish flowers.[1]

It is native to the Mediterranean region and western Asia. The oil is produced in Tunisia, France, Corsica, Spain, Morocco and Italy.[2]

Myrtle should not be confused with the wax myrtle *Myrica cerifera* or bog myrtle *Myrica gale*, whose essential oils are toxic.[1]

Schnaubelt recommends using the Corsican variety of *M. communis*. This oil has a brilliant green colour and has a high 1,8-cineole content.[3]

Method of Extraction

Myrtle essential oil is produced by steam distillation of the leaves and twigs of *M. communis*, and in some places, the flowers, which are highly fragrant, are also included. This may explain the significant difference between the myrtle oils from various regions.[2]

Essential Oil Characteristics

Myrtle oil is a pale-yellow to orange-yellow mobile liquid with a fresh, camphoraceous, spicy and floral-herbaceous odour.[2]

Historical and Traditional Uses

The ancient Persians regarded myrtle as a holy plant. Myrtle was a symbol of love and peace to the Jews and the Greeks regarded it as sacred. Dioscorides prescribed extracts of the leaves for lung and bladder infections.[1]

An extract of the leaves is used in north Africa to alleviate coughs and chest infections. In the 16th century the leaves and flowers were the major ingredients of a skin lotion known as 'angels' water'.[1] The berries are used in bitters and certain liqueurs.[1]

Chemical Composition

A typical chemical composition of myrtle is reported as follows:

α-pinene (8.18%), β-pinene (0.19%), limonene (7.58%), 1,8-cineole (29.89%), α-terpinen-4-ol (0.22%), myrtenol (0.58%), geraniol (0.3%), linalyl acetate (0.53%), myrtenyl acetate (35.9%), carvacrol (0.6%).[4]

Therapeutic Actions

Anticatarrhal, antiseptic, astringent, balsamic, bactericidal, expectorant.

Pharmacology and Clinical Studies

Myrtle is reported to be effective for treating head lice and their eggs.[5]

Indications

Respiratory System

Myrtle is beneficial for chronic conditions of the respiratory system such as bronchitis, catarrhal conditions and chronic coughs.[3,6,7,8]

It has an unobtrusive odour and is well tolerated by young children. It is slightly sedative (unlike eucalyptus oil) which has a stimulating odour, and is recommended as a chest rub or inhalation or oil burner at night.[6]

Urinary System

The oil has been used as an antiseptic for the treatment of urinary tract infections. For bladder infections or infections of the ureter, a sitz bath is recommended.[8]

Skin Care

Myrtle may be used for the treatment of acne, oily skin and open pores.[7,8] Schnaubelt describes green myrtle as a gentle oil which is regenerating, astringent and anti-allergenic.[9] Myrtle oil is astringent and has been used to treat haemorrhoids.[6,8]

Personality Profile

Myrtle is recommended for people with an addictive or self-destructive behaviour:

> *Myrtle is helpful for people whose body seems draped in a gray brown veil from smoking, drug abuse, or emotions like anger, greed, envy or fear. In such cases myrtle oil helps to cleanse the person's delicate inner being to dissolve disharmony.*[8]

Subtle Aromatherapy

Myrtle carries a deep inner wisdom and may serve as a companion for the dying.[8] Worwood says that the spirit of myrtle is energetic truth and forgiveness, giving support to the unsupported and teaching us that divine love embraces all living beings.[10]

Mode of Administration

Topical application — massage, compress, bath, sitz bath, douche, ointment, skin care; Inhalation — direct inhalation, diffuser, oil vaporiser, steam inhalation.

Safety

Myrtle oil is non-toxic, non-irritating and non-sensitising.

References

1. Weiss EA. *Essential oil crops*. CAB International, UK, 1997.
2. Arctander S. *Perfume and flavour materials of natural origin*. Allured Publishing, USA, 1994.
3. Lavabre M. *Aromatherapy workbook*. Healing Art Press, USA, 1997.
4. Lawrence B. *Myrtle oil*. Perfumer and Flavorist, 1977; 2(3): 53.
5. Gauthier R et al. *The activity of extracts of Myrtus communis against Pediculus humanis capitis*. Planta Med Phytother., 1989; 23(2): 95–108. Cited in the Aromatherapy Database, Bob Harris, Essential Oil Resource Consultants, UK, 2000.
6. Davis P. *Aromatherapy: An A–Z*. 2nd edn. The C.W. Daniel Company Limited, Great Britain 1999.
7. Lawless J. *The encyclopaedia of essential oils*. Element Books Limited, Great Britain, 1992.
8. Fischer-Rizzi S. *Complete aromatherapy handbook*. Sterling Publishing Company, USA, 1990.
9. Schnaubelt K. *Advanced aromatherapy*. Healing Art Press, Canada, 1995.
10. Worwood V. *The fragrant spirit*. Doubleday, Great Britain, 1999.

Neroli

Citrus aurantium var. *amara*

Synonyms

Orange flower, Orange blossom, neroli bigarade

Family

Rutaceae

Botany and Origins

Bitter orange is an evergreen tree with long but not very sharp spines and very fragrant flowers. It is a native of southern China and India.[1]

Neroli oil is produced from the flowers of several citrus species. The oil obtained from bitter orange is called neroli bigarade oil or orange flower oil, the oil sweet orange flowers is called neroli Portugal and the oil from lemon flowers is called — neroli citronier.[2]

Neroli bigarade is produced in the south of France, Italy, Tunisia, Morocco, Haiti, Guinea and Algeria.[3]

Neroli oil is often difficult to obtain and is expensive, thus a number of synthetic substances which should be avoided in aromatherapy are available.[2]

As neroli oil is slightly water-soluble, the water remaining after the distillation of neroli essential oil contains traces of neroli oil. This is sold as orange flower water which is used in cosmetics and in food flavouring. Orange flower water is often solvent-extracted to recover the oil which is known as orange flower water absolute. This oil has dark to brownish-yellow colour with a intense floral odour. It is used in perfumery.[2]

Method of Extraction

Neroli essential oil is obtained from the freshly picked flowers of *C. aurantium*, subspecies *amara* by steam distillation.

Essential Oil Characteristics

Neroli oil is a pale-yellow mobile oil which tends to become darker and more viscous with age. It has a powerful, light and refreshing floral top note with very little tenacity.[3]

Historical and Traditional Uses

The bitter orange was first cultivated in the Mediterranean by Arabs in the 10th and 11th centuries. The oil was first distilled in the early 16th century.[2] Neroli is named after the 17th century Italian Princess of Nerola, Anna Maria de La Tremoille, who wore the oil in her gloves.[4]

Neroli oil is one of the key essential oils in the classic Eau de Cologne, along with lavender, bergamot, lemon and rosemary oils. This cologne was valued as a gentle tonic to the nervous system.

The flowers and the oil have been traditionally used for gastrointestinal complaints, nervous conditions, gout, sore throat, as a sedative and for sleeplessness.[1]

Orange blossom water has traditionally been used in Europe in cooking and in skin care preparations. It is especially soothing and anti-inflammatory and has a calming and uplifting effect similar to the essential oil.[5]

Chemical Composition

A typical chemical composition of neroli is reported as follows:

α-pinene (4.26%), camphene (5.5%), sabinene (2.55%), β-pinene (8.67%), myrcene (2.15%), δ-3-carene (2.46%), limonene (22.43%), terpinene (4.14%), α-terpineol (1.87%), linalool (2.52%), linalyl acetate (0.87%), geraniol (1.02%), nerol (6.97%), citronellol (1.87%), citral (2.41%), β-citral (1.87%), methyl anthranilate (1.89%).[2]

Therapeutic Actions

Antidepressant, antiseptic, antispasmodic, bactericidal, carminative, cicatrisant, cordial, deodorant, digestive, nervine.

Pharmacology and Clinical Studies

The oil is reported to exhibit antifungal and antimicrobial activities *in vitro*.[1]

Neroli was effective in diminishing the amplitude of heart muscle contraction, benefiting people who suffer from palpitations or other types of cardiac spasms. The oil was found to reduce the symptoms associated with post-cardiac surgery patients.[6]

Indications

Children's Remedy

Holmes recommends using orange flower water for babies and infants. It may be used in a humidifier, in their bath water or by adding a teaspoon to the feeding bottle. It makes a very soothing, digestive, carminative remedy for infant's colic and its sedative action will help them sleep.[7]

Cardiovascular System

Neroli is beneficial for the heart since it regulates heart rhythm and helps to reduce cramp-like nervous heart conditions.[4] The oil is indicated for the treatment of hypertension and palpitations.[5,8]

Digestive System

Neroli oil may be used to relieve spasms of the smooth muscles of the digestive system. It is beneficial in the treatment of chronic diarrhoea, especially when it arises from nervous tension.[9]

Nervous System

Neroli oil is regarded as one of the most effective sedative and antidepressant remedies and is recommended for the treatment of insomnia and states of anxiety and depression.[8,9]

Fischer-Rizzi describes the therapeutic benefits of the sweet scent of neroli oil as:

> *... reaching down into the soul to stabilise and regenerate. It provides relief and strength for long standing psychological tension, exhaustion, and seemingly hopeless situations.*[4]

Mojay recommends neroli for individuals who are emotionally intense and who are sometimes unstable and are easily alarmed and agitated.[10] Holmes describes neroli as promoting clarity, sensitivity and space and describes it as enhancing the 'lightness of being'.[7]

Skin Care

In skin care, neroli oil is regarded as being non-allergenic and is recommended to reduce redness and irritation. It is beneficial for all skin types, especially dry sensitive skin with broken capillaries.[5,9]

The oil is reputed to have a rejuvenating effect on the skin as it has an ability to stimulate the growth of healthy new cells.[9]

Energetics

Neroli oil clears heat, relaxes the nerves and uplifts the spirits.[7,10] Mojay describes neroli oil as one of the best oils to calm and stabilise the heart and mind:

> *Neroli is particularly beneficial for hot, agitated conditions of the heart characterised by restlessness, insomnia and palpitations, and is indicated for hypertension.*[10]

Personality Profile

The neroli personality is described as being one of the most spiritual personalities. Worwood says that whatever the age, there is a built-in wisdom that extends far beyond that of worldly knowledge. She describes neroli as a personality that seems to have found a way to be ageless, forever young in a spring-like way.[11]

Subtle Aromatherapy

Neroli oil is associated with purity. It brings us in touch with our higher selves, it facilitates all spiritual work and is recommended for enhancing creativity.[12]

Mode of Administration

Topical application — massage, compress, bath, ointment, skin care; Inhalation — direct inhalation, diffuser, oil vaporiser.

Safety

Neroli oil is non-toxic, non-irritating and non-sensitising.

References

1. Leung A, Foster S. *Encyclopedia of common natural ingredients used in food, drugs and cosmetics*. 2nd edn, John Wiley and Sons Inc, USA, 1996.
2. Weiss EA. *Essential oil crops*. CAB International, UK, 1997.
3. Arctander S. *Perfume and flavour materials of natural origin.* Allured Publishing, USA, 1994.
4. Fischer-Rizzi S. *Complete aromatherapy handbook.* Sterling Publishing Company, USA, 1990.
5. Lavabre M. *Aromatherapy workbook.* Healing Art Press, USA, 1997.
6. Stevenson C. *Orange blossom evaluation*. The International Journal of Aromatherapy, 1992; 4(3): 22–4.
7. Holmes P. *Neroli — The lightness of being*. The International Journal of Aromatherapy, 1995; 7(2): 14–17.
8. Lawless J. *The encyclopaedia of essential oils.* Element Books Limited, Great Britain, 1992.
9. Davis P. *Aromatherapy: An A–Z.* 2nd edn. The C.W. Daniel Company Limited, Great Britain, 1999.
10. Mojay G. *Aromatherapy for healing the spirit.* Hodder and Stoughton, UK, 1996
11. Worwood V. *The fragrant mind.* Doubleday, Great Britain, 1995.
12. Davis P. *Subtle aromatherapy.* The C.W. Daniel Company Limited, Great Britain, 1991.

Niaouli

Melaleuca quinquenervia

Synonyms

Broad-leaf tea tree, broad-leaved paperbark, paperbark

Arctander states that niaouli is steam-distilled from the leaves of *M. viridiflora*. However, Lassak says that the names *M. leucadendron* var. *viridiflora* and *M. viridiflora* have been misapplied to this species.[2,3] Weiss also confirms this and says that the source of confusion is because *M. quinquenervia* has several cultivars which produces oils of differing composition.[1]

Family

Myrtaceae

Botany and Origins

Niaouli is a shrub or small tree up to 25 m high with a papery bark. It grows well in swampy ground. In Australia, it is commonly found along the coastal strip of New South Wales, all the way up to the northern tip of Queensland.[3]

Niaouli oil is produced on the island of New Caledonia, where it is referred to as Gomenol.[1,2]

Niaouli has also been introduced to Madagascar. The oil from Madagascar is preferred in aromatherapy as the oil from New Caledonia is often obtained by fractional distillation and is cut.[4,7]

Method of Extraction

Niaouli essential oil is produced by steam distillation of the leaves and twigs of *M. quinquenervia.*

Essential Oil Characteristics

Niaouli oil is a pale-yellow to greenish or almost colourless oil with a strong, fresh, sweet-camphoraceous odour reminiscent of eucalyptus and cardamom.[2]

The 1,8-cineole oil has an odour similar to that of eucalyptus, while the nerolidol and linalool chemotype have a distinct sweetish floral odour.

Historical and Traditional Uses

Niaouli oil is used in medicinal preparations, in cough drops, vaporiser liquids, mouth sprays, gargles and to flavour toothpaste.[2]

Lassak says that the young leaves were bruised in water and a liquid drunk to relieve headaches and colds and during general sickness. The oil is used for coughs and colds and applied externally for neuralgia and rheumatism. The oil was used as a vermifuge.[3]

In France, numerous pharmaceuticals containing niaouli were made up to the 1980s, such as a syrup for respiratory tract infections and suppositories for vaginal infections.[4]

Chemical Composition

There are three principal chemotypes of *M. quinquenervia*. One is rich in 1,8-cineole and the other in nerolidol or linalool.[1,3]

The chemical profile of niaouli is variable. The typical constituents found in niaouli include: oxides: 1,8 cineole (40–50%); monoterpene hydrocarbons: α-pinene, β-pinene, α phellandrene, α-terpinene, limonene (15–20%); monoterpene alcohols: α-terpineol (5–10%), terpinen-4-ol (2–3%); sesquiterpene alcohols: viridiflorol (7–10%), nerolidol (3–4%); sesquiterpene hydrocarbons: β-caryophyllene, viridiflorene (2–3%).[4]

Therapeutic Actions

Analgesic, antirheumatic, antiseptic, bactericide, cicatrisant, decongestant, febrifuge, insecticide, stimulant, vermifuge, vulnerary.

Pharmacology and Clinical Studies

The oil is reported to exhibit antimicrobial activities *in vitro*.[5]

Indications

Integumentary System

Niaouli is recommended for cleaning minor wounds and burns. Davis recommends using 5–6 drops of niaouli in 250 mL of boiled and cooled water to wash and clean a burn wound. It is antiseptic and a vulenerary and will therefore help healing.[6]

Musculoskeletal System

Niaouli oil is recommended for muscular aches and pain and for the relief of arthritis.[9]

Reproductve System

As niaouli is well tolerated by the skin and mucous membranes it is suitable as a vaginal douche for the treatment of cystitis and other urinary tract infections.[6,7,9]

Respiratory System

Niaouli is recommended for acute and chronic bronchitis and sinusitis.[4] Schnaubelt says that niaouli is an excellent expectorant and it also has antiallergenic and antiasthmatic properties.[7,8]

Skin Care

Davis says that because niaouli oil is non-irritant, it is well suited to skin care application. It is recommended for the treatment of acne and boils.[6]

Mode of Administration

Topical application — massage, compress, bath, ointment, skin care; Inhalation — direct inhalation, diffuser, oil vaporiser.

Safety

Niaouli oil is non-toxic, non-irritating and non-sensitising.

References

1. Weiss EA. *Essential oil crops*. CAB International, UK, 1997.
2. Arctander S. *Perfume and flavour materials of natural origin*. Allured Publishing, USA, 1994.
3. Lassak E, McCarthy T. *Australian medicinal plants*. Methuen Australia, Australia, 1983.
4. Collin P, Price L. *Niaouli*. The Aromatherapist, 1997; 4(2): 15–19.
5. Beylier MF, Givaudan SA. *Bacteriostatic activity of some Australian essential oils*. Perfumer and Flavorist, 1979; 4: 23–25. Cited in the Aromatherapy Database, Bob Harris, Essential Oil Resource Consultants, UK, 2000.
6. Davis P. *Aromatherapy: An A–Z*. 2nd edn. The C.W. Daniel Company Limited, Great Britain, 1999.
7. Schnaubelt K. *Medical aromatherapy*. Frog Ltd, USA, 1999.
8. Schnaubelt K. *Advanced aromatherapy*. Healing Art Press, Canada, 1995.
9. Lawless J. *The encyclopaedia of essential oils*. Element Books Limited, Great Britain, 1992.

Nutmeg

Myristica fragans

Synonyms

M. officinalis, M. moschate, M. aromatica, M. amboinensis

Family

Myristicaceae

Botany and Origins

Nutmegs are the dried kernels of the seeds of *M. fragrans*, an evergreen tree to 15 m with dark green leaves, yellow flowers without petals and large yellowish fruit. All parts of the tree are aromatic.[1]

Nutmeg is a native to Banda and Amboina islands in the Moluccas, Indonesia, and is seldom found as a wild plant, because of its popularity as a spice. Nutmeg is commercially cultivated in Indonesia, Grenada and Sri Lanka.[1]

The dried finger-like husk which surrounds the nutmeg seed inside the shell of the fruit is known commercially as mace. Dried, pulverised mace is a well-known household spice.[2]

Method of Extraction

Nutmeg oil is produced by steam-distillation or steam and water distillation of the freshly comminuted, dried nutmegs.[2]

Essential Oil Characteristics

Nutmeg oil is a pale-yellow mobile liquid with a light, fresh, warm-spicy and aromatic odour. The undertone and dry-out remains warm and sweet with a slightly woody aroma.[2]

Historical and Traditional Uses

The use of nutmeg as a food flavouring and a medicine has a long history. It was recorded in the Sanskrit as *jai phal* and probably arrived by trade from the Hindu colonists of Java.[1]

Nutmeg was not known to the Greeks or Romans. The first record of nutmeg in Europe was in 540 AD by Actius of Constantinople. It is believed that Arab traders brought it to Europe from the Moluccas via Java and India and, as with other spices, the Arabs hid the true source to avoid competition.[1]

By the 12th century it was well known in Europe and in 1191, when Emperor Henry VI entered Rome for his coronation, the streets were fumigated with nutmegs and other strewn aromatics.[1]

In search for a route to the spice islands, Vasco da Gama reached the Moluccas, the source of the nutmeg trade. The Portuguese dominated the nutmeg trade for nearly a century. Then the Dutch controlled the trade of nutmegs in the 17th century for another 200 years.[1]

Nutmegs have long been known for their narcotic affect. The first recorded hallucinogenic effect was by Lobelius in 1576. The physiologist JE Purkinje in 1829 ate three nutmegs and described the effects as similar to cannabis intoxication, including disorientation, hallucinations and later a deep sleep. The response to nutmeg intoxication is extremely varied. It appears that freshly grated nutmegs produce the most profound intoxication.[1]

Nutmeg has been used in herbal medicine for gastrointestinal ailments such as diarrhoea, gastric spasms and flatulence. Mace has been used as an antiparasitic and is externally used for the treatment of rheumatism.[3]

Chemical Composition

A comparison in chemical composition of the East Indian and West Indian nutmeg oil is as follows:[5]

Constituent	East Indian Nutmeg	West Indian Nutmeg
α-pinene	18.0–26.5%	10.6–13.2%
camphene	0.3–0.4%	0.2%
β-pinene	9.7–17.7%	7.8–12.1%
sabinene	15.4–36.3%	42.0-50.7%
myrcene	2.2–3.7%	2.5–3.4%
α-phellandrene	0.4–1.0%	0.4–0.7%
α-terpinene	0.8–4.0%	0.8–4.2%
limonene	2.7–3.6%	3.1–4.4%
1,8-cineole	1.5–3.2%	2.5–4.2%
γ-terpinene	1.3–6.8%	1.9–4.7%
linalool	0.2–0.9%	0.3–0.9%
terpinen-4-ol	2.0–10.9%	3.5–6.1%
safrole	0.6–3.2%	0.1–0.2%
methyl eugenol	trace–1.2%	0.1–0.2%
myristicin	3.3–13.5%	0.5–0.9%

Therapeutic Actions

Analgesic, antirheumatic, antiseptic, antispasmodic, carminative, digestive, emmenagogue, prostaglandin inhibiter, stimulant, tonic.

Pharmacology and Clinical Studies

Nutmeg is reported to have psychotropic properties.[3,6] Nutmeg extracts have been found to inhibit the biosynthesis of prostaglandins in animal studies.[3] The anti-inflammatory activity of mace was confirmed in carrageenan-induced oedema in rats.[3] Myristicin is toxic to humans and large doses of nutmeg or its oil may cause convulsions.[4]

Indications

Digestive System

Nutmeg oil is useful as a digestive stimulant, helping people who cannot assimilate food. It may be useful for the treatment of flatulence, nausea, chronic vomiting and diarrhoea.[7,8,9]

Musculoskeletal System

It is an excellent oil to add to a massage oil because of its warming property for muscular aches and pains as well as rheumatism.[7,8,9]

Nervous System

It is classified as a tonic and stimulant and an aid for general fatigue.[7,8,9]

Mode of Administration

Topical application — massage, compress, bath, ointment, skin care; Inhalation — direct inhalation, diffuser, oil vaporiser.

Safety

Nutmeg oil is non-toxic, non-irritating and non-sensitising.

The psychotropic effects associated with nutmeg are believed to be due to the myristicin and elimicin found in the nutmeg. It is believed that myristicin and elimicin are metabolised to TMA and MMDA both of which are hallucinogenic substances.[10]

However closer investigation has revealed the following:[10]

Component	Psychotropic effect
whole nutmeg	highly active
whole nutmeg less the essential oil	no activity
nutmeg oil	weakly active
myristicin on its own	no activity

It appears that the psychotropic properties are due not only to the myristicin and elimicin but to other constituents found in nutmeg.

While ground nutmeg is moderately to strongly psychotropic when taken in high oral doses, the effect of the essential oil is very weak and it appears that non-oral doses will not have any affect at all.

References

1. Weiss EA. *Essential oil crops.* CAB International, UK, 1997.
2. Arctander S. *Perfume and flavour materials of natural origin.* Allured Publishing, USA, 1994.
3. Leung A, Foster S. *Encyclopedia of common natural ingredients used in food, drugs and cosmetics.* 2nd edn, John Wiley and Sons Inc, USA, 1996.
4. Evans WC. *Trease and Evans pharmacognosy.* 15th edn. WB Saunders, 15th edn, UK, 2002.
5. Lawrence B. *Nutmeg oil.* Essential Oils: 1976–1978, Allured Publishing, USA, 1979: 51.
6. Bruneton J. *Pharmacognosy.* Lavoisier Publishing Inc, France, 1999.
7. Lawless J. *The encyclopaedia of essential oils.* Element Books Limited, Great Britain, 1992.
8. Lavabre M. *Aromatherapy workbook.* Healing Art Press, USA, 1997.
9. Valnet J. *The practice of aromatherapy.* The C.W. Daniel Company Limited, Great Britain, 1980.
10. Tisserand R, Balacs T. *Essential oil safety.* Churchill Livingstone, UK, 1995.

Orange, Sweet

Citrus sinensis

Synonyms

Orange oil, *C. aurantium* var. *dulcis*

Family

Rutaceae

Botany and Origins

There are numerous varieties of sweet orange such as Navel, Jaffa and Valencia. It is a smaller tree than the bitter orange tree, less hardy and with few or no spines and the fruits are smaller with a sweet pulp and non-bitter membrane.[1]

The orange tree is believed to be a native of the region between the Himalayas and south-western China. It was not until the early 16th century that the Portuguese explorers introduced the fruit to Europe.[2]

It was introduced to the Americas by Columbus and was primarily grown in the West Indies and Florida. Most of the essential oil produced today comes from Israel, Brazil, North America and Australia.[2]

Method of Extraction

Sweet orange essential oil is cold-pressed from the ripe or almost ripe outer peel of the orange fruit.

Essential Oil Characteristics

Sweet orange oil is a rich yellow-orange to dark-orange-coloured mobile liquid with a sweet, fresh citrus odour, distinctly reminiscent of the odour from a scratched orange peel.

Historical and Traditional Uses

The therapeutic properties of orange were first recognised in ancient China, where the dried peel had been used for centuries to treat coughs, colds and anorexia.[1]

Sweet orange oil is extensively used in food flavouring.[1] The *d*-limonene serves as an important starting material for the synthesis of *l*-carvone, an important source of synthetic spearmint flavour. The price of *l*-carvone from sweet orange oil is usually two-thirds the cost of spearmint.[2]

Chemical Composition

The major constituent of orange oil is limonene, a monoterpene hydrocarbon. A typical chemical composition of sweet orange is reported as follows:

α-pinene (0.54%), myrcene (2.08%), linalool (0.25%) limonene (95.37%), neral (0.06%), citronellal (0.10%), decanal (0.06%), geranial (0.12%).[2]

Therapeutic Actions

Antidepressant, antiseptic, therapeutic, antispasmodic, carminative, cholagogue, digestive, sedative, stomachic, digestive tonic, lymphatic stimulant.

Pharmacology and Clinical Trials

Sweet orange oil has been reported to exhibit antifungal and antibacterial properties.[1,3]

A blind, randomised clinical trial involving 120 children undergoing dental extraction under sevoflurane anaesthesia investigated the effects of sweet orange oil on induction and in recovery. It was found that the children exposed to the sweet orange were more relaxed and cooperative during induction.[4]

Indications

Children's Remedy

Children love the sweet fresh scent of sweet orange. It can be used to help them sleep and to alleviate tummy upsets.

Digestive System

Sweet orange oil helps to settle the digestive system, it prevents and eases spasms and relieves cramps. It is excellent for treating constipation, flatulence and irritable bowel.[6,7] It appears to have a normalising effect on the peristaltic action of the intestines and is recommended for constipation or diarrhoea.[5]

Sweet orange oil is known as a hepatic and cholagogue and may be used to improve the flow of bile and improve the metabolism of fats.[7]

Lymphatic System

Sweet orange oil is known to stimulate lymph fluids, which assists in treating swollen tissue.[6,8,9] This makes it useful in blends for the treatment of cellulite.

Nervous System

The properties of sweet orange oil are said to overlap with those of neroli. It is considered to have a mildly sedative and antidepressant effect.[5] It is recommended in the treatment of anxiety, nervousness and insomnia and may be used with similarly relaxing oils such as lavender, neroli and sandalwood.

Skin Care

Sweet orange oil is beneficial for soothing dry, irritated or acne-prone skin. It is considered to have regenerative properties and can be used for treating aging skin and rough or calloused skin.[9]

Energetics

According to TCM, sweet orange oil helps to circulate stagnant *Qi*, especially when it accumulates in the liver, stomach and intestines. It is considered to be one of the best all-round oils for the digestive system.[7]

Personality Profile

The refreshing, cheerful and sensual nature of sweet orange gives warmth and joy to all who are around it, adults and children alike. It is ideal when we take life too seriously and forget how to laugh. It reduces self-doubt and fears of the unknown and allows one to take on new challenges.[9]

Worwood describes sweet orange personalities as cheerful and optimistic, openhearted, witty, honest and they embrace ideas and suggestions as easily as they embrace people. They have a carefree, friendly smile and joy in their eyes, with faith and understanding which seems to exude from every pore in their body.[10]

Mode of Administration

Topical application — massage, compress, bath, ointment, skin care; Inhalation — direct inhalation, diffuser or oil vaporiser, steam inhalation.

Safety

Sweet orange oil is non-toxic, non-irritating and non-sensitising. The oil is not considered to be phototoxic. However, bitter orange oil has a distinct phototoxic effect.[1]

References

1. Leung A, Foster S. *Encyclopedia of common natural ingredients used in food, drugs and cosmetics.* 2nd edn, John Wiley and Sons Inc, USA, 1996.
2. Weiss EA. *Essential oil crops.* CAB International, UK, 1997.
3. Singh G, et al. *Chemical and fungitoxic investigations on the essential oil of Citrus sinesis.* J Plant Dis Protect, 1993; 100(10): 69–74. Cited in the Aromatherapy Database, by Bob Harris, Essential Oil Resource Consultants, UK, 2000.
4. Mehta S, Stone DN, Whitehead HF. *Use of essential oils to promote induction of anaesthesia in children.* Anaesthesia, 1998; 53(7): 771. Cited in the Aromatherapy Database, by Bob Harris, Essential Oil Resource Consultants, UK, 2000.
5. Davis P. *Aromatherapy: An A–Z.* 2nd edn. The C.W. Daniel Company Limited, Great Britain, 1999.
6. Lawless J. *The encyclopaedia of essential oils.* Element Books Limited, Great Britain, 1992.
7. Mojay G. *Aromatherapy for healing the spirit.* Hodder and Stoughton, UK, 1996.
8. Lavabre M. *Aromatherapy workbook.* Healing Art Press, USA, 1997.
9. Fischer-Rizzi S. *Complete aromatherapy handbook.* Sterling Publishing Company, USA, 1990.
10. Worwood V. *The fragrant mind.* Doubleday, Great Britain, 1995.

Palmarosa

Cymbopogon martini

Synonyms

Palmarosa oil, commonly referred to as East Indian geranium oil, and gingergrass are obtained from two varieties of *C. martini*. It is known in India as rosha or russa grass.[1]

Family

Gramineae

Botany and Origins

Palmarosa is a tufted perennial grass with numerous stiff stems. The grass grows wild in India, particularly north-east of Bombay towards the Himalaya Mountains. The Dutch introduced palmarosa to Java in the 1930s. The grass is also cultivated in the Seychelles Islands and the Comoro Islands.[1]

Method of Extraction

Palmarosa oil is steam-distilled from wild growing, fresh or dried grass of the plant *C. martini*.

Essential Oil Characteristics

Palmarosa oil is a pale-yellow or pale-olive-coloured oil with a sweet, floral-rosy odour and various undertones or top notes according to the quality and age of the oil.[2]

Historical and Traditional Uses

There is no record to when palmarosa oil was first distilled in India, but bruised leaves were used to perfume bath water and provide poultices to relieve pain of neuralgia, lumbago, sciatica and rheumatic pain.[1]

The oil was traded between India and Persia and then shipped to Constantinople, where it became known to European traders as Turkish or Indian Geranium oil.[1]

It is extensively used in perfumery and for scenting soaps. In India the oil is massaged into the joints to alleviate lumbago and rheumatism, and it is taken internally to relieve stomach disorders.[2]

Chemical Composition

A typical chemical composition of palmarosa is reported as follows:

Myrcene (0.13–0.28%), linalool (2.26–3.91%), geraniol (76.3–82.8%), geranyl acetate (5.09–11.8%), limonene (0.15–2.16%).[3]

Therapeutic Actions

Antiseptic, bactericide, cytophylactic, digestive, febrifuge, hydrating, tonic.

Pharmacology and Clinical Studies

Palmarosa oil has been reported to exhibit excellent antifungal and antibacterial properties.[4,5,6]

Palmarosa essential oil was found to give almost complete protection against *Anopheles cullicifacies* (a principal malaria carrier) for up to eleven hours. Palmarosa oil was considered comparable with synthetic repellents such as dimethyl and dibutyl phthalate.[7]

Indications

Digestive System

Acts as a tonic to the digestive system and is reputed to have a beneficial effect on pathogens in the intestinal flora.[8,9] It is reputed to be a digestive stimulant and is recommended for loss of appetite and a sluggish digestion.[8]

Nervous System

It has a calming yet uplifting effect on emotions and may be used to alleviate stress, restlessness and anxiety.[8,9,10]

Skin Care

Palmarosa is extensively used in skin care. It is antiseptic, has hydrating properties, helps to balance sebum production and is reputed to stimulate cellular regeneration.[8,9,11]

It is recommended for all skin types, especially acne, dermatitis, minor skin infections and is also helpful for dry, undernourished skin conditions.[8,9]

Personality Profile

At an emotional level palmarosa encourages free-flowing adaptability and a feeling of security.[10] Palmarosa is recommended for people who have suffered from nervousness and insecurity, and the frequent absence of intimate loved ones.[10]

Energetics

Palmarosa is cooling and moistening. It clears heat and strengthens the yin energy.[10]

Mode of Administration

Topical application — massage, compress, bath, ointment, skin care; Inhalation — direct inhalation, diffuser, oil vaporiser.

Safety

Palmarosa oil is non-toxic, non-irritating and non-sensitising.

References

1. Weiss EA. *Essential oil crops*. CAB International, UK, 1997.
2. Arctander S. *Perfume and flavour materials of natural origin*. Allured Publishing, USA, 1994.
3. Lawrence B. *Palmarosa oil*. Perfumer and Flavorist, 1987; 12(5): 54.
4. Misra N, Batra S, Mishra D. *Antifungal efficacy of essential oil of Cymbopogon martini against Aspergilli*. Int J. Crude Drug Res, 1988; 26(2): 73–76. Cited in the Aromatherapy Database, Bob Harris, Essential Oil Resource Consultants, UK, 2000.
5. Srivastava S. Naik SN, Maheshwari RC. *In vitro studies on antifungal activities of palmarosa and eucalyp-*

tus oils. Indian Perfum, 1993; 37(3): 277–279. Cited in the Aromatherapy Database, Bob Harris, Essential Oil Resource Consultants, UK, 2000.

6. Pattnaik S, Subramanyam VR, Kole CR, Sahoo S. *Antibacterial activity of essential oils from cymbopogon: Inter- and intra-specific differences*. Microbios, 1995; 84: 239–245. Cited in the Aromatherapy Database, Bob Harris, Essential Oil Resource Consultants, UK, 2000.
7. Ansari MA, Razdan RK. *Relative efficacy of various oils in repelling mosquitoes*. Indian J. Malariol, 32(3): 104–111. Cited in the Aromatherapy Database, Bob Harris, Essential Oil Resource Consultants, UK, 2000.
8. Davis P. *Aromatherapy: An A–Z*. 2nd edn. The C.W. Daniel Company Limited, Great Britain, 1999.
9. Lawless J. *The encyclopaedia of essential oils*. Element Books Limited, Great Britain, 1992.
10. Mojay G. *Aromatherapy for healing the spirit*. Hodder and Stoughton, UK, 1996.
11. Lavabre M. *Aromatherapy workbook*. Healing Art Press, USA, 1997.

Patchouli

Pogostemom cablin

Synonyms

P. patchouly, *P. heyneanus*, Patchouly oil

Family

Labiatae or Lamiaceae

Botany and Origins

Patchouli is an aromatic, perennial shrub with erect stems, large green leaves and small white-pink flowers. The common name patchouli is probably derived from the Tamil *paccilai* and the species name from the Philippine vernacular *cablin*.[1]

P. cablin is the prime source for the production of patchouli oil, but several other species, *P. commosum, P. hortensis, P. heyneasus* and *P. plectranthoides* are cultivated for their oils, which are also referred to as patchouli oil. These are, however, considered to be inferior to the oil produced from *P. cablin*.[1]

Patchouli is a native of tropic regions of Asia and is now extensively cultivated in Indonesia, Philippines, Malaysia, China, India, Mauritius, some Caribbean countries, West Africa and Vietnam.[2]

Method of Extraction

To extract patchouli oil it is necessary to rupture the cell walls of the leaf before steam distillation. This is done by controlled, light fermentation, by scalding with superheated steam, or by stacking or baling the dried leaves, thus 'curing' them by fermentation. This is said to produce the best quality patchouli oil.[2]

Essential Oil Characteristics

Patchouli oil is a dark-orange or brownish-coloured, viscous oil with an extremely rich, sweet herbaceous, aromatic spicy and woody balsamic odour.

The odour should remain sweet at all stages of evaporation. The body should display a rich root-like note with a delicate earthiness which should not include 'mould-like' or 'musty' dry odours.[3]

Historical and Traditional Uses

The oil is widely used in Asia for incense, body and garment perfumes, insect repellents and sprinkled in temples. Arabs used it to perfume carpets, Indians textiles and the Chinese produced a perfumed ink for use on scrolls.[4]

The West's fascination with patchouli began in the first decades of the 19th century. In the 19th century there was an enormous amount of trade between India, the Middle East and Europe. Among the most popular goods from the East were the carpets, fabrics, clothes and woven accessories. Many of these, if not all, had layers of crushed or coarse-ground patchouli herb liberally sprinkled amongst them. This was not for aesthetic purposes but for commercial purposes. Patchouli had always been used in Asia as a repellent to moths and small insects. The popularity of the patchouli scent grew to a stage that domestically produced garments, if they were to sell at all, also had to carry the scent of patchouli.[5]

Patchouli became the signature scent for the hippies in the 1960s. Its scent was used to mask the tarry odour of marihuana. It has become one of the most overused social scents of the recent decades, reminding us of the psychedelic 1960s.[4]

In Asia, patchouli herb had long served as a deodorant and insect repellent. Patchouli has for centuries been part of the traditional systems of medicine in Malaysia, China and Japan. The herb is used in Chinese medicine to treat colds, headaches, nausea, vomiting, diarrhoea and abdominal pain.[2]

The oil is extensively used in perfumery, cosmetics and soaps.[2]

Chemical Composition

A typical chemical composition of patchouli oil is reported as follows: monoterpene hydrocarbons (1.0%), sesquiterpene hydrocarbons (62%), oxygenated constituents (37%), patchouli alcohol (33.5%), norpatchoulenol (1.1%).[1]

Of these constituents, it is interesting to note the high percentage of sesquiterpene hydrocarbons which accounts for patchouli's anti-inflammatory properties.

The leaves contain 1.5–4% volatile oil that is composed mainly of patchouly alcohol (ca. 32–40%) and other sesquiterpenes such as busnesol, norpatchoulenol (ca. 2.2%), α-guaiene, α-bulnesene and β-patchoulene. Other compounds found in the oil include cyloseychellene (a tetracyclic sesquiterpene), patchoulipyridine, epiguaipyridine, and guaipyridine (sesquiterpene alkaloids); eugenol, cinnamaldeyde and benzaldehyde; pogostone or dhelwangine (a lactone) and oxygenated sesquiterpenes.[2]

Therapeutic Actions

Antidepressant, anti-inflammatory antiphlogistic, antiseptic, aphrodisiac, astringent, cicatrisant, cytophylactic, deodorant, diuretic, febrifuge, fungicide, insecticide, sedative.

Pharmacology and Clinical Studies

Pogostone, a constituent found in patchouli, is reported to having antimicrobial activities and is responsible for the bactericidal properties of patchouli oil.[2]

Indications

Integumentary System

It is recommended for treating conditions such as sores, fissures, injuries, scars, skin inflammations, eczema and fungal and parasitic skin infections.[6,7,8]

Nervous System

Patchouli is beneficial for alleviating depression, anxiety and stress-related conditions.[6,7]

Skin Care

Patchouli oil is best known in skin care and for topical applications because of its regenerating, disinfecting, moistening and cooling of tissues.

Energetics

Mojay says that patchouli's most valuable therapeutic use is mainly energetic and psychological. Patchouli oil is good for those who, due to excessive mental activity and nervous strain, feel 'out of touch' with their body and their sensuality.[9]

Patchouli's warm and sweet qualities may be used for people with a deficiency of *Qi* in the spleen and pancreas, who, as a result, suffer from fatigue, loose stools and abdominal distension.[9]

Personality Profile

Patchouli's sweet aroma is responsible for its soothing, calming and somewhat hypnotising scent. Patchouli's earthy notes are responsible for its grounding, centring and sensualising effects which are in keeping with its base note. The grounding effect can help heal negative detachment from our body and our environment.[5]

Patchouli oil is suited to the mentally active and tense individual who easily feels divorced from both sensual pleasure and creative expression.[9]

Patchouli personalities are grounded, they often give the impression that they may be slow or sluggish. There is an elderly quality about patchouli personalities, no matter how old they are.[10]

Subtle Aromatherapy

Patchouli oil has a harmonising and stabilising effect on the mind when over-thinking and worrying tend to destabilise one's self-confidence. It is recommended for 'dreamers' and people who tend to neglect or feel detached from their bodies. This may be beneficial for people who are engaged on a spiritual path and are placing an undue share of importance on their mental/psychic experiences to the detriment of their physical wellbeing.[11]

Mode of Administration

Topical application — massage, compress, bath, ointment, skin care; Inhalation — direct inhalation, diffuser, oil vaporiser.

Safety

Patchouli oil is non-toxic, non-irritating and non-sensitising.

References

1. Weiss EA. *Essential oil crops*. CAB International, UK, 1997.
2. Leung A, Foster S. *Encyclopedia of common natural ingredients used in food, drugs and cosmetics*. 2nd edn, John Wiley and Sons Inc, USA, 1996.
3. Arctander S. *Perfume and flavour materials of natural origin*. Allured Publishing, USA, 1994.
4. Morris E. *Fragrance: The story of perfume from Cleopatra to Chanel*. Products of Nature and of Art, USA, 1984.
5. Holmes P. *Patchouli oil*. The International Journal of Aromatherapy, 1997; 8(1): 18.
6. Lawless J. *The encyclopaedia of essential oils*. Element Books Limited, Great Britain, 1992.
7. Davis P. *Aromatherapy: An A–Z*. 2nd edn. The C.W. Daniel Company Limited, Great Britain, 1999.
8. Lavabre M. *Aromatherapy workbook*. Healing Art Press, USA. 1997.
9. Mojay G. *Aromatherapy for healing the spirit*. Hodder and Stoughton, UK, 1996.
10. Worwood V. *The fragrant mind*. Doubleday, Great Britain, 1995.
11. Davis P. *Subtle aromatherapy*. The C.W. Daniel Company Limited, Great Britain, 1991.

Peppermint

Mentha x piperita

Family

Labiatae or Lamiaceae

Botany and Origins

Peppermint is native to southern Europe and was brought to the USA in the early 19th century.[1] The United States is the major producer of peppermint.[1,2] Peppermint is also cultivated in Argentina, Brazil, France, Italy, Morocco, Bulgaria, Holland, Spain, Germany, England, India and Australia.[1]

Peppermint is a perennial herb, growing to the height of 30 to 100 cm. *M. piperita* belongs to a genus consisting of some 20 varieties and hybrids.[2]

M. x *piperita* is, as implied by the written botanical name, a hybrid species from two plants, *M. spicata* and *M. aquatica*.[3]

The various mints used to produce the mint oils are as follows:[4]

Name	Botanical Name	Main Constituent	%
peppermint	*M. piperita*	menthol	29–46%
native spearmint	*M. spicata*	carvone	50–70%
scotch spearmint	*M. gracilis*	carvone	50–70%
cornmint	*M. arvensis*	menthol	70–95%
pennyroyal	*M. pulegium*	pulegone	60–90%
bergamot mint	*M. citrata*	linalyl acetate	57–63%

The major components of the different mints are menthol and pulegone. Cornmint, also referred to as Japanese mint, is cheaper to produce than peppermint and spearmint and is often used as a 'blender' in mint flavours and as an adulterant in peppermint oil. Cornmint is considered more toxic than peppermint oil as it has a higher pulegone content.[4]

Method of Extraction

Peppermint oil is steam-distilled from the partially dried herb of *M. piperita*.

Essential Oil Characteristics

Peppermint oil is a pale-yellow or pale-olive-coloured liquid with a fresh, strong grassy-minty odour with a deep balsamic-sweet undertone and a sweet, clean dry-out note.[1]

Historical and Traditional Uses

Pliny tells us that the Greeks and Romans crowned themselves with peppermint at their feasts, and that peppermint was used to flavour their sauces and wines.[3]

Culpeper was well aware of peppermint's excellent effect on the digestive system:

> *It is useful for complaints of the stomach, such as wind, vomiting ... for which there are few remedies of greater efficacy.*[3]

The mints have been utilised for their medicinal properties for thousands of years, but the oil itself may not have been used as a medicine much before the 16th century, when distillation reached England.[4] Peppermint oil is extensively used in food flavouring, as a fragrance component in toothpastes, mouthwashes, soaps, detergents and perfumes.[2]

Chemical Composition

A typical chemical composition of peppermint is reported as follows:

Menthol (40.0%), menthone (18.7%), 1,8-cineole (7.3%), methyl acetate (3.8%), methofuran (3.0%), isomenthone (2.5%), limonene (2.5%), β-pinene (1.8%), α-pinene (1.4%), germacrene-d (1.3%), trans-sabinene hydrate (1.0%), pulegone (0.8%).[5]

Therapeutic Actions

Analgesic, anaesthetic, antiphlogistic, antiseptic, antispasmodic, astringent, carminative, cephalic, cholagogue, cordial, decongestant, emmenagogue, expectorant, febrifuge, hepatic, nervine, stimulant, stomachic, sudorific, vasoconstrictor, vermifuge.

Pharmacology and Clinical Studies

The choleretic activity of peppermint oil has been confirmed. Peppermint oil and two common essential oil constituents, limonene and geranyl acetate, were tested for their effect on the bile secretion in rats. The results indicated that peppermint exhibited the strongest choleretic activity.[6]

The action of peppermint on morphine-induced contraction and blockage of Oddi's sphincter in guinea pigs was investigated. Peppermint was found to exhibit a pronounced spasmolytic effect.[7]

Balacs cites research which found that peppermint oil exerts its inhibitory effect by interfering with the mobilisation of calcium ions into the tissue.[8] Calcium was implicated in the relaxant effect of peppermint in isolated human gut, and that menthol was responsible. Menthol reduces the calcium influx through voltage-dependent channels.[8,12]

The antispasmodic properties of peppermint have been confirmed in clinical trials. In one trial peppermint was found to be beneficial in helping reduce colonic spasm during endoscopy.[9,12]

Clinical trials involving patients who have just had a colostomy found that peppermint oil helped to reduce much of the distress associated with a colostomy. Patients were given oral doses of enteric-coated capsules containing peppermint. Peppermint was chosen as it not only had an odour that would mask the odour from the colostomy bag, but also because of its effect on the smooth muscle of the bowel. It was found to reduce colonic pressure and prevent foaming, all of which helped to reduce post-operative colic and the frequency of bag change.[10]

Menthol has been presented as a nasal decongestant. This is linked to the cool sensation thought to be due to the stimulation of the nasal cavity thermoreceptors.[11]

Menthol vapours inhibit respiration and may cause very transient apnoea in very young children. The risk is said to be minimal, yet direct application of peppermint oil or menthol on the nasal mucosa of very young children is discouraged.[11,12]

Peppermint oil exhibited a significant antibacterial and antifungal effect in clinical studies.[12]

A topical preparation of peppermint oil in ethanol significantly reduced headache intensity and it was concluded that peppermint oil is an acceptable and cost-effective alternative to oral analgesics in the treatment of tension headaches.[12]

Indications

Analgesic Properties

Peppermint oil is used in liniments for the relief of muscle pain, lumbago, bruises and contusions, joint pain and insect bites. The local anaesthetic action of peppermint is significant. The oil is recommended for myalgia and neuralgia.[13,14]

Digestive System

Peppermint is one of the most effective essential oils for the digestive system. It relieves dyspepsia, nausea, stomach pains, diarrhoea and flatulence.[14,15,16,17,18]

It is an effective remedy for nausea and vomiting and is good for relieving travel sickness. The German Commission E Monographs recommend peppermint oil for obstructions of the bile ducts, gall bladder inflammations and severe liver damage.[13]

Lymphatic System

Gumbel says that peppermint oil has a special affinity with the blood and lymph and that peppermint's refreshing effect on all the tissues lies in the liberating influence on the lymphatic system.[19] He says that the oil's vasoconstrictive effect increases blood flow to the spleen, stimulating the regenerative activity of the spleen in the development of new blood corpuscles.[19]

The lymphatic system is activated in its function through accelerated lymph and tissue fluid circulation.[19]

Nervous System

Peppermint oil helps people become clear-headed and may be beneficial for people who are unable to concentrate or who have mental fatigue. Peppermint oil prevents congestion of blood supply to the brain, helps to clear up any circulatory congestion that exists, stimulates circulation thus strengthening and calming the nerves.[15,17]

Cold compresses of peppermint oil may be applied to the forehead and temples to relieve headaches and migraines. [14,15,16,17]

Respiratory System

Peppermint oil is beneficial for colds and influenza associated with fever and headaches. It is recommended at the onset of a cold to alleviate the symptoms of cold.[17] It is beneficial for sinus congestion, infection or inflammation.[14,15,16]

Skin Care

Peppermint can be used to relieve any kind of skin irritation or itching, but it should be used in a dilution of 1% or less or the irritation may be made worse.

Davis recommends a steam treatment with peppermint to cleanse and decongest the skin.[17] It cools by constricting the capillaries and is a very refreshing skin tonic.

Personality Profile

Worwood describes the peppermint personality as difficult to forget. Some may find them brash and overpowering. They have a fearless spirit and are swift and quick thinkers. They are friendly people who are concerned about the fate of others. Whatever work they take on, they are always dynamic and get totally involved.[20]

Energetics

Peppermint oil often raises a contradiction concerning its warming and cooling effects. It is often listed as having a cooling action. However, Holmes clearly states that it has a warming effect.[21]

Mills attributes this contradictory effect to menthol, a monoterpene alcohol whose physical properties impart a noticeable cooling effect to the skin (vasoconstriction), later followed by pronounced vasodilation and rubefacient effect. This is also accompanied by a slight anaesthetic action (due at least in part to an excitation of cold receptors).[22]

Subtle Aromatherapy

Davis says that peppermint acts on the ego, dispelling pride. She recommends using it to help overcome feelings of inferiority. It is associated with cleanliness and assists people who wish to live an ethical life.[23]

Mojay says that while peppermint oil enhances concentration it works on another level to facilitate the digestion of new ideas. He says that it is the type of oil that enhances our receptive capacities on mental and spiritual levels and would be beneficial for those in need of inspiration and insight.[18]

Mode of Administration

Topical application — massage, compress, bath, ointment, skin care; Inhalation — direct inhalation, diffuser, oil vaporiser, steam inhalation.

For irritable colon the German Commission E Monogaphs for peppermint oil recommend internal daily dose of 0.6 mL in an enterically coated capsule.[13]

Safety

Peppermint oil is non-toxic, non-irritant and may occasionally be sensitising.

The German Commission E Monogaphs recommend that preparations containing peppermint oil should not be used on the face, particularly the nose, of infants and small children.[13]

The only concern regarding the use of peppermint oil is to select peppermint oils with a lower percentage of menthone and pulegone. Tisserand suggests that levels of both these two constituents in peppermint oil are unlikely to produce any toxic effects when the oil is used externally, but caution may be required regarding oral use.[4]

References

1. Arctander S. *Perfume and flavour materials of natural origin.* Allured Publishing, USA, 1994.
2. Leung A, Foster S. *Encyclopedia of common natural ingredients used in food, drugs and cosmetics.* 2nd edn, John Wiley and Sons Inc, USA, 1996.
3. Le Strange R. *A history of herbal plants.* Angus and Robertson, Great Britain, 1977.
4. Tisserand R. *Mint family matters.* The International Journal of Aromatherapy, 1992; 4(1): 20.
5. Lawrence B. *Peppermint oil.* Perfumer and Flavorist, 1986; 11(1): 29.
6. Trabace L et al. *Choleretic activity of some typical components of essential oils.* Planta Med, 1992; 58: Suppl 1:a 650–51. Cited in the Aromatherapy Database, Bob Harris, Essential Oil Resource Consultants, UK, 2000.
7. Giachetti D et al. Pharmacological activity of essential oils on Oddi's sphincter. Planta Med, 1988; 54(5): 38992. Cited in the Aromatherapy Database, Bob Harris, Essential Oil Resource Consultants, UK, 2000.
8. Balacs T. *Peppermint pharmacology.* The International Journal of Aromatherapy, 1992; 4(1): 22.
9. Leicester R et al. *Peppermint oil to reduce colonic spasm during endoscopy.* The Lancet, Oct 30 1983: 989.
10. Gallacher M et al. *A sweet smell of success.* Nursing Times, July 5, 1989; 85(27): 48.
11. Bruneton J. *Pharmacognosy.* 2nd edn. Lavoisier Publishing Inc, France, 1999.
12. Mills S, Bone K. *Principles and practice of phytotherapy.* Churchill Livingstone, UK, 2000.
13. Blumenthal M. et al. *The complete German commission E monographs: Therapeutic guide to herbal medicine.* American Botanical Council USA, 1998.
14. Lavabre M. *Aromatherapy workbook.* Healing Art Press, USA, 1997.
15. Lawless J. *The encyclopaedia of essential oils.* Element Books Limited, Great Britain, 1992.
16. Schnaubelt K. *Medical aromatherapy.* Frog Ltd, USA, 1999.
17. Davis P. *Aromatherapy: An A–Z.* 2nd edn. The C.W. Daniel Company Limited, Great Britain, 1999.
18. Mojay G. *Aromatherapy for healing the spirit.* Hodder and Stoughton, UK, 1996.
19. Gumbel D. *Principles of holistic skin therapy with herbal essences.* Karl F Haug Publishers, Germany, 1986.
20. Worwood V. *The fragrant mind.* Doubleday, Great Britain, 1995.
21. Holmes P. *The energetics of western herbs Vol. I.* Artemis Press, USA, 1989.
22. Mills S. *The essential book of herbal medicine.* Arkana Penguin Books, England, 1991.
23. Davis P. *Subtle aromatherapy.* The C.W. Daniel Company Limited, Great Britain, 1991.

Petitgrain

Citrus aurantium subsp. amara.

Synonyms

C. bigaradia, petitgrain bigarade

Family

Rutaceae

Botany and Origins

Petitgrain oil is produced from the leaves of the bitter orange. It is an evergreen tree with long but not very sharp spines and very fragrant flowers. It is a native of southern China and north-eastern India.[1] The tree is cultivated in mild temperate, semitropical and tropical areas of the world such the south of France, Italy, Algeria, Tunisia, Morocco, Spain, West Africa and in Paraguay.[2]

The word petitgrain is derived from the French word meaning 'little seed', referring to the small unripe fruits from which the oil was originally obtained. The name was retained when the leaves and twigs became the main source.[3] Oils obtained from the leaves of other citrus species such as lemon, bergamot and mandarin may also be labelled petitgrain.[3]

The oil produced from Paraguay is referred to as *petitgrain Paraguay* while the oil from France is referred to as *petitgrain bigarade*.[2]

It has been suggested that the oil from France is of a superior quality. This is because the French producers are careful to use only the leaf and not include any of the wooden branches, nor any small unripe fruit.[4]

During the distillation it is important to ensure that the leaf matter is distilled rapidly with wet steam to prevent hydrolysis of linalyl acetate, the most important constituent of petitgrain.[4]

Method of Extraction

Petitgrain is steam-distilled from the leaves of *C. aurantium.*

Essential Oil Characteristics

Petitgrain bigarade oil is a pale-yellow or amber-coloured liquid of pleasant, fresh-floral, sweet odour, reminiscent of orange flowers with a slightly woody-herbaceous undertone and very faint but sweet-floral dry-out.[2]

Petitgrain Paraguay oil is very similar to petitgrain bigarade oil. However, its top note is slightly harsh, quickly giving way to a heavy and sweet body note of a typical petitgrain character.[2]

Historical and Traditional Uses

Most of the petitgrain oil available today comes from Paraguay. The plant was introduced to Paraguay in the 18th century by Spanish Jesuits.[3]

Petitgrain is an important raw material for perfumery, especially for *Eau de Cologne* and for scenting soaps.[1,2]

Chemical Composition

A typical chemical composition of petitgrain is reported as follows:

Geraniol (2.33%), linalool (27.95%), nerol (1.01%), α-terpineol (7.55%), geranyl acetate (2.61%), linalyl acetate (44.29%), myrcene (5.36%), neryl acetate (0.55%), trans-ocimene (3.32%).[5]

The most important constituent of petitgrain and that which defines its quality is linalyl acetate.[2]

Petitgrain Paraguay oil has a lower ester and higher alcohol content than petitgrain bigarade of French origin.[5]

Therapeutic Actions

Antidepressant, antispasmodic, deodorant, digestive, sedative, stomachic.

Pharmacology and Clinical Studies

Petitgrain has been found to be effective against certain classes of bacteria.[6]

Indications

Digestive System

Petitgrain is a digestive and antispasmodic and is recommended for the treatment of dyspepsia.[9,10]

Nervous System

Petitgrain oil has a stabilising effect on the nervous system.[6] It is uplifting and refreshing and is recommended for nervous exhaustion and stress-related conditions.[6,9] It is similar to neroli in its action though the latter is considered more effective with serious states of depression.[7,10] It is relaxing and may be used for the treatment of insomnia.[7,9,10]

Petitgrain is recommended for people with insomnia stemming from anguish due to solitude, from a refusal of celibacy and from emotional shortcomings that generate increasing troubles.[8]

Respiratory System

Petitgrain may be used to control nervous asthma in people with irritability, anxiety and depression.[8]

Skin Care

Petitgrain has a tonic effect on the skin and is helpful for acne, skin blemishes and helps to reduce overactive sebaceous glands.[7,8] It is used in bath preparations and has deodorising properties.[7]

Personality Profile

The petitgrain personality is closely associated with neroli, and to a lessor extent, the orange personality. The qualities associated with a petitgrain personality are revitalising, balancing, restoring and clarifying. Petitgrain personalities are the providers of comfort and emotional nourishment.[11]

Subtle Aromatherapy

Davis suggests that while neroli activates the highest psychic or spiritual levels of the mind, petitgrain relates to the conscious, intellectual aspect of the mind.[12]

Mode of Administration

Topical application — massage, compress, bath, ointment, skin care; Inhalation — direct inhalation, diffuser, oil vaporiser.

Safety

Petitgrain oil is non-toxic, non-irritating and non-sensitising.

References

1. Leung A, Foster S. *Encyclopedia of common natural ingredients used in food, drugs and cosmetics.* 2nd edn, John Wiley and Sons Inc, USA, 1996.
2. Arctander S. *Perfume and flavour materials of natural origin.* Allured Publishing, USA, 1994.
3. Weiss EA. *Essential oil crops.* CAB International, UK, 1997.
4. Guenther E. *The essential oils.* Robert E. Krieger Publishing Company, USA, 1982.
5. Lawrence B. *Petitgrain oil.* Perfumer and Flavorist, 1977; 1(6): 31.
6. Schnaubelt K. *Advanced aromatherapy.* Healing Art Press, Canada, 1995.
7. Davis P. *Aromatherapy: An A–Z.* 2nd edn. The C.W. Daniel Company Limited, Great Britain, 1999.
8. Mailhebiau P. *Portraits in oils.* The C.W. Daniel Company Limited, Great Britain, 1995.
9. Lawless J. *The encyclopaedia of essential oils.* Element Books Limited, Great Britain, 1992.
10. Lavabre M. *Aromatherapy workbook.* Healing Art Press, USA, 1997.
11. Worwood V. *The fragrant mind.* Doubleday, Great Britain, 1995.
12. Davis P. *Subtle aromatherapy.* The C.W. Daniel Company Limited, Great Britain, 1991.

Pine

Pinus sylvestris

Synonyms

Pine needle, Scotch pine, Norway pine, forest pine.

Family

Pinaceae

Botany and Origins

Scotch pine is a tree with leaves in two-leaved fascicles (clusters), deep fissured bark and up to 40 m high.[1]

The essential oil produced from the Scotch pine, (*P. sylvestris*) is the most widespread variety and commonly used essential oil in aromatherapy.

P. sylvestris is widely grown all over Europe, the Baltic states, Russia, central Europe and southern European countries. The best quality *P. sylvestris* comes from Tyrol, Austria.[2]

Other species which produce pine oil include the eastern white pine (*P. strobus*) from the eastern USA and Canada, the dwarf pine (*P. mugo* var. *pumilio*) grown in central and southern Europe, and the black pine (*P. nigra*) from Austria.[2]

A pine oil is also obtained by steam distillation of the heartwood and stump wood of *P. palustris* and other *pinus* species. The oil is then fractionally distilled under vacuum to yield pine oil. The lighter fractions from this distillate are known as wood turpentine. Production of this oil takes place mainly in the USA.[2]

Method of Extraction

P. sylvestris oil is steam-distilled from the needles, young branches and cones of the Scotch pine tree.

Essential Oil Characteristics

P. sylvestris oil is a clear mobile liquid with a characteristic pine, fresh top note with a distinct sweetness.

Historical and Traditional Uses

Pines are amongst the most important commercial trees. Most of them have straight, unbranched, cylindrical trunks, which furnish large amounts of excellent timber.[3]

Pine needle oil is extensively used in pharmaceutical preparations for cough and cold medicines, vaporising fluids, nasal decongestants and analgesic ointments.[1]

Marguerite Maury considered pine useful for rheumatic conditions such as gout, and an effective diuretic as well as a treatment for pulmonary infections.[4] The oil is also used for room fresheners, disinfectants, soaps and detergents.[2]

Chemical Composition

Scotch pine needle oil contains 50–97% monoterpene hydrocarbons composed mostly of α-pinene with lesser amounts of 3-carene, dipentene, β-pinene, *d*-limonene, α-terpinene, γ-terpinene, *cis*-β-ocimene, myrcene, camphene, sabinene and terpinolene. Other compounds present include borneol acetate (3 to 3.5%), borneol, 1,8-cineole, citral, terpineol, caryophyllene, butyric acid, valeric acid, caproic acid and isocaproic acid.[1]

Therapeutic Actions

Antimicrobial, antineuralgic, antirheumatic, antiseptic, antiviral, bactericidal, balsamic, deodorant, diuretic, expectorant, insecticidal, rubefacient, tonic.

Pharmacology and Clinical Studies

Dwarf pine oil and Scotch pine oil have varying degrees of antimicrobial activities. Limonene, dipentene and bornyl acetate have been reported as the main constituents responsible for the antiviral and antibacterial properties.[1]

Indications

Musculoskeletal System

Pine oil has a stimulating effect on the circulation and may be used in a liniment to relieve the pain of rheumatism and arthritis and for muscular aches from over-exertion.[11]

Nervous System

Pine oil is regarded as a tonic to the lungs, kidneys and the nervous system.[5,6] Mojay says that pine oil is just as effective as rosemary and thyme for combating fatigue and nervous exhaustion.[5]

Pine oil is recommended during times of convalescence or following an illness that leaves one feeling weak or with severe psychological stress.[7] Schnaubelt considers it a tonic and adrenal stimulant and recommends that it be used topically over the kidney area for adrenal support.[8]

Respiratory System

It has excellent expectorant, balsamic and antiseptic properties, thus making it very useful for a wide variety of pulmonary complaints. It is considered one of the best oils to clear cold phlegm from the lungs. It can be used for sinus and bronchial congestion, coughs, asthma, and bronchitis.[5,9,10]

Urinary System

The antiseptic properties of pine indicate its usefulness for conditions such as cystitis and pyelitis.[5,6,9]

Energetics

The energetic qualities of pine oil are warming and drying and it tonifies *Qi*. It is one of the best oils to clear cold phlegm and is recommended for bronchial congestion, coughing and asthmatic breathing.[5,10]

Personality Profile

Pine is recommended for persons who often feel responsible not just for their own actions but for the mistakes and suffering of others. Pine oil instils positivity and restores self-confidence, replacing undue guilt with forgiveness and self-acceptance.[5]

Pine has been described as a symbol of an uncompromising will to live, endurance, strength, and a free spirit that refuses to conform or live in servitude. The oil awakens one's spirit and it is good for people who lack courage, perseverance, self-confidence and patience.[7]

Subtle Aromatherapy

Pine oil may be used to clear a meditation space, especially if the room or space cannot be devoted exclusively for this purpose.[12]

Mode of Administration

Topical application — massage, compress, bath, ointment, skin care; Inhalation — direct inhalation, diffuser, oil vaporiser, steam inhalation.

Safety

Scotch pine oil is non-toxic, non-irritating and non-sensitising. Dwarf pine oil has been reported to be a dermal irritant and dermal sensitiser to certain individuals.[1,9] While dwarf pine is considered a dermal irritant, it is very likely that all pine oils are potential irritants if oxidised, but not when fresh.[13]

References

1. Leung A, Foster S. *Encyclopedia of common natural ingredients used in food, drugs and cosmetics.* 2nd edn, John Wiley and Sons Inc, USA, 1996.
2. Arctander S. *Perfume and flavour materials of natural origin.* Allured Publishing, USA, 1994.
3. Grieve M. *A modern herbal.* Penguin, England, 1931.
4. Maury M. *Marguerite Maury's guide to aromatherapy.* The C.W. Daniel Company Limited, Great Britain, 1994.
5. Mojay G. *Aromatherapy for healing the spirit.* Hodder and Stoughton, UK, 1996.
6. Lavabre M. *Aromatherapy workbook.* Healing Art Press, USA, 1997.
7. Fischer-Rizzi S. *Complete aromatherapy handbook.* Sterling Publishing Company, USA, 1990.
8. Schnaubelt K. *Medical aromatherapy.* Frog Ltd, USA, 1999.
9. Lawless J. *The encyclopaedia of essential oils.* Element Books Limited, Great Britain, 1992.
10. Holmes P. *The energetics of western herbs Vol I.* Artemis Press, USA, 1989.
11. Davis P. *Aromatherapy: An A–Z.* 2nd edn. The C.W. Daniel Company Limited, Great Britain, 1999.
12. Davis P. *Subtle Aromatherapy.* The C.W. Daniel Company Limited, Great Britain, 1991.
13. Tisserand R, Balacs T. *Essential oil safety.* Churchill Livingstone, England, 1995.

Rock Rose

Cistus ladaniferus

Synonyms

Cistus oil, labdanum

Family

Cistaceae

Botany and Origins

Rock rose, also known as cistus or labdanum, is a resinous exudate from *C. ladaniferus*, a small, wild growing shrub, up to 3 m with lance-shaped leaves that are viscid above and densely white woolly beneath.[1,2]

The plant originates in the mountainous coastal regions of the eastern Mediterranean countries and the Middle East.[2] Spain is the major producer of cistus gum, while France is the major producer of the absolute.[2]

Method of Extraction

The gum is obtained by boiling the leaves and twigs in water. The oil is then obtained from the gum by distillation.[1,2]

A concrète is produced by hydrocarbon solvent extraction of the dried plant material. An absolute is then produced from the concrète.[2]

Essential Oil Characteristics

Cistus oil is a pale-orange-coloured oil with a sweet, warm-herbaceous, musky-like odour. The absolute has a sweet herbaceous balsamic odour.

Historical and Traditional Uses

Rock rose was imported into Ancient Egypt from Crete. The resin was extensively used in Egypt as a perfume and as an incense.[3]

At the time of Christ, an incense was made using frankincense and myrrh from Arabia, galbanum and 'onycha'. The later has been identified as gum labdanum, which is exuded from the leaves of rock rose.[3]

The oil has been used in Europe since the Middle Ages. The oil was used in ointments and compresses to treat infected wounds and skin ulcers.[4] The oil is also used as a fixative in many perfumes.[2]

Chemical Composition

A typical profile of cistus oil is reported to contain at least 170 compounds, including α-pinene, β-pinene, camphene, sabinene, myrcene, α-phellandrene, α- and β-terpinenes, limonene, p-cymene, 1,8-cineole, borneol, nerol, linalool, geraniol, *cis*-3-hexen-1-ol, trans-2-hexen-1-ol, terpinen-4-ol, eugenol, 2,2,6-trimethylcyclohexanone, fenchone, α-thujone, isomenthone, acetophenone, ledol, diacetyl, benzaldehyde, *cis*- and *trans*-citral, bornyl acetate and geranyl acetate.[2]

While α-pinene is reported to be the major constituent, no other single constituent predominates.[2]

Therapeutic Actions

Antimicrobial, antiseptic, astringent, emmenagogue, expectorant, sedative, vulnerary.

Pharmacology and Clinical Studies

Cistus essential oil is reported to have antimicrobial activities against *Staphylococus aureus, Escherichia coli* and *Candida albicans*.[2]

Indications

Integumentary System

The oil is well known for its wound healing and is recommended for the treatment of ulcers and wounds.[7] Mailhebiau recommends blending rock rose with *salvia officinalis* and *lavandula officinalis* for the treatment of bedsores. He recommends a blend of rock rose, cypress and lavender for varicose ulcers.[6] The oil has been effectively used for treating chronic skin disorders such as eczema and psoriasis.[4] Rock rose is considered one of the fastest, acting oils to stop bleeding from an open wound.[8]

Lymphatic System

Rock rose is beneficial in a massage oil for increasing lymphatic drainage. For swollen lymph nodes in the neck, Fischer-Rizzi recommends a hot compress with rock rose.[4]

Skin Care

The oil is antiseptic, astringent and tonic and is highly recommended for treating acne or oily skin.[4] It is also recommended for mature skin and wrinkles.[5]

Personality Profile

Fischer-Rizzi says that the warm, deep, spicy and soothing scent of rock rose conveys a warmth that deeply affects the soul. Rock rose is recommended for patients who feel, after a traumatic event, cold, empty or numb.[4]

Subtle Aromatherapy

Rock rose is recommended as an aid to meditation. It is centring and aids in visualising spiritual experiences and bringing them to consciousness.[4,7]

Mode of Administration

Topical application — massage, compress, bath, ointment, skin care; Inhalation — direct inhalation, diffuser, oil vaporiser.

Safety

Rock rose oil is non-toxic, non-irritating and non-sensitising.

References

1. Arctander S. *Perfume and flavour materials of natural origin.* Allured Publishing, USA, 1994.
2. Leung A, Foster S. *Encyclopedia of common natural ingredients used in food, drugs and cosmetics.* 2nd edn, John Wiley and Sons Inc, USA, 1996.

3. Morris, E., *Fragrance: The story of perfume from Cleopatra to Chanel.* Products of Nature, USA, 1984.

4. Fischer-Rizzi S. *Complete aromatherapy handbook.* Sterling Publishing Company, USA, 1990.

5. Lawless J. *The encyclopaedia of essential oils.* Element Books Limited, Great Britain, 1992.

6. Mailhebiau P. *Portraits in oils.* The C.W. Daniel Company Limited, Great Britain, 1995.

7. Lavabre M. *Aromatherapy workbook.* Healing Art Press, USA, 1997.

8. Schnaubelt K. *Advanced aromatherapy.* Healing Art Press, Canada, 1995.

Rose

The two major species of rose used for essential oil production are *Rosa damascena* and *R. centifolia.*

Synonyms

R. damascena is commonly known as Bulgarian Rose, Turkish rose or rose otto. *R. centifolia* is known as rose maroc, French rose, attar of rose or rose absolute.[1]

Family

Rosaceae

Botany and Origins

The *rosa* species are small prickly shrubs 2.4 m high. It is considered a native of Europe and Western Asia.[1]

It has been suggested that the Mediterranean *R. gallica* is one of the species from which modern rose cultivars are derived. *R. gallica* is a vigorous spreading shrub to 1.5 m, with dense foliage and few thorns. It has fragrant, semi-double light red flowers with yellow stamens.[2]

The birthplace of the cultivated rose *R. damascena* was probably northern Persia, or Faristan on the Gulf of Persia. It then spread across Mesopotamia, Palestine and across to Asia Minor and Greece.[3]

The European name for the Damascus rose dates from the Crusades, but it is now incorporated in its botanical name.[2]

While there are thousands of rose varieties, there are three varieties which are typically used for rose oil production. They are:

- Damask rose from *R. damascena*
- Cabbage or May rose produced from *R. centifolia.*
- *R. gallica*[2]

Cultivation of *R. damascena* and production of rose oil was introduced to Bulgaria, then part of the Turkish Empire in the 15th century.[2]

Commercial rose growing to produce rose oil was well established in the Kazanlik region of Bulgaria by the end of the 17th century. It is the Bulgarian rose oil which today is still considered the most prized of all rose oils. The Bulgarian rose industry is confined to one mountain district, having for its centre the town of Kazanlik.[3]

The major rose oil producing countries are France, Bulgaria, Morocco, Turkey, Italy and China.[1]

Method of Extraction

Three main products are obtained from roses: an essential oil, a concrète and an absolute. The essential oil is obtained by steam distillation of the whole flowers, the concrète by solvent extraction of the leaves and flowers and an absolute by further extracting the concrète.[2]

The three products vary from different cultivars or species and also vary from the same cultivar or species grown in geographically separate areas.[2]

Rose otto is generally accepted to apply to the oil distilled from *R. damascena* and it is usually prefixed by the country of origin.[2]

The flowers are generally picked manually and to minimise loss of oil harvesting needs to be done between 5 and 10 am as this is the period that the flowers are open and the oil content is highest.[2]

Flowers must be promptly transported to the distillery before being distilled. Rose oil is produced by a two-stage distillation process. It is a common practice to redistill the distilled water, a process known as cohobation.[4]

The yield of cohobation oil is several times higher than that from the first distillation of the flowering material. The oils from the two distillations are then blended. The phenyl ethyl alcohol in *rose otto* is derived almost exclusively from cohobation water.[4]

According to Grieve, 4,000 kg of flowers yield 1 kg of rose oil, of which one-third comes from the first distillation, and the remaining two-thirds is a result of redistilling the waters.[3]

Rosewater is the aqueous portion of the steam distillation after rose oil has been removed.

Rose absolute is obtained by solvent extraction. Holmes refers to the solvent extraction process as 'dry-cleaning' the plant. Solvent extraction produces a more complete plant extract. However, Holmes suggests that contact with the solvent, which is usually a petroleum ether, may result in minute traces of solvent in the final absolute. He suggests that from an energetic perspective that this may devitalise the essential oil through contact with a 'dead chemical substance'.[5]

Wabner suggests that rose absolute produced by solvent extraction is superior to the distilled rose otto because rose otto actually contains synthetic constituents that are not found in nature.[6]

He proved this by doing a headspace analysis of a live rose and comparing the constituents with that of rose absolute of the same flower and rose otto of the same flower. While the chemical constituents of the rose absolute and live rose were the same the rose otto oil contained several constituents such as rose oxide and damascenone that were a by-product of distillation.[6]

Essential Oil Characteristics

Rose absolute from *R. centifolia* is an orange-yellow to brown-orange viscous liquid with a sweet, deep-rosy, very tenacious odour. The spicy notes are usually less pronounced, while the honey-like notes are similar to that of *R. damascena*.[4]

Rose absolute from *R. damascena* is a orange-yellow to brown-orange viscous liquid with a rich, warm, spicy-floral and very deep rose odour with a pronounced honey undertone.[4]

Rose otto obtained from *R. damascena* from Bulgaria is a pale-yellow or slightly olive-yellow liquid which has a warm, deep-floral, slightly spicy odour and immensely rich with traces of honey.[2]

Rose otto obtained from *R. centifolia* is colourless to pale-yellow, sometimes with a greenish tinge when fresh. It has a deep, sweet, warm, rich, but less spicy odour than Bulgarian or Turkish rose otto oils.[2]

When cooled to a temperature of 20°C, rose otto separates into off-white or colourless blades of crystals (stearopten), which when further cooled congeals to a translucent soft mass.[2] When it is heated with the warmth of the hands the oil will liquefy.

Historical and Traditional Uses

No other flower has been exalted in literature, mythology and used for so many sacred purposes as the rose.

In ancient art and literature the rose was the predominant flower symbol. Its blossom symbolises beauty, love, youth, perfection and immortality.[7]

The word *rosa* comes from the Greek word *rodon* (red), and the rose of the ancients was a deep crimson colour, which probably suggested the Greek fable of its springing from the blood of Adonis. According to Islam, rose originated from the sweat of Mohammed.

It was prized in Babylon, Assyria, China, Rome and Greece. These cultures were aware of the healing properties of rose. Pliny in his book *Natural Senses* discusses at great length the scent of rose; the lands and climate which produce the best scented roses, the best season, time of the day and weather for picking a rose in order to preserve its scent, the point in a rose's life when it smells strongest, the perfume of freshly gathered rose as compared to a faded rose, the use of rose perfume and so on.[10]

Generally, therapeutic remedies containing rose have a cooling and soothing influence. It is interesting to note that the fields of application of rose oil in ancient medicine are almost identical with those of modern aromatherapy.

In Chinese and Sanskrit manuscripts rose was highly praised. Li Shin-Chen tells us of a highly fragrant rose, *R. rugosa*, which is cultivated in China:

> *Its nature is cooling, its taste is sweet with a slight bitterishness, and it acts on the spleen and liver, promoting the circulation of the blood. It is prescribed in the form of an extract for haematemesis, and the flowers are used in all diseases of the liver, to scatter abscesses, and in blood diseases generally.. Essence of rose is made by distilling the flowers of Rosa rugosa. Its medicinal action is upon the liver, stomach, and blood. It drives away melancholy.*[9]

Ancient Rome had an insatiable appetite for roses and rosewater. During festivals and banquets rose petals were strewn over the floor and along the streets. Self-indulgent Romans wore rose garlands at their feasts, as a prevention against drunkenness. To them, the rose was a sign of pleasure, the companion of mirth and wine, but it was also used at their funerals.[11]

The first preparation of rosewater was by Avicenna in the 10th century.[3] Although rose was highly esteemed in ancient civilisations, it is believed that the oil was first distilled in the early 1600s.[2]

Grieve says that rose oil was first discovered at a wedding feast of the princess Nour Djihan to the Grand Mogul Djihanguyr. A canal circling the whole garden was dug and filled with rose water. They noticed a scum had formed on the water and was floating on the surface. The scum turned out to be oil that the heat of the sun had caused to separate from the water.[3]

Rose and rose products were employed extensively in English medicine, notably by the well-known physician Nicholas Culpeper, who used rose oil as an anti-inflammatory agent.[3]

An ointment of roses was used to soothe headaches, a syrup to 'comfort the heart', and rose leaves mixed with mint were applied externally as a poultice to 'quiet the over-heated spirits'.[3]

Nowadays, rose oil and rosewater are extensively used as fragrance components in skin care preparations, perfumes, soaps and in food flavouring.[1]

Chemical Composition

Rose is one of the most complex essential oils known. It contains more than 300 chemical compounds, of which the greater part is still unidentified. The table below identifies 86% of the rose composition. The remaining 14% of the volatile part of the oil represents about 300 substances.

A typical chemical composition of Bulgarian rose otto and Turkish rose otto is as follows:[2]

Constituent	Bulgaria	Turkey
ethanol	1.43%	5.14%
pentanal	0.07%	0.05%
3-hexenal	0.26%	0.16%
α-pinene	0.73%	0.50%
camphene and heptanal	0.14%	0.07%
β-pinene	0.03%	0.02%
myrcene and hexanol	0.50%	0.30%
heptanol	0.02%	0.01%
hexyl acetate	0.01%	0.01%
methyl heptenone	0.04%	0.02%
octanol	0.07%	0.01%
linalool	2.18%	0.54%
cis-rose oxide and nonanal	0.43%	0.33%
trans-rose oxide	0.17%	0.18%
nonanol	0.09%	0.07%
phenylethyl alcohol, decanol and terpinen-4-ol	1.45%	1.88%
citronellol	33.40%	45.04%
nerol	5.90%	3.60%
geraniol and neral	18.47%	11.87%
geranial and carvone	0.72%	0.57%
citronellyl acetate	0.53%	0.72%
neryl acetate	0.06%	0.04%
cinnamaldehyde and C15 paraffin	0.21%	0.3%
geranyl acetate	1.60%	1.23%
eugenol and trans β-damascenone	1.20%	1.19%
methyl eugenol and C16 paraffin	2.37%	3.26%
octanal	0.05%	0.02%
benzaldehyde	0.10%	0.03%

A typical chemical composition of rose absolute from Morocco and Turkey is as follows:[2]

Constituents	Morocco	Turkey
ethanol	0.38%	ni
camphene + heptanal	0.01%	0.02%
β-pinene	0.03%	ni
linalool	0.40%	0.28%
phenylethyl alcohol + decanal + terpinen-4-ol	74.06%	72.28%
citronellol	8.77%	—
nerol	2.52%	—
citronellol+nerol	—	14.04%
geraniol + neral	5.18%	4.1%
citronellyl acetate	0.23%	0.10%
neryl acetate	0.10%	0.17%
geranyl acetate	0.38%	0.15%
eugenol+ trans-b-damascenone	0.89%	0.53%
trans-trans-farnesol	1.30%	0.20%
unidentified	5.70%	ni

ni: not identified under compound name

Therapeutic Actions

Antidepressant, antiphlogistic, antiseptic, antispasmodic, antiviral, aphrodisiac, astringent, bactericidal, choleretic, cicatrisant, depurative, emmenagogue, haemostatic, hepatic, laxative, sedative (nervous system), stomachic, tonic (heart, liver, stomach, uterus).

Pharmacology and Clinical Studies

Wabner cites a study which demonstrated that rose oil can reduce high blood pressure and arrhythmia of the heart. The same study discussed the spasmolytic effect of rose oil and its ability to act as a protective against gastrointestinal ulceration.[7]

The combination of rose and melissa on *Herpes zoster* and *H. simplex* has also been confirmed. According to Wabner the oil is to be applied pure without dilution, two or three times a day for several days.[7]

A clinical trial involving animals found that rose oil exhibited antianxiety effect. It was concluded that rose oil has a pharmacological activity similar to non-benzodiazepine anxiolytic drugs.[8]

Indications

Rose oil has the most diverse therapeutic properties of all essential oils. Most aromatherapists agree that rose oil is effective in all levels of life, for the soul, spirit and body.[9,14,19]

Nervous System

Rose oil has been assigned to the heart. The essential oil of rose has a profound psychological effect.

> *The rose, queen of flowers! Her fragrance, captured in the essential oil, is the most precious of all heavenly scents. It refreshes the soul; its fragrant poetry brings joy to the heart.*[14]

It is referred to as a gentle but potent antidepressant.[12]

Rose may be used as a sedative for the nerves, it is useful for the treatment of palpitations, irritability and insomnia. It helps to release anger, despair and frustration.[5]

It opens the heart and soothes feelings such as anger, fear and anxiety. Rose comforts in times of sorrow; dissolves psychological pain, refreshes a sad heart, and opens doors to love, friendship, and empathy.[14]

Reproductive System

Rose oil is valuable for the treatment of gynaecological problems. Maury comments that rose oil has an astonishing effect on the female sexual organs as a purifying and regulating agent.[13]

Rose oil is considered a tonic of the uterus.[12,17] It regulates menstruation and relieves menstrual cramps and excessive menstrual bleeding.[12,14,15,17]

Rose is recommended for functional infertility.[5] It is beneficial when it is difficult to predict ovulation dates because of an irregular cycle.[12]

Skin Care

Rose oil has excellent emollient, softening and hydrating properties which, accompanied by its stimulating and antiseptic qualities, make it ideal for all skin care, especially for mature, dry or sensitive skin.[12,14,15,16] Rose oil has a tonic and astringent effect on the capillaries and can be used for the treatment of broken capillaries, redness and inflammation of the skin.[12,15] Rosewater is also used in skin care for its soothing and mildly astringent properties.

Energetics

Rose oil is classified as cool and moist in nature, and is recommended for clearing heat and inflammation and for alleviating anxiety and depression.[17]

It may be beneficial for hot conditions involving the liver and gall bladder that result in tension, irritability, headache and constipation.[17]

Personality Profile

Worwood describes the character of *R. centifola* absolute represents passion of the spirit with a deep, hypnotic personality — vivacious and alive, while the spirit of *R. damascena* epitomises the gentleness of the female spirit. She describes rose otto as perfection personified.[19]

Mailhebiau refers to rose as a miracle of nature:

> *... to simply smell it will refine our sensitivity, take us into an unknown world and disperses the shadows of our worries, anxieties and sorrows. It shows us love, not only human love which is a gift as it is — possibly the finest — from existence, but spiritual love, and we would even say divine, were this term not over-used.*[18]

Subtle Aromatherapy

At a subtle level, Mojay says that the power of rose may be symbolised by its traditional classification as a herb of love. The compassion of rose is revealed in its ability to heal emotional wounds. Mojay says that when rejection or loss has injured one's capacity for self-love and nurturing, rose oil brings a sweet, gentle comfort, restoring the trust that makes love possible again.[17]

Davis associates rose as the supreme oil of the heart chakra which is the centre of love, whether that be love for one person or universal love. It will help the heart chakra to open when grief has caused it to close down.[20] She also associates rose with the sacral chakra which is the centre of creativity and sex. She describes rose as a gentle aphrodisiac which helps to spiritualise sexual relationships.[20]

Mode of Administration

Topical application — massage, compress, bath, ointment, skin care; Inhalation — direct inhalation, diffuser, oil vaporiser.

Safety

Rose absolute and rose otto are non-toxic, non-irritating and non-sensitising.

References

1. Leung A, Foster S. *Encyclopedia of common natural ingredients used in food, drugs and cosmetics.* 2nd edn, John Wiley and Sons Inc, USA, 1996.
2. Weiss EA. *Essential oil crops.* CAB International, UK, 1997.
3. Grieve M. *A modern herbal.* Penguin, Great Britain, 1931.
4. Arctander S. *Perfume and flavour materials of natural origin.* Allured Publishing, USA, 1994.
5. Holmes P. *Rose — The water goddess.* The International Journal of Aromatherapy, 1994; 6(2): 8–11.
6. Wabner D. *A rose is a rose is a rose oil.* 2nd Australasian Aromatherapy Conference, Sydney, 1998.
7. Wabner D. *Rose oil: Its use in therapy and cosmetics.* The International Journal of Aromatherapy Winter 1988/Spring 1989; 1(4): 28.
8. Umezu T. *Anticonflict effect of plant-derived essential oils.* Pharmacol Biochem Behav, 1999; 64(1): 35–40. Cited in the Aromatherapy Database, Bob Harris, Essential Oil Resource Consultants, UK, 2000.
9. Tisserand R. *The art of aromatherapy.* The C.W. Daniel Company Limited, Great Britain, 1977.
10. Classens C. *World of sense.* Routledge, Great Britain, 1993.
11. Morris E. *Fragrance: The story of perfume from Cleopatra to Chanel.* Products of Nature, USA, 1984.
12. Davis P. *Aromatherapy: An A–Z.* 2nd edn. The C.W. Daniel Company Limited, Great Britain, 1999.

13. Maury M. *Marguerite Maury's guide to aromatherapy.* The C.W. Daniel Company Limited, Great Britain, 1994.
14. Fischer-Rizzi S. *Complete aromatherapy handbook.* Sterling Publishing Company, USA, 1990.
15. Lawless J. *The encyclopaedia of essential oils.* Element Books Limited, Great Britain, 1992.
16. Lavabre M. *Aromatherapy workbook.* Healing Art Press, USA, 1997.
17. Mojay G. *Aromatherapy for healing the spirit.* Hodder and Stoughton, UK, 1996.
18. Mailhebiau P. *Portraits in oils.* The C.W Daniel Company Limited, Great Britain, 1995.
19. Worwood V. *The fragrant mind.* Doubleday, Great Britain, 1995.
20. Davis P. *Subtle aromatherapy.* The C.W. Daniel Company Limited, Great Britain, 1991.

Rosemary

Rosmarinus officinalis

Synonyms

R. coronarium

Family

Labiatae or Lamiaceae

Botany and Origins

Rosemary is a small evergreen shrub with thick aromatic, linear leaves, which grows up to 2 m in height. It is a native of the Mediterranean region. The plant grows wild in abundance in Spain, France, Corsica, Italy, Sardinia and Tunisia. Most of the essential oil is produced in Spain, France and Tunisia.[1]

There are three principal chemotypes of *R. officinalis*:

- camphor-borneol (Spain)
- 1,8-cineole (Tunisia)
- verbenone (France)

Method of Extraction

Rosemary oil is steam-distilled from the leaves, flowers and twigs of *R. officinalis* and the numerous subvarieties.

Essential Oil Characteristics

Rosemary oil is a pale-yellow to almost colourless mobile liquid with a strong, fresh, woody-herbaceous top note with a clean-woody-balsamic body note which fades into a dry herbaceous base note.[2]

Mailhebiau describes the odour of the Spanish chemotype as strong and rather camphoraceous, the French chemotype as gentle and the Tunisian chemotype as having an odour reminiscent of eucalyptus, giving it a fresher aroma.[3]

Historical and Traditional Uses

The generic name *Rosmarinus* is derived from the Latin *ros*, meaning dew, and *marinus*, meaning sea, referring to its habit of growing near the coast.[4]

Rosemary is probably one of the best-known and most used of aromatic herbs. The ancient Egyptians favoured it and traces of it have been found in the first dynasty tombs. To the Greeks and Romans it was considered a sacred plant. They believed rosemary symbolised love and death.[4]

Rosemary has been used medicinally for centuries. Theophrastus and Dioscorides recommended it as a powerful remedy for stomach and liver problems; Hippocrates said rosemary should be cooked with vegetables to overcome liver and spleen disorders and Galen prescribed it for jaundice.[4]

In place of more costly incense the ancients used rosemary in their religious ceremonies. It was a custom to burn rosemary with juniper berries to purify the air and prevent infections.[4]

Rosemary was known to have a stimulating effect on the mind and as a useful aid to the memory. Consequently, the herb became known as a symbol of remembrance.[4]

Culpeper recommended the herb for the treatment of diseases of the head and brain, such as giddiness and swimmings therein, drowsiness or dullness, the dumb palsy, or loss of speech, the lethargy and the falling sickness.[4]

The oil was used externally as a rubefacient and was added to liniments as a fragrant stimulant. It was used to prepare Hungary water, which was used to restore the vitality of paralysed limbs. Hungary water was first prepared for the Queen of Hungary and was considered very effective in the treatment of gout.[5]

Rosemary oil is extensively used in hair lotions as it is reputed to renew hair growth and prevent premature baldness. It is used for the prevention of dandruff.[5]

Rosemary oil is extensively used as a fragrance component in cosmetics, soaps, detergents and perfumes.[1]

Chemical Composition

There are three principal chemotypes of *R. officinalis* growing in Europe: camphor, borneol and verbenone. A comparative major component composition of various rosemary oils is as follows:[6]

Compound	Tunisian	Spanish	French
α-pinene	10.3–11.6%	19.1–26.9	10.4%
borneol	2.8–4.2%	2.4–3.4%	3.1%
β-pinene	4.9–7.7%	4.3–7.7%	7.6%
camphor	9.9–12.5%	12.7–20.7	–
bornyl acetate	1.0–1.2%	0.4–1.6%	13.2%
camphene	4.0–4.3%	7.0–9.9%	4.2%
1,8-cineole	40.1–44.45	17.0–25.1%	49.1%
camphene	4.0–4.3%	7.0–9.9%	4.2%
limonene	2.0–4.8%	2.9–4.9%	2.1%

Due to the differences in composition, these oils can be applied for different purposes to achieve maximum efficiency. The camphor-borneol chemotype rosemary is best used as a general stimulant and is considered the most specific heart tonic of all the rosemary oils.[3] It is also suitable for muscular aches and pains.[3,7]

The cineole chemotype rosemary is best used for the treatment of respiratory ailments such as bronchitis, asthma and sinusitis.[3,7] It is also used to facilitate elimination from the liver and the kidneys.[7]

The verbenone chemotype is the most appropriate to strengthen liver and gall bladder.[3] The verbenone rosemary is considered the most gentle non-irritant essence and is excellent for high quality skin care preparations.[7]

Therapeutic Actions

Analgesic, antidepressant, astringent, carminative, cephalic, cholagogue, cordial, digestive, diuretic, emmenagogue, hepatic, hypertensive, nervine, rubefacient, stimulant, sudorific, tonic.

Pharmacology and Clinical Studies

Rosemary oil is reported as having antimicrobial activities.[1,12] It was also found to stimulate locomotor activity of mice when administered orally or by inhalation. 1,8-cineole is believed to be the active principle.[8]

In animal experiments, rosemary oil induced tonicoclonic convulsions. The oil inhibited oxygen consumption and the electrolyte gradients of sodium and potassium.[9]

Rosemary oil has an inhibiting action on muscle contraction when tested on contractile electro-induced response of guinea pig ileum. The constituent borneol was found to have the greatest spasmolytic activity.[10]

Rosemary oil is reported as having hyperglycaemic and insulin release inhibitory effects in a study involving rabbits.[11]

Indications

Cardiovascular System

Rosemary oil is considered a tonic of the heart.[13] It is said to benefit cardiac fatigue, palpitations, low blood pressure and circulatory problems of the extremities.[14]

Digestive System

Rosemary is recommended as a tonic for the liver and gallbladder.[13] It may be used in the treatment of gallbladder infections, biliary colic and gallstones.[7,14,15] For this purpose Fischer-Rizzi recommends warm compresses of rosemary.[14]

Mailhebiau recommends *R. officinalis* ct. *bornyl acetate, verbenone* for people who are very tired, with an overloaded liver, fetid breath and a grey complexion. He describes it as a 'remarkable regulator of the liver'.[3]

Musculoskeletal System

It makes a good analgesic and should be used for treating rheumatism, arthritis and tired, stiff and overworked muscles.[7,13,15]

Nervous System

Rosemary oil is well known for its stimulating effect on the central nervous system (CNS). It is reputed to be a brain stimulant and is used for poor concentration and nervous debility.[13,14,15]

Mailhebiau recommends blending rosemary ct. 1,8-cineole with peppermint and lavender as an excellent treatment for alleviating headaches.[3]

Respiratory System

Rosemary ct. 1,8-cineole is recommended for catarrhal conditions and respiratory ailments such as bronchitis, asthma and sinusitis.[3,7,15] Rosemary ct. verbenone is recommended for its mucolytic properties.[3,7,13]

Skin Care

Rosemary has traditionally been used in skin and hair care.[13] It is extensively used in hair care products as it is reputed to stimulate hair growth and prevent premature baldness. It is also used for the prevention of dandruff.[5]

Energetics

Mojay refers to rosemary as one of the most valuable and invigorating essential oils, describing it as an excellent tonic for the body's yang energy, promoting the circulation of *Qi* and blood.[16]

Personality Profile

Rosemary personalities are young at heart and have found the elixir of youth. They are imaginative, happy, sensitive people with determination. They love security and aim to be in a secure position in love and life because it's within a secure environment that they can express themselves fully. Rosemary has a spirit that vibrates at an astonishing level, others often find it difficult to keep up with rosemary personalities. They have the ability to perform several tasks at once. They love a challenge and set high standards for themselves.[17]

Mailhebiau provides us with a character profile of each chemotype of rosemary. He describes *R. officinalis* ct. *1,8-cineole* as a cheerful, youthful and sincere character while *R. officinalis* ct. *bornyl acetate, verbenone* is a superhuman being whose stability, strength and equilibrium have no equal in love, justice and light. On the other hand *R. officinalis* ct *camphor* is an elderly man, essentially characterised by the temperament of an old moaner.[3]

Subtle Aromatherapy

Davis describes rosemary as a psychic protector. She recommends using the oil first thing in the morning before exposing oneself to all the external influences. Rosemary oil is associated with clear thought and is helpful wherever there is a need for clarity. It is therefore associated with the third eye or brow chakra.[18]

Mode of Administration

Topical application — massage, compress, bath, ointment, skin care; Inhalation — direct inhalation, diffuser, oil vaporiser.

Safety

Rosemary oil is non-toxic, non-irritating and non-sensitising. However, it should not be used during pregnancy and by persons suffering from epilepsy or high blood pressure.[13,14,15]

References

1. Leung A, Foster S. *Encyclopedia of common natural ingredients used in food, drugs and cosmetics.* 2nd edn, John Wiley and Sons Inc, USA, 1996.
2. Arctander S. *Perfume and flavour materials of natural origin.* Allured Publishing, USA, 1994.
3. Mailhebiau P. *Portraits in oils.* The C.W. Daniel Company Limited, Great Britain 1995.
4. Le Strange R. *A history of herbal plants.* Angus and Robertson, Great Britain, 1977.
5. Grieve M. *A modern herbal.* Penguin, England, 1931.
6. Lawrence B. *Rosemary oil.* Perfumer and Flavorist, April/May 1986, 11(2): 75.
7. Lavabre M. *Aromatherapy workbook.* Healing Art Press, USA, 1997.
8. Kovar KA et al. *Blood levels of 1,8-cineole and locomotor activity of mice after inhalation and oral administration of rosemary oil.* Planta Medica, 1987, 53(4): 315–318. Cited in the Aromatherapy Database, Bob Harris, Essential Oil Resource Consultants, UK, 2000.
9. Steinmetz MD et al., *Actions of essential oils of rosemary and certain of its components on the cerebral cortex of the rats in vitro.* J. Toxicology Clin Exp, 1987, 7(4): 259–271. Cited in the Aromatherapy Database, Bob Harris, Essential Oil Resource Consultants, UK, 2000.
10. Taddei I et al. *Spasmolytic activity of peppermint, sage and rosemary essences and their major constituents.* Fitoterapia, 1988, 59(6): 463–468.
11. Al-Hader AA et al. *Hyperglycaemic and insulin release inhibitory effects of Rosmarinus officinalis.* J. Ethnopharmacology, 1994, 43: 217–221. Cited in the Aromatherapy Database, Bob Harris, Essential Oil Resource Consultants, UK, 2000.
12. Soliman FM et al. *Analysis and biological actvity of the essential oil of Rosmarinus officinalis from Egypt.* Flavour Fragrance Journal, 1994, 9: 29–33. Cited in the Aromatherapy Database, Bob Harris, Essential Oil Resource Consultants, UK, 2000.
13. Davis P. *Aromatherapy: An A–Z.* 2nd edn. The C.W. Daniel Company Limited, Great Britain, 1999.
14. Fischer-Rizzi S. *Complete aromatherapy handbook.* Sterling Publishing Company, USA, 1990.
15. Lawless J. *The encyclopaedia of essential oils.* Element Books Limited, Great Britain, 1992.
16. Mojay G. *Aromatherapy for healing the spirit.* Hodder and Stoughton, UK, 1996.
17. Worwood V. *The fragrant mind.* Doubleday, Great Britain, 1995.
18. Davis P. *Subtle aromatherapy.* The C.W. Daniel Company Limited, Great Britain, 1991.

Rosewood

Aniba rosaeodora

Synonyms

Bois de Rose oil

Family

Lauraceae

Botany and Origins

The tree is a tropical, medium-sized, wild growing evergreen from the Amazon basin.[1]

Method of Extraction

Rosewood is oil is steam-distilled and occasionally water-distilled from the chipped wood of *A. rosaeodora*.

Essential Oil Characteristics

Rosewood oil is a colourless to pale-yellow liquid of a refreshing, sweet-woody, somewhat floral-spicy odour. The top note varies considerably with the origin and quality of the oil. It is usually camphoraceous and peppery with a hint of cineole.[1]

Historical and Traditional Uses

The commercial interest in rosewood is because of the linalool which is an important aromatic chemical used in the fragrance industry. However, with the advent of synthetic linalool and cheaper sources of linalool from ho leaf oil from China, the production of rosewood oil has declined.[1]

While the *A. rosaeodora* species is not threatened, as a result of heavy exploitation of the trees very few trees exceeding a 30 cm girth can be found within 20 km of river banks of navigable rivers. This is the only means of bulk transportation in the Amazon region.[2]

Shawe also says that the production of rosewood is not efficient. Young branch wood provides high oil yields, but is rejected on site in favour of the more readily portable trunk wood. This means that up to 60% of the wood biomass is left on site and therefore wasted. Further losses occur in sawing and chipping the wood prior to distillation, and owing to outdated equipment, oil recovery is inefficient.[2]

While substantial stands of *A. rosaeodora* still remain because they are in inaccessible parts of the Amazon, producers are now harvesting smaller trees than before, including species of *Aniba* that had previously been left untouched.[2]

Trees with an acceptable trunk diameter for distillation take 10 years to produce. A project investigated the possibility of using the leaf to produce a rosewood leaf oil. The results look promising. The leaf oils contain about 73–78% linalool, about 10% less than the wood, and a differing qualitative composition in minor constituents — sesquiterpenes. The benefit is that it contains no camphor, often found in ho leaf oil.[3]

Chemical Composition

The major constituent of rosewood oil is linalool (80–90%). The oil is also made up of 1,8-cineole, α-terpineol, geraniol, citronellal, limonene, α-pinene, β-pinene, p-elemene, *cis*- and *trans*-linalool oxides and sesquiterpenes.[4]

Therapeutic Actions

Antidepressant, antiseptic, bactericide, cephalic, cytophylactic, deodorant, insecticide, stimulant.

Pharmacology and Clinical Studies

Linalool, the main constituent in rosewood, has been reported to have anticonvulsant activity in mice and rats, and spasmolytic activity on isolated guinea pig ileum.[4] Rosewood is reported to have antimicrobial properties.[5]

Indications

Nervous System

Rosewood's uplifting and enlivening properties are reputed to have an overall balancing effect. It is a wonderful oil to use for people who are feeling stressed, depressed and dragged down by the burdens of life.[8] The oil is also recommended for alleviating headaches and anxiety.[6,7,8]

Skin Care

It is an antiseptic and cytophylactic oil and is beneficial for treating acne, dermatitis, sensitive skin, aged skin and damaged skin.[6,7] It is a very safe oil to use on the skin and its antiseptic properties make it an excellent oil to use in a deodorant.[6,8]

Subtle Aromatherapy

Davis suggests using rosewood for meditation or in preparation for any spiritual healing. It has a calming effect without inducing any drowsiness. It is associated with the crown chakra.[9]

Mode of Administration

Topical application — massage, compress, bath, ointment, skin care; Inhalation — direct inhalation, diffuser, oil vaporiser.

Safety

Rosewood oil is non-toxic, non-irritating and non-sensitising.

References

1. Arctander S. *Perfume and flavour materials of natural origin.* Allured Publishing, USA, 1994.
2. Shawe K. *Conservation and aromatherapy — What you need to know.* The World of Aromatherapy III Conference Proceedings, NAHA, 2000; 27–32.
3. Santana A et al. *Brazilian rosewood oil.* The International Journal of Aromatherapy, 1997; 8(3): 16–20.
4. Leung A, Foster S. *Encyclopedia of common natural ingredients used in food, drugs and cosmetics.* 2nd edn, John Wiley and Sons Inc, USA, 1996.
5. Lobato AM et al. *Antimicrobial activity of essential oils from the Amazon.* Acta Amazonica, 1989; 19: 355–363. Cited in the Aromatherapy Database, by Bob Harris, Essential Oil Resource Consultants, UK, 2000.
6. Lawless J. *The encyclopaedia of essential oils.* Element Books Limited, Great Britain, 1992.

7. Lavabre M. *Aromatherapy workbook.* Healing Art Press, USA, 1997.

8. Davis P. *Aromatherapy: An A–Z.* 2nd edn. The C.W. Daniel Company Limited, Great Britain, 1999.

9. Davis P. *Subtle aromatherapy.* The C.W. Daniel Company Limited, Great Britain, 1991.

Sage

Salvia officinalis

Synonyms

Common sage, Garden sage, Dalmatian sage

Family

Lamiaceae or Labiatae

Botany and Origins

S. officinalis is a small, evergreen shrubby perennial with woody stems near the base and herbaceous ones above. It grows up to 0.8 m high and is a native of the Mediterranean region. It is cultivated worldwide.[1]

Sage oil, usually known as Dalmatian sage oil, is produced in Bosnia. It is also produced in the USA, Bulgaria, Turkey, Malta, France and Germany.[2] *S. lavandulaefolia* is closely related to *S. officinalis*. It grows wild in Spain and south-western France.[2]

Method of Extraction

Sage oil is distilled from the dried leaves of *S. officinalis*.

Essential Oil Characteristics

Sage oil is a pale-yellow, mobile liquid with a fresh, strong, warm-herbaceous and camphoraceous odour.[2]

Historical and Traditional Uses

The generic name *Salvia* is derived from the Latin *salvare*, meaning 'to save', which refers to its medicinal properties.

16th century herbalist Gerard tells us that sage:

> *is singularly good for the head and brain, it quickenethe the senses and memory, strengtheneth the sinews, restoreth health to those who have palsy, and taketh away shaky trembling of the members.*[3]

According to Culpeper, sage was reputed to provoke urine, bring down women's courses, stops the bleeding of wounds and cleanses foul ulcers and sores.[3]

Nowadays, sage is used as a tonic, digestive, astringent and antispasmodic. It is used as a tea or infusion, it is used to reduce perspiration, to stop the flow of milk, to treat nervous conditions, dysmenorrhea, diarrhoea, gastritis and sore throat. Sage is commonly used as a flavour ingredient in food products.[1]

Chemical Composition

A typical chemical composition of sage is reported as follows:

α-pinene (1.7–5.9%), camphene (3.1–7.5%), β-pinene (0.3–1.6%), myrcene (0.5–0.8%), limonene (1.1–2.0%), 1,8-cineole (6.9–11.2%), α-thujone (17.0–21.6%), β-thujone (1.7–3.7%), camphor (23.1–27.3%), linalool (0.5–0.7%), bornyl acetate (1.1–2.8%), borneol (3.7–4.5%).[4]

Therapeutic Actions

Anti-inflammatory, antibacterial, antiseptic, antispasmodic, astringent, digestive, diuretic, emmenagogue, febrifuge, hypertensive, stomachic, tonic.

Pharmacology and Clinical Studies

Sage oil has been reported as having antispasmodic effects. Small doses of the essential oil inhibited isolated guinea pig ileum contractions induced by electrical stimulation.[5] A clinical trial identified sage as exhibiting significant hypoglycaemic activity.[6]

Sage oil is reported to have significant antimicrobial activity on oral bacteria responsible for the development of dental disease.[7] A clinical trial also identified that the ketone components of *S. officinalis* (thujone and camphor) are responsible for an increase in epileptiform seizures.[8]

Indications

Digestive System

Sage strengthens and promotes digestion.[11] It is recommended where there is a loss of appetite.

Musculoskeletal System

Mailhebiau recommends sage for treating rheumatism and arthritis.[9] Davies says that sage is very warming and could be used by male athletes who are undergoing intensive training.[10]

Nervous System

The oil is recommended for general nervous debility.[13]

Reproductive System

Sage oil has a beneficial effect on the female reproductive system. It is said to imitate the hormone oestrogen, thereby regulating the menstrual cycle.[11,13,14] It is particularly beneficial for treating delayed, scanty or no menstruation with cramp and for menopausal problems, particularly sweating.[11,13] Mailhebiau describes sage as the 'saving' herb — he says that it is a remarkable oil that brings rapid relief in the case of painful periods. He does warn us that in excessive doses it is toxic.[9]

Respiratory System
Sage has expectorant and mucolytic properties.[9]

Skin Care
Sage is reputed to be highly regenerative in skin care. Schnaubelt recommends a blend of sage, everlasting and rosehip oil for slow-healing wounds. He suggests two applications per day for 10 days on a recent wound or for 3 to 6 months for old scars.[14]

Lavabre says that sage is a regulator of seborrhoea and recommends using it for the treatment of acne, dermatitis, eczema, dandruff and hair loss.[11] Valnet recommends using sage for atonic wounds, sores, ulcers, insect bites and eczema.[18] Mailhebiau recommends sage for regulating sweating.[9]

Energetics

The energetics of sage are mainly drying and astringent. It is very effective for treating deficiencies of *Qi*. It is recommended for nervous exhaustion and a tonic during convalescence.[13]

Personality Profile

Mailhebiau describes the archetype of sage:

> *the essence which saves ... mature in age, which does not necessarily signify advanced in years, prompted by certain wisdom and authority, she addresses women, appealing more to their intelligence than their hearts. Salvia officinalis exerts her vigour against the tide in these times of emotional crisis where sexuality triumphs over conscience and love, her crises and emotional illusions, which she has skilfully turned to account to build up her exceptional character.*[9]

Subtle Aromatherapy

Davis suggests using sage in conjunction with meditations or visualisations to develop wisdom.[15]

Mode of Administration

Topical application — massage, compress, bath, ointment, skin care; Inhalation — direct inhalation, diffuser or oil vaporiser.

Safety

In spite of the therapeutic value of sage oil, I recommend that *S. officinalis* essential oil be used only by professional aromatherapists.

Tisserand and Lawless recommend that sage oil not be used in aromatherapy.[12,16] The oil contains a high percentage of thujone and camphor which have been identified as provoking epileptic seizures.

While the thujone content of sage is marginally lower than that of tansy and thuja, it is similar to that of wormwood, and therefore it has been suggested that sage oil is equally as toxic as these oils.[16] However, Schnaubelt says that sage is one of the safest of all the oils having a high thujone content and that sage oil is less toxic than the thujone content alone would suggest.[14]

The German Commission E Mongraphs state that alcoholic extracts of sage and sage essential oil are contra-indicated in pregnancy and that their prolonged use may cause epileptiform convulsions.[17]

Sage oil should be used only with great caution and should not be used during pregnancy, for young children or anyone suffering from epilepsy.[10,11]

Davis cites cases where individuals have used only a few drops in a massage oil or bath and the oil induced moderate to severe uterine contractions and caused excessive menstrual bleeding.[10]

References

1. Leung A, Foster S. *Encyclopedia of common natural ingredients used in food, drugs and cosmetics.* 2nd edn, John Wiley and Sons Inc, USA, 1996.
2. Arctander S. *Perfume and flavour materials of natural origin.* Allured Publishing, USA, 1994.
3. Le Strange R. *A history of herbal plants.* Angus and Robertson, Great Britain, 1977.
4. Lawrence B. *Sage oil.* Perfumer and Flavorist, 1984, 9(5): 87.
5. Bruneton J. *Pharmacognosy.* 2nd edn, Lavoisier Publishing Inc, France, 1999.
6. Essway GS et al. *The hypoglycaemic effect of volatile oil of some Egyptian oils.* Vet Med J Giza, 1995; 43(2): 167–172. Cited in the Aromatherapy Database, Bob Harris, Essential Oil Resource Consultants, UK, 2000.
7. Shapiro S et al. *The antimicrobial activity of essential oils and essential oil components towards oral bacteria.* Oral Microbiol Immunol, 1994; 9(4): 202–208. Cited in the Aromatherapy Database, Bob Harris, Essential Oil Resource Consultants, UK, 2000.
8. Steinmetz MD et al. *The activity of essential oils of sage, thuja, hyssop and certain components on the respiration of cerebral cortex slices in vitro.* Plantes Med Phytother, 1985; 19(1): 35–37. Cited in the Aromatherapy Database, Bob Harris, Essential Oil Resource Consultants, UK, 2000.
9. Mailhebiau, P., *Portraits in oils.* The C.W. Daniel Company Limited, Great Britain, 1995.
10. Davis P. *Aromatherapy: An A–Z.* 2nd edn. The C.W. Daniel Company Limited, Great Britain, 1999.
11. Lavabre M. *Aromatherapy workbook.* Healing Art Press, USA, 1997.
12. Lawless J. *The encyclopaedia of essential oils.* Element Books Limited, Great Britain, 1992.
13. Holmes P. *The energetics of western herbs Vol. I.* Artemis Press, USA, 1989.

14. Schnaubelt K. *Advanced aromatherapy*. Healing Art Press, Canada, 1995.

15. Davis P. *Subtle aromatherapy*. The C.W. Daniel Company Limited, Great Britain, 1991.

16. Tisserand R, Balacs T. *Essential oil safety*. Churchill Livingstone, UK, 1995.

17. Blumenthal M et al. *The complete German commission E monographs: therapeutic guide to herbal medicine*. American Botanical Council, USA, 1998.

18. Valnet J. *The practice of aromatherapy*. The C.W. Daniel Company Limited, Great Britain, 1980.

Sandalwood

Santalum album

Synonyms

East Indian sandalwood oil, white sandalwood oil

Family

Santalaceae

Botany and Origins

The sandalwood oil of commerce is mainly obtained from East Indian sandalwood, *S. album*. Other oils sold as sandalwood are derived from other *Santalum* species or trees that are not members of the Santalaceae family.[1] In this monograph the designation sandalwood will refer to *S. album*.

Other *Santalum* species producing a timber and/ or oil are listed below.

Common Name	Botanical name	Product
East Indian Sandalwood	*S. album*	T/O
Australian Sandalwood	*S. spicatum*	O
Northern Sandalwood	*S. lanceolatum*	T/O
Polynesian Sandalwood	*S. freycinetianum*	T/O
Hawaiian Sandalwood	*S. ellipticum*	O
Chilean Sandalwood	*S. fernandezianum*	T/O
Fijian Sandalwood	S. *yasi*	O

Santalum species producing 'sandalwood' timber (T) or oil (O).[1]

Other species which produce an oil incorrectly referred to as sandalwood oil, or the oil is used to adulterate genuine sandalwood oil are listed in the table below.

Common Name	Botanical name	Product
Bastard sandalwood	*Eremophila mitchelli*	O
East African Sandalwood	*Osyris tenuifolia*	O
Red Sandalwood	*Pterocarpus santalinus*	T
Bead tree	*Adenanthera pavonia*	T
Candlewood	Amyris balsamifera	O

Non-*Santalum* species producing 'sandalwood' timber (T) or oil (O).[1]

S. album is a small evergreen tree up to 9 m. It is native to and cultivated in the tropical regions of Asia such as India, Sri Lanka, Malaysia, Indonesia and Taiwan. India is the main producer of sandalwood oil.[2]

The tree is a root parasite. A sandalwood seedling can survive only by becoming attached to the roots of other plants. Once the roots are well attached to an adjoining plant, the sandalwood tree is then also able to obtain nutrients directly from the soil.[1] Over 30 species can nourish sandalwood; these include teak, clove, bamboo and the tropical guava tree.[3]

The essential oil is principally contained in the heartwood and larger roots. Heartwood formation accelerates rapidly from 20 years and is at its prime in trees 30 to 60 years old.[1]

Harvesting sandalwood for timber and oil involves felling the tree by uprooting, not cutting the trunk. Only mature trees are harvested. The Indian government has strict regulations governing harvesting of sandalwood.[1]

To manufacture the oil, only the heartwood of trees over 30 years old should be used. If younger trees are used, not only do you end up with an inferior oil, but the yield is considerably less. The Indian government has set a standard which specifies that the oil must contain a minimum of 90% santalols.[4]

Method of Extraction

The oil is steam-distilled or water-distilled from the coarsely powdered heart wood and the major roots of *S. album*.

Essential Oil Characteristics

Sandalwood oil is a pale-yellow to yellow, viscous liquid having an extremely soft, sweet-woody and almost animal-balsamic odour, presenting little or no particular top note, and remaining uniform for a considerable length of time due to its outstanding tenacity.

Historical and Traditional Uses

Sandalwood is one of the oldest known aromatic materials, and has at least 4,000 years of history of use. It is believed that the oil was known in Sri Lanka over 1,000 years ago, but it is only in the last 100 years that the oil has become an important aromatic oil. The use of sandalwood and its products became an integral part of Brahmin, Buddhism and other religious rituals. Sandalwood sawdust and oil, gum arabic and other materials were moulded into incense sticks.[1]

Sandalwood's common name is derived from the Sanskrit *chandana*.[4] Sandalwood is considered one of the finest woods for carving and the highest quality heartwood is often reserved for this use. It is generally used for ornamental objects and furniture.[2]

The sawdust is used in incense sticks or further powdered for use in sachets to scent stored clothes. A paste of the sandalwood powder is applied to the forehead at religious ceremonies by Hindus.[2]

The perfume industry uses sandalwood oil extensively. It is widely used for its tenacious base note, which acts as a fixative, and its ability to blend and harmonise with other essential oils.[2]

Sandalwood was rarely mentioned in medieval European herbals. It was not until the 18th century that sandalwood became well known and highly prized in Europe.[1] It was recommended for the treatment of gonorrhoea and urinary tract infections.[5]

Chemical Composition

A typical chemical composition of sandalwood is reported as follows.[4]

	Age of tree (years)	
	10	30
oil percentage	0.9%	4.0%
santalols	74.6%	89.2%
santyl acetate	5.4%	3.5%
santalenes	4.9%	2.3%

Therapeutic Actions

Anti-inflammatory, antiphlogistic, antiseptic, antispasmodic, astringent, carminative, demulcent, diuretic, emollient, expectorant, sedative, tonic.

Pharmacology and Clinical Studies

Sandalwood oil is reported to have diuretic and urinary antiseptic properties.[2] Clinical trials have identified that α-santalol and β-santalol have a sedative effect.[6] The oil has also been reported to significantly decrease the incidence of papillomas.[7]

Indications

Lymphatic System

Sandalwood is beneficial for treating venous and lymphatic stasis such as varicose veins and swollen lymph nodes. Holmes suggests that this may be due to the sesquiterpene alcohols which have an anti-inflammatory effect.[8]

Nervous System

Sandalwood oil has a relaxing effect on the nerves and may be used for hot, agitated emotional states that lead to conditions such as headache, insomnia and nervous tension.[9]

Respiratory System

Sandalwood is recommended for the treatment of respiratory tract infections, especially when its soothing, demulcent effects are required.[9] It is recommended for chronic bronchitis involving a chronic dry cough.[9,10,11,12]

Urinary System

Sandalwood oil has traditionally been used for the treatment of genitourinary tract infections such as cystitis and gonorrhoea.[9,10,11,12,16] Sandalwood is an astringent and helps to resolve mucous congestion. Sandalwood oil helps to restore the mucous membrane and minimise the risk of infection.[12]

Skin Care

Applied to the skin, sandalwood oil is soothing, cooling and moisturising and primarily used for dry skin conditions caused by loss of moisture and skin inflammations.[9] It may be used to relieve eczema and psoriasis and for the treatment of oily skin and acne.[9,10,11]

Energetics

The qualities of sandalwood oil are *cooling*. It is primarily indicated for conditions of a hot, inflammatory and catarrhal nature — particularly where the skin, intestines, genitourinary system and the lungs are involved.[9]

Personality Profile

Sandalwood personalities are serene and in charge of their emotions, fully aware of their direction in life.[13]

Fischer-Rizzi suggests that sandalwood aids people who want to make human contact and overcome isolation. She says that it is an ideal remedy for nervous depression, fear, stress and a hectic daily tempo.[14]

When you react to others with aggression and irritation, it is time to reach for sandalwood.[14]

Subtle Aromatherapy

Sandalwood has long been considered the wood and oil of choice for meditation. It is reputed to quieten mental chatter that can distract a person meditating.[9,15] It is also recommended for the preparation of healing work.[15]

Sandalwood has a prominent effect in the facilitation of spiritual development closely associated with the crown chakra. However, its greatest virtue lies in linking the base and crown chakra.[15]

Mode of Administration

Topical application — massage, compress, bath, sitz bath, douche, ointment, skin care; Inhalation — direct inhalation, diffuser, oil vaporiser, steam inhalation.

For bronchial problems and sore throats a very low dilution may be used as a gargle.[9]

Safety

Sandalwood oil is non-toxic, non-irritating and non-sensitising.

References

1. Weiss EA. *Essential oil crops*. CAB International, UK, 1997.
2. Leung A, Foster S. *Encyclopedia of common natural ingredients used in food, drugs and cosmetics*. 2nd edn, John Wiley and Sons Inc, USA. 1996.
3. Morris E. *Fragrance: The story of perfume from Cleopatra to Chanel*. Products of Nature and of Art, USA, 1984.
4. Chana J. *Sandalwood Production*. The International Journal of Aromatherapy 1994; 6(4): 11–13.
5. Squire P. *Squire's companion to the British pharmacopoeia*. 13th edn, Churchill Livingstone, UK 1885.
6. Okugawa H et al. *Effect of a-santalol and b-santalol deom sandalwood on the central nervous system of mice*. Phytomed, 1995; 2(2): 119–126. Cited in the Aromatherapy Database, Bob Harris, Essential Oil Resource Consultants, UK, 2000.
7. Dwivedi C et al. *Chemopreventive effects of sandalwood oil on skin papillomas in mice*. European Journal Cancer Prevention. 6(4): 399–401. Cited in the Aromatherapy Database, Bob Harris, Essential Oil Resource Consultants, UK, 2000.
8. Holmes P. *The wisdom of being*. The International Journal of Aromatherapy, 1994; 6(4): 14–17.
9. Mojay G. *Aromatherapy for healing the spirit*. Hodder and Stoughton, UK, 1996.
10. Davis P. *Aromatherapy: An A–Z*. 2nd edn. The C.W. Daniel Company Limited, Great Britain, 1999.
11. Lawless J. *The encyclopaedia of essential oils*. Element Books Limited, Great Britain, 1992.
12. Holmes P. *The energetics of western herbs Vol. II*. Artemis Press, USA, 1989.
13. Worwood V. *The fragrant mind*. Doubleday, Great Britain, 1995.
14. Fischer-Rizzi S. *Complete aromatherapy handbook*. Sterling Publishing Company, USA, 1990.
15. Davis P. *Subtle aromatherapy*. The C.W. Daniel Company Limited, Great Britain, 1991.
16. Lavabre M. *Aromatherapy workbook*. Healing Art Press, USA, 1997.

Sandalwood, Australian

Santalum spicatum

Family

Santalaceae

Botany and Origins

Several oils designated sandalwood oil or distilled from *Santalum spp*. have been produced in Australia. However, only the oil produced from *S. spicatum* has achieved commercial importance.[1]

Two other Australian oils, incorrectly referred to as sandalwood, are distilled from the wood of *S. lanceolatum* and *Eremophila mitchelli*.[1]

S. spicatum is a small evergreen tree, 3–8 m in height when mature. The bark is rough, fibrous and furrowed on the lower trunk and greyish or bluish and smooth on the upper trunk and branches. The sapwood is pale, the heartwood dark brown.[1]

S. spicatum grows in the drier inland regions of Western and South Australia. The tree is parasitic — it needs to grow in association with other trees and shrubs. Two common local hosts are *Acacia acuminata*. and *A. aneura*.[1]

Sandalwood is harvested by pulling out the trees and roots, and the trunk and branches above 2.5 cm diameter are used. The tree is slow-growing and it takes up to 50 to 100 years to reach legal felling size. The Western Australian government has declared large reserves, with regeneration encouraged by seeding and protection against grazing.[1]

At commercial size it takes about 90 pulled trees to produce a tonne of wood (including roots and stump). The roots and the butt of the trunk have a higher percentage of essential oil.[2]

The future of *S. spicatum* is very promising. It has a chemical profile similar to that of *S. album*. As the supply of *S. album* becomes more restrictive and costly, the popularity of Australian sandalwood in aromatherapy will increase.

Method of Extraction

The essential oil is obtained by a combination of solvent extraction and steam distillation of the wood of *S. spicatum*.[3,4]

Essential Oil Characteristics

Australian sandalwood oil is a pale-yellow to yellow, viscous liquid with a soft, woody and extremely tenacious odour.[3] It differs from *S. album* in having a rather dry-bitter slightly resinous top note. On drying out the odour is similar to that of *S. album*.[3]

Historical and Traditional Uses

Sandalwood has been exported since 1845 when 4 tons was shipped to Colombo. Between 1908 and 1930 the annual average was about 8,000 tons, reaching a maximum of 15,000 tons in 1920. Harvesting of existing sandalwood is now controlled by the Western Australian government through a system of licensed contractors and quotas.[1]

The aborigines made a cough medicine by soaking or boiling the inner bark in water.[5] The ground under wild trees is usually littered with past seasons' seeds, known as quandong nuts, and are used by Australian aborigines to alleviate colds and stiffness.[5]

Chemical Composition

A typical analysis of *S. spicatum* essential oil by gas-phase chromatography is compared to *S. album*:[4]

Component	*S. spicatum*	*S. album*
β-santalene	2%	2%
cis-α-santalol	37%	50%
trans-β-santalol	1%	1%
cis-α-bisabolol	4%	0%
β-bisabolol	3%	0%
cis-trans-alpha-bergamatol	5%	3%
epi-cis-β santalol	3%	4%
cis-β- santalol	19%	20%
cis-nuciferol	5%	1%
trans-nuciferol	2%	2%
cis-lanceol	2%	2%

Therapeutic Actions

Anti-inflammatory, antiseptic, antispasmodic, astringent, carminative, demulcent, diuretic, emollient, expectorant, sedative, tonic.

Pharmacology and Clinical Studies

The chemical composition of Australian sandalwood indicates that it would have similar properties to *S. album*.

Beylier obtained good results with Australian sandalwood against *Staphylococcus aureus* whereas *S. album* was reported to have negligible activity.[5]

Australian sandalwood oil was found to have antiviral activity against human papilloma virus and *Herpes simplex* I and II.[6]

Australian sandalwood oil was found to have anti-inflammatory effect on UV-induced inflammation. It was found to inhibit enzymes responsible for an inflammatory response.[7]

Indications

Integumentary System

Clinical trials demonstrate that Australian sandalwood is active against *Herpes simplex* viruses I and II. The oil also has considereable antimicrobial effects and is recommended for bacterial and fungal skin infections.

Australian sandalwood contains α-bisabolol, which is known to have an anti-inflammatory effect.[4,7] The oil appears to be effective in the management of conditions such as psoriasis, dermatitis, eczema and various scalp irritations.[8]

Nervous System

It can be assumed from the chemical profile of Australian sandalwood that it will have a very similar effect on the nervous system as that of *S. album*.

Respiratory System

The anti-inflammatory and antiseptic properties of Australian sandalwood will assist in alleviating the symptoms of colds such as dry cough, bronchitis, sore throat, tonsillitis, earache and sinusitis.[7,8] The oil can also be used to alleviate the symptoms of asthma by relaxing muscles which spasm during an attack, and reduce swelling and irritation.[7]

Skin Care

Applied to the skin, Australian sandalwood oil is soothing, cooling and moisturising and primarily used for dry skin conditions caused by loss of moisture and skin inflammations. It may be used to relieve eczema and psoriasis and for the treatment of oily skin and acne.

Personality Profile

Kerr says that Australian sandalwood has a similar personality profile to that of *S. album*.[4]

Subtle Aromatherapy

Australian sandalwood can be used in subtle aromatherapy in the same way as *S. album*.

Mode of Administration

Topical application — massage, compress, bath, sitz bath, douche, ointment, skin care; Inhalation — direct inhalation, diffuser or oil vaporiser, steam inhalation.

Safety

Australian sandalwood oil is considered non-toxic, non-irritating and non-sensitising.

References

1. Weiss EA. *Essential oil crops*. CAB International, UK, 1997.
2. Denham R. *Sandalwood at a glance*. www.agric.wa.gov.au, Agriculture Western Australia, 1998.
3. Arctander S. *Perfume and flavour materials of natural origin*. Allured Publishing, USA, 1994.
4. Kerr J. *Essential oil profile — Australian sandalwood*. Aromatherapy today, 2000; 15: 8–12.
5. Lassak EV, McCarthy T. *Australian medicinal plants*. Methuen Press, Australia, 1983.
6. Dwiredi C, Abu-Ghazaleh A. *Chemopreventive effects of sandalwood oil on skin papillomas in mice*. European Journal of Cancer Prevention, 1977; 6:

399–401. Cited in Australian Sandalwood Oil Product Data Sheet, Australian Sandalwood Company.

7. *Australian sandalwood oil product data sheet.* Australian Sandalwood Company.
8. Webb M. *Bush sense.* Australia, 2000.

Spearmint

Mentha spicata

Synonyms

M. viridis, common spearmint

Family

Lamiaceae

Botany and Origins

Spearmint is a hardy branched perennial herb with bright green, lance-shaped leaves with finely toothed edges and a smooth surface.[1]

Although it is a native to Europe, it is now common to much of North America and western Asia. The USA is the major producer of spearmint. Smaller quantities of spearmint oil are produced in Europe.[2] In some countries the use of *mint* as a culinary herb and herbal tea does not differentiate between spearmint and *M. viridis*, known as 'The Garden Mint'.[2]

Method of Extraction

Spearmint oil is produced by steam distillation of the fresh flowering tops of *M. spicata*.

Essential Oil Characteristics

Spearmint oil is a pale-olive or pale-yellow mobile liquid with a warm, slightly green, herbaceous, penetrating odour reminiscent of the odour of the crushed herb.[2]

Historical and Traditional Uses

The use of spearmint dates back to the ancient Greeks who used it in their bath water. The Romans introduced spearmint into Britain where it was used to stop milk from curdling. In medieval times it became a feature in oral hygiene and was used to heal sore gums and for whitening teeth.[1]

Spearmint has been used in Western and Eastern cultures as an aromatic, stomachic, stimulant, antiseptic, local anaesthetic and antispasmodic in treating indigestion.[3] Spearmint oil is primarily used as a flavouring in toothpastes, chewing gum, candy, and mouthwashes.[2,3]

Chemical Composition

A typical chemical composition of spearmint is reported as follows:

α-pinene (0.7%), β-pinene (2.3%), carvone (63.3%), 1,8-cineole (0.8%), linalool (1.1%), limonene (20.2%), myrcene, caryophyllene (0.3%), menthol (0.5%).[4]

Therapeutic Actions

Antiseptic, antispasmodic, carminative, cephalic, emmenagogue, insecticide, restorative, stimulant.

Pharmacology and Clinical Studies

Spearmint is reported as having antimicrobial properties.[5]

Indications

Digestive System

Spearmint shares similar properties to peppermint. It has only a trace amount of menthol so it is less harsh on the skin. This makes spearmint an excellent choice for children with digestive problems, such as nausea, flatulence and constipation and diarrhoea.[1]

Spearmint oil is recommended for indigestion, hepatobiliary disorders and it relieves flatulence, hiccups and nausea.[6,7,8]

Nervous System

Spearmint oil has an uplifting effect, reducing mental strain and fatigue, stress and depression.[6,7]

Respiratory System

Used as an inhalation it can be used to decongest sinus problems, catarrhal conditions and asthma.[6,7,8]

Skin Care

Spearmint is recommended for the treatment of acne, dermatitis and congested skin.[6]

Mode of Administration

Topical application — massage, compress, bath, ointment, skin care; Inhalation — direct inhalation, diffuser, oil vaporiser.

Safety

Spearmint oil is non-toxic, non-irritating and non-sensitising.

References

1. Grieve M. *A modern herbal.* Penguin, Great Britain, 1931.
2. Arctander S. *Perfume and flavour materials of natural origin.* Allured Publishing, USA, 1994.
3. Leung A, Foster S. *Encyclopedia of common natural ingredients used in food, drugs and cosmetics.* 2nd edn, John Wiley and Sons Inc, USA, 1996.
4. Lawrence B. *Spearmint oil.* Perfumer and Flavorist, Dec/Jan 1977; 1(6): 31.
5. Montes MA. *Antibacterial activity of essential oils from aromatic plants growing in Chile.* Fitoterapia, 1998; 69(2): 170–172. Cited in the Aromatherapy

Database, Bob Harris, Essential Oil Resource Consultants, UK, 2000.

6. Lawless J. *The encyclopaedia of essential oils.* Element Books Limited, Great Britain, 1992.
7. Lavabre M. *Aromatherapy workbook.* Healing Art Press, USA, 1997.
8. Holmes P. *The energetics of western herbs Vol. I.* Artemis Press, USA, 1986.

Tangerine

Citrus reticulata blanco var. *'tangerine'*

Synonyms

C. nobilis var. *delicosa*

Family

Rutaceae

Botany and Origins

The botanical origins of tangerine and mandarin are similar. They are both considered to be varieties of the same species.[1]

The tangerine fruit is much larger than the mandarin, almost globoid, and its peel is usually yellow or pale-yellow to reddish. The tangerine represents a lower stage of horticultural development of the mandarin, and with intensive cultivation and after a sufficient period of time evolved into a mandarin.[2]

Method of Extraction

Tangerine oil is cold-pressed from the peel of the ripe fruit of *C. reticulata.*

Essential Oil Characteristics

The oil is orange-coloured, mobile and with a fresh, sweet odour, reminiscent of bitter orange and Valencia orange oil, rather than mandarin. It completely lacks the characteristic dryness and note of mandarin oil and it also has a much 'thinner' body.[3]

The amine note of freshly expressed mandarin note, due to N-methylanthranilates, a nitrogen-containing ester, is not present in tangerine oil.[3]

Historical and Traditional Uses

Apart from its use in aromatherapy, tangerine oil is extensively used in flavours, where it gives interesting modifications with sweet and bitter orange oils, grapefruit, and lime oil in flavour compositions for soft drinks, candy and liqueurs.[3]

Chemical Composition

A typical chemical composition of tangerine is reported as follows:

α-pinene (1.00%), myrcene (2.03%), limonene (91.23%), γ-terpinene (3.09%), and trace amounts of citronellal, linalool, neral, neryl acetate, geranyl acetate, geraniol, thymol and carvone.[4]

Therapeutic Actions

Antiseptic, antispasmodic, cytophylactic, digestive, depurative, sedative, stomachic, tonic.

Pharmacology and Clinical Studies

No clinical studies or pharmacological studies were available.

Indications

Therapeutically, tangerine oil has similar properties to mandarin and orange oil.

Digestive System

Tangerine has a tonic effect on the digestive system, and it may be used for calming the intestines and relieving flatulence.[5]

Pregnancy

It is a safe oil to use during pregnancy and is recommended in a massage blend to prevent stretch marks. For this purpose it should be blended with essential oils such as lavender and neroli and carrier oils such as wheatgerm and apricot kernel. It should be used daily from about the fifth month of pregnancy.

Skin Care

Tangerine oil is recommended for acne, congested and oily skin.[4]

Mode of Administration

Topical application — massage, compress, bath, sitz bath, douche, ointment, skin care; Inhalation — direct inhalation, diffuser, oil vaporiser, steam inhalation.

Safety

Tangerine oil is non-toxic, non-irritating and non-sensitising.

References

1. Weiss EA. *Essential oil crops.* CAB International, UK, 1997.
2. Guenther E. *The Essential oils. Vol. III.* Robert E. Krieger Publishing Company, USA, 1982.
3. Arctander S. *Perfume and flavour materials of natural origin.* Allured Publishing, USA, 1994.
4. Lawrence B. *Tangerine oil.* Perfumer and Flavorist, 1980; 5(6): 27.
5. Lavabre M. *Aromatherapy workbook.* Healing Art Press, USA, 1997.

Tea Tree

Melaleuca alternifolia

Synonyms

Ti-tree, narrow-leaved paperbark

Family

Myrtaceae

Botany and Origins

M. alternifolia is a shrub or small tree which grows up to 5–7 m, usually with a single trunk but may have multiple stems originating from a common rootstock. The trees coppice quickly and vigorously. *M. alternifolia* is confined to the warmer, wetter, east coast of Australia. It naturally prefers swampy areas, drainage lines and river banks. Most of the oil available nowadays is from commercial plantations.[1]

The name *Melaleuca* is derived from the Greek word *melos* (dark, black) and *leukon* (white). This name was apparently given to the first species described, *M. leucadendron*, which had white papery bark on the higher stems and branches and a black lower trunk. The common name of paperbark refers to the paper-like bark which can often be peeled from the larger trees in broad strips.[1]

Method of Extraction

Tea tree oil is water- or steam-distilled from *M. alternifolia*.

Essential Oil Characteristics

Tea tree oil is a pale-yellowish green to almost clear mobile liquid with a warm spicy, aromatic odour.

Historical and Traditional Uses

The Australian aborigines have long recognised the virtues of tea tree. The leaves were simply crushed in the hand and the volatile oil inhaled to relieve colds and headaches. The name tea tree was first used by Captain Cook in 1777, when the leaves of *melaleuca* or *leptospermum* were brewed to make a tea to prevent scurvy. The common name of tea tree applies to a number of species of *leptospermum* and *melaleuca*.[1]

Tea tree oil was first distilled in Australia in the 1920s. The medicinal properties of the oil were soon identified:

> *An essential oil extracted from a variety of tea tree growing in profusion on the North coast of New South Wales was brought to my notice about twelve months ago. Analysis by Mr. W.R. Penfold, Curator and Economic Chemist of the Sydney Technological Museum, showed that it was non-toxic, non-irritating and eleven to thirteen times stronger than carbolic as a germicide (Rideal-Walker coefficient).*
>
> *Dirty wounds, such as the result of street accidents, may be washed or syringed out with a 10% watery lotion, the solvent properties will loosen and bring away the dirt which is usually ground in, and the tissues will remain fresh and retain their natural colour. Dressings dipped in a 2.5% solution may then be applied, changed every twenty four hours and healing will readily take place.*
>
> *The pus solvent properties led me to try the lotion for perionychia which is usually so disheartening and so frequently results in the loss of the nail or deformity. Here the results were excellent. Infections which resisted treatment of various kinds for months, were cured in less than a week. The fingers were dressed with lint soaked in 10% solution and changed every twenty four hours.*
>
> *Twenty drops in a tumbler of warm water used as a gargle quickly clear up a sore throat in the early stages; it should be an excellent prophylactic for many infective conditions which gain entrance to the body through the naso-pharynx.*[2]

Chemical Composition

A typical chemical composition of tea tree is reported as follows:

α-pinene (2.1%), β-pinene (0.4%), sabinene (0.2%), myrcene (0.4%), α-phellandrene (0.8%), α-terpinene (7.1%), limonene (1.4%), 1,8-cineole (3.0%), γ-terpinene (15.7%), p-cymene (6.2%), terpinolene (3.4%), linalool (0.2%), terpinen-4-ol (45.4%), α-terpineol (5.3%).[1]

The Australian Standard for tea tree oil (AS 2782 — 1985) requires that the 1,8-cineole content shall not exceed 15% and the terpinen-4-ol content shall be at least 30%.[3] There has been much research done on the microbiological activity of the essential oil with regards to the terpinen-4-ol to cineole ratio.[1]

Maintaining quality control when harvesting from the bush has been a problem because physically identified trees of *M. alternifolia* may produce oil with cineole content ranging from 0–65%.[1]

There has been no evidence to support the fact that tea tree oil with lower levels of 1,8-cineole is considered superior to tea tree oil with higher levels of 1,8-cineole (5–15%). Southwell says that the antifungal and anthelmintic activities may actually be enhanced by 1,8-cineole. It was also identified that the antimicrobial properties of tea tree oil did not vary when the terpinen-4-ol content was maintained constant and the 1,8-cineole content varied from 20% to 1.5%.[4]

However, another study tested the major components of tea tree oil including 1,8-cineole, terpinen-4-ol, p-cymene, linalool, α-terpinene, γ-terpinene, α-terpineol and terpinolene. The constituents were tested against a range of micro-organisms and only terpinen-4-ol inhibited all of the micro-organisms. In a previous study the whole oil failed to inhibit *pseudomonas* — one of the test organisms.[5]

Therapeutic Actions

Antimicrobial, antifungal, antiseptic, bactericide, cicatrisant, expectorant, fungicide, immunostimulant, insecticide, stimulant, sudorific.

Pharmacology and Clinical Studies

The antibacterial and antifungal properties of tea tree oil are well documented through clinical studies.[6,8,9]

Comparative tests have also shown its potential benefits in treating acne (*vs.* benzoylperoxide) and onychomycosis (*vs.* clotrimazole).[6,10] Onychomycosis is a common cause of nail disease which is caused by *Trichophyton rubrum* and *Candida* species. A double-blind trial compared 1% clotrimazole and 100% tea tree by applying them directly to the toenails twice daily for six months. The results showed similar improvement in clinical assessment, nail appearance and symptomatology. Both preparations were comparable in efficacy and cost.[7]

It has also been successfully tested for vaginal infections.[6]

Indications

Antimicrobial Properties

Tea tree is considered unusual in that it has a broad spectrum antimicrobial activity against bacteria, viruses and fungi.[8,16]

Genitourinary System

Tea tree oil is recommended for the treatment of thrush, vaginitis, cystitis and pruritis.[13,14,15,16]

Immune System

Davis says that tea tree oil is a very powerful immunostimulant, so when the body is threatened with any infection, tea tree increases its ability to respond. She recommends tea tree oil for debilitating illnesses such as glandular fever, and for people who repeatedly succumb to infections or who are very slow to recover from any illness.[11]

Respiratory System

Tea tree oil is recommended for the treatment of asthma, bronchitis, catarrh, coughs, sinusitis and whooping cough.[13,14,15]

Skin Care

Tea tree is recommended for the treatment of acne, athlete's foot, blisters, burns, cold sores, dandruff, herpes, insect bites, oily skin rashes, verrucae, warts and wounds.[14,15,16] Davis recommends placing a single drop of neat tea tree oil on the centre of the wart every day and covering it with plaster.[11]

Energetics

Holmes recommends tea tree for dispersing wind cold conditions. Wind cold is characterised as the onset of respiratory tract infections with aches and pains, chills and a dislike for cold.[12]

According to Mojay, tea tree oil strengthens the defensive *Qi*. It can be used to eradicate harmful pathogens and prevent the recurrence of infections.[13]

Personality Profile

Mojay says that the strong, bittersweet spiciness of tea tree essential oil invigorates the heart and mind, uplifting the spirit and building confidence.[13]

Subtle Aromatherapy

Tea tree oil is recommended for physically delicate individuals who struggle not only with their bodies, but with the feelings of victimisation and doom that often accompany chronic ill-health.[13]

Mode of Administration

Topical application — massage, compress, bath, sitz bath, douche, liniment, skin care; Inhalation — direct inhalation, diffuser, oil vaporiser, steam inhalation.

Safety

Tea tree oil is non-toxic, non-irritant and possibly sensitising to some individuals.

Researchers found that tea tree oil that had been stored in clear glass bottles changed significantly. Most interesting was a rapid increase in the levels of para-cymene, one of the minor components of tea tree oil. The para-cymene content had increased from 3% to over 30% in the light-exposed oil in clear glass bottles. Terpinen-4-ol, the primary antimicrobial fraction of the oil, was oxidised to trihydroxymenthane.

This dramatic oxidation effect was barely apparent in the oil protected by amber glass bottles, which maintained a composition nearly identical with the control throughout the trial.[17]

Para-cymene has been identified as a potent skin irritant which causes painful episodes of erythema and oedema of the skin. Oxidised tea tree oil with high para-cymene content caused slow healing and extensive chemical burns when applied to the skin.[17]

References

1. Weiss EA. *Essential oil crops.* CAB International, UK, 1997.

2. Morris H. *A new Australian germicide*. Medical Journal of Australia, 26 January 1930: 417.
3. *Australian Standard 2782 — 1985, Essential oils — oil of melaleuca, terpinen-4-ol type*. Standards Association of Australia, Australia, 1985.
4. Southwell IA et al. *Is cineole detrimental to tea tree oil?* Perfumer and Flavorist, 1996; 21(5): 7–10.
5. Carson CF, Riley TV. *Antimicrobial activity of the major components of the essential oil of Melaleuca alternifolia*. Journal of Applied Bacteriology, 1995; 78(3): 264–269.
6. Bruneton J. *Pharmacognosy*. 2nd edn, Lavoisier Publishing Inc, France, 1999.
7. Buck DS et al. *Comparison of two topical preparations for the treatment of onychomycosis: Melaleuca alternifolia oil and clotrimazole.* Journal of Family Practice, 1994; 38(6): 601–605. Cited in *Australian Tea Tree* by C. Dean, The 2nd Australasian Aromatherapy Conference Proceedings, Australia, 1998.
8. Hammer KA et al. *In vitro activity of essential oils, in particular Melaleuca alternifolia oil and tea tree oil products against Candida spp*. Journal of Antimicrobial Chemotherapy. 1998; 42(5): 591–595. Cited in *Australian Tea Tree* by C. Dean, The 2nd Australasian Aromatherapy Conference Proceedings, Australia, 1998.
9. Carson CF et al. *In vitro activity of the essential oil of Melaleuca alternifolia against Streptococcus spp*. Journal of Antimicrobial Chemotherapy. 1996; 37(6): 1177–1181. Cited in *Australian Tea Tree* by C. Dean, The 2nd Australasian Aromatherapy Conference Proceedings, Australia, 1998.
10. Bassatt I et al. *A comparative study of tea tree oil vs benzoylperoxide in the treatment of acne.* Medical Journal of Australia, 1990; 153(8): 455–458.
11. Davis P. *Aromatherapy: An A–Z.* 2nd edn. The C.W. Daniel Company Limited, Great Britain, 1999.
12. Holmes P. *The energetics of western herbs Vol. I.* Artemis Press, USA, 1986.
13. Mojay G. *Aromatherapy for healing the spirit.* Hodder and Stoughton, UK, 1996.
14. Lawless J. *The encyclopaedia of essential oils.* Element Books Limited, Great Britain, 1992.
15. Lavabre M. *Aromatherapy workbook.* Healing Art Press, USA. 1997.
16. Schnaubelt K. *Advanced aromatherapy*. Healing Art Press, Canada, 1995.
17. Dean C. *Australian tea tree oil.* Australasian Aromaherapy Conference, Sydney, 1998.

Thyme

Thymus vulgaris

Synonyms

Red thyme

Family

Lamiaceae or Labiatae

Botany and Origins

There are more than 300 different varieties of thyme. The most common species is *T. vulgaris,* known as garden or common thyme. Other species include *T. serpyllum,* known as creeping thyme or mother thyme, *T. zygis*, known as Spanish thyme, and *T. citrodorus*, known as lemon thyme.

The essential oil industry distinguishes between two types of thyme oil — red and white. White thyme is a rectified red thyme oil which is often compounded with pine oil fractions, rosemary fractions and eucalyptus fractions.

There are six different chemotypes of *T. vulgaris*. The two most common ones are located close to the Mediterranean sea, at a low altitude: the thymol type and the carvacrol type.[1]

The *Thymus vulgaris* c.t. *linalool* prefers the sun and south-exposed slopes.[2]

The geraniol chemotype is rare and mixed with the linalool type. It is mainly located in high altitudes, on well exposed slopes at an altitude of 1,000–1,200 metres. The thuyan-4-ol chemotype is very rare and located between the thymol-carvacrol one and that of linalool. The composition of the thuyan-4-ol chemotype is very similar to that of *Origanum marjorana*.[2]

The last chemotype is mainly found in the eastern Mediterranean area and is the α-terpinyl acetate one.[2]

Method of Extraction

Thyme oil is produced by water and steam distillation of the dried or partially dried leaves and flowering tops of thyme.[3]

Essential Oil Characteristics

Red thyme oil is a brownish-red, orange-red coloured liquid with an intense warm herbaceous odour that is somewhat spicy and distinctly aromatic.[4]

Wild thyme, distilled from *T. serpyllum,* is a pale-yellow, mobile liquid with a fresh, somewhat sharp-terpene, woody-herbaceous odour with a spicy-phenolic undertone.[4]

Historical and Traditional Uses

The name originates from the Greek word *thymon*, meaning 'to fumigate'. Others derive the name from the Greek word *thumus*, meaning courage — as the plant was associated with bravery.[5]

The Roman soldiers bathed in a bath infused with the herb before entering battle, and in the Middle Ages sprigs of thyme were woven into the scarves of knights departing for the Crusades. In the Middle Ages, St Hildegarde prescribed thyme for plague and paralysis, leprosy and body lice. Thyme was a strewing herb in Britain and was included in the posies carried by judges and kings to protect them from disease in public.[5]

Culpeper described the properties of thyme:

> *A noble strengthener of the lungs, as notable a one as grows, nor is there a better remedy growing for whooping cough. It purgeth the body of phlegm, and is an excellent remedy for shortness of breath. It is so harmless you need not fear the use of it. An ointment made of it takes away hot swelling and warts, helps sciatica and dullness of sight and takes away any pains and hardness of the spleen: it is excellent for those that are troubled with the gout and the herb taken anyway inwardly is of great comfort to the stomach.*[5]

Thymol is the principal active constituent of thyme oil. It is a powerful antiseptic for internal and external uses; it was extensively used to medicate gauze and wool for surgical dressings. It resembles carbolic acid in its action, but it is less irritating to wounds and its germicidal action is greater.[5]

Thyme was used, along with clove, lemon and chamomile essential oils, as a disinfectant and antiseptic in hospitals until the First World War, as it could kill yellow fever organisms and was seven times stronger than carbolic acid. It was sprayed onto the clothes of soldiers during the Crimean War to protect against disease and lice.[5]

The antioxidant property of thyme oil can be utilised to prevent a number of pathological disorders such as atherosclerosis, cancer, inflammation and rheumatoid arthritis. It is also used to prevent rancidity and preservation of foods.[3]

Chemical Composition

A typical chemical composition of *T. vulgaris* and *T. zygis* is reported in the table below.[2]

Actions

Antirheumatic, antiseptic, antispasmodic, bactericide, cardiac, carminative, cicatrisant, diuretic, emmenagogue, expectorant, hypertensive, insecticide, stimulant, tonic, vermifuge.

Pharmacology and Clinical Studies

Thyme oil is reported to have antispasmodic, expectorant and carminative properties. It also has excellent antimicrobial activity.[3]

Thymol, one of the major constituents of thyme oil, is reported to have strongly fungicidal and anthelmintic properties as well as being mildly irritating.[1] The antioxidant properties of thyme oil have been well researched.[3,6]

Indications

Digestive System

Thyme oil is a digestive stimulant and a carminative. It promotes appetite, eases abdominal distension and relieves flatulence.[7,8] Mojay says that the strong antimicrobial properties of thyme can help to counteract intestinal putrefaction, gastroenteritis and candidiasis.[8]

Immune System

Thyme oil is recommended for all infections. It stimulates the production of white blood corpuscles, so it strengthens the body's immune system.[9] Mailhebiau says that the *T. vulgaris* ct. *thymol* is an excellent immunostimulant, particularly where there have been repeated infectious pathologies.[1]

Musculoskeletal System

Thyme oil is used to ease gout, rheumatic pain and arthritis and sporting injuries. It is recommended for fixed pain of a contracted or cramping nature.[7]

Constituent	T. vulgaris			T. serpyllum
	Thymol chemotype	Carvacrol chemotype	Linalool chemotype	
α-thujone	4.6%	4.9%	0.26%	1.53%
α-pinene	0.75%	4.3%	0.3%	0.7%
camphene	0.3%	0.8%	0.27%	0.2%
β-pinene	0.34%	0.35%	—	0.17%
p-cymene	26.0%	33.9%	2.0%	25.0%
α-terpinene	24.0%	44.85%	0.28%	4.85%
linalool	4.2%	4.2%	77.5%	3.4%
borneol	0.65%	0.8%	0.2%	—
β-caryophyllene	3.55%	2.5%	2.85	2.5%
thymol	34.0%	5.5%	2.2%	8.3%
carvacrol	4.7%	24.5%	trace	14.2%
geraniol	—	—	—	9.0%

Nervous System
It is considered a nerve tonic and an intellectual and mental stimulant which is beneficial in cases of nervous depression and mental fatigue.[7,10] It is also recommended for headaches and stress-related complaints.[7]

Respiratory System
As a respiratory tonic, antiseptic and expectorant, thyme may be used for any cold condition involving weakness, congestion and/or infection of the lungs. It will benefit chronic fatigue, shallow breathing, catarrhal coughs and bronchitis, especially when there is copious, clear or white catarrh.[7,9]

T. vulgaris ct. *linalool* has excellent infection-fighting properties. It has a higher percentage of monoterpene alcohols and is considered more gentle and very safe to use with children. When blended with myrtle, it helps calm spasmodic coughing fits.[1]

T. vulgaris ct. *thymol* has excellent bronchopulmonary and immunostimulant properties and is ideal for treating colds, coughs, sore throats, bronchitis, whooping cough and asthma.[1]

According to Valnet an aqueous solution of 5% thyme kills typhus bacillus in 2 minutes. It can kill colon bacillus in 2–8 minutes, staphylococcus in 4–8 minutes and streptococcus and diphtheric bacillus in 4 minutes.[11]

Tonic
Thyme oil is particularly effective for people who are fatigued, depressed or lethargic. It is very useful during convalescence and it stimulates the appetite. It helps to revive and strengthen the body and mind and is reputed to stimulate the brain and improve memory. It stimulates the circulation and may be used to raise low blood pressure.[7,9,11]

Skin Care
Schnaubelt recommends using *T. vulgaris* ct. *linalool* for skin infections, as it is non-irritating.[12]

Energetics
Thyme increases *Qi*, stimulates and warms the lungs and dispels wind cold. It is indicated for the onset of infections with stiff muscles, aches and pains, chills and fatigue.[13]

Thyme will dispel any cold condition involving weakness, congestion and/or infection of the lungs. It is particularly beneficial for chronic fatigue, shallow breathing, catarrhal coughs and bronchitis.[8] It also tonifies the yang *Qi* of the heart, strengthening the heartbeat and improving circulation.[8]

Personality Profile
According to Mailhebiau *T. vulgaris* ct. *thymol* corresponds to a strong and stocky man, living close to nature. He is a very physical person whose mind is healthy and clear. He works hard and never gets lost in sterile intellectualism. He lives simply in a world he does not understand well, while relying on simple and sure values.[14]

On the other hand he describes *T. vulgaris* ct. *linalool* as an introverted young man, with a difficult temper, who may look outwardly as fragile as he is strong in his deep self.[14]

The linalool chemotype is helpful for children suffering psychic problems due to parental lack of understanding and conflicts and who are unbalanced by family disharmony, due to its strong antidepressive and stimulating effect on the psyche.[14]

Subtle Aromatherapy
Mojay describes the subtle effects of thyme as energising and dispelling despondency. He suggests that the oil will restore morale at the deepest level. Thyme seeks to imbue spiritual fortitude and bodily vigour.[8]

Cunningham says that thyme has the effect of closing down the psychic mind in favour of the conscious intellectual mind. This may be particularly beneficial for people who tend to be dreamy, detached or immersed in their spiritual life to the detriment of their physical wellbeing.[15]

Mode of Administration
Topical application — massage, compress, bath, liniment, skin care; Inhalation — direct inhalation, diffuser, oil vaporiser.

Safety
Thyme oil is non-toxic, non-irritating and a possible sensitiser in some individuals.

References

1. Mailhebiau P. *Portraits in oils*. The C.W. Daniel Company Limited, Great Britain, 1995.
2. Soulier J. *The thymus genus*. Aromatherapy Records, No. 1, September 1995: 38–49.
3. Leung A, Foster S. *Encyclopedia of common natural ingredients used in food, drugs and cosmetics*. 2nd edn, John Wiley and Sons Inc, USA, 1996.
4. Arctander S. *Perfume and flavour materials of natural origin*. Allured Publishing, USA, 1994.
5. Grieve M. *A modern herbal*. Penguin, Great Britain, 1931.
6. Youdim KA, Deans SG. *The antioxidant properties of thyme (Thymus zygis L.) essential oil: An inhibitor of lipid peroxidation and a free radical scavenger.* Journal of Essential Oil Research, 2002; 14: 210–215.

7. Lawless J. *The encyclopaedia of essential oils.* Element Books Limited, Great Britain, 1992.
8. Mojay G. *Aromatherapy for healing the spirit.* Hodder and Stoughton, UK, 1996.
9. Davis P. *Aromatherapy: An A–Z.* 2nd edn. The C.W. Daniel Company Limited, Great Britain, 1999.
10. Lavabre, M. *Aromatherapy workbook.* Healing Art Press, USA, 1997.
11. Valnet J. *The practice of aromatherapy.* The C.W. Daniel Company Limited, Great Britain, 1980.
12. Schnaubelt K. *Medical aromatherapy.* Frog Ltd, USA, 1999.
13. Holmes P. *The energetics of western herbs Vol. I.* Artemis Press, USA, 1989.
14. Mailhebiau P. *Approach to the characterology of thymes.* Aromatherapy Records, 1995; 1: 57–60.
15. Cunningham S. *Magical aromatherapy.* Llewellyn Publications Inc., USA, 1989.

Vetiver

Vetiveria zizanoides

Synonyms

Andropogon muricatus, vetivert.

Family

Poaceae or Gramineae

Botany and Origins

V. zizanoides is a tall, densely tufted perennial grass which is native to India. The main root stock is a stout, branching rhizome developing an extensive but not deeply penetrating fibrous mat of aromatic roots.[1]

Vetiver is used to prevent soil erosion, since its abundant lacework of rootlets will prevent the loss of soil on mountainous slopes against excessive erosion which occurs during the wet season.[2]

Most Indian, Sri Lankan and Malaysian oil is produced from wild plants. Vetiver is grown commercially for oil in Java, the Seychelles, Reunion, Brazil, Haiti and Japan.[1] In India, oil produced from vetiver collected in the wild and cultivated vetiver is differentiated by calling the former Khus oil and the latter vetiver oil.[2]

The finest quality vetiver is referred to as *Bourbon vetiver* and originates from the Reunion Islands.[1]

Method of Extraction

Vetiver oil is steam-distilled from cleaned and washed rootlets which are dried, cut and chopped, then soaked in water before distillation.

Essential Oil Characteristics

Vetiver oil is an amber- to brownish-coloured viscous oil whose odour is sweet and very heavy, woody, earthy, reminiscent of the roots and wet soil. The oil produced from rootlets that are too young tends to display some 'green' potato peel-like or asparagus-like top notes.[2]

Historical and Traditional Uses

Vetiver has long been valued in India for its aromatic properties. In Sri Lanka, it is known as *Oil of Tranquillity*. In India, the dried, thin, wiry roots are woven into fans, screens and mats to scent the houses. As the hot, dry breeze enters through the verandas, the vetiver screens are wet — refreshing, cooling and fragrancing the house.[1]

A drink is made from the fresh rhizomes and is taken as a stimulant and tonic. In Ayurvedic medicine, vetiver is used to alleviate thirst, heat-stroke, fever and headaches. The oil is applied as part of a liniment to relieve inflammatory disorders of the joints and skin, and it has been used for rheumatoid arthritis.[3]

Vetiver oil is extensively used in perfumery as a fixative and as an odour contributor in bases such as fougere, chypre, oriental, moss and wood bases and modern woody-aldehydic bases.[2]

Chemical Composition

The chemical composition of vetiver is considered complex.[1] The main constituent in vetiver oil is vetiverol (50–75%). Three carbonyl compounds, α-vetivone, β-vetivone and khusimone are considered to be the primary odour-influencing constituents.[1]

Therapeutic Actions

Antiseptic, nervine, sedative, mild rubefacient, tonic.

Pharmacology and Clinical Studies

V. zizanoides was reported to have antimicrobial activity against cultures of *Trichomonas vaginalis*.[4]

Indication

Musculoskeletal System

Vetiver oil is a mild rubefacient and may be used for arthritis, rheumatism and muscular pain.[6,7,8]

Nervous System

Vetiver oil is relaxing and is beneficial for anyone experiencing stress, anxiety, insomnia or depression.[6,7]

Vetiver oil is recommended for physical, mental and emotional burnout which results from total exhaustion.[3]

Reproductive System

Vetiver is reputed to regulate hormonal secretions of oestrogen and progesterone.[3,5,9] This makes vetiver an ideal oil to use during menopause, where the hormones need supplementing and its grounding and cooling effects will help to reduce the symptoms of hot flushes.

Holmes suggests that vetiver is useful for PMS because of endocrine and emotional reasons.[3] Vetiver is recommended for PMS caused by oestrogen deficiency that often displays weepiness and depression and PMS associated with progesterone deficiency that typically presents feelings of unworthiness.[3,9]

Skin Care

Vetiver oil assists in strengthening the body's connective tissue. It is beneficial for weak, loose or simply fatigued skin. Holmes suggests using it during and after childbirth to minimise stretch marks.[3]

Gumbel says that vetiver oil mainly influences the subcutis. Its application is especially recommended where the skin has become atrophic and slack and where there is too little adipose tissue built up. The resorptive power of the skin is stimulated, so that tissue development will be strengthened and vitalised.[10]

Energetics

Vetiver is cool and moist. It clears heat, nourishes, calms and uplifts.[3,9]

It nourishes and supports yin *Qi*, which is the body's restorative and metabolic function. It is for this reason that Mojay recommends using vetiver for poor appetite, weight loss, anaemia and malabsorption.[9]

Personality Profile

Vetiver is grounding, centring, visionary and wisdom. Vetiver personalities are often strong and intellectual, and are aware of their surroundings. They are very interested in the esoteric side of life, particularly the journeys of the shamans and voyages to uncover the earth's mysteries.[10]

Subtle Aromatherapy

Fischer-Rizzi describes the qualities of vetiver:

> *This essential oil connects us to earth's energies. It is a source of vital energy and regeneration. The earthy fragrance of the oil supports all of those who have lost touch with the earth and their roots. Vetiver nourishes people who have cold feet or have their heads in the clouds. When we lose contact with the ground beneath us, with reality, we pay the price of a weakened immune system. When in touch with the earth, we breathe fresh air, enjoy the magic of an open fire, and feel the wind blow through our hair.*[5]

Mojay also refers to vetiver's ability to reconnect us to mother earth:

> *Whether mentally exhausted from overwork, or out of touch with our body and its needs, vetiver sedates and yet restores us — centres and reconnects us — closing the gap between spirit and matter.*[9]

Vetiver is beneficial for anyone who needs to be brought into close contact with the earth, to ground and centre their energies.[11] Vetiver relates to the root chakra.[8,11]

Davis recommends vetiver as protection against oversensitivity and may be applied to the solar plexus to prevent becoming a 'psychic sponge'. To do this, apply one drop of vetiver oil on the fingertips and gently massage it to the solar plexus in an anticlockwise direction.[12]

Mode of Administration

Topical application — massage, compress, bath, ointment, skin care; Inhalation — direct inhalation, diffuser, oil vaporiser.

Safety

Vetiver oil is non-toxic, non-irritating and non-sensitising.

References

1. Weiss EA. *Essential oil crops.* CAB International, UK, 1997.
2. Arctander S. *Perfume and flavour materials of natural origin.* Allured Publishing, USA, 1994.
3. Holmes P. *Vetiver oil.* The International Journal of Aromatherapy, 1993; 5(3): 13–15.
4. Viollon C et al. *Antagonistic activities, in vitro, of some essential oils and natural volatile compounds in relation to the growth of Trichomonas vaginalis.* Filoterapia, 67(3): 279–281. Cited in the Aromatherapy Database, Bob Harris, Essential Oil Resource Consultants, UK, 2000.
5. Fischer-Rizzi S. *Complete aromatherapy handbook.* Sterling Publishing Company, USA, 1990.
6. Davis P. *Aromatherapy: An A–Z.* 2nd edn. The C.W. Daniel Company Limited, Great Britain, 1999.
7. Lawless J. *The encyclopaedia of essential oils.* Element Books Limited, Great Britain, 1992.
8. Lavabre M. *Aromatherapy workbook.* Healing Art Press, USA, 1997.
9. Mojay G. *Aromatherapy for healing the spirit.* Hodder and Stoughton, UK, 1996.
10. Gumbel D. *Principles of holistic skin therapy with herbal essences.* Karl Haug Publishers, Germany, 1986.
11. Worwood V. *The fragrant mind.* Doubleday, Great Britain, 1995.

12. Davis P. *Subtle aromatherapy.* The C.W. Daniel Company Limited, Great Britain, 1991.

Yarrow

Achillea millefolium

Synonyms

Milfoil, common yarrow

Family

Asteraceae or Compositae

Botany and Origins

Yarrow is a perennial creeping herb, growing to a height of 10 to 60 centimetres, with erect stems, lace-like leaves divided into feathery leaflets, and a composite lead of numerous, tiny, daisy-like flowers, white or pink in colour. It grows wild all over Europe, western Asia and the United States. It is mostly cultivated in Germany, Belgium, Hungary and Yugoslavia.[1]

Method of Extraction

Yarrow oil is steam-distilled from leaves and flowering tops of *A. millefolium.*

Essential Oil Characteristics

Yarrow oil is a dark-blue or greenish-blue to dark-olive-coloured oil with a sharp, somewhat camphoraceous odour, drying out in a sweeter, faint and pleasant note. The bluish colour is due to the presence of azulenes.[1]

Historical and Traditional Uses

The common name for the plant 'yarrow' is a corruption of its Anglo-Saxon name, *gearwe*, while its specific name, *millefolium*, refers to its finely divided, feathery leaves.[2]

Yarrow was esteemed as a vulnerary, and its old names of Soldier's Wound Wort and Knight's Milfoil testify to this. The term *Achillea* originates from Achilles, the legendary Greek warrior who apparently made an ointment from the leaves, using it to treat his warriors wounded in the siege of Troy.[2]

By the 1450s, yarrow was extensively used for its therapeutic properties. Herbalist Gerard recommended the herb for headaches, to stop nose bleed and for toothaches. Culpeper informed us that yarrow is 'drying and binding'. He recommended a poultice for treating piles and an ointment of the leaves to cure wounds.[2]

The herb is still prescribed for its diaphoretic, stimulant and tonic effects, mainly in warm infusions as a way of opening the pores to induce perspiration in the treatment of colds and influenza.[2]

The herb is recommended for lack of appetite, stomach cramps, flatulence, gastritis, enteritis, internal or external bleeding of all kinds, wounds, sores and skin rashes.[3,4]

Chemical Composition

A typical chemical composition of yarrow is reported as follows:

Tricyclene (0.27%), α-pinene (9.41%), camphene (6.02%), β-pinene (7.13%), sabinene (12.35%), borneol acetate (2.10%), 1,8-cineole (9.59%), γ-terpinene (3.71%), limonene (1.71%), isoartemisia ketone (8.6%), borneol (2.55%), camphor (17.79%). Traces of chamazulene have also been identified.[5]

Therapeutic Actions

Anti-inflammatory, antirheumatic, antiseptic, antispasmodic, astringent, carminative, cicatrisant, diaphoretic, digestive, emmenagogue, expectorant, haemostatic, stomachic, tonic.

Pharmacology and Clinical Studies

Yarrow extracts are reported to have hypotensive, astringent, antibacterial and choleretic properties.[3]

Indications

Circulatory System

Yarrow oil is beneficial for treating varicose veins and haemorrhoids. For this purpose it should be blended with cypress oil and used in a compress or in a liniment.[9]

Digestive System

Yarrow oil may be used to alleviate stomach cramps and gall bladder pain.[6,7]

Integumentary System

Yarrow oil is highly valued for its treatment of wounds. Its antiseptic, astringent, styptic and anti-inflammatory properties contribute to its excellent affinity with skin problems and it may be used to soothe irritated skin, help heal infections and used in compresses may also be excellent for eczema and allergic skin reactions.[6,7,8,9]

Reproductive System

For infections of the pelvic region, yarrow is recommended in a sitz bath or compress. For vaginal infections and irritations, a douche is recommended.[7] It is also recommended to help alleviate menstrual pain because it is an emmenagogue.[7,8]

Yarrow is recommended as a balancing remedy during menopause. During hormonal system changes the oil helps keep psychological equilibrium intact and supports reorganisation of shifting energies.[7]

Energetics

According to TCM, yarrow is cooling and drying. It is recommended inflammatory conditions.[8]

Yarrow also stimulates the liver and regulates the flow of *Qi*, making it beneficial for indigestion, intestinal colic and releasing stagnant *Qi* and the blocked emotions that go with it.[8]

Personality Profile

Mojay compares yarrow to everlasting oil which is ideal for deeply repressed anger and bitterness. Yarrow is considered most appropriate for people whose feelings of anger and rage are subconsciously linked to vulnerability and emotional wounds. It is therefore beneficial to help such people release the bitterness of hidden rage and relinquish their tears.[8]

Subtle Aromatherapy

Yarrow helps to balance yin and yang energies. Fischer-Rizzi says that yarrow helps us reconcile opposing forces. This makes the oil a perfect companion in times of major life changes such as mid-life crisis, menopause or other times of transition.[7]

Mode of Administration

Topical application — massage, compress, bath, ointment, skin care; Inhalation — direct inhalation, diffuser, oil vaporiser.

Safety

Yarrow oil has been reported to be non-toxic and non-irritating.[6] Asteraceae containing sesquiterpene lactones such as yarrow are frequently responsible for dermatitis od allergic origin.[4]

References

1. Arctander S. *Perfume and flavour materials of natural origin.* Allured Publishing, USA, 1994.
2. Le Strange R. *A history of herbal plants.* Angus and Robertson, Great Britain, 1977.
3. Leung A, Foster S. *Encyclopedia of common natural ingredients used in food, drugs and cosmetics.* 2nd edn, John Wiley and Sons Inc, USA, 1996.
4. Bruneton J. *Pharmacognosy.* 2nd edn, Lavoisier Publishing, France, 1999.
5. Lawrence B. *Yarrow oil.* Perfumer and Flavorist, 1984; 9(4): 37.
6. Lawless J. *The encyclopaedia of essential oils.* Element Books Limited, Great Britain, 1992.
7. Fischer-Rizzi S. *Complete aromatherapy handbook.* Sterling Publishing Company, USA, 1990.
8. Mojay G. *Aromatherapy for healing the spirit.* Hodder and Stoughton, UK, 1996.
9. Schnaubelt K. *Advanced aromatherapy.* Healing Art Press, Canada, 1995.

Ylang Ylang

Cananga odorata var. *genuina*

Synonyms

Cananga oil

Family

Annonaceae

Botany and Origins

Ylang ylang originates from South-East Asia, although it is now native in Burma, Malaysia, Papua New Guinea and other Pacific Islands. It was introduced to the tropical countries of Africa, Asia, the Caribbean and the French colonies of the Indian Ocean.[1]

Ylang ylang essential oil is primarily produced in Indonesia and Madagascar, with smaller amounts from Reunion, Comoros Islands and the Philippines.[1]

Cananga is a fast-growing, tall evergreen tree which grows up to 35 m; however, under cultivation it is pruned to about 3 m. The tree bears numerous, large, yellow-green, strongly scented flowers. It flowers all year round. However, the main flower harvests are in the early dry season.[1]

Two types of oil are produced from the flowers of *C. odorata*: cananga oil from forma *macrophylla* and ylang ylang oil from forma *genuina*. Cananga oil has a higher sesquiterpene content but is low in alcohols and esters; conversely, ylang ylang contains a proportion of alcohols and esters.[1]

Method of Extraction

Ylang ylang essential oil is produced by steam and water distillation of the freshly picked flowers from *C. odorata.*

Distillation is carried out in small stills since the flowers would suffer considerably by the weight and pressure of a heavy charge of flowers.[2]

Madagascan distilleries produce four and often five fractions or grades of ylang ylang: premier, extra, first, second and third the quality and price decreasing in the same order.[1]

The fractions are usually separated by controlling the specific gravity of the distillate. By controlling the specific gravity, producers make the interruptions at the moment when they feel that the oil can be classified within one of these groups.

A *ylang ylang complete* oil is often available. While the name suggests that the oil should be the natural distillate from the uninterrupted water-and-steam distillation of the *C. odorata* flowers, the *complete* is made by blending ylang ylang extra, grade 1 and grade 2 fractions.[2]

Essential Oil Characteristics

Ylang ylang extra is a pale-yellow oil with a powerful floral and intensely sweet odour. The base note becomes more pleasant, softer and sweet.[2]

Ylang ylang complete is usually a yellowish, somewhat oily liquid with a powerful and intensely sweet, but soft balsamic floral odour with a floral woody undertone.[2]

Ylang ylang third grade is a yellowish oily liquid with a sweet-floral odour and balsamic-woody base note.[2]

Cananga oil is a yellow to orange-yellow rather viscous liquid with a sweet, fresh-floral odour with a characteristic woody-leathery base note. The odour is considered more harsh than ylang ylang.[1]

Historical and Traditional Uses

Ylang ylang has long been considered one of the most important essential oils in perfumery. The higher grades are generally used in perfumes while the lower grades are used for soaps and detergents.[3]

In Java, the flowers are strewn on the bridal bed of newly weds and the oil is blended with coconut oil to alleviate skin conditions, and as a base in cosmetics and hair care products. Cananga oil is extensively used in soaps, where its tenacity is highly valued. It was the main ingredient in Macassar hair dressing, popular in Victorian England.[1]

Chemical Composition

Typical chemical compositions of the various grades of ylang ylang are reported as follows:[4]

constituents	extra	1st grade	2nd grade	3rd grade
linalool	13.6%	18.6%	2.8%	1.0%
geranyl acetate	5.3%	5.9%	4.1%	3.5%
caryophyllene	1.7%	6.0%	7.5%	9.0%
p-cresyl methyl ether	16.5%	7.6%	1.8%	0.5%
methyl benzoate	8.7%	6.4%	2.3%	1.0%
benzyl acetate	25.1%	17.4%	7.0%	3.7%
benzyl benzoate	2.2%	5.3%	4.7%	4.3%
other sesquiterpenes	7.4%	28.8%	54.5%	97.0%

Therapeutic Actions

Antidepressant, antiseptic, aphrodisiac, hypotensive, sedative.

Pharmacology and Clinical Studies

Ylang ylang oil is reported to exhibit good antibacterial properties against *Stap. aureus*.[5]

Ylang ylang was found to be one of the most popular choices of essential oils in a clinical trial using essential oils to control epileptic seizures.[11]

Indications

Circulatory System

Ylang ylang is recommended for treating palpitations and reducing high blood pressure.[7,8,9,11]

Nervous System

Ylang ylang is known for its ability to slow down over-rapid breathing and over-rapid heart beat. These symptoms are usually associated with shock, anxiety and anger.[6,9,10]

The oil is renowned as an antidepressant and is particularly beneficial for treating nervous depression, feelings of anger, rage and frustration.[7] Ylang ylang is commonly classified as an aphrodisiac. This is undoubtedly due to ylang ylang's ability to reduce stress and anxiety, often associated with sexual inadequacy.[6,8,11]

Reproductive System

Ylang ylang has proven beneficial for treating PMS, especially associated with extreme mood swings that occur just before the onset of menstruation.[7] For this purpose, Fischer-Rizzi recommends blending ylang ylang with clary sage and neroli. This blend should be used in a bath, massage oil or in a vaporiser.

Skin Care

Added to a skin care preparation, ylang ylang oil is beneficial in softening and balancing the moisture in the skin. It is recommended in hair care to treat split ends.[7] It can be used in a shampoo base or massaged into the tips of the hair after shampooing with a base oil such as apricot kernel or jojoba oil.

Ylang ylang is recommended for dry and oily skin, and is reputed to have a balancing action on sebum production.[6,9,10]

Energetics

Ylang ylang is cooling, clearing heat from the heart, when severe nervous tension leads to palpitations, hypertension and tachycardia.[8]

Personality Profile

Fischer-Rizzi best describes the ylang ylang personality:

> *The spirit of ylang ylang usually fits the person naturally drawn to it. Upon inhaling ylang ylang with its heavy seductive, sweet aroma one can imagine a fiery, temperamental, passionate and erotic person with an awesome radiance and confidence never losing her balance. She would also dress in bright and colourful clothing and loves to wear jewellery.*[7]

Therefore, ylang ylang can be used for the woman who does not allow herself to live, who hides her femininity, dresses drably, and does not care what she looks like. She lacks self-confidence, may be extremely frustrated and appears nervous, depressed and tense.[7]

Fischer-Rizzi recommends using ylang ylang for men to become less harsh towards themselves and others. It allows them to get intouch with their feminine side and nurtures their understanding and intuition. Many men may find the rich floral scent of ylang ylang overwhelming. If this is the case ylang ylang should be blended with sweet orange, bergamot or sandalwood.[7]

The ylang ylang person is extremely passionate and feminine, charismatic, erotic and sensual. Male or female ylang ylang personalities are not happy alone, flourishing best when they have an audience to applaud their achievements.[12]

Subtle Aromatherapy

Ylang ylang helps to create a feeling of peace and dispels anger which is often a hindrance to meditation, healing and all spiritual activities.[13]

Mode of Administration

Topical application — massage, compress, bath, ointment, skin care; Inhalation — direct inhalation, diffuser, oil vaporiser.

Safety

Ylang ylang oil is non-toxic, non-irritating and non-sensitising. Excessive use may cause nausea or headaches.[6,9]

References

1. Weiss EA. *Essential oil crops.* CAB International, UK, 1997.
2. Arctander S. *Perfume and flavour materials of natural origin.* Allured Publishing, USA, 1994.
3. Leung A, Foster S. *Encyclopedia of common natural ingredients used in food, drugs and cosmetics.* 2nd edn, John Wiley and Sons Inc, USA, 1996.
4. Lawrence B. *Ylang ylang oil.* Perfumer and Flavorist, 1986; 11(5): 195.
5. Ontengco DC et al. *Screening for the antibacterial activity of essential oils from some Philippine plants.* Acta Manilana, 1995; 43:19–23. Cited in the Aromatherapy Database, by Bob Harris, Essential Oil Resource Consultants, UK, 2000.
6. Davis P. *Aromatherapy: An A–Z.* 2nd edn. The C.W. Daniel Company Limited, Great Britain, 1999.
7. Fischer-Rizzi S. *Complete aromatherapy handbook.* Sterling Publishing Company, USA, 1990.
8. Mojay G. *Aromatherapy for healing the spirit.* Hodder and Stoughton, UK, 1996.
9. Lawless J. *The encyclopaedia of essential oils.* Element Books Limited, Great Britain, 1992.
10. Lavabre M. *Aromatherapy workbook.* Healing Art Press, USA, 1997.
11. Betts T. *Practical experience of using aromatherapy in people with epilepsy.* Aroma'95 Conference, July 1995, Guilford, UK.
12. Worwood V. *The fragrant mind.* Doubleday, Great Britain, 1995.
13. Davis P. *Subtle aromatherapy.* The C.W. Daniel Company Limited, Great Britain, 1991.

Exotic Essential Oils

Objectives

After careful study of this chapter, you should be able to:

- state the botanical origins for a range of exotic essential oils
- identify the organoleptic properties for a range of exotic essential oils
- outline the historical and traditional uses for a range of exotic essential oils
- state the method of extraction for a range of exotic essential oils
- identify the chemical constituents for a range of exotic essential oils
- discuss the therapeutic properties for a range of exotic essential oils
- state the safety requirements for a range of exotic essential oils.

Introduction

I have titled this chapter 'Exotic Essential Oils'. This does not imply that the oils are rare or difficult to get, even though this may be correct in some cases, it simply infers that the essential oils are not commonly used in mainstream aromatherapy.

Ambrette Seed

Botanical Name

Abelmoschus moschatus

General Description and Origins

The plant belongs to the mallow family and is found in Central and South America, Indonesia and India.[1] It is an evergreen shrub about 1.5 m high bearing large single yellow flowers with a purple centre. The seed pod has the shape of a five-cornered pyramid, containing greyish-brown, kidney-shaped seeds which have a musky odour.[1]

Extraction

Whole ambrette seeds are distilled to yield an essential oil that also contains small amounts of palmitic acid. The crushed seeds yield a solid essential oil that is high in palmitic acid. This is similar to a concrete.[1]

Characteristics

Ambrette seed absolute has a floral, musk-like, slightly sweet odour. Ambrette seed oil should be allowed to age for several months before being used in perfumery. By then, the initial fatty note is subdued, and a rich, sweet, floral-musky, distinctly wine-like or brandy-like odour is developed with a bouquet and roundness rarely found in any other essential oils.[2] Adulteration with synthetic ambrettolide (a natural constituent of ambrette seed) is common.[1]

Chemical Composition

A typical chemical composition of ambrette seed absolute is reported as follows:

Ambrettolide (7-hexadecen-16-olide), decyl acetate, dodecyl acetate, 5-dodecenyl acetate (0.01%), 5-tetradecenyl acetate (0.4%), and α-macrocyclic lactone 5-tetradecen-14-olide.[3]

Traditional Uses

Ambrette seed has been used as a stimulant to ease indigestion, cramp and nervous dyspepsia. In Chinese medicine the seeds have been used to treat headaches. The seeds are commonly used as a spice in the East.[1]

Properties

Antispasmodic, aphrodisiac, carminative, nervine, stimulant, stomachic.[1,4]

Aromatherapy Uses

Ambrette is considered to have a powerful effect on the adrenal glands and could be used when the adrenals need to be stimulated. Ambrette may be used for treating anxiety, depression, nervous tension and stress-related conditions.[4]

Other Uses

Employed by the cosmetic and perfumery industries in oriental-type perfumes and for the adulteration of musk. Also used as a musk substitute.[1]

Precautions

Ambrette seed oil is non-toxic, non-irritant and non-sensitising.[4]

Asafoetida

Botanical Name

Ferula asa-foetida

General Description and Origins

A large branching perennial herb that grows up to 3 m, with a thick fleshy root system and pale-yellow green flowers. It is a native to Eastern Iran and Western Afghanistan.[1] It is also known as devil's dung.[1,4]

Extraction

The oleoresin is obtained by making incisions into the root and above-ground parts of the plant. The essential oil is obtained from the resin by steam distillation.[2]

Characteristics

Asafoetida oil is a pale yellow or orange-yellow coloured liquid having an almost obnoxious and acrid garlic-like odour.[2]

Chemical Composition

A typical chemical composition of asafoetida oil is reported as follows:

Dimethyl trisulphide, 2-butyl methyl disulphide, 2-butyl methyl trisulphide, di-2-butyl disulphide, di-2-butyl trisulphide, di-2-butyl tetrasulphide, di-1-butyl trisulphide.[5]

The sulphides present in asafoetida are responsible for the strong characteristic odour.

Traditional Uses

In traditional Chinese medicine it has been used as a nerve stimulant for treating neurasthenia. It has also been recommended for the treatment of asthma, bronchitis, convulsions, coughs, flatulence and hysteria.[1] It is listed in the British Herbal Pharmacopoeia for the treatment of intestinal flatulent colic.[6]

Properties

Carminative, spasmolytic, expectorant.[1,4]

Aromatherapy Uses

The oil is not commonly used due to its strong garlic-like odour. However, it is beneficial for the treatment of asthma, bronchitis and whooping cough as well as nervous exhaustion and fatigue.[4]

Other Uses

Dried asafoetida root is commonly used as a condiment and spice in cooking.[1,4]

Precautions

Asafoetida oil is non-toxic and non-irritant.[4]

Balsam, Peru

Botanical Name

Myroxylon balsamum var. pereirae

General Description and Origins

It is a large and beautiful tree that is valued for its wood. Every part of the tree abounds in a resinous juice. It also has extremely fragrant flowers. The balsam is a pathological exudate obtained from the exposed lacerated wood, after strips of the bark have been removed.[2]

The name 'Balsam of Peru' is derived from the fact that it was shipped from Peru. Peru balsam is produced almost exclusively in El Salvador.[2]

Extraction

The crude balsam is collected from the trees. In its crude form it solidifies into a dark-brown semi-solid mass. An essential oil is obtained from the crude by distillation or a resin-free oil is produced from the crude balsam by high vacuum dry distillation.[2]

Characteristics

The oil has a rich, sweet, balsamic, 'vanilla-like' odour.[2]

Chemical Composition

Peru balsam oil consists mainly of balsamic esters such as benzyl benzoate, benzyl cinnamate and cinnamyl cinnamate and a small amount of nerolidol, benzyl alcohol and free benzoic and cinnamic acids.[1]

As Peru balsam is semi-solid at room temperature, it is often diluted and adulterated with benzyl benzoate, benzyl alcohol and other low-cost solvents.[2]

Traditional Uses

Peru balsam has been used extensively in topical preparations for the treatment of wounds, indolent ulcers, scabies, haemorrhoids, pruritus, and bed sores.[1]

Properties

Antiseptic, antibacterial, anti-inflammatory, balsamic, expectorant, parasiticide, promotion of granulation process, stimulant.[1,4,7]

Aromatherapy Uses

Peru balsam is recommended for the treatment of scabies, for infected and poorly healing wounds and for skin diseases such as pruritus, prurigo and in the later stages of acute eczema.[1]

The balsam is a common contact allergen, which may cause dermatitis. It is not commonly used in aromatherapy but it has been suggested for dry and chapped skin, eczema, rashes, sores and wounds, asthma, bronchitis, nervous tension, stress. Like other balsams it has a warming, opening, comforting quality.[4]

Other Uses

The balsam is used extensively in topical medicinal preparations.[1,4,7] It is used as a fixative and fragrance component in soaps, detergents, creams, lotions and perfumes.[1,4] It is used in dentistry for treating dry socket (post-extraction alveolitis) and as a component in certain dental impression materials.[1]

Precautions

The crude balsam is well known to cause allergies and sensitisations.[1,4,7] The distilled oil is free of allergens.[4]

Benzoin

Botanical Name

Styrax spp.

General Description and Origins

The benzoin-producing styrax species are small to medium trees that grow in tropical Asia.[1]

Sumatra benzoin is a resin produced from trees that grow in the Malay peninsula, Sumatra and Java, while Siam benzoin is produced from trees growing in Laos, Vietnam, Cambodia, China and Thailand.[1]

Siam benzoin resinoid is considered to be of a higher quality and is preferred in fine perfumery.[2]

Extraction

Benzoin absolute is prepared by solvent extraction. Benzoin tincture is prepared by 20 parts by weight of Siam benzoin macerated with alcohol.[2]

Characteristics

Benzoin resinoid comes in various sizes of pebble-like and tear-shaped pieces. The tincture has a sweet, balsamic-vanillin-like odour. Benzoin absolute has a delicate balsamic odour, which is free from any harsh resinous and acid notes.[2]

Chemical Composition

Sumatra benzoin contains approximately 90% resinous matter, which is principally composed of sumaresinolic acid and coniferyl cinnamate, 1% vanillin and traces of cinnamyl acetate, styrene and benzaldehyde.[1]

Traditional Uses

Benzoin tincture has long been used in skin care as an antiseptic and a styptic for cuts. The tincture is recommended for dentistry to treat inflammation and oral herpatic lesions.[1]

Properties

Anti-inflammatory, antiseptic, astringent, carminative, deodorant, expectorant, sedative, styptic, vulnerary.[1,4]

Aromatherapy Uses

Benzoin is recommended for treating asthma, bronchitis, coughs and laryngitis.[4] It is used in skin care preparations for its skin-healing properties and its preservative effect.[1,2]

Other Uses

Benzoin tincture is extensively used in perfumery because it makes an excellent fixative.[1,2]

Precautions

Benzoin is non-toxic and non-irritant. However, the tincture is a possible sensitiser.[4]

Caraway Seed

Botanical Name

Carum carvi

General Description and Origins

Caraway is a delicate biennial which grows to 60 cm high with pale-green finely defined leaves on hollow stems bearing while umbel-shaped flowers.[10]

The plant is native to Europe and Western Asia. Caraway is cultivated in Holland, Denmark, Poland, Russia, Hungary, Germany, England, Spain, Tunisia, India and Pakistan.[2]

Extraction

The oil is steam-distilled from the dried, crushed ripe seeds.

Characteristics

Caraway oil is a pale-yellow to brownish, mobile liquid with an intensely spicy odour reminiscent of caraway seeds.[2]

Chemical Composition

A typical chemical composition of caraway seed oil is reported as follows:

Myrcene (0.4%), limonene (43.9–45.7%), dihydrocarvone (0.2–0.5%), carvone (51.9–53.9%), dihydrocarveol (0.6–1.2%), carveol (0.2–0.7%).[11]

Traditional Uses

The seeds have been extensively used as a domestic spice, especially in bread, cakes and cheeses.[4] It has traditionally been used for dyspepsia, intestinal colic, menstrual cramps, poor appetite and bronchitis.[1] It is listed in the British Herbal Pharmacopoeia for the promotion of breast milk and for flatulent colic in children.[6]

Properties

Antimicrobial, antiseptic, antispasmodic, aperitif, astringent, carminative, diuretic, digestive, emmenagogue, expectorant, galactagogue, stimulant, spasmolytic, stomachic, tonic, vermifuge.[4]

Aromatherapy Uses

Carvone, a principal component, has been implicated in chemopreventative activity. Carvone induces the detoxifying enzyme glutahione S-transferase (GST) in several mouse target tissues.[1] Leung says that compounds that induce an increase in the activity of GST detoxification are considered potential inhibitors of carcinogenesis.[1]

Caraway oil is principally used as a carminative and stomachic. It has a calming effect on stomach disorders and is recommended to settle the digestion and stimulate the appetite. It gives relief from diarrhoea and general bowel complaints.[1,4]

As an expectorant it is beneficial for bronchitis and bronchial asthma.[4] It is also used for relieving menstrual discomforts and promoting milk secretions.[1]

The German Commission E Monographs suggest using 3–6 drops of caraway seed essential oil internally for the treatment of dyspeptic problems such as mild, spastic conditions of the gastrointestinal tract, flatulence, bloating and fullness.[7]

Other Uses

Caraway seeds are often used in pharmaceutical products as a flavour ingredient for carminative, stomachic and laxative preparations. The oil is also used as a fragrant component to toothpaste, mouthwash products, cosmetics and perfumes. The seeds are extensively used as a flavouring ingredient, especially condiments.[4]

Precautions

Caraway seed oil is non-toxic and non-sensitising. However, it may cause dermal irritation in concentration.[4]

Cassie Absolute

Botanical Name

Acacia farnesiana

General Description and Origins

Acacias are small trees which grow in warm temperate and semi-tropical regions of the world.[2]

There are over 400 known species of acacia. It is believed to be a native of the West Indies, now widely cultivated in tropical and semi-tropical regions throughout the world, mainly southern France and Egypt.[2]

Extraction

The concrete is obtained via solvent extraction of the flowers. A further extraction of the concrete yields the absolute.[1]

Characteristics

Cassie absolute is a dark-yellow or pale-brown viscous liquid, which may be clear at room temperature but separating waxy flakes at reduced temperatures. It possesses an extremely warm, powdery, herbaceous, floral (almost violet) top note with a tenacious cinnamic-balsamic dry out.[2]

Chemical Composition

A typical chemical composition of cassie absolute is reported as follows:

β-pinene (0.3%), myrcene (0.34%), eugenol (0.6%), o-cresol (8.2%), benzaldehyde (0.3%), methyl heptenone (0.8%), linalool (1.04%), α-terpineol (1.26%), geraniol (11.8%), β-ionone (4.7%), farnesol (13.5%), nerolidol (0.42%), methyl salicylate (18.5%).[12]

Traditional Uses

An infusion of the flowers is used as an antispasmodic, aphrodisiac and insecticide. The flowers are used in a bath for dry skin. In India an infusion of the leaves is used to treat gonorrhoea and the roots are chewed for sore throat.[1]

Properties

Antiseptic, antirheumatic, aphrodisiac, antispasmodic, balsamic, insecticide, stimulant.[1,4]

Aromatherapy Uses

It is recommended for depression, nervous exhaustion, stress-related conditions and for dry and sensitive skin.[4]

Other Uses

Cassie absolute is used in fine perfumery, because it blends well with other natural fragrances such as jasmine and rose.[1]

Precautions

No available data on toxicity.

Champa Absolute

Botanical Name

Michelia champaca

General Description and Origins

Also known as champaka. *Michelia champaca* is a tall, slender evergreen tree with fragrant deep-yellow to orange flowers. It is related to the magnolia. The tree is native to the Philippines and Indonesia. Champa is also cultivated in India, south-east China and Reunion Island.[2]

Extraction

Champa absolute is obtained by solvent extraction of the yellow flowers of *Michelia champaca*.

An attar is also prepared using sandalwood.[2] An essential oil is also extracted from the wood.[9]

Characteristics

Champa absolute is a dark-yellow or brownish-orange viscous liquid. It has a delicate dry floral odour reminiscent of orange blossom, ylang ylang, carnation and tea rose.[2]

Chemical Composition

The chemical composition of champa absolute is very complex. It is reported to contain approximately 240 constituents, including phenyl ethyl alcohol, methyl anthranilate, indole, linalool, benzyl acetate, eugenol, cinnamic alcohol, benzoic acid and phenyl acetic acid.[9]

Traditional Uses

All parts of the tree have therapeutic value. The flowers are used in combination with the seeds as an antidote to scorpion and snake bites. The juice of the leaves is blended with honey and used for treating colic. An infusion of the flowers and fruit is used for reducing fever.[9]

Champa flowers are used in India as an offering to the gods and goddesses. In Indian folklore it is considered to be an incarnation of Laxmi, the goddess of wealth and prosperity.[8]

Properties

Aphrodisiac, antidepressant, diuretic, emollient, emmenagogue, stimulant, stomachic and tonic.[8,9]

Aromatherapy Uses

The attar is highly esteemed as a perfume, but it also has excellent therapeutic uses. It is used for treating gout, rheumatism, amenorrhoea and dysmenorrhoea.[9]

Lind describes the exotic sensual scent of champa as warming, indulging and gratifying, enhancing self-esteem and confidence.[9] It is cooling and moisturising on the skin and is recommended for fever. Irani recommends champa for anger, manic depression and for its grounding effect.[8]

Other Uses

Champa absolute is extensively used in perfumery.

Precautions

Champa absolute is non-toxic and non-irritant.

Coriander

Botanical Name

Coriandrum sativum

General Description and Origins

Coriander is a strong-smelling herb, up to 0.8 m high, with bright green delicate leaves with a profusion of small, umbrella-shaped, pale-pink to whitish flowers which produce the seeds.[10]

Coriander leaves are also referred to as cilantro. They have an intense, fresh green aroma. Upon drying, the seeds are small and almost spherical, 5 mm in diameter.[10]

Coriander is a native of Europe and Western Asia. It is now cultivated throughout the world. Most of the essential oil is produced in Russia, Poland, Hungary, Holland, France and England.[2]

Extraction

An essential oil is obtained by steam distillation of the crushed seeds. An essential oil is also obtained by steam distillation of the leaves.

Characteristics

Coriander seed oil is a colourless to pale-yellow liquid with a sweet, somewhat woody-spicy aromatic aroma with a peppery-woody base note.[2]

Chemical Composition

A typical chemical composition of coriander seed oil is reported as follows:

α-pinene (9.3–11.0%), camphene (1.4–1.6%), β-pinene (0.8–0.9%), sabinene (0.7–0.8%), myrcene (1.9–2.0%), limonene (3.4–3.5%), g-terpinene (11.4–12.1%), p-cymene (6.9–7.1%), linalool (56.9–58.4%), camphor (0.9–1.1%), α-terpineol (0.9–1.3%), geraniol (1.7%–2.2%), geranyl acetate (0.8–1.1%).[13]

An essential oil is also produced from the fresh leaves. It contains a high proportion of decyl aldehyde — which imparts an intense green aroma.[2]

Traditional Uses

The leaves are commonly used as a garnish and domestic spice in cooking.[1,4,10]

The German Commission E Monographs recommend coriander seed for dyspeptic complaints and loss of appetite.[7] In traditional Chinese medicine coriander seeds are used as a stomachic, the treatment of measles, dysentery and haemorrhoids.[1]

Properties

Analgesic, aperitif, antispasmodic, bactericidal, depurative, digestive, carminative, stimulant, stomachic.[1,4]

Aromatherapy Uses

Coriander seed oil is recommended for the treatment of arthritis, gout, muscular aches and pains and rheumatism. It alleviates dyspepsia, flatulence, nausea and may be used for debility and nervous exhaustion. It stimulates the appetite and is recommended for the treatment of anorexia nervosa.[4,14]

Other Uses

Coriander seed oil is used as a fragrance component in soaps, cosmetics and perfumes. It is also used in flavouring tobacco.[1]

Precautions

Coriander seed oil is non-toxic, non-irritant and non-sensitising.[4]

Dill

Botanical Name

Anethum graveolens

General Description and Origins

Dill is an annual or biennial herb with a smooth erect stem, growing up to 1 m high. It is a native of the Mediterranean region, but is now cultivated worldwide. Dill seed oil is mainly produced in Europe.[1]

Extraction

Dill seed essential oil is steam-distilled from the crushed, dried seeds of *Anethum graveolens*.[2]

Characteristics

Dill seed oil is a pale-yellow to colourless oil with a fresh, warm-spicy aroma.[2]

Chemical Composition

A typical chemical composition of dill seed oil is reported as follows:

α-pinene (trace), camphene (trace), β-pinene (trace), myrcene (0.3%), α-phellandrene (0.4-1.1%), limonene (39.5–39.6%), β-phellandrene (1.2–1.3%), cis-ocimene (trace–0.1%), p-cymene (trace–0.1%), terpinolene (trace), carvone (54.6–54.8%), myristicin (trace–0.4%).[16]

Traditional Uses

The ancient Romans regarded dill as a symbol of vitality. Culpeper was aware of dill's excellent carminative action:

> *... it stays the hiccough, being boiled in wine, and but smelled unto being tied in a cloth. The seed is more use than the leaves, and more effectual to digest raw and vicious humours, and is used in medicines that serve to expel wind, and the pains proceeding there from...*[17]

Dill seeds are used as a carminative and a flavour. Dill seeds are also used in gripe water for infants.[4,15,17] The German Commission E Monographs recommend dill seeds for the treatment of dyspepsia.[7]

Properties

Antispasmodic, bactericidal, carminative, digestive, emmenagogue, galactagogue, hypotensive, stimulant, stomachic.[1,4]

Aromatherapy Uses

Dill seed oil is used as an aromatic carminative for the relief of colic, dyspepsia, flatulence and indigestion.[1,4] It is also recommended for the treatment of bronchial asthma, dysmenorrhoea and for promoting lactation.[1,4]

Other Uses

Dill seed is extensively used as a culinary spice. The seeds are extensively found in breads, condiments and relishes and meats.[1,4,10]

Precautions

Dill seed oil is non-toxic, non-irritant and non-sensitising.[4]

Elemi

Botanical Name

Canarium luzonicum

General Description and Origins

A tropical tree which grows up to 30 m tall and yields a resinous exudate which is used to produce the essential oil. Elemi is native to the Philippines and the Moluccas, where it is also cultivated.[1]

Extraction

The resin is extracted with a solvent to form the resinoid. Elemi oil is obtained by the steam distillation of the resin.[2]

Characteristics

Elemi oil is a colourless or pale-yellow mobile liquid with a fresh, lemon-like, peppery odour that dries out into a balsamic, slightly green-woody and sweet-spicy, pleasant note.[2]

Chemical Composition

A typical chemical composition of elemi oil is reported as follows:

α-pinene (5.4%), β-pinene (1.0%), sabinene (1.3%), limonene (26.9%), β-phellandrene (1.6%), p-cymene (7.7%), myrcene (1.0%), α-phellandrene (4.3%), elemol (10.65%).[18]

Traditional Uses

Elemi resin was used by the Egyptians for embalming.[14] The resin has been used in the manufacture of incense, soaps and is used to improve the toughness of varnishes. Elemi gum has been used as a stomachic and as an expectorant.[1]

Properties

Antiseptic, balsamic, cicatrisant, expectorant, stimulant, stomachic, tonic.[4]

Aromatherapy Uses

Catarrhal conditions respond well to elemi oil. It eases congestion of the lungs and controls excess mucus.[4,14]

Elemi oil is recommended in skin care for aged skin, infected cuts and wounds, inflammations and wrinkles. It is drying and cooling to the skin. It may also be beneficial for the treatment of chronic skin conditions such as ulcers, fungal growths and infected wounds.[4,14]

Worwood says that elemi oil can be used in emotional healing to encourage soothing, calm, stillness, contentment, compassion and peace.[19]

Other Uses

The resinoid and oil are primarily used as fixatives and fragrance components in soaps, detergents, cosmetics and perfumes. Elemi oil is occasionally used as a flavouring ingredient in food products, alcoholic and soft drinks.[1]

Precautions

Elemi oil is non-toxic, non-irritant and non-sensitising.[4]

Galangal

Botanical Name

Alpinia officinarum

General Description and Origins

Galangal is a reed-like plant with long, narrow leaves, reaching the height of about 1 m with ginger-like rhizomes.[10] It is a native to south-east China. Cultivated in China, Indonesia, Thailand and Japan.[2] It is belongs to the same plant family as ginger.

Extraction

The essential oil is steam-distilled from the roots of *Alpinia officinarum.*

Characteristics

Galangal oil is a yellowish to olive-brown, occasionally pale-olive or pale-yellow liquid possessing a fresh, spicy-camphoraceous and spicy-woody odour reminiscent of laurel leaf, cardamom and ginger oil.[2]

Chemical Composition

A typical chemical composition of galangal oil is reported as follows:

Tricyclene (trace), α-pinene (7.1%), α-thujene (6.2%), α-fenchene (0.1%), camphene (0.3%), β-pinene (11.5%), sabinene (0.9%), 1,8-cineole (47.3%), β-phellandrene (0.3%), γ-terpinene (2.1%), cis-β-ocimene (trace), p-cymene (0.3%), terpinolene (1.1%), borneol (0.4%), isoborneol (0.4%), neral (trace), geranial (0.11%), β-thujone (trace), geraniol (trace), citronellol (trace), linalool (0.8%), γ-3-carene (trace), myrcene (1.4%), δ-terpinene (1.1%), limonene (4.3%), terpinen-4-ol (6.0%), α-terpineol (4.7%), trans-sabinene hydrate (trace), cis-p-menth-2-en-1-ol (0.1%), trans-p-menth-2-en-1-ol (0.4%), geranyl acetate (1.8%), bornyl acetate (0.4%), α-fenchyl alcohol (0.3%).[20]

Traditional Uses

Galangal root was known to ancient Indians for its medicinal and culinary purposes. It has been used as a spice for over a thousand years, especially in curries.[4] The root is currently listed in the British Herbal Pharmacopoeia for the treatment of dyspepsia, flatulence, colic, nausea and vomiting.[6]

Properties

Antiseptic, bactericidal, carminative, diaphoretic, stimulant and stomachic.[4]

Aromatherapy Uses

Galangal oil is especially beneficial for digestive complaints such as flatulence, dyspepsia and nausea.[4]

Other Uses

Galangal root is used as a spice and flavour ingredient.[4,10]

Precautions

No safety data available.

Galbanum

Botanical Name

Ferula galbaniflua

General Description and Origins

Several species of Ferula are used as a source of galbanum. *Ferula galbaniflua* is a large perennial with a smooth stem, shiny ovate leaves and small flowers. It contains resin ducts that exude an oleoresin. The dried resinous exudate is collected by making incisions at the base of the stem.[4]

Galbanum is native to the Middle East and western Asia. Cultivated in Iran, Turkey and Afghanistan. Normally the resin is distilled either in Europe or the USA.[1]

Extraction

Galbanum oil is obtained by steam distillation of the root exudation of *Ferula galbaniflua*.

Characteristics

Galbanum is a clear to pale-yellow or green, olive-brown, mobile liquid which possesses a powerful green, leaf-like odour with a woody, pine-needle-like and balsamic undertone.[2]

Chemical Composition

A typical chemical composition of galbanum oil is reported as follows:

Tricyclene (0.5–1.0%), α-pinene (10–20%), camphene (0.5–1.0%), β-pinene (45–50%), myrcene (0.5–1.0%), δ-3-carene (10–20%), limonene, cis-ocimene, trans-ocimene, terpinolene, α-fenchyl acetate, linalyl acetate, bornyl acetate, α-terpinyl acetate, α-fenchyl alcohol, guaiol, γ-eudesmol, bulnesol, α- and β-eudesmol.[21]

Traditional Uses

It was used by ancient civilisations as incense, and in Egypt for cosmetics and in the embalming process.[4,14] Leung says that it is often used in a similar way to asafoetida for the treatment of wounds, inflammations and skin disorders and for respiratory, digestive and nervous system ailments.[1]

Properties

Anti-inflammatory, antimicrobial, antiseptic, aphrodisiac, balsamic, carminative, cicatrisant, emmenagogue, expectorant, hypotensive, restorative, tonic.[1,4]

Aromatherapy Uses

Although galbanum oil is not commonly used in aromatherapy, it has been recommended in skin care for the treatment of abscesses, acne, boils, cuts and inflammations that are slow to heal.[4,14]

It is beneficial for alleviating asthma, bronchitis, catarrh and chronic coughs. It may be useful for reducing stress-related conditions and nervous disorders.[4]

Worwood says that galbanum oil can be used to induce feelings of calm, stability, direction, concentration, fortitude and focus.[19]

Other Uses

It is used extensively as a green component, especially in floral, herbaceous and conifer perfumes. It is used as a flavour component in many food products.[1]

Precautions

Galbanum oil is non-toxic, non-irritant and non-sensitising.[4]

Guaiacwood

Botanical Name

Bulnesia sarmieti

General Description and Origins

A small, wild tropical tree which grows up to 4 m tall and is a native of South America, growing in Brazil, Paraguay and Argentina.[2]

Extraction

Guaiacwood oil is steam- and occasionally water-distilled from the wood.

Characteristics

Guaiacwood oil is a soft or semi-solid mass, yellowish to greenish yellow or pale amber in colour. It is often described as having a delicate sweet, 'tea rose' odour.[2]

Chemical Composition

Guaiacwood oil contains guaiol (42–72%), bulnesol, δ-bulnesene, β-bulnesene, α-guaiene, β-patchoulene and guaioxide.[1]

Traditional Uses

The wood is extensively used for ornamental carving.[2,4] It was used for the treatment of rheumatism and gout.[4] It is listed in the British Herbal Pharmacopoeia as a specific for rheumatism and rheumatoid arthritis.[6]

Properties

Anti-inflammatory, antioxidant, antirheumatic, antiseptic, diaphoretic, diuretic.[4]

Aromatherapy Uses

Guaiacwood oil may be used for the treatment of arthritis and gout.[4] The German Commission E Monographs recommend guaiacwood for the treatment of rheumatic complaints.[7]

Other Uses

The oil is used as a starting material for the synthesis of guaiazulene, which Leung cites as having anti-inflammatory properties.[1] The oil is a low-cost fixative and modifier, an excellent blender in woody-floral perfumes, in soap compounds as well as high-class perfumes. It has often been used as an adulterant for rose absolute, amyris oil, sandalwood oil, costus oil and oakmoss resin.[1]

Precautions

Guaiacwood oil is non-toxic, non-irritant and non-sensitising.[4]

Ho Leaf/Wood

Botanical Name

Cinnamomum camphora

This monograph will discuss the linalool chemotype.

General Description and Origins

Cinnamomum camphora is a tall evergreen, growing up to 30 m. It is widely cultivated in Taiwan, Japan and China. Guenther says that there are three distinct chemotypes of *C. camphora* exit. They are as follows:

- hon sho — camphor chemotype
- ho sho — linalool chemotype
- yu sho — cineole chemotype.[24]

Guenther says that the three chemotypes are morphologically identical and can only be identified by the oil yield.[24]

Ho leaf oil used in aromatherapy comes from the ho sho tree. Burfield and Sheppard-Hanger say that ho wood is often a blend of essential oils produced from the steam distillation of the wood of the *Cinnamomum* species such as *C. camphora L. var. linaloolifera* and *C. camphora Seib. var. glavescens Hayata.*[23] They state that the more sweet camphoraceous leaf and branch oils of these species often have a linalool content as low as 15%. However, they are often fractionated and rectified to produce oils with a high *l*-linalool and negligible camphor content.

Burfield and Sheppard-Hanger state that the Chinese authorities have introduced a ban on tree-felling of certain species of *Cinnamomum* because of climatic concerns.[23] This has caused the price of ho oils to increase. They also state that there are potential problems of exhaustion of the *Cinnamomum* species as there is no policy of tree replanting.[23]

Extraction

Ho oil is steam-distilled from the leaf or the wood of *C. camphora*. The leaf oil is less expensive than the wood oil.

Characteristics

Ho leaf oil is a clear oil with a clean, sweet, floral-woody and delicate odour.

Ho wood oil is a pale yellow or almost colourless oil with a sweet, camphoraceous, somewhat woody-floral odour. Arctander says that there are several grades of ho wood oil, the best ones being free of the camphoraceous notes.[2]

Chemical Composition

The chemical composition of the three chemotypes of ho oil are as follows:[22]

	Yu Sho 1,8-cineole Chemotype	Hon Sho Camphor Chemotype	Ho Sho Linalool Chemotype
Monoterene hydrocarbons	18.5%	14.0%	trace
1,8-cineole	21.6%	4.6%	0.2%
Camphor	33.3%	45.6%	97.5%
Linalool	trace	trace	trace
Terpineol	19.3%	9.9%	—
Safrole	0.8%	18.1%	—
sesquiterpenes	3.0%	6.2%	trace
Resinous compounds	1.7%	0.4%	—
Other constituents	1.8%	1.2%	—

It is interesting to note that the linalool found in rosewood oil is *d*-linalool, and the linalool found in ho leaf oil is *l*-linalool, which is the same type as found in lavender oil.

Traditional Uses

The camphor and cineole chemotypes have long been used in traditional medicine; however, there are no traditional therapeutic uses for the linalool chemotype.

Properties

Burfield and Sheppard-Hanger cite Franchomme and Pénöel who state that *C. camphora Seib. var. glavescens Hayata* is a powerful anti-infectious, antibacterial, antiviral tonic, general stimulant and useful against respiratory, digestive and genital infections. They also cite research that indicates that ho leaf oil has antifungal and antimicrobial properties.[23]

Aromatherapy Uses

Kerr say that ho leaf oil has an uplifting and enlivening effect, which is helpful to balance the emotions.[22] He recommends using it when one is feeling weary and over-burdened with problems and says that it has an overall calming effect without inducing any drowsiness. Kerr suggests that ho leaf is a tissue regenerator, making it beneficial for treating aged skin. He also states that it is ideal for people with dry, sensitive and inflamed skin.[22]

Other Uses

The camphor and cineole chemotypes have been produced since the 13th century. According to Kerr the linalool chemotype was not considered of any importance as there was no use for it until the 1920s.[22] It was then produced as a source of linalool for the perfume industry. Recently it has become popular in aromatherapy as a substitute for rosewood oil.

Precautions

There are no contra-indications for ho leaf or ho wood oil. Some texts may have confused camphor oil with ho leaf oil, which comes from the same species.

Jonquil Absolute

Botanical Name

Narcissus jonquilla

General Description and Origins

This very fragrant narcissus species originated in Asia Minor; it is cultivated in the Grasse region of southern France and in Morocco for the purpose of extracting perfume oil.[2]

Extraction

Jonquil is extracted from the flowers with petroleum ether to yield a concrete which in turn is processed to an absolute.[2]

Characteristics

Jonquil absolute is a viscous, dark-brown or dark-orange to olive-brown liquid with a heavy, honey-like, deep-sweet floral odour with a strong green undertone and a very tenacious dry-out.[2]

Chemical Composition

A typical chemical composition of jonquil absolute is reported as follows:

(E)-β-ocimene (35.2%), methyl benzoate (23.4%), linalool (17.8%), benzyl acetate (1.0%), indole (1.7%), methyl (E)-cinnamate (7.8%), prenyl benzoate (1.8%), (E,E)-α-farnesene (0.6%), benzyl benzoate (4.4%), prenol, isoprenol, (Z)-3-hexanol, prenyl acetate, isoprenyl acetate, methyl (Z)-3-hexenoate.[25]

Traditional Uses

Jonquil absolute is traditionally used in fine perfumery.

Properties

Antispasmodic, aphrodisiac, narcotic, sedative.[4]

Aromatherapy Uses

Jonquil absolute can be used in emotional healing to encourage inspiration, creativity, stillness and inner vision.[19]

Other Uses

Jonquil absolute is used in expensive perfumes of the narcotic/floral type.

Precautions

Jonquil absolute is non-toxic, non-sensitiser. However, it may be a mild irritant.[4]

Lemon Myrtle

Botanical Name

Backhousia citriodora

General Description and Origins

Lemon myrtle is an evergreen tree native to Southern Queensland, with glassy, green, aromatic leaves. It grows to a height of 15 m.

The plant is native to Australia. It is considered a rare plant, restricted to Queensland. The genus *Backhousia* is named after a British botanist, James Backhouse (1794–1869). The species name *citriodora* 'lemon-scented', is a neo-Latin formation (citrus and odour).[26]

Lemon myrtle oil was first distilled in 1890 by a German doctor who sent it home to be used in the essential oil industry. The most recent commercial production of lemon myrtle oil commenced in 1993.[26]

Extraction

Lemon myrtle oil is steam-distilled from the leaves of *Backhousia citriodora.*

Characteristics

Lemon myrtle oil has an intensely fresh lemon-like odour with a sweet undertone.[2]

Chemical Composition

A typical analysis of *Backhousia citriodora* essential oil is as follows:[27]

Component	Typical Range
β-pinene	trace–0.5%
Linalool	trace–0.4%
β-carophylene	trace–0.4%
Neral	35.0–40.0%
Geranial	55.0–60.0%
Citronella	0.01–1.0%
Methyl heptonone	trace–0.4%
Cyclocitral	trace–0.5%
Myrcene	trace–0.5%

Traditional Uses

Lemon myrtle was traditionally used in as a source of citral-rich essential oil for lemon flavouring and fragrance. However, it was supplanted by more economical sources of essential oils rich in citral such as may chang and lemongrass.[26]

Properties

Antibacterial, antifungal, sedative, carminative.[29]

Aromatherapy Uses

Research has found lemon myrtle to have potent antimicrobial activity.[28] Lemon myrtle's antimicrobial activity indicates that it is beneficial for conditions such as influenza, bronchitis and *herpes simplex*.[29]

Webb recommends lemon myrtle for improving concentration as well as being relaxing and emotionally uplifting.[29]

Other Uses

Lemon myrtle leaves have now become very popular in Australian cuisine. It imparts an exquisite lemon tang to seafood and chicken dishes. It has replaced the traditional kaffir lime leaves often used in South East Asian dishes.

Precautions

Lemon myrtle oil is non-toxic. However, as it has a high citral content it is a dermal irritant and dermal sensitiser.[28,29]

Mastic

Botanical Name

Pistacia lentiscus

General Description and Origins

Mastic is a natural oleoresin, produced from a small bushy tree, *Pistacia lentiscus*. When incisions are made into the trunk a natural oleoresin is excreted which then hardens into brittle pea-sized lumps.[2]

Mastic is produced in various Mediterranean countries, but most of the world's production comes from the small Greek island of Chios, just offshore from Izmir in Turkey.[2]

Extraction

Mastic oil is produced by steam distillation of the oleoresin.[2]

Characteristics

Mastic oil is a pale-yellow, mobile liquid with a turpentine-like, fresh balsamic odour.[2]

Chemical Composition

A typical chemical composition of mastic oil is reported as follows:

α-pinene (58.86–77.10%), camphene (0.75–1.04%), β-pinene (1.26–2.46%), myrcene (0.23–12.27%), limonene (0.41–0.95%), γ-terpinene (trace), terpinolene (trace), linalool (0.48–3.71%), pinocarveol (0.29–2.14%), α-terpineol (0.31–0.35%), β-caryophyllene (0.70-1.47%).[30]

Traditional Uses

Mastic has traditionally been used in the East for the manufacture of confectionery and cordials. It is still used for the treatment of diarrhoea. In the West it is used in the same way as turpentine.[4]

Properties

Antiseptic, astringent, diuretic, expectorant, stimulant.[4]

Aromatherapy Uses

Mastic oil is not commonly used in aromatherapy. However, it is indicated for the treatment of arthritis, gout, muscular aches and pains, rheumatism and sciatica. It may be used to relieve bronchitis, catarrh and in skin care it may be utilised to repel insects.[4] Mastic is beneficial for its vasoconstrictive action, especially for the treatment of varicose veins.[31]

Other Uses

Mastic is used extensively in pharmaceutical and technical preparations such as varnishes for dentists.[4]

Precautions

Mastic oil is non-toxic, non-irritant. However, it may be sensitising on some individuals.[4]

Opopanax

Botanical Name

Commiphora erythraea

General Description and Origins

Opopanax oleoresin is extracted from a tall tropical tree that is closely related to myrrh, which contains a natural oleoresin.

Opopanax oil, sometimes known as Bisabolol myrrh, is produced from *Commiphora erythraea*, which grows wild in Somalia and Ethiopia.[4]

Extraction

Opopanax oil is obtained from steam or water distillation of the oleoresin.

Characteristics

Opopanax oil is an orange-coloured, pale-yellow or olive-yellowish to dark amber-greenish liquid with a sweet-balsamic, spicy, warm, animal-like odour. It resinifies on exposure to air.[2]

Arctander compares opopanax with myrrh oil:

> *... the difference between the two oils is obvious: the vegetable-soup-like, slightly animal-sweet odour of opopanax is entirely different from the medicinal-sharp freshness of myrrh oil.*[2]

Chemical Composition

A typical chemical composition of opopanax oil is reported as follows:

δ-elemene, α-cubebene, α-copaene, cis-α-bergamotene, β-elemene, α-santalene, trans-α-bergamotene, caryophyllene, epi-β-santalene, α-humulene, γ-humelene, α-muurolene, trans-α-bisabolene, ar-curcumene, δ-cadinene.[32]

Traditional Uses

Opopanax gum has traditionally been used as an ingredient in incense.[4]

Properties

Antiseptic, antispasmodic, balsamic, expectorant.[4]

Aromatherapy Uses

Lawless says that opopanax essential oil has similar properties to myrrh.[4]

Other Uses

Opopanax oil is used as a fixative and fragrance component in high-class perfumery as a base for woody, heavy floral, leather, oriental, chypre, fougere and fantasy perfume types. It is also used in liqueurs to give body and wine-like notes.[4]

Precautions

Opopanax oil is non-toxic, non-irritant and non-sensitising.[4] The oil is phototoxic.[42]

Ravensara

Botanical Name

Ravensara aromatica

General Description and Origins

Ravensara is a tree that grows up to 20 m high with a reddish-grey bark. It is indigenous to Madagascar. It is also cultivated on the island of Reunion and in Mauritius.[33]

Extraction

The oil is distilled from the leaves and twigs.

Characteristics

Ravensara oil combines the freshness of 1,8-cineole found in oils such as eucalyptus and cajeput with the gentle warmth of the monoterpene alcohols such as those found in tea tree and rosewood.[33]

Chemical Composition

A typical chemical composition of *Ravensara aromatica* oil is as follows: α-terpineol (10.8%), α-pinene (5.35%), α-humulene (0.82%), 1,8-cineole (55%), α-phellandrene (3.2%), myrcene (10.72%), p-cymene (2.2%), linalool (0.78%), terpinen-4-ol (4.2%).[33]

Therapeutic actions

Antiseptic, antimicrobial, antiviral, expectorant, immunomodulant.[14,31,34]

Traditional therapeutic uses

Schnaubelt says that ravensara oil is extremely well tolerated, whether inhaled or applied topically.

Its tolerability and strong antiviral action make it the oil of choice for the treatment of influenza.[31]

Ravensara oil has excellent antiviral properties, particularly for the flu. Mailhebiau recommends diluting it in a carrier oil with *Eucalyptus radiata* and using it as a massage rub. It is one of the first essential oils one should turn to as a preventative at the first signs of chills, shivers or tiredness. It is highly effective in cases of bronchitis, rhinitis and sinusitis, and for more serious pathologies such as whooping cough, especially when blended with cypress.[34]

Ravensara is a nerve tonic and a mental and physical stimulant and can be used to revitalise people suffering from physical and nervous fatigue.[34] Mailhebiau suggests blending it with *Mentha piperita* and *Laurus nobilis* for people who no longer enjoy life and doubt everything and no longer know where they are through lack of aims or ideals.[34]

Lunny recommends using ravensara for the treatment of *herpes zoster*. Gently apply the oil on a cotton swab, using a different swab every time to avoid cross-infection or the spread of the virus. This treatment should alleviate the pain and irritation. When there is already a great deal of inflammation ravensara should be blended with Roman chamomile.[33] Lunny recommends blending ravensara with neroli, rosewood and myrtle for the treatment of chronic fatigue syndrome.[33]

Cautions and Contra-indications

Ravensara oil is non-toxic, non-irritant and non-sensitising.

Spikenard

Botanical Name

Nardostachys jatamansi

General Description and Origins

Spikenard is also known as 'false' Indian valerian root.[2] It is a tender aromatic herb with a pungent rhizome root.

Spikenard oil, sometimes known as nard oil, is obtained from the roots of two species of *Nardostachys,* erect perennial members of the *Valerianaceae* family. The first of these is *Nardostachys jatamansi,* which can be found in the Himalayan region of India.[2]

Another species of which very little is known is *Nardostachys chinensis*, an ancient Chinese medicinal plant from which a Chinese spikenard oil is obtained. This latter oil is of very little interest because very little is available commercially.

Extraction

Spikenard oil is steam-distilled from the dried and crushed roots and rhizomes.

Characteristics

Spikenard oil is a pale-yellow to amber-coloured liquid with a heavy, sweet-woody, spicy-animal odour similar to valerian oil.[2]

Chemical Composition

A typical chemical composition of spikenard oil is reported as follows:

α-pinene (0.1%), camphene (trace), β-pinene (0.1%), limonene (0.1%), 1,8-cineole (0.2%), β-patchoulene (0.7%), α-gurjunene (0.6%), β-gurjunene (29.8%), α-patchoulene (29.8%), seychellene (1.7%), 3,4-dihydro-β-ionone (trace), β-ionone (1.4%), patchouli alcohol (6.0%), 1-hydroxyaristolenone (6.2%), aristolenone (0.7%).[35]

Traditional Uses

Spikenard was regarded as one of the most costly and precious of all aromatics in ancient times. A detailed account of Mary Magdalene's use of spikenard is found in the Bible:

> *Mary brought in a pound of a very costly ointment, pure nard, and with it anointed the feet of Jesus, wiping them with her hair; the house was full of the scent of the ointment.*[4]

Like frankincense and myrrh, the biblical association of spikenard makes it very special and mystical. Traditional therapeutic uses include tonic, cooling, antipyretic and laxative properties. It was used for the treatment of skin diseases, throat troubles, ulcers, leprosy and diseases of the blood.

Dioscorides suggests that the herb is 'warming and drying', good for nausea, flatulent indigestion, menstrual problems, inflammations and conjunctivitis.[4]

Properties

Anti-inflammatory, bactericidal, deodorant, fungicidal, laxative, sedative and tonic.[4]

Aromatherapy Uses

Gumbel describes spikenard as the ultimate essential oil to find inner balance in the emotional, spiritual and physical interplay of energies. He suggests that in skin care spikenard is balancing, soothing and rejuvenating. It has also been suggested that spikenard may have similar sedative properties to that of valerian.[36] Schnaubelt recommends rubbing spikenard over the heart or the solar plexus to provide a sedative effect.[31]

Worwood says that spikenard may be used to encourage forgiveness, reduce fearfulness and to instil calm and balance.[19]

Other Uses

It has very little use, apart from sometimes being used as a substitute for valerian oil.

Precautions

Spikenard oil is non-toxic, non-irritating and non-sensitising.[4]

Spruce

Botanical name

Tsuga canadensis

General Description and Origins

Spruce is a large evergreen tree up to 50 m tall, also known as hemlock spruce. Spruce is native to the east coast of the USA.

Extraction

Spruce oil is steam-distilled from the needles and twigs of *Tsuga canadensis.*

Characteristics

Spruce oil is a pale-yellow to colourless oil with a very pleasant, balsamic-fresh odour with a slightly fruity undertone.[2]

Chemical Composition

A typical chemical composition of spruce oil is α-pinene, β-pinene, limonene, bornyl acetate, tricyclene, phellandrene, myrcene, thujone, dipentene and cadinene.[4]

Traditional Uses

The British Herbal Pharmacopoeia recommends an infusion or decoction of hemlock bark for the treatment of diarrhoea, cystitis, leucorrhoea, stomatitis and gingivitis.[6]

Properties

Antimicrobial, antiseptic, antitussive, astringent, diaphoretic, diuretic, expectorant, nervine, rubefacient, tonic.[4]

Aromatherapy Uses

Spruce oil is recommended for the relief of muscular aches and pain, poor circulation and rheumatism. It is very effective for the treatment of asthma, bronchitis, colds and flu, coughs and respiratory weakness.[4] Schnaubelt recommends spruce oil for restoring depleted adrenal glands.[31]

Other Uses

Spruce oil is extensively used for scenting room fresheners, perfumes, bath products and household cleaning products.[2]

Precautions

Spruce oil is non-toxic, non-irritating and non-sensitising.[4]

Tagetes

Botanical Name

Tagetes minuta

General Description and Origins

A strongly scented herb about 0.3 to 1 m high with bright orange, daisy-like flowers and soft green oval leaves.[1]

Tagetes is native to South America and Mexico. It grows wild in South Africa, Europe, Asia and North America. The oil is produced in South Africa, France, Argentina and Egypt.[2]

Extraction

Tagetes oil is produced from the steam distillation of the fresh flowering herb. An absolute is obtained by solvent extraction from the fresh flowering herbs.[2]

Characteristics

The essential oil of tagetes is a mobile, dark-yellow to orange-yellow coloured liquid that solidifies on exposure to air, daylight and moisture. The odour is intensely herbaceous-green, with a sweet-fruity undertone and a somewhat bitter herbaceous dry-out.[2]

Chemical Composition

A typical chemical composition of tagetes oil is reported to be:

dihydro-tagetone (17.74%), ocimene (40.42%), (E)-tagetone (1%), (Z)-tagetone (10%), (E)-tagetone (5.3%), germacrene (3.5%).[37]

Traditional Uses

The flowers have been used in decoctions for the treatment of whooping cough, colds, colic, mumps, sore eyes and mastitis.[1]

Properties

Anthelmintic, antispasmodic, bactericidal, carminative, diaphoretic, emmenagogue, fungicidal and stomachic.[4] Leung reports that tagetes has hypotensive, bronchodilator, spasmolytic and anti-inflammatory properties.[1]

Aromatherapy Uses

Tagetes oil is recommended for the treatment of bunions, calluses, corns and fungal infections.[4,14]

Other Uses

Tagetes oil finds limited use in perfumery and is often used for flavouring tobacco and in many other food substances. Tagetes extract is approved for use in chicken feed to give the characteristic yellow colour to egg yolks and the yellow colour of chickens' skin.[1]

Precautions

Tagetes oil should be used with caution on the skin as it is possible that it may cause dermal sensitisation.[4]

Tarragon

Botanical Name

Artemisia dracunculus

General Description and Origins

It grows wild in many European and Asian countries.

Extraction

Tarragon oil is steam-distilled from the whole above-ground part of the herb.

Characteristics

Tarragon oil is a colourless to very pale yellow liquid with a sweet-anisic, green-spicy aroma.[2]

Chemical Composition

A typical chemical composition of tarragon oil is reported as follows:

α-thujene (0.01%), α-pinene (1.44%), camphene (0.11%), sabinene (0.14%), β-pinene (0.19%), myrcene (0.25%), limonene (4.65%), ocimene (13.54%), γ-terpinene (17.01%), α-thujone (0.09%), linalool (0.03%), β-thujone (0.09%), menthone (0.14%), methyl chavicol (60.46%), bornyl acetate (0.14%), eugenol (0.3%), methyl eugenol (0.51%), cinnamyl acetate (0.14%).[38]

Traditional Uses

The herb is used as a stomachic, diuretic, hypnotic, emmenagogue and treating toothache.[1] It is commonly used as a culinary herb and used extensively in vinegars, pickles and seasonings.[2]

Properties

Anthelmintic, antiseptic, antispasmodic, aperitif, carminative, digestive, diuretic, emmenagogue, stimulant, stomachic.[4]

Aromatherapy Uses

Schnaubelt says that tarragon oil is one of aromatherapy's strongest antispasmodics.[31] Therefore it is not surprising that tarragon is recommended for dyspepsia, flatulence, hiccoughs, intestinal spasm, nervous indigestion and sluggish digestion. It is also recommended for amenorrhoea, dysmenorrhoea and PMT.[4]

Other Uses

Tarragon oil is used as a fragrance component in soaps, detergents and perfumes.[1]

Precautions

Because of the high methyl chavicol content, tarragon oil is not recommended for use in aromatherapy as it is potentially hepatotoxic and carcinogenic.[42] Lawless says that tarragon is moderately toxic and should be used in moderation. She recommends avoiding tarragon during pregnancy.[4]

Tuberose Absolute

Botanical Name

Polianthes tuberosa

General Description and Origins

Tuberose is a tender, tall, slim, perennial that grows up to 50 cm high, with long, slender leaves, a tuberous root and large fragrant white, lily-like flowers. It is a native of Central America and is cultivated in France, India, Morocco, Egypt and on the Comoro Islands.[2]

Extraction

The concrete or absolute is prepared from the hand-picked flowers by effleurage or solvent extraction.[2]

Characteristics

Tuberose absolute has a very heavy, honey-like, sweet floral odour with narcotic undertones.[2]

Chemical Composition

A typical chemical composition of tuberose absolute is reported as follows:

N-formyl methyl anthranilate (trace), methyl anthranilate (trace), N-methyl methyl anthranilate (trace), methyl nicotinate, ethyl nicotinate, 2,5-diethylprazine, skatole, indole (0.02%).[39]

Traditional Uses

The double-flowered variety is grown for ornamental purposes and for use by the cut flower trade.[2]

Properties

According to Lawless tuberose absolute has a narcotic effect.[4]

Aromatherapy Uses

Tuberose absolute is not often used in aromatherapy. It is extensively use in perfumery. Worwood describes the character profile of tuberose:

> *The tuberose personality is daring, attractive, hypnotic, charming, extroverted and spontaneous. Tuberose should be used to promote enthusiasm, sensuality, expressiveness, sensitivity and motivation.*[40]

Other Uses

Tuberose absolute is used extensively in floral fine fragrances.[2]

Precautions

No safety data available. It is often subject to extensive adulteration.

Turmeric

Botanical Name

Curcuma longa

General Description and Origins

Turmeric, also known as curcuma, is a perennial tropical herb that belongs to the ginger family. It grows up to 1 m high with a thick rhizome root.[1]

It is a native of south Asia where it has been known and used for thousands of years as a spice and common medicinal plant. It is cultivated extensively in India, China, Indonesia and other tropical countries, and it no longer grows wild.[1]

Extraction

Turmeric oil is produced by steam distillation from the dried rhizome.

Characteristics

Turmeric oil is a yellow to dark-orange liquid with a fresh, spicy odour reminiscent of ginger and galangal.[2] The yellow colour of turmeric is due to curcuminoids (0.3–5.4%), the main one being curcumin.[41]

Chemical Composition

A typical chemical composition of turmeric oil is reported as follows:

Tumerone (30.0%), ar. turmerone (23.6%), zingiberone (25%), 1,8-cineole (1.0%), α-phellandrene (1.0%), sabinene (0.6%), borneol (0.5%).[41]

Traditional Uses

Turmeric is a common remedy in traditional Chinese and Indian medicine. In China it has been used to treat conditions such as flatulence, colic, abdominal pain, postpartum abdominal pain, liver disorders, amenorrhoea, dysmenorrhoea, haemorrhage, bruises and sores, toothache, chest pain and shoulder pain. It is also used as a poultice to relieve pain and itching of sores and ringworms.[1,42]

The German Commission E Monographs recommend turmeric rhizome for the treatment of dyspeptic conditions.[7]

Properties

Analgesic, antiarthritic, anti-inflammatory, antioxidant, bactericidal, cholagogue, digestive, diuretic, hypotensive, rubefacient, stimulant.[1,4]

Aromatherapy Uses

The choleretic action of turmeric essential oil is attributed to tolmethyl carbinol, while its anti-inflammatory activity is attributed to curcumin and the volatile oil.[1]

Turmeric oil is recommended for the treatment of arthritis and rheumatism and for digestive problems and liver congestion.[4]

Other Uses

The ground roots of turmeric are extensively used as a spice and for making curry powder. Turmeric is also used as an antioxidant in capsules and tablets.[1,4]

Precautions

Turmeric oil is non-toxic, non-irritant and non-sensitising.[4]

Valerian

Botanical Name

Valeriana officinalis

General Description and Origins

Valeriana officinalis is a perennial herb with deeply dissected leaves, which grows up to 1.5 m high. It is a native of Asia, and it grows in most parts of Asia and Europe. The plant is cultivated in Russia, the Baltic states, Belgium, Germany and France.[2]

An essential oil is also produced from *Valeriana wallichii*, commonly known as Indian valerian. This plant grows wild and is cultivated in the northern mountainous regions of India. It is generally considered to have a poorer odour to the European valerian oil.[2]

Extraction

Valerian essential oil is steam-distilled from the rhizomes of *Valeriana officinalis.*

Characteristics

Valerian oil is an olive-green to olive-brown coloured liquid with a warm, earthy odour and a distinct musk-like character of great tenacity.[2]

Chemical Composition

A typical chemical composition of valerian oil is reported as follows:

α-pinene (2.5%), β-pinene (4.8%), isobornyl acetate (31.5%), caryophyllene (7.6%), bornyl isovalerate (1.5%).[43]

Traditional Uses

Valerian oil is commonly used as a herbal tincture, tea or tablet for insomnia and as a sedative.[1] The German Commission E Monographs recommend an infusion or a tincture of valerian for restlessness and sleeping disorders of a nervous nature.[7]

Properties

Antispasmodic, bactericidal, carminative, hypnotic, sedative.[4]

Aromatherapy Uses

Valerian oil is recommended for insomnia, nervous indigestion, migraine and nervous tension.[4]

Other Uses

Valerian oil is used in perfumery for its musky-woody aroma. It is sometimes used for tobacco flavouring.[2]

Precautions

Valerian oil is non-toxic, non-irritating and possibly sensitising.[4]

Verbena

Botanical Name

Lippia citriodora or *Aloysia triphylla*

General Description and Origins

The plant grows up to 2 m high, with light green lancet-shaped leaves with small white blossoms at the tips of the branches. Originally from Chile and Argentina, lemon verbena is nowadays cultivated in southern France, Algeria, Morocco, Tunisia and Italy.[2]

Extraction

Verbena oil is produced by steam distillation of the leaves.

Characteristics

Verbena oil is a pale-yellow to yellow or olive-greenish coloured liquid with an intensely fresh, lemony fruity-floral fragrance.[2]

Chemical Composition

Verbena oil contains 11 monoterpene hydrocarbons, 14 sesquiterpene hydrocarbons and 29 oxygenated compounds. The major compounds were found to be geranial (26%), neral (12%), geraniol (6.0%), limonene (4.2%), 1,8-cineole (3.0%), heptenone (1.75%), citronellal (1.0%), copaene (1.0%), caryophyllene (3.0%), neryl acetate (4.0%), germacrene D (1.8%), α-farnescene (4.8%), gernyl acetate (1.8%), citronellol (1.0%), curcumene (4.5%), nerolidol (1.3%), spathulenol (2.5%), and nerol (5.2%).[44]

Traditional Uses

Lemon verbena has been traditionally used in herbal medicine for nervous conditions that manifest as digestive complaints.[4]

An infusion of lemon verbena makes a refreshing and cooling summertime drink. It has also been recommended for all kinds of digestive upsets and for congestion of the liver.[14]

Properties

Antiseptic, antispasmodic, carminative, detoxifying, digestive, febrifuge, sedative, stomachic.[4]

Aromatherapy Uses

Fischer-Rizzi says that the fragrance of lemon verbena oil is like the morning when everything seems fresh, new and promising.[45]

The oil may be used to relieve tiredness and overcome apathy, listlessness and disinterest.[45] Fisher-Rizzi suggests that the essential oil is ideal for people who continue to live in the past or who miss opportunities and the beauty of the present moment. It is recommended for the treatment of anxiety, insomnia, nervous tension and stress-related conditions.[4,45]

Other Uses

Commonly used in perfumery and citrus colognes.[1,4]

Precautions

Verbena oil is non-toxic. However, it is a potential dermal irritant and dermal sensitiser. It is reported to be photosensitising.[4] True verbena oil is expensive and is subject to extensive adulteration with oils such as lemongrass, lemon and citronella.

Violet Leaf Absolute

Botanical Name

Viola odorata

General Description and Origins

A small, tender, perennial plant with dark green, heart-shaped leaves and fragrant violet-blue flowers. The plants are cultivated mainly in Italy and France.[2]

Extraction

The concrete is obtained by solvent extraction of the leaves and an absolute by further extraction of the concrete.

Characteristics

The leaf absolute is an intense dark green viscous liquid with a strong green-leaf odour and delicate floral undernote.[2]

Chemical Composition

A typical chemical composition of violet leaf absolute is reported as follows:

2-trans-6-cis-nonadien-1-al, n-hexanol, n-octen-2-ol-1, benzyl alcohol, tertiary octenol, heptenol, octenal and traces of eugenol.[46]

Traditional Uses

The leaf and flowers have been used in traditional herbal medicine for congestive pulmonary conditions and sensitive skin conditions such as weak capillaries.[4]

The British Herbal Pharmacopoeia lists the dried flowers and leaf as a specific for eczema and skin eruptions with serious exudate, particularly associated with rheumatic conditions.[6]

Properties

Analgesic (mild), anti-inflammatory, antiseptic, decongestant, diuretic, expectorant.[4]

Aromatherapy Uses

Violet leaf absolute is used for the treatment of skin problems such as acne, eczema, thread veins and wounds.[4,14] The oil has also been suggested for dizziness, headaches, insomnia, nervous exhaustion.[4] Arcier recommends violet leaf oil for the treatment of fluid retention and as an effective expectorant of the respiratory tract.[47]

Other Uses

Used in expensive perfumery to bring about a green violet note.[2]

Precautions

Violet leaf absolute is non-toxic, non-irritant, possibly sensitising to some individuals.[4]

References

1. Leung A, Foster S. *Encyclopedia of common natural ingredients used in food, drugs and cosmetics.* John Wiley & Sons Inc, USA, 1996.
2. Arctander S. *Perfume and flavour materials of natural origin.* Allured Publishing, USA, 1994.
3. Lawrence B. *Ambrette seed.* Perfumer and Flavorist 1978; 3(4): 54.
4. Lawless J. *The Encyclopaedia of essential oils.* Element Books Limited, Great Britain, 1992.
5. Lawrence B. *Asafoetida.* Perfumer and Flavorist 1985; 10(1): 43.
6. *British herbal pharmacopoeia.* British Herbal Medicine Association, England, 1987.
7. Blumenthal M, et al. *The complete German commission E monographs: Therapeutic guide to herbal medicine.* American Botanical Council USA, 1998.
8. Irani F. *The magic of ayurveda aromatherapy.* Subtle Energies, Australia, 2001.
9. Lind E. *Discovering champaka oil.* Aromatherapy Quarterly 1997; 55: 9–11.
10. Hemphill I. *Spice notes.* Pan MacMillan, Australia, 2000.

11. Lawrence B. *Caraway oil.* Perfumer and Flavorist 1985; 10(1): 43.
12. Lawrence B. *Cassie absolute.* Perfumer and Flavorist 1984; 9(3): 35.
13. Lawrence B. *Coriander seed.* Perfumer and Flavorist 1991; 16(1): 49.
14. Davis P. *Aromatherapy A–Z.* 2nd edn, The C.W. Daniel Company Limited, Great Britain 1999.
15. Evans WC. *Trease and Evans pharmacognosy.* WB Saunders, 15th edn, UK, 2002.
16. Lawrence B. *Dill seed.* Perfumer and Flavorist 1985/1986; 10(6): 29.
17. Grieves M. *A modern herbal.* Penguin, England, 1931.
18. Lawrence B. *Elemi.* Perfumer and Flavorist 1984; 9(3): 35.
19. Worwood VA. *The fragrant heavens.* Transworld Publishing, Great Britain, 1999.
20. Lawrence B. *Galangal.* Perfumer and Flavorist 1986; 11(1): 29.
21. Lawrence B. *Galbanum.* Perfumer and Flavorist 1978; 3(4): 54.
22. Kerr J. *Ho leaf/rosewood.* Aromatherapy Today, 1998; 7: 6–9.
23. Burfield T, Sheppard-Hanger S. *Substituting for rosewood oil ... a look at other high linalol containing oils.* Aromatherapy Today, 2003; 26: 30–37.
24. Guenther E. *Volume IV: The essential oils.* Krieger Publishing Company, USA, 1950.
25. Lawrence B. *Jonquil and its extracts.* Perfumer and Flavorist 1995; 20: 45.
26. Taylor R. *Lemon Myrtle the essential oil.* CSIRO Rural Research 172, Spring 1996: 18–19.
27. *Product specification sheet for Backhousia citriodora.* The Good Oil Plantation Pty Ltd, Australia.
28. Ryan T, Cavanagh H, Wilkinson J. *Antimicrobial activity of Backhousia citriodora oil.* Simply Essential, 2000; 138: 6–8.
29. Webb M. *Bush sense.* Australia, 2000.
30. Lawrence B. *Lentisque or mastic gum tree oils and absolute.* Perfumer and Flavorist 1992; 17(1): 45.
31. Schnaubelt K. *Advanced aromatherapy.* Healing Art Press, Canada, 1995.
32. Lawrence B. *Opopanax.* Perfumer and Flavorist 1983; 8(5): 19.
33. Lunny V. *Essential oil of ravensara.* Aromatic Thymes, Winter 1998: 24–25.
34. Mailhebiau P. *Portraits in oils.* The C.W. Daniel Company Limited, Great Britain 1995.
35. Lawrence B. *Spikenard oil.* Perfumer and Flavorist 1985/1986; 10(6): 29.
36. Gumbel D. *Principles of holistic skin therapy with herbal essences.* Karl F. Haug Publishers, Germany, 1986.
37. Lawrence B. *Tagetes oil.* Perfumer and Flavorist 1992; 17(5): 131–3.
38. Tateo F. *Basil oil and tarragon oil: Composition and genotoxicity evaluation.* Journal of Essential Oil Research 1989; 1(3): 111–118.
39. Lawrence B. *Tuberose absolute.* Perfumer and Flavorist 1995; 20: 42.
40. Worwood V. *The fragrant mind.* Doubleday, Great Britain, 1995.
41. Balacs T. *Turmeric oil.* The International Journal of Aromatherapy 1994; 6(1): 12–15.
42. Balacs T, Tisserand R. *Essential oil safety.* Churchill Livingstone, UK, 1995.
43. Lawrence B. *Valerian oil.* Perfumer and Flavorist 1985; 10(5): 93.
44. Lawrence B. *Lemon verbena.* Perfumer and Flavorist 1976; 1(2): 17.
45. Fisher-Rizzi S. *Complete aromatherapy handbook.* Sterling Publishing Company, USA, 1990.
46. Lawrence B. *Violet leaf oil.* Perfumer and Flavorist 1978; 3(1): 29–32.
47. Arcier M. *Aromatherapy.* Hamlyn Publishing Group, UK, 1990.

Vegetable Oils

Objectives

After careful study of this chapter, you should be able to:

- Describe fatty acids and explain their functions.
- Explain the process for extracting vegetable oils.
- Define a cold pressed oil.
- List a range of carrier oils recommended for use in aromatherapy.
- Explain the therapeutic properties of a range of carrier oils.
- Explain the therapeutic properties of a range of infused oils.

Introduction

In aromatherapy vegetable oils are often referred to as 'carrier oils'. This often implies that the vegetable oils are of very little value and simply serve as a carrier for the essential oils. This is far from the truth. As you will soon find out, vegetable oils have many benefits in aromatherapy and skin care.

Vegetable oils extracted from nuts and seeds have played an important role in many cultures as medicines, beauty treatments and food supplements.

What is a Vegetable Oil?

All vegetable oils are defined as lipids, and are largely composed of fatty acids which are composed of two parts, one fatty and the other acid. Linked together, they are referred to as a fatty acid.

Fatty acids are the major building blocks of fat in human bodies and foods and are important sources of energy for the body. They are also major structural components of the membranes which surround subcellular organelles and are therefore important in the building and maintenance of healthy cells.

A fatty acid molecule contains a non-polar, fatty and water-insoluble carbon chain of variable length, made entirely of carbon and hydrogen atoms, ending in a methyl ($-CH_3$) group. The other end of the molecule is a weak organic acid called a carboxyl ($-COOH$) group.

There can be any number of carbon atoms in the fatty carbon chain, but the most common lengths vary between 4-carbons (butyric acid, found in butter) and 24-carbons (found in fish oil).

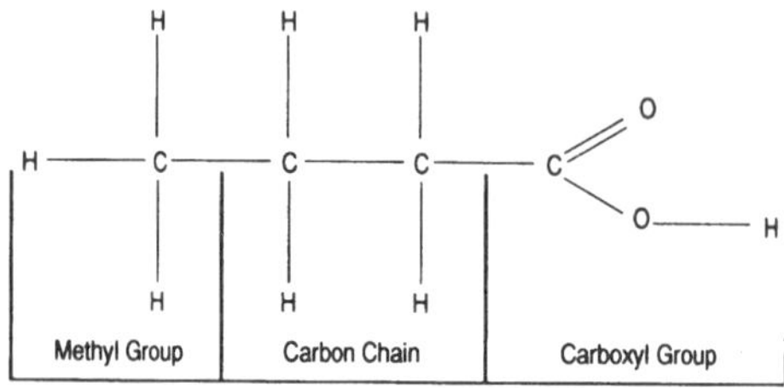

Basic structure of a fatty acid.

Fatty acids may be saturated or unsaturated. To determine whether a fatty acid is saturated or unsaturated check the number of double bonds that occur in its structure. These double bonds result in fewer hydrogen atoms in the molecule. Fewer hydrogen atoms in a structure means less saturated. Since there can be many double bonds, or only a few, in a long chain fatty acid, the terms *mono-unsaturated* (one double bond), or *polyunsaturated* (two or more bonds) have come into general use.

Chemists assign numbers to the carbon atoms in fatty acid chains to simplify them. The numbering system is referred to the omega system. This system numbers the carbon atoms in sequence, starting from the methyl end.

Double bonds can occur in the fatty carbon chain at any point. This is very important from a nutritional point of view as it changes the properties and biological functions of the fatty acid.

Saturated Fatty Acids

Mono-unsaturated Fatty Acids

Polyunsaturated Fatty Acids

Examples of saturated, mono-unsaturated and polyunsaturated fatty acids.

Function of Fatty Acids

Fatty acids have many different functions as part of the body fat under the skin and around the organs, being used for insulation and shock absorption. All fatty acids can be used for energy production while others are used for more important functions.

Fatty acids containing fewer than 16 carbon atoms and all saturated fatty acids are oxidised in the body to produce energy, calories and heat. The shorter the saturated fatty acid the more readily it oxidises and the easier it is to digest. This is important for people who suffer from a weak or diseased liver. Since one of the important functions of the liver is to metabolise fats, a symptom of liver malfunction is the difficulty in digesting fatty foods, and a feeling of tiredness or heaviness after eating a fat-rich meal. Shorter chain fatty acids are less demanding on the liver and are preferable in diets of people with liver disorders.

Unsaturated fatty acids can be lengthened or more double bonds inserted and the highly unsaturated molecules which result are used for special functions in the most active tissues such as brains, sense organs, adrenal glands and sexual organs. Some unsaturated fatty acids, the essential fatty acids, can be partially oxidised and in this process, which is enzyme-controlled, the fatty acids are changed into prostaglandins, which regulate many functions of all tissues in a hormone-like way.

Saturated Fatty Acids

Saturated fatty acids have no double bonds. Each carbon atom is linked to hydrogen atoms by single bonds. Saturated fatty acids are mostly of animal origin such as red meat and dairy produce and are easy to identify because they tend to be solid at room temperature (e.g., lard, butter or cheese). The longer the carbon chain in a saturated fatty acid, the higher its melting point and the harder it is.

Name of Fatty Acid	Number of Carbon Atoms	Melting Point (°C)
butyric	4	–8
caproic	6	03
caprylic	8	17
capric	10	32
lauric	12	44
myristic	14	54
palmitic	16	63
stearic	18	70
arachidic	20	75
behenic	22	80
lignoceric	24	84

Chain length, structural formula and boiling points of saturated fatty acids.[1]

Short chain saturated fatty acids with up to 10 carbon atoms are found in butter and milk fat, and also in coconut oil. The human body uses saturated fatty acids up to 14 carbons in length as:

- a source of energy for the body to burn
- an insulator to keep the body warm.[1]

The three most common saturated fats in food are myristic, palmitic and stearic acids. These longer chained saturated fatty acids appear to be the most potent elevators of cholesterol and low-density lipoproteins (LDL) that encourage deposits in the arteries and raise the risk of heart attacks and thrombosis.[1]

This is a problem in cardiovascular diseases and other diseases of fatty degeneration, which plague those populations whose diet is high in beef and dairy foods.

Unsaturated Fatty Acids

Unsaturated fatty acids differ from the simpler saturated fatty acid in only one respect. They contain one double bond or more between carbon atoms in their fatty carbon chain. Physically, they are liquid at room temperature.

The mono-unsaturated fatty acid oleic acid is found abundantly in olive oil, while poly-unsaturated fatty acids are found in a number of vegetable oils, including safflower seed, sunflower seed, sesame, soybean, wheatgerm and corn. Indeed, polyunsaturated fatty acids are characteristic of vegetable oils, with the notable exceptions of palm and coconut oils, which are high in saturated fat.

Examples of polyunsaturated fatty acids are linoleic, linolenic and arachidonic acids. These are collectively known as the 'essential fatty acids', because they are essential for life.

None of these are produced by the body, although linolenic and arachidonic acids may be synthesised from other nutrients. Linoleic acid, however, must be obtained from diet. By eliminating all fats and oils from daily intake, people run the risk of precipitating deficiency disease.

Oleic acid is the most important mono-unsaturated acid in nutrition. It is found in olive oil, almond oil, other seed oils, in the membranes of plant and animal cell structures, and in the fat deposits of most land animals. It is not an essential fatty acid as the body can make its own. However, it is a valuable addition to the diet. In excess, it can interfere with the metabolism of essential fatty acids.

Essential Fatty Acids

The most important fatty acids in human nutrition and health are two acids with 18 carbon links:

- linoleic acid
- linolenic acid.

Linoleic Acid and the Omega-6 Family

Linoleic acid can be metabolised to produce two useful fatty acids: gamma linolenic acid (GLA), and dihomogamma-linolenic acid (DGLA). These are obviously names, which the chemists have had fun with. For our purposes they will be called GLA and DGLA. Collectively, these are called the omega-6 fatty acids because of their structures.

Linoleic acid is the main omega-6 polyunsaturated fatty acid found in most cold-pressed vegetable oils such as safflower seed, sunflower seed, walnut, pumpkin seed, sesame seed and linseed oils. A deficiency of linoleic acid can lead to a variety of disorders such as; eczema like skin eruptions, loss of hair, liver degeneration, excessive sweating with thirst, susceptibility to infections, poor wound healing, sterility in males, miscarriage in females, arthritis, heat and circulatory problems and growth retardation.[2]

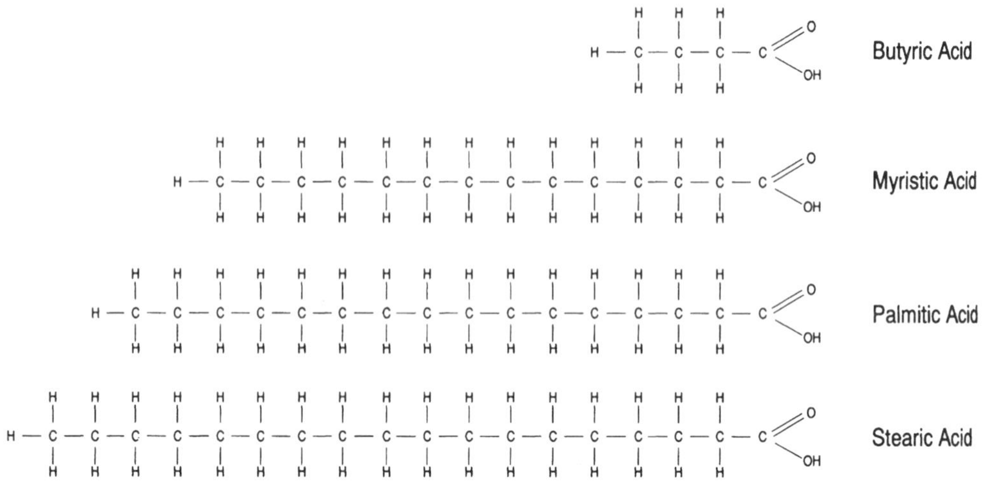

Butyric Acid

Myristic Acid

Palmitic Acid

Stearic Acid

Chain length and structural formula of essential fatty acids.

GLA has a few natural sources, in particular evening primrose oil and borage seed oil. These fatty acids are vital and have been very successful in the experimental treatment of a number of conditions such as premenstrual tension, atopic eczema, psoriasis, heart and vascular disease, rheumatoid arthritis and multiple sclerosis.[3]

Linolenic Acid and the Omega-3 Family

Linolenic acid, otherwise known as alpha linolenic acid is found in high concentrations in vegetable oils such as linseed and canola, and in the oils from cold water fish such as salmon, sardines, mackerel and tuna. When it is metabolised in the body, linolenic acid forms a number of members of the omega-3 fatty acid family, with the most important ones being eicosapentaenoic acid (EPA), and docosahexanoic acid (DHA).

A deficiency of linolenic acid is known to cause a variety of disorders including retardation of growth, muscular weakness, lack of co-ordination, tingling of arms and legs, disturbances of vision and behavioural changes. The omega-3 fatty acids do not have the broad spread of actions of the omega-6 fatty acids. Their effect is on the cardio-vascular system.[1] Research into the omega-3 fatty acids has shown that they can.

- prevent blood clots
- prevent dangerous abnormalities in heart rhythm, which are a common feature in sudden heart attack
- reduce elevated serum levels of complex fats known as triglycerides and to improve their balance, to help lower cholesterol
- stop certain cells sticking to the walls of the arteries
- prevent some inflammatory reactions in the body such as rheumatoid arthritis
- help lower blood pressure
- provide immunity to certain diseases.[4,5]

Since these are many of the causes of heart disease in Western countries, it is not surprising that the use of the omega-3 family has increased around the world, for its use in heart disease alone. An adult requires about 5 gm of each essential fatty acid each day.[5] A deficiency may result in rough or dry skin, dull hair, or abnormal nails. Polyunsaturated fatty acids are also important because of the role they play in reducing fatty deposits within the body.[1]

Polyunsaturates

Omega-6		Omega-3
High linoleic	**GLA Oils**	**High linolenic**
Corn Cotton seed Soya bean Safflower Sunflower	Borage Evening primrose	Linseed Fish oils such as salmon, mackerel, tuna and anchovy

Food sources of polyunsaturated fatty acids.

Toxic Fatty Acids

Several natural oils contain toxic fatty acids, and are not good oils for human consumption. Cotton seed oil contains from 0.6 to 1.2% of a cyclopropene fatty acid with 19 carbon atoms, which has toxic effects on the liver and gall bladder. This fatty acid also slows down sexual maturity. On a biochemical level, this fatty acid destroys the desaturase enzymes which are responsible for metabolising the unsaturated fatty acids. It also enhances the ability of aflatoxins to cause cancer.[1]

Cotton seed oil also has the highest content of pesticide residue. The cotton farmers overspray their crops in order to keep cotton pests under control. Refining removes part of the toxic fatty acids and pesticides. However, cotton seed oil is not recommended to use for human or animal consumption.[1]

Canola oil (formerly known as rapeseed) contains erucic acid, a 22-carbon chain fatty acid. Until 1974 rapeseed oil produced in Canada contained up to 40% erucic acid. In response to government concerns over the results of rat studies which showed erucic acid causes fatty degeneration of the heart, kidneys, adrenals and thyroid, geneticists have bred new varieties of rape seed, whose content of erucic acid is lower. According to some government standards less than 5% erucic acid is permissible.[1]

Another toxic fatty acid is the hydroxy fatty acid ricinoleic acid, which makes up 80% of the fatty acid content of castor oil. This fatty acid stimulates the secretion of fluids in the intestine and for this reason is used as a purge in medicine. Apart from causing very powerful intestinal contractions, castor oil has no harmful effects.[1]

Extracting Vegetable Oils

The process for extracting vegetable oils is described below.

Cleaning and Cooking

The seeds are initially mechanically cleaned, crushed and cooked for up to 2 hours at varying temperatures depending on the seed being used. An average temperature used is 120° C. This process makes the next step easier by destroying the cells which contain the oil.[1]

Expeller Pressing

The crushed seeds are pressed in an expeller press, which is a continually rotating spiral-shaped augur which moves the seed forward and pushes the seed against a metal press head. The pressure generated in the head of an expeller press reaches several tonnes per centimetre.[1]

The turning auger further crushes the seed and creates friction in the seed mass, which produces heat in the press head. The heat and pressure force the oil out of the seed and the oil runs out through slots or holes in the side of the press head, while the oil cake, the solid remainder of the seed mash, is pushed out through slits at the end of the press head. This pressing process usually takes a few minutes at temperatures around 85° C.[1]

The oil is then filtered and then bottled and sold as cold pressed oil. However, most commercial manufacturers will then treat this 'unrefined oil' by several processes such as degumming, refining, bleaching and deodorising.

Solvent Extraction

Solvent extraction has been described as a more efficient, but less healthy way of extracting the oil from the seed by using solvents such as hexane or heptane.[1] This same method is often used to get the last oil remaining in the oil cake after expeller pressing, thus increasing the yield of the oil from the seed. Once the oil-solvent mixture has been separated from the seed meal, the solvent is evaporated off at a temperature of about 150° C.[1]

Degumming

In this process, gums and complex carbohydrates called polysaccharides are taken out of the oil. Lecithin, well known for its health benefits, is also isolated and sold separately for its health benefits. Degumming is carried out at 60° C, with water and phosphoric acid.[1]

Refining

In this process the oil is mixed with sodium hydroxide and sodium carbonate. This removes free fatty acids from the oil. Free fatty acids form soap with sodium hydroxide, which then dissolves in the watery part of the mixture. Phospholipids, protein-like substances, and minerals are also further removed in this process. The refining temperature is around 75° C. At this stage the oil still contains pigments.[1]

Bleaching

Acid-treated clays and Fuller's Earth are used to remove the pigments of chlorophyll and betacarotene and the remaining traces of soap. Bleaching takes place at 110° C. During bleaching toxic peroxides and conjugated fatty acids are formed from the essential fatty acids present in the oil.[1]

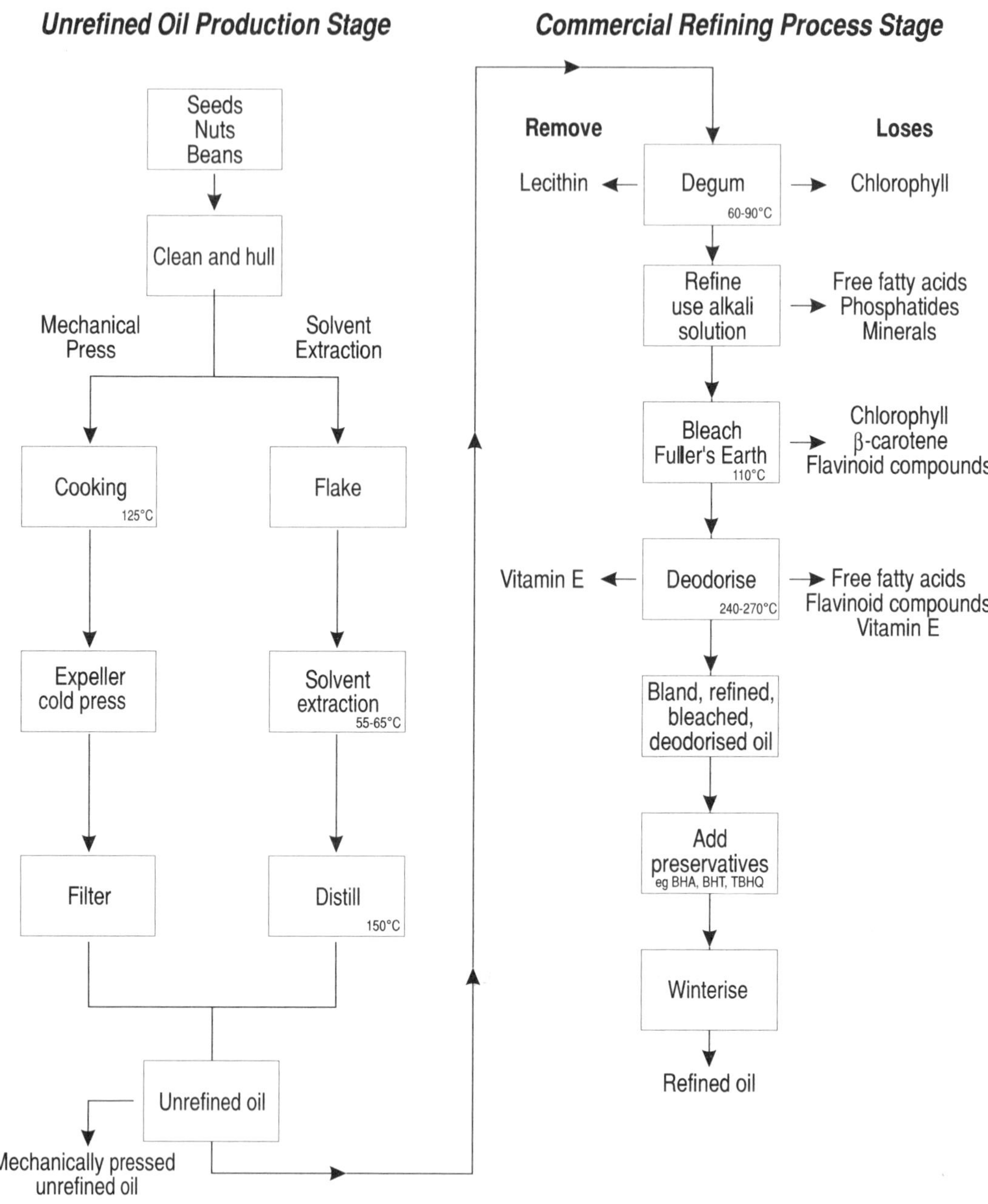

Schematic of the steps involved in the processing of vegetable oils.

Deodorisation

This involves steam distillation under pressure and exclusion of air to remove aromatic oils. This removes more free fatty acids, pungent odours and unpleasant tastes, which are not present in the natural oil in the seed before the processing began. Deodorisation takes place at the incredibly high temperature of 240° C to 270° C for 30 to 60 minutes.[1]

The peroxides produced in the refining step are removed. Vitamin E, phytosterols and some pesticide residues and toxins are also removed by deodorisation.[1]

The oil is finally odourless, tasteless and cannot be distinguished from oils derived from other sources which have been similarly treated.[1] Believe it or not this oil can still be sold as *cold-pressed*, because no external heat was applied during the pressing of the oil.

Preservative and Winterisation Stage

Before distributing the refined oil to the supermarkets, several antioxidants will be added to it. These may include butylated hydroxytoluene (BHT), butylated hydroxyanisole (BHA), propyl gallate, tertiary butylhydroquinone (TBHQ) or citric acid, to replace the natural antioxidants beta-carotene and vitamin E which were destroyed in the refining process. Defoamers may also be added, and the oil is bottled and sold.[1]

Winterisation is the process whereby an oil is cooled and filtered again to prevent it from developing turbidity when is cooled in the refrigerator.[1]

What are Cold-pressed Oils?

Most people are surprised when they hear that there is no such thing as a 'cold-pressed oil'. The term implies (incorrectly) that no heat is used, thus it must be nutritionally superior. In reality it means that no external heat has been applied to the seed while it is being pressed. It does not guarantee that no heat has been applied before or after the actual pressing process. The expeller method describe previously is usually used to extract oils and the temperature would rarely exceed 100° C. The unsaturated fatty acids contained in the oil begin to change their molecular arrangement from the natural cis-configuration to the unnatural trans-configuration (which is a toxic substance) once the temperature begins to exceed 160° C. Thus the heat produced during pressing is not really a problem, and the term we ascribe to 'cold-pressed' is not entirely based on fact and does not really exist.

It would therefore be more appropriate to search for unrefined oils that have been mechanically pressed as opposed to chemically extracted.

Commonly Used Vegetable Oils

The seeds of most plants contain oil, which serve as the high energy starter for the seedling. Just like the chicken's egg, the plant seed has to contain enough energy to sprout a whole plant. The tougher the environmental condition, the more oil the seed needs to store. The colder the climate, the more of the unsaturated fatty acids it contains in its oil to increase its metabolic rate. For this reason, the amounts of the various fatty acids contained in the oil from different seeds vary greatly.

The amount of oil found in the different seeds varies from 4% for corn oil to over 70% for pecans.

Sweet Almond Oil

Prunus amygdalus

The almond tree is a native of the Middle East. There are two varieties, the sweet almond *(dulcis)* and bitter almond *(amara)*. It is the sweet almond that is widely used, as the bitter almond contains traces of amygdalin that can be hydrolysed or distilled to produce the deadly hydrocyanic acid.[6]

The earliest use of almond oil dates back to the Romans who used it extensively in skin care preparations.[7]

Almond oil is highly nutritious, being a good source of trace minerals and rich in the polyunsaturated fatty acid linoleic acid. It is an excellent emollient for chapped hands and is extensively used in skin care preparations.[6]

A typical analysis of sweet almond is as follows:

Fatty Acid	Name	Percentage
C14	Myristic	0.1
C16	Palmitic	6.6
C16:1	Palmitoleic	0.5
C17	Heptadecenoic	0.1
C17:1	9-Heptadecenoic	0.1
C18	Stearic	1.3
C18:1	Oleic	64.6
C18:2	Linoleic	26.3
C18:3	Linolenic	0.2
C20	Arachidic	0.1
C20:1	Eicosenoic	0.1

Apricot Kernel Oil

Prunus armeniac

Apricot kernel oil is a good source of polyunsaturated fatty acids. It has a light texture, making it very easily absorbed into the skin. The light texture of this oil makes it especially suitable for facial massage blends. It is good for the treatment of mature, dry, sensitive or inflamed skins.[8]

A typical analysis of apricot kernel oil is as follows:

Fatty Acid	Name	Percentage
C16	Palmitic	4.9
C16:1	Palmitoleic	0.9
C17	Heptadecenoic	—
C17:1	9-Heptadecenoic	0.1
C18	Stearic	1.0
C18:1	Oleic	62.0
C18:2	Linoleic	30.6
C18:3	Linolenic	0.2
C20	Arachidic	0.1
C20:1	Eicosenoic	0.1

Avocado Oil

Persea americana

The avocado tree was first found growing in South American swamp lands where it was nicknamed 'alligator pear'. Technically, avocados are a fruit because they have a stone.[8]

The oil is extracted from the flesh which contains up to 30% pure oil — a figure rivalled only by olive and palm fruit.[8] Crude avocado oil is produced by mechanical pressing on hydraulic presses, followed by centrifugal extraction.

The oil is rich in many nutrients including vitamin A and D, lecithin and potassium. The oil is rich in chlorophyll, the reason for its dazzling green colour. Although the oil is mono-unsaturated, it is not as stable as olive oil at high temperatures, so is not suitable for cooking.[8]

Avocado oil can be used to soothe the skin, being useful for conditions such as nappy rash and eczema. It is moisturising to the skin and is ideal for dry, mature skin and assists in the treatment of climate-damaged and undernourished or aged skin.[6,8]

A typical analysis of avocado oil is as follows:

Fatty Acid	Name	Percentage
C16	Palmitic	12.0–16.0
C16:1	Palmitoleic	4.3–6.8
C18	Stearic	2.0
C18:1	Oleic	60.0–72.0
C18:2	Linoleic	8.0–15.03
C18:3	Linolenic	2.0 maximum

Canola Oil

Brassica napus

Also known as rapeseed oil. This oil has been extensively used in commercial food preparation. Canola belongs to the cabbage family and grows 1.5 to 1.8 metres high with vivid yellow flowers. The seeds contain 35-40% pure oil, and the young leaves can be served as a vegetable. Because of its rather unfortunate name, rapeseed, the Canadians decided to register the name Canola for the oil produced from the rapeseed.[1]

Canola oil has the highest percentage of unsaturated fats of any oil. It contains over 90% mono- and polyunsaturated fatty acids and is a light oil with very little flavour. It is unstable at high temperatures and will produce more toxic effluents when cooked.[1]

A typical analysis of canola oil is as follows:

Fatty Acid	Name	Percentage
C16	Palmitic	3.0–4.5
C16:1	Palmitoleic	0.2–0.3
C18	Stearic	1.3–1.7
C18:1	Oleic	56.0–62.0
C18:2	Linoleic	19–24
C18:3	Linolenic	8.2–13.0
C22:1	Erucic	0.2–1.8

Evening Primrose Oil

Oenothera biennis

The evening primrose is a tall, spiky plant that blooms only in the evening, hence its common name. The North American Indian medicine men were the first to recognise its potential as a healing agent and used to brew the seed pods to make an infusion for healing wounds.

Evening primrose oil is rich in fatty acids, one in particular, GLA. The GLA found in evening primrose oil is biologically important as it affects much of the enzyme activity in the body. Every process that takes place in the body is triggered by the action of various enzymes, including the production of prostaglandins. These hormone-like substances regulate bodily functions such as:

- lowering blood pressure
- inhibiting thrombosis
- inhibiting cholesterol
- inhibiting inflammation
- inhibiting platelet aggregation
- regulating production of saliva and tears.
- regulating oestrogen, progestogen and prolactin in the luteal phase of the menstrual cycle.[1,6]

Prostaglandins are the end result of a chemical chain reaction which starts with essential fatty

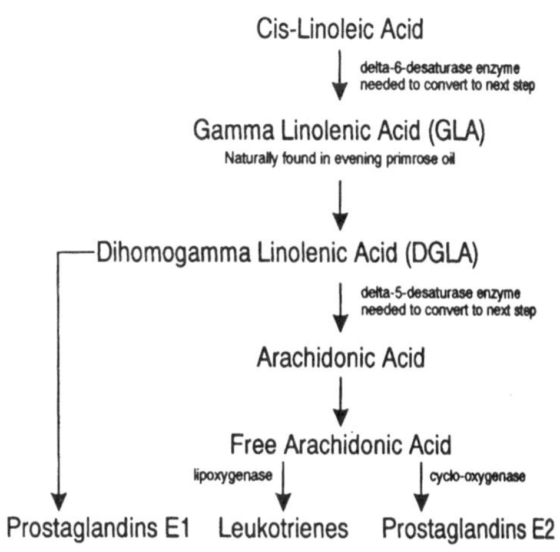

Prostaglandin synthesis from linoleic acid.

acids — notably linoleic acid which is found in cold-pressed oils. These essential fatty acids are not manufactured by the body, they can only be obtained from the diet. The flow chart on this page shows the synthesis of prostaglandins from linoleic acid.

Linoleic acid is converted into GLA, the substance found in evening primrose oil, and then to DGLA and then to arachadonic acid. The latter two are present in all cell structures and are the precursors of prostaglandins. It is assumed that this conversion process is efficiently dealt with in the body. However, certain factors inhibit the production of GLA. Research shows that the following factors inhibit the production of GLA:

- a diet rich in saturated fats
- a diet rich in processed vegetable oils
- consumption of alcohol
- diabetes
- aging process
- lack of zinc, magnesium and vitamin B — all of which are necessary for GLA formation
- viral infections, radiation, cancer
- stress.

This is why evening primrose oil is beneficial. It has been found that the GLA from this oil is a more efficient precursor of arachidonic acid than the linoleic acid found in sunflower seed oil. Studies in evening primrose have found that it may be beneficial for:

- improving certain kinds of eczema
- improving the condition of the hair, nails and skin
- relieving premenstrual tension
- reducing the production of cholesterol
- enabling insulin to work more effectively
- preventing inflammation and controlling arthritis.[1]

Evening primrose oil can be used externally as a massage oil. It has been found to be effective for the treatment of eczema and psoriasis, premenstrual tension, rheumatoid arthritis and weight reduction.[5]

A typical analysis of evening primrose oil is as follows:

Fatty Acid	Name	Percentage
C16:1	Palmitolic	6.1
C18:1	Oleic	1.9
C20:0	Arachidic	0.3
C22:0	Behenic	0.1
C18:1w9	Oleic	6.3
C18:1w7	Oleic	0.6
C20:1w9	Eicosenoic	0.2
C22:1w9	Erucic	—
C24:1w9	Tetracosenoic	—
C18:2w6	Linoleic	65.0–73.9
C18:3w6	Gamma linolenic	8.5–11.5
C18:3w3	Alpha linolenic	0.2

Jojoba Oil

Simmondsia chinensis

The jojoba plant was first recorded by British botanist HF Link in 1822, when he landed at Baja California in Northern Mexico and observed the wild shrub in its natural context. Link named the plant *Simmondsia chinensis*, after a fellow British botanist and explorer, TW Simmonds.[8]

Jojoba oil (pronounced ho-ho-ba) is unique because the oil is not composed of fat but of liquid wax. In scientific terms, waxes are esters of long-chain fatty acids with long-chain monohydroxyl alcohols, whereas fats are esters of long-chain fatty acids with glycerine. Being composed of mostly wax esters, it means that there is very little likelihood of deterioration of the oil.[7]

Jojoba oil is ideal for use in cosmetics because of its molecular stability and its natural moisturising and healing properties. Jojoba's resistance to oxidation means that it does not require additional chemical preservatives. It is suitable for all skin types, whether dry, oily or sensitive.[7,8]

When applied to the scalp as a treatment, jojoba oil acts to regulate and remove the sebum layer. Research also indicates that jojoba oil is beneficial in the treatment of certain dry scalp and skin problems such as psoriasis and eczema. The oil is an excellent emollient for the skin, rendering it soft and smooth.[7]

A typical fatty acid profile of jojoba is:

Fatty Acid	Name	Percentage
C16:0	Palmitic	1.5
C16:1	Palmitoleic	0.4
C18:1	Stearic	13.9
C18:2	Oleic	0.3
C18:3	Linoleic	0.2
C19:0	Linolenic	trace
C20:0	Nonadecenoic	—
C20:1	Eicosenoic	0.1
C22:0	Behenic	0.2
C22:1	Erucic	11.2
C24:0	Lignoceric	0.1
C24:1	Nervonic	0.9

Linseed Oil

Linum usitatissumum

Linseed oil takes it name from Latin — 'most useful' and is extracted from the flax plant. Flax is an annual crop with rich blue flowers and tiny brownish seeds. There are several varieties, each with different uses. The long stemmed variety is grown for its lengthy fibres that are woven into linen, while the seeds of the short-stemmed varieties are commonly used for oil production.[8]

The use of linseed oil can be traced back to Hippocrates who recorded that it was a useful treatment for stomach and skin disorders. Linseed is valued by herbalists for its mucilage properties, meaning it contains a slimy material that is not absorbed but passes straight through the body.[8]

Linseeds are a very effective and gentle bulking agent and can be used as a laxative when swallowed whole with plenty of water. The mucins and water-binding substances in linseed work by increasing the volume of the stool. This then presses against the intestinal walls and triggers the peristalsis movement. In addition, the mucins form a protective and gliding film, which covers the sensitive mucous membranes. This can be useful for healing intestinal wall irritations. Linseeds can be crushed and used as a poultice to draw out excess fluid from body tissues.[1]

Linseed oil contains mainly omega-3 fatty acids normally found in fish oil and is therefore recommended for vegetarians who prefer not to take fish oils. Linseed oil is beneficial in the treatment of major degenerative conditions such as cancer, cardiovascular disease, diabetes, multiple sclerosis and arthritis.[1]

One of the drawbacks of linseed oil is that it needs to be used fresh as it spoils much faster than other oils. So keep it in a refrigerator and a tightly sealed amber bottle.

A typical analysis of linseed oil is as follows:

Fatty Acid	Name	Percentage
C16	Palmitic	5.5
C16:1	Palmitoleic	—
C18	Stearic	3.5
C18:1	Oleic	19.1
C18:2	Linoleic	15.3
C18:3	Linolenic	56.6

Macadamia Oil

Macadamia integrifolia or M.ternifolia

Macadamia oil is high in palmitoleic acid, a monounsaturated fatty acid not commonly found in many other vegetable oils. Palmitoleic acid is also found in sebum, thus macadamia oil has been often recommended for older skin which starts to dry as the sebum production diminishes. It is a highly nourishing and emollient oil recommended for dry and mature skin.[8]

A typical fatty acid profile of macadamia oil is:

Fatty Acid	Name	Percentage
C14	Myristic	0.6–1.6
C16	Palmitic	7.0–11.0
C16:1	Palmitoleic	18.0–25.0
C18	Stearic	2.0–4.0
C18:1	Oleic	55.0–62.0
C18:2	Linoleic	1.0–4.0
C20	Arachidic	2.0–4.0
C20.1	Eicosenoic	2.0–4.0

Neem Oil

Azadirachta indica

Neem is native to the Indian subcontinent. It is a deciduous tree which grows up to 15 metres. It is a graceful spreading tree with clusters of fragrant white flowers. All parts of the neem tree can be used. The twigs are used for toothbrushes in Asia, the bark and the leaves are commonly used for their medicinal properties and the oil pressed from the seed is renowned as an anti-fruit fly agent and is considered insecticidal and antiseptic.[9]

The following compounds have been found in neem oil: 0.2% myristic acid, 16.2% palmitic acid, 14.6% stearic acid, 3.4% archidic acid, 56.6% oleic acid and 9.0% linoleic acid. It is quite rich in tocopherols. The most important constituent is azadirachtin.[9]

Traditionally, neem oil was cold-pressed. However, because of the low yield of oil, much of the oil available today is obtained by solvent extraction, using hexane as a solvent. The oil dissolved in the solvent is filtered and the mixture of hexane and neem oil is subjected to distillation to separate the volatile hexane from the fatty oils.[9]

Neem has been used for centuries in India and is extensively used in Ayurvedic medicine to treat a multitude of ailments and conditions.

Neem oil is used in soaps, shampoos and skin care preparations. It has antibacterial and antifungal properties and can be used for inhibiting viral and fungal infections such as warts, athlete's foot, ringworm, candida and staph.[9] Neem oil is also effective for the treatment of skin disorders such as rashes, eczema, scabies and ringworm. In skin care, you can add neem oil to facial and body creams. In hair care preparations neem oil can be used in scalp preparations; to prevent any itching and dandruff. It has been traditionally used as an effective head lice treatment.[9]

Neem oil is used in toothpaste. It inhibits gum infection and inflammation, receding gums, tooth decay and mouth ulcers. It is used to repel house flies and fleas. Applied to the skin, neem oil acts as an insect repellent; it keeps mosquitoes, fleas and sandflies from biting.[9]

Olive Oil

Olea europaea

The olive is traditionally regarded as a symbol of peace. The ancient Greeks wore garlands of olive leaves in their hair as they prayed for peace. Even in modern political setting, an olive branch within a dove's beak which is depicted as a symbol of peace on the blue and white flag of the United Nations.[7]

The best oil comes from the fruit which is nearly fully ripe and hand picked. The oil itself comes from the pulp, not the kernel, and mills crush the fruit gently so that the stone does not fracture. The oil is separated by centrifuging, and filtered for purity. This is true 'virgin olive oil', but there are various grades of virgin oil, depending on the aroma and degree of acidity.[7]

Olive oil is extensively used for the manufacture of soaps, ointments and cosmetics. Many people find olive oil a little heavy for massage, but it may be blended with less viscous vegetable oils for this purpose.

The oil is highly nutritious and is extensively used in salads and is ideal for cooking. It can be applied externally to sprains, bruises and insect bites and can be used as a treatment for dandruff, especially if it is blended with rosemary oil.[7]

A typical analysis of olive oil is as follows:

Fatty Acid	Name	Percentage
C16	Palmitic	11.0
C16:1	Palmitoleic	1.2
C18	Stearic	2.7
C18:1	Oleic	75.5
C18:2	Linoleic	8.0
C18:3	Linolenic	0.7

Rosehip Oil

Rosa rubiginosa

Rosehip oil is produced in Chile and has recently become a popular oil, particularly in regenerative skin care. The oil is obtained by solvent extraction or cold-pressing.

It is extracted from the seeds of a rose bush which grows wild in the southern Andes. Clinical trials have found rosehip oil to be extremely beneficial in tissue regeneration for conditions such as burns, facial wrinkles and the treatment of scars following surgery.

The oil has been used to reduce wrinkles and signs of premature aging.[10] It also helps to counter the drying effects of the sun which are usually noticed by the fine wrinkles or crow-feet around the eyes and mouth. The oil can be used to attenuate scars (both surgical and accidental), by reducing the redness or hyperpigmentation, reducing the formation of keloid scar tissue formed and loosening up fibrous cords.

It is believed that these important functions in the regeneration and repair of skin tissue are due to the high levels of linoleic (47.4%) and linolenic (33.0%) fatty acids.[10] Recent research indicates the presence of retin A or retinoic acid this may account for the effects that rosehip oil has on the skin.[11]

Safflower Oil

Carthamus tinctorius

Safflower is also known as American saffron, belong to the sunflower family. The oil is extracted from the seeds of the plant and has a bland, slightly nutty flavour. Among the natural vegetable oils it is one of the least expensive and also has the highest percentage of unsaturated fatty acids.[7]

Safflower oil becomes rancid if it is not stored in a refrigerator and is not suitable for deep frying because its flavour and nutritional properties are unstable at high temperatures.[7]

A typical analysis of safflower oil is as follows:

Fatty Acid	Name	Percentage
C16	Palmitic	6.0–7.5
C16:1	Palmitoleic	trace–0.1
C18	Stearic	2.0–2.5
C18:1	Oleic	11.0–13.5
C18:2	Linoleic	76.0–80.0
C18:3	Linolenic	trace– 0.1

Sesame Seed Oil

Sesamum indicum

Sesame, also known as *benne*, is one of the oldest herbs grown specifically for its seeds. The Chinese cultivated sesame some 5,000 years ago, the Egyptians ground it to produce flour, and Roman soldiers mixed sesame seeds with honey to give them extra strength for their long arduous military campaigns. Sesame oil can be extracted from normal seeds, or seeds that have been roasted prior to being pressed. The latter oil is dark and smoky red and is often used in Chinese cooking. The natural oil is light in colour and slightly nutty to taste.[7]

Sesame oil contains 41% mono-unsaturated fatty acids, and 44% polyunsaturated, but contains only 42% linoleic acid. This combination means that sesame seed oil is comparatively stable and does not turn rancid on contact with the air. The oil is also high in vitamin E, calcium, magnesium and phosphorus. It is a good source of vegetable protein and comparatively rich in lecithin. The oil can be used in skin care as a natural moisturiser.[7]

A typical analysis of sesame oil is as follows:

Fatty Acid	Name	Percentage
C16	Palmitic	5.5–9.5
C16:1	Palmitoleic	—
C18	Stearic	4.0–6.0
C18:1	Oleic	33.5–46.0
C18:2	Linoleic	41.0–51.0
C18:3	Linolenic	trace–1.0

Soyabean Oil

Glycine max

Soyabean oil comes from the soya plant, which belongs to the pea or legume family. It can be traced back 5,000 years to its first recorded cultivation in mainland China. The oil is extracted from the smooth egg-shaped beans, which have an oil content of approximately 20%.[7]

Cold-pressed soyabean oil is the second best source of vitamin E (87 mg per 100 ml) after wheatgerm oil. It contains more lecithin than any other vegetable oil. The oil is comparatively high in unsaturated fatty acids. It can be used in massage, being suitable for all skin types.[7]

A typical analysis of soyabean oil is as follows:

Fatty Acid	Name	Percentage
C16	Palmitic	10.4
C16:1	Palmitoleic	0.1
C18	Stearic	4.1
C18:1	Oleic	23.9
C18:2	Linoleic	53.5
C18:3	Linolenic	6.8

Sunflower Oil

Helianthus annus

Sunflowers were prized by the South American Indians who ground the seeds of the flower in a mortar and pestle to make meal. Sunflower seeds contain vitamins A, D and E and are also rich in minerals such as calcium, zinc, potassium, iron and phosphorus.[7]

The oil from the seeds of sunflower resembles that of safflower, to which it is related.[7] Sunflower is an inexpensive oil to use for massage and may be blended with other cold-pressed oils.

A typical analysis of sunflower oil is as follows:

Fatty Acid	Name	Percentage
C16	Palmitic	6.4
C16:1	Palmitoleic	0.1
C18	Stearic	4.2
C18:1	Oleic	14.2
C18:2	Linoleic	73.5
C18:3	Linolenic	0.2

Wheatgerm Oil

Triticum durum, T. aestivum

Wheat is the most widely cultivated cereal grain in the world and is derived from a hybrid wild wheat that grew in the Middle East 10,000 years ago. Most varieties of cultivated wheat belong to two basic types: *T. durum* and *T. aestivum*. The latter is used to produce bread, while *T. durum* is a harder type of wheat used to make semolina, spaghetti and other forms of pasta.[7]

Wheat grain consists of three parts: the bran, or outer husk, representing 12% of the grain by weight; the germ (around 3%) and the starchy endosperm (85%). Milling of white flower separates the wheatgerm. Unfortunately it is the wheatgerm that contains 25% of the protein and a vast array of vitamins and minerals.[7]

Wheatgerm oil is extracted by warm pressing or solvent extraction from the 'germ' of wheat. It is an extremely valuable source of vitamin E (190 mg per 100 gm) and essential fatty acids. Because of its vitamin E content it is a natural antioxidant and is well protected from the elements that usually break down vegetable oils, such as light and heat. It promotes the formation of skin cells, improving blood circulation, and helps relieve symptoms of dermatitis.[8]

It has antioxidant properties which help to remove cholesterol deposits from the arteries and are thus of vital importance in combating heart disease.[7]

A typical fatty acid profile of wheatgerm oil is:

Fatty acid	Name	Percentage
C14:0	Myristic	less than 0.1
C16:0	Palmitic	15.77
C16:1	Palmitoleic	0.2
C18:0	Stearic	1.02
C18:1	Oleic	19.15
C18:2	Linaleic	53.9
C18:3	Linolenic	7.07
C20:0	Arachioic	0.19
C20:1	Ecisadenoic	1.54
C20.2	Eicosadinoic	0.14
C22:0	Behenic	0.13
C24:0	Lionoceric	0.4
C24:1	Nervonic	less than 0.1

Macerated Oils

Macerated oils include arnica, calendula, carrot and hypericum oils, but almost any plant can be macerated. To make a macerated oil place freshly harvested herbs loosely in a transparent, wide-mouthed glass jar and add a cold-pressed vegetable oil such as sweet almond or apricot kernel. Seal the jar so that it is airtight and leave it for four to eight weeks, shaking vigorously once a day. At the end of the period, the oil is drained and filtered and is ready to use as a macerated oil. Store the oil in a dark bottle.

Arnica

Arnica montana

Arnica grows almost exclusively in the high mountainous regions of Northern Europe. The German folk name for arnica literally means 'mountain well-being'. The flowering heads of the plant are used for the preparation of either a macerated oil or a tincture of arnica and the root stock is usually employed for homoeopathic preparations.

Arnica oil or the tincture should be used for external applications only. The German Commission E Monographs recommend arnica oil (extract of 1 part herb and 5 parts fatty oil) for external use in injuries in which the skin is not broken such as bruises, rheumatic muscle and joint problems, contusions, haemorrhages and swellings, including bone fractures.[12]

Calendula

Calendula officinalis

Calendula is a native of the Mediterranean region and the whole flower blossom, not the petals alone, is employed for medicinal purposes.

Calendula has anti-inflammatory properties and vulnerary properties, making it useful for stubborn wounds, skin inflammations and varicose veins.[6] It is effective in treating skin problems such as rashes and, in particular, chapped and cracked skin and makes an excellent base oil for treating abrasions, sunburn, superficial and limited burns, insect bites and eczema.[13]

Calendula oil has also been used for treating venous complaints. In cases of venous inflammation the ointment should be lightly applied, blending it with cypress and lemon essential oils. When applied consistently, calendula decreases the symptoms of varicose veins and venous congestion by inhibiting inflammation, toning tissue and promoting enhanced blood supply to tissue.

The wound healing properties of calendula have been documented in many studies and it was found that a combination of lipophilic extracts (oil extracts) and hydrophilic extracts (containing flavonoids and saponins) promoted healing and skin repair and had anti-inflammatory properties.[14,15,16]

Hypericum

Hypericum perforatum

Hypericin is believed to be the principal active constituent of hypericum, which is also known as St John's wort. Hypericin is contained in the viscid oily substance in the glands on the leaves, petals and stems of the plant. Research has found that the hypericin concentration varies in different parts of the plant. The lowest is in the main stem (120 ppm), leaves (290,380 ppm) and flowers and buds (2150 ppm).[16]

Hypericin is known as a psychotropic activator of neuronal metabolism. This possibly accounts for its antidepressant and mood-lifting properties.[17]

Studies have shown that hypericin is a potent anti-viral drug, especially against enveloped viruses. Studies have confirmed hypericin's activity against the AIDS viruses in laboratory tests.[18]

The oil is used topically for mild burns, bruises, haemorrhoids, varicose veins, wounds, sores and ulcers. It has also been indicated for nerve pain such as neuralgia, sciatica and for some rheumatic pain.[6,12,13,15]

Hypericum oil is prepared by infusing the flowers in a fixed oil such as sweet almond oil for approximately three weeks. This is then pressed and strained. The oil which is bright red can be used externally for massage purposes to treat many of the conditions indicated previously.

There is one side effect that is associated with hypericin. It increases photosensitivity so it should not be used before going into the sun.[6,12,15]

References

1. Erasmus, Udo. *Fats and oils: The complete guide to fats and oils in health and nutrition.* Alive Books, Canada, 1986.
2. Krause BS et al. *Food, nutrition and diet therapy.* WB Saunders Company, USA, 1979.
3. Graham J. *Evening primrose oil.* Thornsons Publishing Company, United Kingdom, 1984.
4. Stanton R. *Eating for peak performance.* Allen & Unwin, Australia, 1994.
5. Pizzorno J, Murray M. *A text book of natural medicine Vol 1.* 2nd edn, Churchill Livingstone, United Kingdom, 1999.
6. Leung A, Foster S. *Encyclopedia of common natural ingredients used in food, drugs and cosmetics.* John Wiley & Sons Inc, USA, 1996.
7. Drury N & S. *Healing oils and essences.* Harper & Row, Australia, 1987.
8. Earle L. *Vital oils.* Ebury Press, United Kingdom, 1991.
9. Puri HS. *Neem: the divine tree.* Harwood Academic Publishers, Singapore, 1999.
10. Price S, Price L. *Aromatherapy for health professionals.* 2nd edn, Churchill Livingstone, United Kingdom, 1999.
11. Dweck A. The role of natural ingredients in anti-aging of the skin. Cosmetics, Aerosols & Toiletries in Australia. 2003; 16(3); 14–22.
12. Blumenthal M, et al. *The complete German Commission E Monographs: Therapeutic guide to herbal medicine.* American Botanical Council, USA, 1998.
13. Bruneton J. *Pharmacognosy.* 2nd edn, Lavoisier Publishing Inc, France, 1999.
14. Bone K. *The real value of herbal preparations in cosmetic products.* 29th Annual conference of the Australian Society of Cosmetic Chemists, May 1994.
15. Varro T. *The honest herbal.* 3rd edn, Pharmaceutical Products Press, USA, 1993.
16. Southwell IA et al. *Hypericin content variation in hypericum perforatum in Australia.* Phytochemistry, 1991; 39: 475–478.
17. *Hypericum perforatum.* ATMS Newsletter, 1993; 6: 18.
18. Castleman M. *The healing herbs.* Rondale Press, USA, 1991.

Hazardous Essential Oils

Objectives

After careful study of this chapter, you should be able to:

- list a range of hazardous essential oils that are not recommended for use in aromatherapy or should be used with caution
- explain why these essential oils should be used with caution or not be used in aromatherapy.

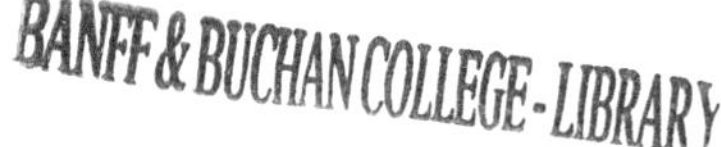

Introduction

Essential oils have been used for centuries and the toxicology of the majority of essential oils is well documented. The purpose of this chapter is to identify the hazards of some of these oils.

Ajowan

Botany and Origins

Ajowan oil is distilled from the fruits or, occasionally, from the whole plant of *Trachyspermum copticum*. The herb is cultivated in India, in the Seychelles Islands and in the West Indies (Montserrat).[1]

Essential Oil Characteristics

Ajowan oil is a yellow-orange to pale brownish liquid with a pungent, herbaceous spicy and medicinal odour reminiscent of red thyme.[1]

Historical and Traditional Uses

Ajowan has been used in India as an Ayurveda herb. Infusion of the seeds may be used to alleviate digestive problems and to treat infections. The seeds are used in curry powders.[2]

Ajowan oil has been used by the pharmaceutical industry for the isolation of thymol. However, since the introduction of synthetic thymol, ajowan oil has ceased to be an important source of thymol as it is not economic to remove natural thymol from the oil.[1]

Typical Constituents

A typical chemical composition of ajowan oil is reported as follows: α-pinene (0.63%), β-pinene (1.56%), camphene (0.63%), limonene (2.25%), γ-terpinene (20.35%), p-cymene (23.78%), thymol (48.5%), carvacrol (6.8%).[3]

Contra-indications and Hazards

Due to the high thymol/carvacrol content, ajowan is classified as a dermal irritant and a mucous membrane irritant.[2,4]

Bitter Almond

Botany and Origins

Bitter almond oil is distilled from the partially de-oleated press-cake of bitter almond kernels from the tree of *Prunus amygdalus* var *amara*.[1] The bitter almond tree is cultivated in the USA, Israel, Syria, Turkey, Morocco, Spain and France.[1]

A fixed oil is produced by separating the kernels from their shells and crushing them in a press. The fixed oil does not contain benzaldehyde or hydrocyanic acid (HCN). The remaining almond meal is macerated in warm water for 12 to 24 hours. During maceration, the naturally occurring glycoside amygdalin is hydrolysed into benzaldehyde and hydrocyanic acid (also known as prussic acid). These constituents are not present in the fixed oil, kernel or in the dry deoleated press-cake.[1]

HCN is extremely toxic as little as 0.02 g of this substance is lethal to the average human being. This amount of HCN can be found in about 8 to 10 drops of the crude unrectified oil.[1]

Before the oil is used for food flavouring the HCN is removed by rectifying and alkali washing.[1]

Essential Oil Characteristics

Bitter almond oil is a colourless liquid with a strong sweet and clean odour, reminiscent of crushed, wet bitter almonds or a high-grade benzaldehyde.[1]

Historical and Traditional Uses

Rectified bitter almond oil is extensively used to make 'almond essence' or as a food flavouring. The odour is familiar to those who enjoy the European candy 'Marzipan'.[1,2]

Bitter almond oil, which is free of HCN, can be regarded as pure benzaldehyde. It is reported to have antipeptic, local anaesthetic and antispasmodic properties.[4] Rectified bitter almond oil is now being replaced by synthetic benzaldehyde in food flavouring.[4]

Typical Constituents

A typical chemical composition of bitter almond oil is reported as follows: benzaldehyde (95%), HCN (2–4%).[5]

Contra-indications and Hazards

Bitter almond oil is considered extremely toxic and should not be used in aromatherapy.[2,4]

Boldo

Botany and Origins

The small tree, *Peumus boldus*, grows wild in Chile, South America. The leaves are collected for pharmaceutical purposes, and the essential oil is steam-distilled from dried leaves.

Essential Oil Characteristics

Boldo oil is yellow and has a strong, spicy odour, somewhat reminiscent of wormseed.[1]

Historical and Traditional Uses

Boldo has long been recognised in South America as a valuable cure for gonorrhoea and for the treatment of genito-urinary inflammation.[2]

The herb is reported to have choleretic, diuretic, stomachic and cholagogic properties.[2,5,8]

An infusion of the dried leaves or an alcoholic extract is recommended for the treatment of gall stones, pain in the liver and gall bladder, cystitis and rheumatism.[6]

Typical Constituents

A typical chemical composition of boldo oil is reported as follows: α-pinene (4.0%), β-pinene (0.8%), camphene (0.6%), limonene (1.6%), δ-terpinene (1.0%), ascaridole (16.1%), 1,8-cineole (16.0%), p-cymene (28.6%), linalool (9.1%).[7]

Contra-indications and Hazards

Boldo oil is considered highly toxic and neurotoxic. It has an LD_{50} of 0.13 g/kg.[4] The toxicity of boldo is due to ascaridole. Boldo essential oil should not be used in aromatherapy.[2,4]

Buchu

Botany and Origins

The essential oil of buchu is steam-distilled from the dried leaves of *Agathosma betulina* or *Agathosma crenulata*, a herb that grows wild and abundantly in South Africa.

Essential Oil Characteristics

Buchu oil is a yellowish to brownish-yellow liquid, oily and somewhat viscous, depending on the age of the oil and the dryness of the plant material prior to distillation. The odour is very peculiar: a strong bitter-sweet somewhat minty-camphoraceous root-like, penetrating odour, reminiscent of pennyroyal.[1]

Historical and Traditional Uses

The first recorded use of Buchu was in 1653. The Bushmen, the Hottentot and other tribes had been using it in traditional ceremonies, as an insect repellent, as a perfume, healing of sores and contusions, for the relief from rheumatism and as a 'pick me up' tonic.[9]

Herbal preparations of buchu are used for the treatment of cystitis, urethritis, nephritis and catarrh of the bladder.[5,6,8]

Buchu oil is used as a component in the flavouring of black currant. *A. betulina* is preferred because of its higher diosphenols that are considered to be more desirable flavour components.[5]

Typical Constituents

Agathosma betulina oil contains sulphurated terpenoid ketones such as 8-mercapto-p, menthane-3-one and 8-acetylthio-p.menthone-3-one.[9] A typical chemical composition of *Agathosma crenulata* oil is reported as follows: d-pulegone (50%), iso-pulegone (10%), diosphenol (1%), 4-diosphenol (1%), iso-menthone (22%), menthone (6%).[9]

Contra-indications and Hazards

As the essential oil from *A. crenulata* contains pulegone, it is likely to have similar toxicity to that of pennyroyal. It is not recommended for use in aromatherapy.[2,4]

Calamus

Botany and Origins

Calamus oil is steam-distilled from the roots of the wild growing or cultivated *Acorus calamus*, a perennial plant that is known in the USA as 'sweet flag'. It is a decorative plant and grows wild all over the swampy areas of the temperate zones in Europe, Asia and America. The roots can be dried without substantial loss of essential oil provided they are kept unpeeled.[1]

Calamus is also known as Acorus or sweet flag root.[1] Certain varieties of *Acorus calamus* have a higher potential for toxicity due to β-asarone than others. Some species are β-asarone free. The table below summarises the β-asarone content in the essential oil of the three most commonly available varieties:[10]

Variety	Origin	β-asarone %
americanus	Nth America	absent
calamus	Europe	< 10%
angustatus	India	Up to 80–96%

Essential Oil Characteristics

Calamus oil is generally a pale-yellow to pale-brown, viscous liquid of a warm, woody-spicy and pleasant odour with great tenacity.[1]

Historical and Traditional Uses

Calamus root is used in herbal medicine as an infusion or tincture for its carminative, spasmolytic and diaphoretic properties.[6]

The antispasmodic activity of calamus is proportional to the amount of β-asarone, with the spasmolytic activity decreasing with higher β-asarone concentrations.[10] It is recommended for the treatment of acute and chronic dyspepsia, gastritis, gastric ulcer, anorexia and intestinal colic.[5,6] The essential oil is used as a fragrance component in soaps, detergents, cosmetics and perfumes.[5]

Typical Constituents

A typical chemical composition of calamus oil is reported as follows: acorenone (8.0%), β-gurjunene (6.7%), isoshyobunone (6.2%), β-asarone (5.2%), calamendiol (3.8%), α-selinene (3.8%), α-calacorene (3.5%), calamusenone (3.2%), camphone (3.2%), shyobunone (2.6%).[9]

Contra-indications and Hazards

Clinical trials involving rodents have demonstrated the carcinogenic activity of calamus.[4,10,11] Calamus oil contains the carcinogenic constituent β-asarone, a compound which belongs to the chemical group known as phenyl propanoids.[10]

β-asarone is a procarcinogen. This means that it must first undergo metabolic hydroxylation in the liver before achieving toxicity. Cytochrome P_{450} in the hepatocytes is responsible for secreting the hydolysing enzymes that convert β-asarone into its genotoxic epoxide structure.[10]

Calamus oil is considered extremely toxic, carcinogenic and hepatotoxic. It should not be used in aromatherapy.[2,4]

Camphor

Botany and Origins

Camphor oil is produced by steam distillation from the wood, root stumps and branches of *Cinnamomum camphora*, also known as Hon-Sho, growing in Formosa and Japan.[1]

Along with the crude oil a solid, partly crystalline mass of crude camphor is extracted. The essential oil is separated from the crude camphor by filter pressing. This yields the crude camphor oil that is subsequently rectified under vacuum, yielding another 50% of crude camphor. The remaining 50% of the filter-pressed crude camphor oil is now free of camphor. It contains light terpenes, cineole, safrole, terpineol and sesquiterpene alcohols.[1] These constituents are separated into various fractions that are referred to as:

- white camphor — the light fraction containing cineole and monoterpenes
- brown camphor — the medium to heavy fraction which contains up to 80% safrole and some terpineol
- blue camphor — the heavy fraction which contains sesquiterpenes.[1]

White camphor has the lowest boiling point and does not contain any safrole. However, it contains around 30 to 50% camphor.[4] This is the oil that is commonly sold in aromatherapy as camphor.

Historical and Traditional Uses

White camphor has a long-standing traditional use in the treatment of respiratory tract infections. It is attributed with antiseptic, bactericidal, diuretic, expectorant, stimulant, rubefacient and vermifuge properties.[2,8]

White camphor is recommended for the treatment of acne, skin inflammations, oily skin, arthritis, muscular aches and pains, rheumatism and for respiratory conditions such as bronchitis, coughs and colds.[2]

Synthetic camphor is prepared from turpentine oil. The action of hydrogen chloride on pinene is converted into bornyl chloride which, on treatment with sodium acetate, yields isobornyl acetate. Hydrolysis of this to isoborneol and subsequent oxidation gives camphor.[12]

Typical Constituents

The chemistry of camphor is very complex. There are five main chemotypes:

- camphor
- cineole
- safrole
- linalool
- sesquiterpenes.

A typical chemical composition of camphor oil is reported as follows: α-pinene (3.7%), camphene (1.64%), β-pinene (1.26%), sabinene (1.47%), phellandrene (0.17%), limonene (2.71%), 1,8-cineole (4.75%), γ-terpinene (0.24%), p-cymene (0.14%), terpinolene (0.3%), furfural (0.16%), camphor (51.5%), linalool (0.68%), bornyl acetate (0.02%), terpinen-4-ol (0.57%), caryophyllene (1.49%), borneol (0.02%), piperitone (2.41%), geraniol (0.63%), safrole (13.4%), cinnamaldehyde (0.08%), methyl cinnamate (0.08%), eugenol (0.12%).[13]

Brown camphor contains approximately 80% safrole and yellow camphor contains 10 to 20% safrole and 15 to 23% camphor.[4]

Contra-indications and Hazards

White camphor — case studies are cited in which one teaspoon of camphorated oil, equivalent to about 1 mL of camphor, was lethal to a 16-month-old child and a 19-month-old child.[4]

The *British Medical Journal* reported an incident involving a man who attempted suicide by ingesting 150 mL of camphorated oil (a camphorated oil is usually 20% camphor essential oil in cottonseed oil). He suffered peripheral circulatory shock, severe dehydration due to vomiting, and three attacks of severe and prolonged grand mal epilepsy. He recovered after intensive supportive treatment. The dosage was believed to be one of the highest to be followed by survival.[9]

Camphor preparations should not be used in the facial region of infants and small children, especially around the nasal area.[8]

As long as white camphor essential oil does not contain safrole it is relatively non-toxic, non-sensitising and non-irritating.[2] However, the camphor content of white camphor suggests that it is convulsant and neurotoxic.[4]

Yellow and brown camphor — safrole has been proven to be a carcinogen in animal trials.[4,10]

Safrole, like estragole and β-asarone, though not directly hepatocarcinogenic, is readily converted by enzymatic activation in the liver to substances which are known to be toxic. Cytochrome P_{450} in the hepatocytes is responsible for secreting the hydolysing enzymes that convert safrole into dihydrodiol and glutathione conjugates and allylic epoxide intermediates which have the potential to generate extensive genetic and cellular toxicity.[10]

The safrole content of yellow and brown camphor indicates that it is carcinogenic and hepatotoxic. Yellow and brown camphor oil should not be used in aromatherapy.[2,4]

Cassia

Botany and Origins

Cassia oil, known as Chinese cinnamon oil, is steam-distilled from the leaves of *Cinnamomum cassia*, a large slender tree that grows in China. The bark is distilled together with the leaves and the stalks, twigs and waste material from the collection of the bark of the cassia tree.

Essential Oil Characteristics

The oil is a dark-brown liquid with a strong, spicy, warm and woody-resinous odour with intensely sweet, somewhat balsamic undertones.[1]

Historical and Traditional Uses

The dried herb is traditionally used as a spice. In traditional medicine it has been used for digestive complaints. It is used in much the same way as cinnamon, mainly for digestive complaints such as flatulence, dyspepsia, colic, diarrhoea and nausea.[6]

Typical Constituents

A typical chemical composition of cassia oil is reported as follows: cinnamic aldehyde (87%), cinnamyl acetate (0.08%), benzaldehyde (4.73%), linalool (0.13%), chavicol (0.33%).[14]

Contra-indications and Hazards

It contains 75–90% cinnamaldehyde that is the cause of the cassia's potent dermal sensitiser and irritant. It is not recommended for use on the skin.[2,4]

Costus

Botany and Origins

Costus oil is steam-distilled from the comminuted dried roots of *Saussurea lappa*, a large plant that is found growing wild in the Himalayan highlands at high altitude.[1]

Essential Oil Characteristics

Costus oil is a pale-yellow to brownish-yellow, very viscous liquid with an extremely tenacious odour, reminiscent of old precious wood and orris oil.[1]

Historical and Traditional Uses

The root has been used in India and China for digestive complaints, respiratory problems such as asthma and coughs and for infections such as cholera and typhoid.[2,5] Costus and its derivatives are used as fixatives and fragrance components in cosmetics and perfumes.[5]

Typical Constituents

The essential oil of costus is predominantly made up of sesquiterpene lactones such as dehydrocostus lactone and costunolide, which together make up approximately 50% of the oil, α- and β-cyclocostunolide, alantolactone, isoalantolactone, dehydrocostus lactone and cynaropicrin.[5]

Contra-indications and Hazards

Costus is non-toxic, non-irritant and a possible sensitiser.[2] Costus is classified as a severe dermal sensitiser.[4,5]

The major constituent in costus oil responsible for the oil's extreme dermal sensitisation properties is costuslactone.[5]

Elecampane

Botany and Origins

An essential oil is extracted by steam distillation from the roots and rhizomes of *Inula helenium*, a tall plant related to the sunflower. Elecampane is cultivated in Belgium, Germany, France and south-eastern Europe.

Essential Oil Characteristics

The oil is dark yellow to brownish-yellow with an odour that has some resemblance to those of calamus and costus.[1]

Historical and Traditional Use

Elecampane root is an expectorant, antitussive, diaphoretic and bactericidal and is indicated for bronchial or tracheal catarrh, cough of pulmonary tuberculosis and irritating cough in children.[5,6]

The German Commission E Monographs recommend elecampane preparations for diseases of the respiratory tract, gastrointestinal tract and the urinary system.[8]

Typical Constituents

Elecampane oil is composed primarily of sesquiterpene lactones such as alantolactone (also called helenin), isoalantolactone, dihydroisoalantolactone and dihydroalantolactone.[5]

Contra-indications and Hazards

The severe dermal sensitisation of elecampane essential oil is due to alantolactone.[3,4,8] The oil is not recommended for use in aromatherapy.[2,4]

Horseradish

Botany and Origins

Horseradish essential oil is obtained by water and steam distillation of the comminuted horseradish root from *Cochlearia armoracia*.

Essential Oil Characteristics

The essential oil is pale yellow to almost colourless and it has an intense sharp odour reminiscent of mustard oil with a lachrymatory effect.[1]

Historical and Traditional Uses

The roots and leaves of horseradish have been universally used as a medicine and condiment. The root is considered a stimulant, rubefacient, diuretic and antiseptic.[2]

Grieve recommends taking horseradish as a condiment with oily fish or rich meat, by itself, steeped in vinegar or in a plain sauce, as it acts as an excellent stimulant of the digestive system. She suggests eating it with meals to get rid of persistent cough following influenza.[16]

Typical Constituents

A typical chemical composition of horseradish oil is reported as follows: allyl isothiocyanate (44.3–55.7%), phenyl ethyl isothiocynanate (38.4–51.3%).[15]

Contra-indications and Hazards

The hazardous constituent found in horseradish oil is allyl isothiocynate. Horseradish oil is considered a severe toxic, severe dermal irritant and a severe mucous membrane irritant. Allyl isothiocynate is extremely toxic and a violent irritant to mucous membranes and the skin. Horseradish essential oil should not be used in aromatherapy.[2,4]

Mustard

Botany and Origins

Mustard seeds come from *Brassica nigra*, known as black mustard; *Brassica juncea*, known as brown mustard; and *Sinapis alba*, known as white mustard. Arctander says that only black mustard yields an essential oil. *Brassica nigra* originates in south-eastern Europe and the eastern Mediterranean countries.[1] However Leung says that an essential oil is also available from the brown mustard. Brown mustard is native to Asia.[5]

The essential oil is produced by steam and water distillation of the enzymatically hydrolysed suspension of comminuted press-cakes of black mustard seed in warm water. A glucoside located in the seed is decomposed by hydrolysis under the influence of an enzyme which is present in other cells of the seed.[1]

Essential Oil Characteristics

Mustard oil is a clear to pale-yellow mobile liquid with an extremely sharp, irritating odour.[1]

Historical and Traditional Uses

White mustard seeds have also been used as poultices to relieve congestion and to alleviate neuralgia and other pains and spasms. An infusion of the seeds is said to relieve chronic bronchitis and the pain of rheumatism.[5,8,16]

Mustard oil is used in very low dilutions (less than 0.2%) as a flavour ingredient in many food products such as meat and meat products, desserts, condiments and relishes.[5]

Typical Constituents

The hazardous constituent found in mustard oil is allyl isothiocynate (approximately 99%).[4]

Contra-indications and Hazards

Mustard oil should not be used in aromatherapy.[2,4] It is considered one of the most hazardous essential oils.[4] The essential oil is not present in the free state in the seed or powdered seed, but in the form of glycosides, so preparations made from these by mechanical means do not contain allyl isothiocyanate.[4]

Inhalation of mustard oil produces extremely unpleasant sensations in the head and irritates the eyes and mucous membranes of the nose and respiratory system. In the skin, mustard oil produces almost instant blistering.[4,5]

Oregano

Botany and Origins

Oregano oil is steam-distilled from the dried, flowering herb of several plant species native to Europe. The most commonly used plants are:

- *Thymus capitus*
- *Origanum vulgare*
- *Origanum smyrnaeceum*
- *Origanum maru.*

Essential Oil Characteristics

Origanum oils have a strong, herbaceous, camphoraceous odour with a dry-woody and phenolic dry-out.[1]

Historical and Traditional Uses

Origanum vulgare is the true oregano of the garden herb, which has a very ancient use as a medicine and a culinary herb.

The oil has traditionally been used as a stimulant, carminative, diaphoretic and a nerve tonic. It is recommended for the treatment of indigestion, rheumatism, headaches, respiratory problems such as asthma, coughing and bronchitis and for influenza.[2,5,17,18]

Typical Constituents

A typical chemical composition of oregano oil is reported as follows: carvacrol (14.0%), thymol (12%), p-cymene (3.0%), cis-ocimene (13.5%), caryophyllene (9.2%), linalool (3.0%).[19]

Contra-indications and Hazards

The main constituents in oregano oil are carvacrol and thymol. Both constituents are phenols that contribute to oregano's skin irritant and mucous membrane irritant properties.[2,4]

Oregano oil is not recommended for use on persons with hypersensitive skin, diseased or damaged skin or children under 2 years of age.[4]

Parsley Seed

Botany and Origins

Parsley seed oil is produced by the steam distillation of the ripe fruit (seed) of *Petroselinum sativum*, the common garden parsley.

Essential Oil Characteristics

The oil is a yellowish to amber-coloured liquid with a warm-woody, spicy, somewhat sweet-herbaceous odour.[1]

Historical and Traditional Uses

Parsley seed oil is mainly used for its depurative and diuretic properties. Hot compresses over the bladder are beneficial for treating cystitis and kidney problems.[20] It is also recommended as a uterine tonic and should be useful for the treatment of amenorrhoea and dysmenorrhoea.[2,20]

It has been recommended for treating bruises as it assists in shrinking the broken blood vessels immediately below the skin.[20]

Apiol is reported to be a spasmolytic, vasodilator and emmenagogue. Apiol may cause vascular congestion and increased smooth muscle contractibility in the bladder, intestine and uterus; damage to the kidney epithelia and heart arrhythmia; may cause fatty liver, emaciation and bleeding of mucous membranes of the gastrointestinal tract.[5,8] Parsley seed has been traditionally used as an abortifacient.[4,8]

Typical Constituents

Three chemotypes of parsley seed oil exist. The typical chemical composition of each of the chemotypes is as follows:[21]

myristicin chemotype — myristicin (49–77%), 2,3,4,5-tetramethyoxyallylbenzene (1–23%) apiol (0 3.0%).

apiol chemotype — myristicin (9–30%), 2,3,4,5-tetramethyoxyallylbenzene (trace–6%) apoil (58–80%).

2,3,4,5-tetramethyoxyallylbenzene chemotype — myristicin (26–37%), 2,3,4,5-tetramethyoxyallylbenzene (52–57%) apoil (0 to trace).

Contra-indications and Hazards

The hazardous constituent in parsley seed is apiol. This is believed to contribute to the oil's abortifacient properties. The oil also contains myristicin. While myristicin is known to be psychotropic, Tisserand reports that parsley seed oil does not exhibit any neurotoxic properties.[4] Parsley seed oil is contra-indicated in pregnancy and inflammatory kidney diseases.[2,4]

Pennyroyal

Botany and Origins

Pennyroyal oil is steam-distilled from the freshly harvested dried herb *Mentha pulegium,* which is also referred to as European pennyroyal. Another plant called American pennyroyal *(Hedeoma pulegeoides)* also produces an essential oil rich in pulegone.[1]

Essential Oil Characteristics

The oil is a pale-yellow to almost colourless mobile liquid of a very fresh, strong herbaceous-minty aroma.[1]

Historical and Traditional Uses

Pennyroyal herb is used for the treatment of flatulence, dyspepsia, intestinal colic, the common cold, delayed menstruation and gout.[6] The essential oil is recommended for the treatment of dyspepsia, nausea, vomiting, amenorrhoea and dysmenorrhoea and is reputed to be an excellent flea and mosquito repellent.[18] Pennyroyal has enjoyed folk status as an abortifacient since ancient times.[22]

Typical Constituents

A typical chemical composition of pennyroyal oil is reported as follows: pulegone (52–63.5%), menthone (0.5–30.8%), iso-menthone (5.2–19.8%), neomenthone (3.0%).[23]

Contra-indications and Hazards

The toxicity of pennyroyal is due to the pulegone content, which is toxic to the liver because it is metabolised to epoxides.[4,10]

Tisserand and Balacs report several fatalities involving the ingestion of pennyroyal oil.[4] One case involves that of an 18-year-old woman who died after ingesting the equivalent of 24 g of pulegone. She was alternately lethargic or agitated, suffered from nausea and abdominal pain, and she developed massive hepatic necrosis and renal insufficiency.[24]

The emergency treatment for pennyroyal poisoning is the administration of N-acetylcysteine, as soon as possible after ingestion (140 mg/kg then 70 mg/kg every four hours). N-acetylcysteine is an antioxidant agent that protects against endotoxemia.[10,11]

Pennyroyal oil is considered toxic and an abortifacient. It is not recommended for use in aromatherapy.[2,4]

Rue

Botany and Origins

Rue oil is steam-distilled from the freshly harvested, blooming or fruit-bearing plant *Ruta montana*.

Essential Oil Characteristics

Rue oil is a yellow to orange-yellow material, liquid at room temperature, but solid at temperatures below 10°C. The odour is sharp-herbaceous, distinctive fruity-orange-like with a characteristic bitter acrid undertone that makes the overall impression an unpleasant one.[1]

Historical and Traditional Uses

Rue oil has been reported as having anthelmintic activities.[5] Rue oil has also been used as a source of natural 2-undecanone, a starting material for the synthesis of methylnonyl acetaldehyde, a valuable perfume chemical.[1] Rue herb has been used as an emmenagogue, uterine stimulant, for the treatment of snake and insect bites and as a hemostatic.[5]

Typical Constituents

A typical chemical composition of rue oil is reported as follows: 2-nonanone (18%), 2-nonyl acetate (11.0%), 2-undecanone (30%), 2-butanone (3.0%), psoralen (1.28%), bergapten and xanthotoxin (7.24%).[25]

Rue oil contains several ketones that contribute to its hazards. It also contains several furanocoumarins, bergapten, xanthotoxin and psoralen, which have phototoxic effects.

Contra-indications and Hazards

When applied to the skin, rue oil may produce a burning sensation, erythema (redness) and vesication (blisters).[5] Rue oil is a potential abortifacient, a neurotoxin, a skin and mucous membrane irritant and phototoxic.[2,4,5] It should not be used in aromatherapy.

Sassafras

Botany and Origins

Sassafras oil is steam-distilled from the roots or root bark of *Sassafras albidum*, a medium-sized North American tree. The essential oil exists in the root bark tissue right beneath the cork, but the root wood itself also contains some essential oil. The roots and stumps are comminuted into chips and steam-distilled.[1]

Very little oil is produced from *Sassafras albidum* in the USA. Most so-called sassafras oils come from *Ocotea pretiosa* in Brazil or *Cinnamomum porrectum* in China.[1]

Essential Oil Characteristics

Sassafras oil is a yellow to pale-brownish-yellow oily liquid of sweet spicy and slightly camphoraceous odour with a long-lasting woody floral and sweet undertone.[1]

Historical and Traditional Uses

It was first exported to England by the early European settlers in the 17th century, who learned of its medicinal properties from the native Americans. It is reported to have diaphoretic and diuretic properties and was used in the treatment of colds, flu and arthritic pains.[10]

Natural root beer, popular in the USA, was made with sassafras. Sassafras is banned as its major constituent, safrole, is now banned as a food additive.[1]

Sassafras was traditionally used in treating bronchitis, high blood pressure of elderly people, rheumatism, gout, arthritis, skin problems and kidney problems. It was also recommended for head lice and cutaneous eruptions.[5,6]

Typical Constituents

A typical chemical composition of sassafras oil is reported as follows: safrole (80–90%), 5-methyoxy-eugenol, asarone, coniferaldehyde, camphone, and traces of menthone, thujone, anethole, apiol, elimicin, myristicin and eugenol.[26]

Contra-indications and Hazards

The hazardous constituent is safrole. According to research cited by Tisserand, safrole is highly toxic on chronic dosing, 95% lethal to rats at 10,000 ppm after 19 days of dosing. When administered orally, safrole is a low-level hepatic carcinogen in rats.[4]

Safrole is readily converted by enzymatic activation in the liver to substances which are known to be toxic. Cytochrome P_{450} in the hepatocytes is responsible for secreting the hydolysing enzymes that convert safrole into dihydrodiol and glutathione conjugates and allylic epoxide intermediates which have the potential to generate extensive genetic and cellular toxicity.[10]

Sassafras oil has been classified as being a potential carcinogenic. The UK and EC 'standard permitted proportion' of safrole in food flavouring is 0.001 g/kg of food. The FDA has banned safrole as a food additive. Sassafras should not be used in aromatherapy.[4]

Savin

Botany and Origins

Savin oil is steam-distilled from the leaves and twigs of a small bush, *Juniperus sabina*. Savin oil may have been confused with *Juniperus communis*. This is why common juniper berry oil is mistakenly reputed to be an abortifacient.

Essential Oil Characteristics

Savin oil is a pale-yellow to almost colourless liquid with a unique, very unpleasant, nauseating odour reminiscent of juniper berry oil and cypress oil.[1]

Historical and Traditional Uses

It was once used as an ointment or dressing for blisters to promote discharge and for syphilitic warts and other skin problems. It is not administered nowadays because of its toxicity.[16]

Typical Constituents

A typical chemical composition of savin oil is reported as follows: sabinyl acetate (37.5–38%), sabinene (26–30%), α-pinene (2.2–6.8%), limonene (0.6–1.2%), terpinen-4-ol (2.0–3.2%), α-cadinene (1.5–4.5%).[27]

Contra-indications and Hazards

Savin oil is toxic and an abortifacient. It should not be used in aromatherapy.[2]

Savory (Summer and Winter)

Botany and Origins

Various species of savory are steam-distilled to produce an essential oil. These are known as summer savory, distilled from *Satureia hortensis*, and winter savory, distilled from *Satureia montana*. In France, *Satureia hortensis* is cultivated and *Satureia montana* grows wild.[1]

Essential Oil Characteristics

Savory oil is a pale-yellow to almost colourless liquid with a fresh medicinal odour, reminiscent of sage and thyme.[1]

Historical and Traditional Uses

Both summer savory and winter savory are used as a tea for the carminative, expectorant and tonic properties.[2,5] Both varieties of savory can be used for treating stomach and intestinal disorders such as cramps, nausea and indigestion. Summer savory oil is reported to have excellent antimicrobial properties.[5]

Typical Constituents

A typical chemical composition of winter savory oil is reported as follows: carvacrol (60–75%), thymol (1.0–5.0%), p-cymene (10–20%), γ-terpineol (2.0–10.0%), 1,8-cineole (3.8%), borneol (12.5%), α-terpineol (2.5%).[28]

Summer and winter savory oils have a high percentage of carvacrol and thymol, phenols which contribute to the oil's skin irritant properties.

Contra-indications and Hazards

Summer and winter savory essential oils are dermal irritants and mucous membrane irritants.[2,4] Persons with sensitive skin and children under the age of two should not use the oil. The oil should not be used in concentrations of more than 1%.[4]

Tansy

Botany and Origins

The essential oil is steam-distilled from the flowering herb *Tanacetum vulgare*.

Essential Oil Characteristics

Tansy oil is a yellowish to orange-olive-coloured liquid with a warm, almost sharp spicy, dry and herbaceous odour.[1]

Historical and Traditional Uses

Traditionally tansy is used to expel worms, to treat colds and fever, to prevent possible miscarriage and to ease dyspepsia and cramping pains. Externally, the crushed leaves were used as a remedy for scabies, bruises, sprains and rheumatism. The herb is an effective vermifuge and anthelmintic.[6,29]

Typical Constituents

A typical chemical composition of tansy oil is reported as follows: thujone (66–81%), isopinocamphone, camphor, boneol, camphone, artemisone, piperitone.[9]

The oil contains a higher percentage of thujone, a ketone which contributes to the oil's toxic and neurotoxic properties.

Contra-indications and Hazards

Tansy oil is toxic and neurotoxic. Tansy oil should not be used in aromatherapy.[2,4]

Thuja

Botany and Origins

Thuja oil is distilled from the leaves and twigs of *Thuja occidentalis*. Thuja oil is also known as cedarleaf oil.

Essential Oil Characteristics

Thuja oil is a pale-yellow to almost colourless, mobile liquid with an intensely sharp, fresh, camphoraceous odour.[1]

Historical and Traditional Uses

Decoctions of the fresh leaves can be used to treat amenorrhoea, rheumatism, cough, bronchial catarrh, fever and gout.[5,6,29] Externally, it is used to treat warts and ringworm.[29]

Typical Constituents

A typical chemical composition of thuja oil is reported as follows: α-thujone (60.0%), β-thujone (9.5%), α-pinene (1.3%), camphene (1.2%), δ-sabinene (1.8%), fenchone (14%), camphone (2.0%), terpinen-4-ol (1.2%) and bornyl acetate (2.3%).[30]

The main constituents found in thuja oil are thujone (40–80%), fenchone (7–15%), camphor (2–3%). All these constituents are ketones.

Contra-indications and Hazards

Due to the high percentage of thujone, the oil is toxic and neurotoxic. Thuja essential oil should not be used in aromatherapy.[2,4,5] Toxic signs of ingestion of thuja oil are convulsions, gastroenteritis, flatulence and hypertension.[4]

Wintergreen

Botany and Origins

Wintergreen oil is derived by water distillation of the leaves of *Gaultheria procumbens*. Prior to distillation, the leaves are exposed to enzymatic action in warm water. During this process methyl salicylate is formed as a decomposition product from a glycoside in the plant material.[1]

Essential Oil Characteristics

Wintergreen oil is a pale-yellow to yellow-pink-coloured liquid with an intense sweet-aromatic odour.

Historical and Traditional Uses

Wintergreen oil is recommended for external application as a liniment because of its anti-inflammatory and antirheumatic properties. It is a specific for rheumatoid arthritis.[6,29]

Salicylates have the ability to suppress the synthesis of prostaglandins, which have an integral role in the management of pain and inflammation.[10]

The oil is extensively used as a flavouring for toothpaste, chewing gum and soft drinks.[2,5]

Typical Constituents

The main constituent found in wintergreen oil is methyl salicylate (98%). Most commercial wintergreen oils are in fact synthetic methyl salicylate.[5]

Contra-indications and Hazards

Numerous cases of methyl salicylate poisoning have been reported. Signs of methyl salicylate poisoning included CNS excitation, rapid breathing, fever, high blood pressure, convulsions and coma.[4] Tisserand cites research which shows that methyl salicylate can be absorbed transdermally in sufficient quantities to cause poisoning in humans.[4]

Studies indicate that compounds containing salicylates such as wintergreen potentiate blood-thinning drugs such as warfarin.[4,10] Wintergreen oil is considered toxic and should not be used in aromatherapy.[2,4] However, the British Herbal Pharmacopoeia recommends using wintergreen externally as a liniment.[6]

Wormseed

Botany and Origins

Wormseed oil is distilled from the dried herb of *Chenopodium ambrosioides*. This plant grows wild in the USA and India. Also known as chenopodium oil.

Essential Oil Characteristics

Wormseed oil is pale yellow to almost colourless with a heavy unpleasant, nauseating odour. The odour is reminiscent of savin.[1]

Historical and Traditional Uses

Wormseed oil is used as an anthelmintic for the treatment of roundworm, hookworms and dwarf tapeworms.[5]

Typical Constituents

A typical chemical composition of wormseed oil is reported as follows: ascaridole (60–80%), cymene, limonene, terpinene, myrcene.[4] The toxic constituent found in wormseed oil is ascaridole.

Contra-indications and Hazards

Wormseed oil is considered to be very toxic. Toxic effects include irritation of skin and mucous membranes, vomiting, headaches, vertigo, kidney and liver damage, temporary deafness and circulatory collapse.[4] Wormseed oil is toxic and neurotoxic. It should not be used in aromatherapy.[2,4]

Wormwood

Botany and Origins

Wormwood oil is steam-distilled from the dried herb (leaves and flowers) of *Artemisia absinthium*. It is a native of central and southern Europe, where it grows wild in abundance.

Essential Oil Characteristics

Wormwood oil is a very dark green, brownish-green or bluish-green coloured liquid with an odour that is intensely herbaceous, green, warm and deep.[1]

Historical and Traditional Uses

Wormwood has traditionally been used as a digestive tonic for the treatment of loss of appetite and indigestion.[6,8,29] It is highly recommended for the treatment of worm infestations such as roundworm and pinworm.[29]

Wormwood was used in the liqueur absinthe. Prolonged consumption of this drink led to a condition known as 'absinthism'. The symptoms included auditory and visual hallucinations, hyperexcitability, intellectual enfeeblement and addiction.[31]

In 1915, France banned the production of absinthe containing wormwood. It was claimed that wormwood acted as a narcotic in higher doses and was habit-forming.[31]

Typical Constituents

A typical chemical composition of wormwood oil is reported as follows: α-thujone (2.76%), β-thujone (46.44%), sabinene (2.76%), myrcene (1.0%), trans-sabinol (3.2%), trans-sabinyl acetate and linalyl acetate (27.78%) and geranyl propionate (1.4%).[32]

Contra-indications and Hazards

The toxicity of wormwood oil is associated with the high thujone content. It has been suggested that thujone interacts with the same central nervous system receptor sites as tetrahydrocannabinol, the psychoactive compound in marijuana.[4,10]

Long-term use or high dosage of products high in thujone can cause restlessness, vomiting, vertigo, tremors, renal damage and convulsions.[10] Wormwood oil is considered toxic and neurotoxic and should not be used in aromatherapy.[2,4]

References

1. Arctander S. *Perfume and flavour materials of natural origin*. Allured Publishing, USA, 1994.
2. Lawless J. *The encyclopaedia of essential oils*. Element Books Limited, Great Britain, 1992.
3. Lawrence B. *Ajowan oil*. Perfumer and Flavorist 1979; 4(2): 53.
4. Tisserand R, Balacs T. *Essential oil safety*. Churchill Livingstone, UK, 1995.
5. Leung A, Foster S. *Encyclopaedia of common natural ingredients used in food, drugs and cosmetics*. John Wiley & Sons Inc, USA, 1996.
6. *British herbal pharmacopoeia*. British Herbal Medicine Association, England, 1983.
7. Lawrence B. *Boldo oil*. Perfumer and Flavorist 1977; 2(1): 3.
8. Blumenthal M, et al. *The complete German commission E monographs: Therapeutic Guide to Herbal Medicine*, American Botanical Council USA, 1998.
9. *A safety guide on the use of essential oils*. Compiled by The International School of Aromatherapy, Nature by Nature Oils Ltd, UK, 1993.
10. McGuffin M, et al. eds. *American Herbal Products Association's botanical safety handbook*. CRC Press, USA, 1997.
11. Bruneton J. *Pharmacognosy*. 2nd edn, Lavoisier Publishing Inc, France, 1999.
12. Evans WC. *Trease and Evans pharmacognosy*. WB Saunders, 15th edn. UK, 2002.
13. Lawrence B. *Camphor oil*. Perfumer and Flavorist 1979; 4(4): 54.

14. Lawrence B. *Cassia oil*. Perfumer and Flavorist 1978; 3(4): 54.
15. Lawrence B. *Horseradish oil*. Perfumer and Flavorist 1981; (.6)1: 45–6.
16. Grieves M. *A modern herbal*. Penguin, England, 1931.
17. Valnet J. *The practice of aromatherapy*. The C.W. Daniel Company Limited, Great Britain, 1982.
18. Lavabre M. *Aromatherapy workbook*. Healing Art Press, USA, 1990.
19. Lawrence B. *Oregano oil*. Perfumer and Flavorist 1989; 14(1): 36–9.
20. Davis P. *Aromatherapy A–Z* 2nd edn, The C.W. Daniel Company Limited, Great Britain, 1999.
21. Lawrence B. *Parsley seed. essential oils*: 1981–1987. Allured Publishing, USA, 1987: 27.
22. Riddle J. *Eve's herbs*. Harvard University Press, England, 1997.
23. Lawrence B. *European pennyroyal oil*. Perfumer and Flavorist 1978; 3(5): 35.
24. Bruneton J. *Toxic plants*. Lavoisier Publishing, France, 1999.
25. Lawrence B. *Rue oil*. Perfumer and Flavorist 1978; 3(2): 45.
26. Lawrence B. *Sassafras oil*. Perfumer and Flavorist 1978; 3(3): 46.
27. Lawrence B. *Savin oil*. Perfumer and Flavorist 1982; 7(4): 41.
28. Lawrence B. *Savory oil*. Perfumer and Flavorist 1981; 6(4): 73.
29. Hoffman D. *A new holistic herbal*. 3rd edn, Element Books Limited, Great Britain, 1990.
30. Lawrence B. *Thuja oil*. Perfumer and Flavorist 1979; 4(1): 48.
31. Turner R. *Absinthe: The green fairy*. The International Journal of Aromatherapy 1992; 17(2): 32.
32. Lawrence B. *Wormwood oil*. Perfumer and Flavorist 1992; 5(2): 6.

Unit IV

Practical Matters

Unit IV provides you with the knowledge and skills required for the practice of aromatherapy such as:

- The requirements for professional practice.
- The importance and role of a consultation before a treatment.
- The skills necessary to select and blend the appropriate essential oils.
- A step by step description of the aromatherapy massage technique.
- The ways in which aromatherapy can be utilised within a health care environment.

Unit IV includes the following chapters:

Requirements for Professional Practice

Objectives

After careful study of this chapter, you should be able to:

- define professionalism
- define the role of professional ethics
- explain how the practice of good ethics helps to build a successful aromatherapy practice
- explain the need for strict sanitary and safety practices
- identify the requirements for setting up a clinic
- develop business skills to establish a successful aromatherapy practice.

Introduction

In health care, practitioners of different modalities are able to perform their duties as prescribed by their occupation and their level of training.

Many occupations and professions have national or state regulatory and training boards to develop and upgrade professional standards and to regulate licensing procedures. However, at the time of publication, no state in Australia has adopted licensing procedures to regulate the practice of aromatherapy. Regardless of this, it is important for aromatherapists to practise within professional boundaries.

Professionalism

According to the Macquarie Dictionary, professionalism means:

> *following an occupation as a means of livelihood or for gain.*[1]

While there may be many definitions of the term 'professional', they all have the same meaning — a person who is focused on and committed to a given profession.

The term 'aromatherapy' has now entered the lingua franca of the health and beauty community. However, it is a concern that the failure to clearly define the term 'aromatherapy' has led to many unhelpful and inaccurate representations of aromatherapy. This may confuse the general public at a time when the real therapeutic values of aromatherapy are becoming more widely known in the community at large.

Aromatherapy is now recognised by many members of the community as a therapy that can offer genuine assistance to the health industry as a whole. Professional aromatherapists now play an important role in health care by:

- Saving taxpayers' money through the promotion and practice of preventative medicine.
- Reducing degenerative and iatrogenic diseases.
- Treating or managing many so-called incurable diseases that have defied the medical system with all its millions of dollars of research, latest technology and hospitals.
- Improving primary health care services offered in hospitals and aged care facilities.

The Professional Aromatherapist

How can you achieve a successful career as a professional aromatherapist?

Knowledge and Training

If you want to be successful in your aromatherapy practice you must prepare for success. Preparation, planning and performance are assets that help you do your job in the most professional manner. You should take every opportunity to pursue new avenues of knowledge.

Attend professional seminars, read trade journals and other publications relating to your business and become active in professional associations where you can exchange ideas with other dedicated people.

Image

To inspire confidence and trust in your client, you should project a well-groomed, professional appearance at all times. In an aromatherapy practice, personal health and good grooming are assets that client admire and are essential for your protection and that of the client.

The first impression is important and will begin with the waiting room. This is where you first greet the client; the room should be light and airy with a soothing décor. If the client has to wait, then have some interesting literature on aromatherapy available. Certificates and diplomas should always be displayed as a further reassurance of your standards. Your business image is important and should be built on good service and truth in advertising. Consistent high standards and good service are the foundations on which successful businesses are built.

Understand Human Relationships

In addition to gaining the necessary technical skills as a professional aromatherapist, you must be able to understand your clients' needs. This is the basis of good human relationships. A pleasant voice, good manners, cheerfulness, patience, tact, loyalty, empathy, and interest in the client's welfare are some of the desirable traits that help to build the client's confidence in you.

Client confidentiality is important as they often confide their personal feelings and they trust you not to betray their confidence. This is why listening is an invaluable asset. Listen with empathy, tactfully changing the subject when necessary.

Respect the therapeutic relationship between the client and the practitioner and refrain from crossing sexual boundaries. Since aromatherapy will involve massage, it is important that your client knows the difference between sensuality and sexuality, intimacy and touch. It is important that you act appropriately to avoid sexual harassment.

The following guidelines for good human relations will help you interact successfully with people from all walks of life:[2]

Tact

Tact is your ability to deal with a client who is overly critical, finds fault, and is difficult to please. It may be that he or she just wants attention. Tact can help you deal with this client in an impersonal but understanding manner. To be tactful is to be most considerate to all concerned.

Cheerfulness

A cheerful attitude and a pleasant nature will make a client feel at ease.

Patience

Patience is the ability to be tolerant under stressful or undesirable conditions. Your patience and understanding will help you deal with people who are ill. Patience will help you change negative feelings into more positive ones.

Honesty

Honesty does not mean you have to be brutally frank with a client. You can answer questions in a factual but tactful manner.

Intuition

Intuition is your ability to have insight into people's feelings. When you genuinely care for people, it is easier to show sympathy and understanding for their problems. People will often confide in you when their intuition tells them you are trustworthy.

Sense of Humour

It is important to have a sense of humour, especially when dealing with difficult people or situations. A good sense of humour helps you remain optimistic, courteous and in control.

Maturity

Maturity does not depend on age, but what you have gained from your life experience. Maturity is the quality of being reliable, responsible, self-disciplined and well adjusted.

Self-esteem

Self-esteem is projected by your attitudes about yourself and your profession. If you respect yourself and your profession, you will be respected by others.

Self-motivation

Self-motivation is your ability to set positive goals and put forth the energy and effort required to achieve those goals. It means making sacrifices when necessary to achieve your goals.

Professional Ethics

The role of professional associations has become increasingly more important as government legislation can often affect the rights of individual therapists. The advantages offered by a professional association may be:[3]

- enhanced professional self-identity
- unity that protects identity
- stronger direct professional representation
- stronger financial base
- enhanced public relations
- maintaining active research programmes.

The public should be confident that a professional association will have policies in areas relating to:

- safety issues
- control of unsatisfactory behaviour by therapists
- a requirement for continuing post-qualification training
- the need for all therapists to have completed accredited courses.

Most professional associations have a code of ethics which ensures that standards are established and maintained for the welfare of individual clients, your reputation and the reputation of the profession you represent.

A therapist who conducts himself or herself ethically gives the client confidence. A satisfied client is your best means of advertising because his or her recommendation helps you maintain public confidence and build a sound business. A code of ethics should include:[2]

- Treat all clients with the same fairness and courtesy.
- Provide the highest quality care for those seeking professional services.
- The consultation and all communication with the client must be confidential.
- The aromatherapist should perform only those services for which qualifications are held and should refer a client to an appropriate practitioner when indicated.
- Respect and cooperate with other ethical health care providers to promote health and wellbeing.
- Be honest in all advertising of services providing such advertising does not bring discredit on the profession of aromatherapy.

- Know and comply with all relevant rules, laws and regulations of your council, state and country.
- A therapist should not discriminate against colleagues or clients.
- A therapist should not deliberately mislead a client seeking advice.
- The clinic must be clean, neat and professionally presented to reflect the profession of aromatherapy.
- Maintain physical, mental and emotional wellbeing.
- All practitioners should maintain active participation in professional associations and should pursue continuing education and training.
- Maintain a professional dress code.

Sanitary Practices

In the health care profession every precaution must be taken to protect the health of the clients as well as the health of the therapist.

The nature of the health care profession determines the procedures for the extent of sanitisation and sterilisation. For example, an acupuncturist will need to ensure that acupuncture needles and equipment are sterilised by autoclaving. A beauty therapist must apply products with sterilised applicators. An aromatherapist does not have the same kind of implements or have a need for the same sanitation procedures; however, appropriate and recommended procedures should be adhered to.

Contagious diseases, skin infections and other problems can be caused by the transfer of infectious material by unclean hands and nails and by unsanitary equipment and supplies. One of the primary precautions in infection control is thorough hand washing. You should wash your hands before and after each aromatherapy session.

You should also ensure that any items that come into contact with a client are clean and sanitised. Supplies such as towels, blankets and sheets should be clean and fresh for each client. After each use, towels should be laundered in hot water. If there is a concern that the towels have been contaminated, add a few drops of lavender or tea tree to the wash water.

Safety Practices

Aromatherapy does not involve the use of hazardous equipment or practices; however, there are still safety issues that the aromatherapist must keep in mind. Safety is an attitude put into practice with the focus on the prevention of situations and the elimination of conditions that may lead to injury of the therapist or the client. Safety considerations should focus on:[2]

- the premises
- equipment
- fire safety
- first aid
- therapist safety
- client safety.

The Premises

The premises includes the building that houses the clinic, the equipment and the space within the clinic. Safety precautions in the premises include:[3]

- keep all halls and walkways clear
- keep all carpets vacuumed and clean
- keep all solid floors cleaned and sanitised
- sanitise all bathing facilities
- make sure all floors in wet areas are slip-proof
- sanitise all equipment that is exposed to the client (table surfaces, linen etc.)
- maintain hand-washing facilities (soap, sanitised towels).

Equipment

- each time a massage table is set up, check all the hinges and check the table for stability
- maintain all equipment
- store equipment and linen properly.

Fire Safety

- be familiar with the location and use of fire extinguishers
- clearly indicate fire exits
- be aware of evacuation procedures
- establish a policy regarding the use of open flames, candles and oil vaporisers.

First Aid

- keep a maintained first aid kit on the premises
- make sure all personnel know the location of the first aid kit
- as many staff as possible should learn first aid and CPR techniques.

Therapist Safety

- When lifting equipment or clients, use proper lifting techniques to prevent muscle strain and injury.[2]
- Maintain a good posture when practising massage to prevent muscle strain and overuse syndromes which may result in back, shoulder or arm injury.[2]
- Use equipment according to manufacturers' instructions and recommendations.[2]
- Know the location of the first aid kit.[2]
- Wash your hands before and after every treatment.[2]
- Know contra-indications for aromatherapy massage and perform procedures that cause no injury and are within your scope of practice.

Client Safety

- Understand the cause of infection and assure clients' protection with sanitary practices such as:[2]
    a. use clean linen with each client
    b. wash hands before and after each client
    c. provide sanitary bathing facilities and restrooms
    d. avoid open wounds and sores
    e. do not practise massage if you have a contagious illness.
- Provide safe, clear entrances and passages by keeping walkways clear and well-lit, providing non-skid walkways and floor surfaces.[2]
- When necessary, assist client on and off the massage table.[2]
- Check to make sure that client is not sensitive or allergic to products that you will be using.
- Use proper procedures in dealing with illness and injury.

Supplies and Equipment

Each room should have the appropriate furnishings and equipment for the treatments to be given. All supplies must be kept in a clean, sanitised condition. Supplies such as oils and linen should be ready before the client enters the room.

The following is a checklist of equipment and supplies generally needed for an aromatherapy clinic.

Room equipment
Supply and linen cabinets
Chairs
Massage table
Stool
Pillows
Sheets
Towels
Bathroom scales
Indirect lighting
Desk or table
Clothes hangers
Small table
Clock
Covered rubbish bin

Therapy equipment
Anatomical charts
Bathroom scales
Foot basin
Cotton for facial cleansing
Cotton-tipped swabs
Client record cards
Alcohol or other sterilising agents
Measuring cylinders
Funnels
Small mixing bowls
Storage cabinet
Bowls for preparing compresses
Tissues
Oil burners

Supplies
Essential oils
Carrier oils
Ointment or cream base
Empty glass and plastic bottles
Glass jars
Blank labels
Floral waters

There may be other items that you wish to add to this list.

Setting up a Clinic

Clinic Space

An aromatherapy treatment room should be approximately 3 metres by 4 metres. This will allow enough space for all needed equipment as well as enough room to move around the table.

It should also allow enough space for a desk, chair and a supply cabinet. It is handy to have a stool in the massage room, because there are times when you can sit down while working on the client's neck, face, feet or hands. Sitting down for a few minutes can provide a much-needed rest when working long hours.

Temperature

The temperature of the treatment room should be comfortable. The room should be warm enough so that the client does not feel a chill. If a client becomes cold, it is very difficult to relax.

The room should also be adequately ventilated. Poor ventilation causes the room to become stuffy and the air may acquire an overwhelming odour. Proper ventilation ensures an abundance of fresh air.

Lighting

It is difficult for the practitioner or the client to be comfortable when lighting in the room is too bright. Reflective or soft natural light is preferred. Dimmer switches will enable you to reduce the intensity of the lighting. Avoid direct overhead lighting or any light that can shine directly into the client's eyes.

Music

Soothing music can provide another sensory dimension to a relaxing aromatherapy massage. While you may find the ambience that the music creates soothing, please remember to ask your client what he or she prefers. Some people find it distracting and prefer absolute quiet. Music may be useful in masking outside noise which is distracting.

The Massage Table

Your massage table should be stable, firm and comfortable. If you travel to do treatments, you may prefer a table that is portable. The table should not shake, rock or squeak.

The table should be the correct height to give you the leverage needed to prevent fatigue of your back, neck, arms, and shoulders. Oneway of testing the optimum height of your table is to place the palm of your hand flat on the table. While doing this, you should be able to hold your arm straight at your side.

Ensure that the width of your table will give enough arm support for larger clients. The padding on the table should be firm so that the pressure applied by the therapist to the client is absorbed by the client's body and not pushed into the table. A face cradle is extremely valuable for the comfort of the client.

Business Skills

Starting your own clinic

As the demand for preventative and holistic medicine increases, there will be many business opportunities for professional aromatherapists. Whether you decide to establish your own clinic or work as an employee, it is important to understand the responsibilities associated with running a business. The therapist who understands sound business practices is more likely to succeed because he or she will be more aware of the responsibilities associated in being self-employed.

Unfortunately, being a good aromatherapist is not good enough to succeed in business. The secret is not knowing how to do aromatherapy treatments, but knowing how to make money doing aromatherapy treatments. All too often people have failed because they have not recognised this very important difference.

Many business failures are the result of management problems. You must be able to recognise your strengths and weaknesses from the start. Take an honest and personal look at yourself, your business idea and the chances of making it in the marketplace. Honesty is the key word because, in the end, if you fool anyone it will be yourself.

Keep an open mind in your thinking. This will not be easy, especially if this has been a lifetime dream. However, you must have a realistic appraisal of your chances of success.

The Profile of a Successful Business Owner

Like most other people in small business you are hoping to earn a better living and enjoy the benefits of being your own boss. However, the money you will make will at times seem insufficient for the responsibility, long hours and hard work that are required in becoming your own boss.

How do you know whether you will succeed in business or not? Are there any personality characteristics that guarantee success? While there is no checklist that, if properly completed, would make failure an impossibility, many studies have shown that certain personality traits are important to anyone in small business. These are just a few:

- desire to achieve
- motivation
- technically competent
- good judgement
- intelligent
- courage
- initiative
- self-confidence

- energetic
- honesty
- emotionally stable.[4]

While few people have all of these traits, if you are to be successful you should at least be able to claim most of them. You can succeed in small business provided you are willing to work hard and prepared to take some challenges/risks.

The Risks Associated in Running Your Own Business

You do not have to like risk taking but you have to accept and look upon risks as a challenge. You will face four kinds of risks:[4]

1. **The risk of financial difficulties or even failure.** Most newcomers to the business field will have their entire life savings invested in the venture or the equity in their home committed. At the very least, you and your family may have to accept a lower standard of living until the business gets on its feet.
2. **The risk of interrupting your career.** Whatever you are doing now, you probably have some sort of job security or career path open to you. If the business does not succeed, will you have difficulties finding another job?
3. **The risk of straining family relationships.** Starting a business makes great demands on energy, emotion and time. What is devoted to the business will not be devoted to the family.
4. **The risk of psychological failure.** This is rarely discussed but it is very important. Failure in business may lead to loss of confidence, feeling inadequate and difficulty in starting to work effectively again or to retain a normal personal life.

It is important that you discuss these risks with those close to you — those who will be most affected by your future business decisions. The tables below highlight the advantages or disadvantages that may apply to your situation.

Self–employed[4]

Advantages	Disadvantages
Personal satisfaction	Many risks to be faced within and outside your control (political, economic and social environment)
Independence of decision	Many more 'bosses' customers, creditors, competitors, and government regulators
Financial reward	Sole responsibility for all decisions — sometimes a lonely feeling.
Sense of achievement	Longer workdays
Social recognition	Fewer holidays
Opportunity for leadership	Few people to talk over your problems with.
Social role in the community	
Job creation	

Working for another[4]

Advantages	Disadvantages
Less financial risk	Financial rewards may be limited
Security, stability	Competition among employees
Regular work	Freedom of action and initiative may be limited
Large organisation fills the need of 'belonging'.	Promotion not always on basis of merit
Status of 'titles'	

Your Financial Needs

In business you are going to have to accept a certain amount of financial risk. The degree of that risk depends on your individual circumstances. You will need to seriously consider the following questions:

- How much do you need to maintain your present lifestyle?
- How much change are you prepared to accept?

Each one of us has different requirements, and to assist you in identifying yours complete the table below. A word of warning! Be realistic! The only person you will fool will be yourself.

Your present monthly commitments	(A) What you spend now	(B) The minimum you need to get by
Mortgage payments or rent		
Food		
Clothing		
Telephone		
Electricity		
Rates		
Insurance		
Education		
Health		
Car costs		
Entertainment		
Loans		
Other		
TOTAL	$	$

If you have difficulty now in making your present monthly income meet the total in column (A), you may have to take a long, hard look at whether or not you can afford to take on additional financial responsibilities of going into business. Be honest, there will be difficulties enough having personal credit problems to worry about.

Column (B) represents the minimum you need. This total, multiplied by 12, should not be less than your anticipated income from your proposed business venture.

Selecting Finance

There are really only two kinds of financing available to you to start and operate your business: your money, called equity, or someone else's, called a loan.

Before we deal with each, it is very important to learn to think of your business as a separate entity, as opposed to your own personal affairs. We are not necessarily talking of a separate legal entity, but about the need to think of your business assets and obligations as if they were those of a separate person. This concept is very important. The money you put into the business becomes capital for the business — and it should not be regarded as being available to you for personal requirements.

Equity is the investment that you make in your business, usually in the form of cash, but it can also be in the value of equipment, buildings or other assets that you are prepared to risk in the business. Risk is the operative word — you must be prepared to accept that it is your equity that will be lost first, if losses are sustained.

The amount of your investment or equity will often determine the extent to which lenders will become involved in your enterprise. After all, if you are not prepared to accept a degree of risk, why should they?

The wages or drawings that you, as the owner-manager, will take from the business should be considered as an expense, so that the real profit of the enterprise is apparent. All too often, the effort and time expended by an owner are not correctly reflected in the financial results, with the result that true profit is often overstated.

Loans, on the other hand, do carry an obligation to repay the principal as well as an additional cost, called interest. It may be helpful to think of this as a rental of the money you need, much in the same way that you rent any other asset for your business.

How Much Finance Will You Need?

The answer to this depends on many factors. The table below will help you determine how much capital you will require to set up your business.

Purchase cost (if buying established clinic)	
Plant, fixtures, equipment	
Renovation costs	
Purchase stock/material	
Repayment loan for first month	
Establishment costs (e.g., solicitor, accountant)	
Advance payment (rent, insurance)	
Initial advertising, marketing expenses	
Operating costs for at least 4 months (wages, electricity, leasing, stationery)	
Personal needs for at least 5 months	
Subtotal (A)	
Margin for contingencies — 10% to 25% of A. (B)	
Capital required (A+B)	

How much should you contribute and how much should you borrow?

In some situations you may not be able to borrow, as lenders are often sceptical of new ventures. But as a general guideline your contribution should not be less than your total borrowings.

Major Expenses Related to Starting an Aromatherapy Practice

The start-up costs for running a business include all the expenses incurred before any revenues are collected. Those costs vary according to the size and complexity of the business being established. Start-up costs are out-of-pocket costs during the planning stage to be recovered during the operation of the business.

The two main reasons why small businesses fail are under-capitalisation and poor management. Most aromatherapists are self-employed. They may work from home, a small office space, a space shared with another practitioner or in conjunction with another health care provider. Regardless of where you locate your practice, there will be certain expenses in setting up your practice.

- *Rent or lease* — May include first and last month's rent.
- *Services/utilities* — Connection fees and deposit for electricity, gas, telephone and internet.
- *Equipment and supplies* — Massage tables, linen, essential oils, base oils and bottles.
- *Furniture* — Desk, chairs, supply cabinet, music system, filing cabinet and lighting.
- *Decorating supplies* — Paint, curtains, plants.

- *Office supplies* — Calculator, computer, pens, stapler, filing supplies, appointment and receipt books.
- *Advertising expenses* — Telephone directory, newspaper advertising.
- *Printing expenses* — Business cards, stationery, information forms and brochures.
- *Insurance and licence costs* — Practitioner liability, public liability, fire, theft and storm damage insurance.
- *Initial operating cost* — Opening business cheque account with enough capital to cover miscellaneous expenses until the business is up and running.

How to Structure Your Business?

There are three basic forms of business organisation:[5]

Single Proprietorship

A sole trader carries on business in his/her own right, as the only proprietor either in his/her own name e.g., Joe Bloggs or under a business name such as 'Healing Hands'. Under the Business Names legislation, the name of the business is required to be registered with the Office of Fair Trading and Business Affairs. In the above example, Joe Bloggs is not required to register his own name, while 'Healing Hands' must be registered.

A sole trader will be required to declare the income from the business in his/her own personal tax return, and to pay income tax at personal tax rates. The sole trader owns the assets and is responsible for the liabilities of the business. Liability is unlimited and will extend to the total personal assets including his/her share of those assets jointly owned with another person.

Partnership

A partnership is formed when two or more people go into business with a view of making a profit. The business may be carried out under the partners' personal names or a registered business name. Partnerships are regulated by the Partnership Act and the agreement between the partners. The agreement should be in writing and prepared on advice of a solicitor.[5]

An important aspect of a partnership is the unlimited liability of each partner for all the financial obligations of the business. This even applies to debts incurred by a partner without the knowledge or consent of other partners. Therefore, a partnership should only be considered where there is a high degree of loyalty, competence and complete understanding between the partners and the business involves a low level of risk.[5]

A partnership is required to lodge an income tax return. However, the profits of the partnership are distributed to the partners in proportions designated by the partnership deed or as agreed from time to time. The partners are thus liable individually for personal income tax on their shares of the profit and they must include their shares of the profit in their individual tax returns along with their income from other sources.[5]

Company

A business may be conducted by a company as an entity in its own right and comes into existence by incorporation under Companies legislation which also regulates the running of the company and sets out the duties of its officers.[5]

It is normal for a solicitor to prepare documents and apply for incorporation. It has a memorandum setting out its powers and articles of association governing the carrying out of these powers. A company has shareholders who are the owners of the company and directors who run the company. The shareholders may also be directors and employees, which is often the case in a small family business.[5]

Shareholders receive a credit towards the tax on dividends equal to the relevant amount of tax paid by the company. The liability of the shareholders is limited to the unpaid calls on their shares in the company and therefore a company structure is advantageous in a high-risk business. However, major creditors may call upon directors to personally guarantee the company's liabilities. Personal liability of directors and employees may also arise out of an offence under the Corporations Law or negligence in the performance of their duties.[5]

Business Regulatory Requirements to Operate an Aromatherapy Practice

There are local, state and federal regulations that must be considered when beginning a business. It is to your advantage to be aware of and to comply with all regulations in the process of organising the business rather than be surprised after the fact and have to pay heavy penalties or restructure and relocate the business. The regulatory requirements may include:

- licensing of premises as a workplace
- registration of business name
- planning and zoning permits: Ensure that your clinic complies with local zoning requirements
- health act requirements, e.g., If you practise beauty therapy or acupuncture your clinic will have to comply with the relevant government health act

- worker's compensation if you are employing staff
- taxation requirements
- superannuation for employees.

Small businesses do not always have the resources to employ people with expertise needed in today's business environment. Specialised assistance is often necessary to overcome specific problems. Specialised help and assistance can be obtained from a variety of sources including:

- accountants
- solicitors
- business advisers
- professional associations
- small business agencies.

The Types of Insurance an Aromatherapist Should Carry

You will need to have adequate insurance against fire, theft and liability. To determine the specific requirements and amount of coverage to cover your business and yourself, consult with one or more insurance agents. If you work from home, review your homeowner's policy concerning the liability of operating a business out of your home. If you lease an office, check the lease to determine which liability responsibilities are yours and which are the landlord's.

Here is a check list of different types of insurance available:

- Public liability insurance covers the cost of injury and litigation resulting from injuries sustained on your property. This is usually a part of a homeowner's policy but it does not usually cover business-related activities.
- Malpractice liability insurance protects you from lawsuits that may be filed by a client because of injury or loss that results from negligence or substandard performance of a professional.
- Fire and theft insurance covers fixtures, furniture, equipment, products and supplies. If you work from home, ensure that your policy is adequate to cover your home clinic.
- Medical/health insurance helps to cover the cost of medical bills, especially hospitalisation, serious injury, or illness.
- Disability insurance protects you from loss of income if you are unable to work due to long-term illness or injury.
- Worker's compensation insurance is required if you have employees. It covers the medical costs of the employees if they are injured on the job.

Setting Your Fees

As a business person offering a service, your income is dependent on the fees you charge for your services. In determining your fee structure, there are several factors to consider.

You are a professional aromatherapist selling a valuable service. Set a fee that compensates you fairly and reflects your credibility. Consider the market and your competition. A little research will tell you what services are offered by other practitioners in the area and what they charge for those services. Set your fees in accordance with others in the area. If you offer a unique service that is in high demand, your fee may be higher.

If you are self-employed and aromatherapy is the sole source of your income, you must consider all the costs of operating your business and determine how many treatments you must do and at what rate to earn a living. If you are working for someone else, you may be working for an hourly rate or for a percentage of each massage you perform. You must determine what you are willing to receive for each treatment you do. The percentage you receive may depend on who furnishes the equipment, supplies and services such as telephone, receptionist, advertising, towels and oils.

Business Planning

Research has shown that businesses that develop and use formal business plans have a greater chance of success and survival than those who do not, irrespective of the size of the business.

Planning involves clarifying your purpose, stating a mission, setting goals and determining priorities.

A *mission statement* is a short general statement of the main focus of your business. Developing a mission statement requires careful consideration. The mission statement expresses the purpose of the business and should be used to promote the public image of your business.[6]

The *purpose* relates to why the business exists. It is important to focus on outcomes and results.[6] You may have several purposes for doing business. Clarifying those purposes allows you to direct your energies toward those purposes. Examples may include:

- to provide a nurturing and healing environment
- to make a positive difference for my clients.

Goals should be specific, attainable, measurable accomplishments that you can set and make a commitment to achieve. The business goals should support your mission statement and reinforce your purpose. Goals clarify your intentions and provide the focus you need to achieve your dreams.

Goals should be short-term and long-term. You can have life long-goals, five-year goals, one-year goals, six-month goals, goals for next week and goals for tomorrow or goals for today. It is necessary to set deadlines with each goal. Keep your goals personalised and in the present tense. Make your goals realistic and attainable but do not hesitate to think big. Ensure the goals are specific:

- I will see five patients a day
- I will attend the next international aromatherapy conference
- I will increase my income by 25% this year.

Once you set your goals, it takes planning and commitment to realise them. List the benefits of attaining your goals, brainstorm possible steps needed to reach the goal. Identify potential obstacles and develop a strategy to overcome them. Then develop a strategic plan to achieve your goals.

Selecting a Location for Your Clinic

Finding the right location for your practice will influence your ability to succeed. A frequent cause of business failure is locating in an area that is not suitable for that particular type of business.

Choose a site that will accommodate your clinic needs, that will be pleasing to your clients, fits your image and is within your budget. The clinic must be easy to locate, with the address clearly visible from the street. It should be easily accessible and relatively quiet. An ideal space should have one or more treatment rooms, a reception/waiting area, an office and bathroom facilities with a shower.

Being near public transport and having adequate parking are important considerations. Before signing a lease on a location, make sure it suits your needs. If you have to remove or replace fixtures, make repairs, change specific structures or install equipment, plumbing or electrical work ensure that this be included as part of the lease or the costs of such work may come as a big shock to you.

Many therapists choose to work from home. This is an inexpensive alternative but may require a special permit from your local council. It is imperative that the portion of the home used as a clinic is kept clean, neat and be used only as your clinic, not doubling up as a rumpus room for the children to play in as well. There will be many tax deductions that can be claimed for having an office in your home. You should confirm the possible claims with your tax accountant.

There are three areas to consider in making your location decision:

- the trading area as a whole
- the town or city
- the actual site.[4]

In selecting	Things to look for	Things to avoid
The trading area	Growing population	Declining population
	Extent of the market competition	Personal preference for a particular climate
The town	Potential for growth	Desire to succeed in one's home town
The site	Accessibility	Personal preference for social environment
	Exposure to customers	
	Occupancy costs	The cost — there may be a reason why the rent is 'cheaper' in one location than another
		Impulsive action

If you are considering leasing the premises, you should at least know the answers to the following questions:[4]

- Who owns improvements that the tenant makes?
- What insurance cover does the landlord hold and what should the tenant cover?
- What are the lease renewal provisions?
- Does the tenant have the right to sublet?
- Are there any options for expansion?
- How is rent determined?
- Are there any restrictions on the use of the property?

Basic Bookkeeping

A good bookkeeping system is essential to the success of a business. You will need to keep client records as well as records of income from services and sale of products. Even though you may hire an accountant, it is still very important for the self-employed aromatherapist to understand the basics of bookkeeping. It is difficult to manage a successful business if you do not understand the principles of sound business administration and management.

Without a proper bookkeeping system you will not be able to determine the progress of the business, especially the cost of doing business in relation to income. Business records are necessary to meet the requirements of government laws pertaining to taxes and employees.

The bookkeeping system should be only as complicated as the business requires. If you have a computer, you may consider an accounting software package which will be a valuable tool in managing your business.

For a self-employed individual, a system that records income and disbursements is sufficient. Once a good system is established and kept current, it reduces the end-of-year tax preparation drudgery and offers an accurate accounting of the business's financial position.

Setting up a Separate Business Account

Setting up your own business cheque account enables you to separate personal and business expenses. Open a separate account under the name of the business. Deposit all business income into the account. Use it whenever making cash disbursements. Pay all business bills through your business account. Do not use the business account to pay personal or non-business expenses. An updated chequebook ledger is a good way to register disbursements and income. Ledgers that are more complete are necessary to track a business's financial standing.

Petty Cash Account

A petty cash fund should be maintained to pay small disbursements for incidentals. Receipts should be kept for each transaction, which should be properly recorded in a petty cash ledger. Occasionally a cheque should be drawn from the business cheque account to bring the petty cash fund back to a desired level.

Bank Statements and Reconciliations

Each month the bank will send a bank statement listing the deposits, payments, cheques and bank fees that have been processed through your account. Reconcile the statement with your cheque book, correcting your mistakes and notify the bank immediately if there are any problems.

Many banks offer internet banking. This allows you to manage your business finances on a daily basis. See if your bank charges a fee for this service and compare this cost with the cost of operating a standard cheque account.

Revenue Records

These include daily receipts and a ledger sheet of all income with information as to the source, type and amount of income. A receipt or invoice should be prepared for each business transaction.

The invoice should include:

- your business name
- the date
- the client's name
- a description of the services given
- amount charged for the services
- a description of the goods sold
- amount charged for the goods sold
- a space to indicate the date paid.

If you provide credit, you must include credit terms. Keep a copy of the invoice for your records and give a copy to your client.

The income ledger is a summary of all sales and cash receipts. There are different ways to set up the income ledger. You should record every income transaction. Income may be categorised as aromatherapy treatments, gift vouchers or retail goods.

Expenses Record

The expense record is a ledger that separates and classifies business expenditure. Each column of the ledger is for a different category of expenditure. All the information posted in the expense ledger comes from the chequebook register. Each entry in the ledger should include the date, cheque number, the payee and the total amount entered into the appropriate column.

List of Business Expenses

Business expenses are partially or totally deductible from business income in determining the profit or loss of the business. These categories can be used when writing cheques and on the disbursement ledger. The following are possible expenses categories:

- accounting expenses
- advertising expenses
- motor vehicle expenses — fuel, maintenance, repayments, registration, insurance and leasing
- bad debts
- bank fees
- cleaning and janitorial expenses
- cost of products sold
- depreciation
- donations to charity
- professional association fees
- education expenses
- entertainment

- equipment expenses
- furnishing and fixtures
- insurance
- interest paid on loans
- office supplies
- postage and freight
- professional, legal and consulting fees
- rent
- repairs and maintenance
- telephone expenses
- travel — business-related expenses
- wages

Business Receipts

Keep receipts of every purchase or expenditure related in any way to the business. After recording transactions, file the receipts. Each month create a new file so the receipts are separated to reflect and support the entries in the monthly disbursement ledger. Ensure that all receipts are kept for the period specified by the tax legislation in your country.

Accounts Receivable

If you extend credit to your clients, you will have to keep an ongoing record of each transaction. This may complicate the bookkeeping process considerably. In private practice it is best to keep it simple, by requesting payment at the time of service.

Accounts Payable

If you buy supplies or services on credit, keep a file for each account or business that extends you credit. Accounts payable records the money you owe to other people or businesses.

Assets and Depreciation Records

Items and equipment purchased for your business are considered assets. Supplies and inventory are not considered assets. You should maintain a current record of business assets that includes an item description, date of purchase and purchase price. Add new items when purchased and remove items when they are sold or retired from use.

For taxation purposes, the cost of the item is depreciated over a number of years. It may be necessary to consult with your accountant to determine the amount of depreciation, as the depreciation schedule may vary according to the type of equipment.

Inventory

Maintaining a good inventory system will ensure that you do not run out of supplies or be overstocked on items that do not sell well. Supplies to be used are generally classified as consumption supplies, and those to be sold should be classified as retail supplies.

Appointment Book

The appointment book is one of the most important documents for organising a successful and prosperous business. It is an important tool in time management. A well-kept appointment book ensures that appointments are not missed and are scheduled so that you can be on time. Keep your appointment book handy and up to date. The appointment book should have enough space to record the time of the appointment, the client's name, phone number and possibly the fee you should receive from each client.

Marketing and Promotions

Marketing is done to promote and increase your business. Common methods of promoting your business include public speaking and appearances, writing articles for newspapers and professional magazines, setting up stands at health fair shows and other public functions.

The objective of marketing is to become known and to be visible to those in the community who may seek your service. It also creates an awareness and desire in potential clients to use your services. Promotional activities in a health care industry are largely educational in nature. Marketing will let your potential clients know who you are, what you do and how your services will benefit them.

Developing Promotional Material

An important part of your promotional activity is having appropriate printed materials to distribute when you meet potential customers. Printed materials include business cards, brochures, stationery and newsletters. Your printed material should appeal to your target market and reflect your professionalism. Always include your name, address and phone number on every piece of promotional material.

Whenever you speak to a group or an individual about your services, be sure to leave them with a card or brochure. Even though you may not get a new client directly from your printed material, it serves as a reminder and contains information on how you can be contacted.

Advertising

This may include magazines, newspapers, telephone listing or direct mailing. Advertising can become important to the success of your business. Plan your advertising budget wisely as it can also become a waste of money if your advertisements do not increase your business profile.

A classified advertisement in a telephone directly is often a good idea. Make sure the listing of your service is under Aromatherapy or Natural Therapies, with your credentials and association affiliations.

Public Relations

Some of the best advertising you can get is free. A feature article in a local paper is an excellent way to gain recognition in your community. Offer to make personal appearances to give talks and demonstrations to various groups. You may offer to speak at social meetings, health clubs, schools or as a guest on a radio or television talk show.

An essential aspect in developing good public relations is networking. Networking is developing personal and professional contacts for the purpose of giving and receiving support and sharing resources and information. Become involved in networking groups such as the Chamber of Commerce or other business groups. Participate in seminars or functions to meet others with whom you may develop networking relationships. Always keep business cards handy when attending these functions and freely distribute them.

Encouraging Referrals

One of the most effective and inexpensive methods of creating new business is through referrals. The two main sources of referrals are current clients and other health care professionals. Satisfied customers are one of your most effective means of advertising. Remember that, in word-of-mouth advertising, the most important mouth is yours. Encourage referrals. Let your clients know that you not only appreciate their business, but that if they appreciate what you do they should tell others. Give them extra business cards and encourage them to tell their friends about your service. Offer them a bonus treatment for every new paid client that they refer to you.

To promote referrals from other health professionals in your area make yourself and what you do known to them. Explain how your services would benefit them and their clients. Write a letter, and then follow up the letter with a phone call. Arrange a meeting with them and offer them a treatment so they can experience firsthand what you have to offer. Always present yourself in a professional manner. When other health care professionals send referrals, confer with them to determine their reasons and goals for sending the client to you. Report back to them about the client's progress as a result of the aromatherapy treatment. A good working relationship between health care professionals will generate more referrals.

Whenever a new client comes in who has been referred, be sure to acknowledge the person who referred him or her with a thank-you note.

Client Retention

Your clients are your most valuable asset. Treat your clients with courtesy and respect. Besides giving a good aromatherapy treatment, make sure your client feels appreciated and cared for. Record each session, paying attention to the client's personal interests, likes and dislikes. Refer to your records before each visit to ensure that you are aware of their idiosyncrasies. Avoid their dislikes, discuss their interests and do those special little things they like. Thank them for coming.

Keep your clients on a mailing list, send them newsletters, birthday or holiday greetings and offer special promotions over slower periods.

Remember, your clients are your reason for being in practice, they are the source of your income, and they deserve the best service you can give.

Customer Service

Unless your clinic is offering a unique service with a product that nobody else has, your client can always go somewhere else for the same treatment. However, it is the little extras that can make a huge difference. Just think about your favourite restaurant. Why is it your favourite? Is the food better than that served in other restaurants? Is it bigger and better than all the rest? The answer is probably no! The simple fact is that it is usually the almost indefinable aspects of the resturant that make it your favourite. This may include the ambiance, the background music, the friendly staff, the candles, the fresh flowers and the freshly baked bread rolls, just to name a possible few. And I bet that all these aspects that ensure that you keep coming back for more are unlikely to be costing the owner much at all.

Fortunately the situation is the same for the natural therapies industry. You don't have to have the biggest or the 'best' clinic to be successful. However, you do have to offer your client an experience that they will want to keep coming back for— again and again.

The following tips will ensure that you make a positive first and lasting impression on your clients.

- Check if your client needs to visit the bathroom before they undress or before lying down if they are in their robe.
- Invest in good quality towelling. Clients notice cheap towels — after all, they're in close contact with them during the treatment.

- Ensure that your client is comfortable before you commence the treatment.
- Play relaxation music rather than the radio.
- Offer non-caffeinated refreshments such as herbal teas, juice and water.
- The treatment room should be set up before your client enters the room. Clients should never walk into a room that has just been vacated by your previous client.
- Provide your client with fresh robes, slippers, towels.
- Make sure the rooms are warm when the client is having a massage.
- Send your client cards to say 'thank you', 'happy birthday'.
- Have your treatment menu printed on good quality paper. Describe the treatments to entice your client to book them.
- Keep a detailed 'client history' for every client. For example, don't ask your client if they would like a peppermint tea on every visit, especially since they have told you on a previous visit that they don't like it!
- Provide newsletters for your client to read.
- Offer a gift certificate or client referral program.
- Open on Sundays and at night — this can be a more convienient time for many clients.

There are many other ways to make your treatment centre extra special – the options open to you are only limited by your imagination and to a certain extent your budget.

References

1. Delbridge A, et al. eds. *Macquarie dictionary.* 3rd edn, Macquarie Library Pty Ltd, Australia, 1997.
2. Beck M. *Milady's theory and practice of therapeutic massage.* Milady Publishing Company, 1994.
3. Heather D. *Professionalism in aromatherapy.* Simply Essential 1993; 11: 10–11.
4. *Starting a small business: Training in management package 1.* Australian Government Publishing Services, Australia, 1996.
5. McLure B. ed, *The small business handbook.* Information Australia, 1998.
6. Humphrey N. *The business startup guide.* Penguin books, Australia, 2001.

The Consultation

Objectives

After careful study of this chapter, you should be able to:

- explain the role of the consultation
- explain the need to establish rapport
- examine a range of communication skills relevant to a consultation
- outline the structure of a consultation
- examine basic counselling skills that can be used in a consultation
- explain the objectives in the management phase
- explain the procedure for preparing a case study and a case history
- determine when it is necessary to make a referral.

The Consultation

The successful outcome of an aromatherapy consultation depends on an array of skills required by the aromatherapist. These skills, collectively called 'consulting skills', include communication skills, clinical skills, diagnostic skills, educative skills, therapeutic skills, manual skills, counselling skills and management skills. These skills will generally apply to anyone working in the health care industry.

Murtagh, Professor of General Practice at Monash University and author of the classic text *General Practice*, says that the consultation is often broken up into three phases:[1]

1. Establishing rapport.
2. Diagnostic phase — the history, the physical examination, and other investigations.
3. Management phase — explanation of treatment strategy, client education, prescribing remedies, referrals and follow-up.

Murtagh cites work done by Pendleton, who outlines the key tasks to a consultation. These may serve as a helpful guideline:[1]

1. To define the reason for the patient's attendance, such as the nature and history of the problem, the aetiology of the problem, the patient's ideas, concerns and expectations.
2. To consider other concerns such as continuing problems and risk factors.
3. To choose, with the patient, an appropriate action for each problem.
4. To achieve a shared understanding of the problems with the patient.
5. To involve the patient in the management and encourage him or her to accept appropriate responsibility.
6. To use time and resources appropriately in the consultation and in the long-term.
7. To establish or maintain a relationship with the patient that helps to achieve the other tasks.

Establishing Rapport

Although rapport building occurs throughout all phases of the consultation the initial encounter with the patient sets the foundation for the professional relationship during the consultation.

The first consultation is the first opportunity for the client and the therapist to meet one another and to clarify their intentions and expectations for an aromatherapy treatment. During the first consultation you will learn about the client's conditions, needs and expectations. The purpose of the consultation is to exchange information regarding the client's conditions and expectations and the services offered by the therapist.

First impressions are lasting impressions. The image that you present will influence your client's respect and confidence. Be prepared by having everything needed for the consultation and treatment organised and ready. Greet the client in a professional and friendly manner. Be courteous and sensitive. Keep the consultation relaxed yet directed towards pertinent information.

The first time a client makes an appointment it is important to determine whether the appointment for an aromatherapy treatment is appropriate. The prospective client may be looking for services that you do not provide, or it may be determined that aromatherapy is contra-indicated for the conditions of the prospective client. Screening prospective clients with a few questions can save valuable time for you and the prospective client as well as eliminating any inappropriate situations. Questions to consider asking include:

- Have you had an aromatherapy treatment before?
- How did you find out about my services?
- What is your main reason for making this appointment?

There is no need to go into detail. However, responses to these questions will clarify if an appointment is desired and appropriate.

During the first consultation you should clearly explain your operational and client interaction policies. When policies concerning missed or late appointments and payment of fees are clearly stated, misconceptions and awkward situations may be avoided. The policies may be printed on the preliminary questionnaire form, on a sign or verbalised. Regardless of how they are expressed, only set policies you are willing to uphold.

You should explain any procedures that you use during the treatment session. It is important to keep the client informed about what is being done and why. During the consultation the client may want to know how the aromatherapy treatment will be beneficial. Being able to answer your client's questions will add credibility to your services as a health professional and helps to build client confidence.

The first consultation is usually the most extensive as an assessment form needs to be completed and treatment strategies developed. Subsequent sessions usually begin with a short question and answer session to determine any changes in conditions or treatment strategy. If this is your patient's second or subsequent consultation, it is important to quickly familiarise yourself with the patient's case history, preferably before the visit.

Murtagh recommends the following rapport-establishing techniques:[1]

- greeting the client with a friendly interested manner
- treating the client with respect and courtesy
- greeting the client with his or her preferred name
- shaking hands if appropriate
- making the client feel comfortable
- being 'unhurried' and relaxed
- being well briefed about prior consultations
- focusing firmly on the client
- listening carefully and appropriately
- making appropriate reassuring gestures.

Communication Skills

Communication skills are fundamental to consulting skills and are the key to the effectiveness of the aromatherapist as a health professional. Communication skills are essential in obtaining a good case history so that you can develop a successful therapeutic outcome for the client.

Mitchell and Cormack say that good communication takes place when there is a respectful and caring therapeutic relationship. They suggest that it is the duty of the practitioner to:[2]

- negotiate an authentic relationship which may change over time and which is suited to the needs of the particular individual
- listen carefully to what the patient wishes to communicate
- offer support, encouragement and realistic hope
- be sensitive to the patient's emotional state and needs.

Murtagh suggests the following communication strategies to improve communication skills:[1]

- avoid jargon
- provide clear explanations
- give clear instructions
- evaluate the patient's understanding
- summarise and repeat.

Effective communication also depends on good listening skills. Listening includes four essential elements:[1]

- checking the facts
- checking feelings
- encouraging
- reflecting.

Murtagh describes the role of listening as follows:

> *One does not listen with just his ears: he listens with his eyes and with his sense of touch. He listens by becoming aware of the feelings and emotions that arise within himself because of the contact with others (that is, his own emotional resonance is another 'ear'), he listens with his mind, his heart, and his imagination. He listens to the words of others but he also listens to the messages that are buried in the words or encoded in all the cues that surround the words. He listens to the context, verbal messages and linguistic pattern, and the bodily movements of others. He listens to the sounds and to the silences.*[1]

Interviewing Techniques

There are a number of basic interviewing techniques that can be used during a consultation. It is important to use the least controlling interview technique before embarking on direct questioning.

The Open-ended Question

The open-ended question is essential in initiating the interview. A question such as 'What kind of troubles have you been having?' says to the patient that you are interested in everything that they feel is important enough to tell you.[1]

The open-ended question gives the patient an opportunity to take temporary control of the consultation and to outline problems and concerns.[1]

Listening and Silence

Silence is a means of encouraging communication. While the patient is communicating freely, the therapist's behaviour of choice should be an interested, attentive and relaxed silence. Silence can encourage communication but one has to be careful that the person does not feel uncomfortable with the process. The therapist must use silence when the patient has stopped speaking from being overwhelmed with emotion.[1]

Facilitation

Facilitation promotes communication by utilising techniques such as manner, gestures or words that do not specify the kind of information that is being sought. Facilitation suggests that you are interested and encourage the patient to continue. It may include a nod of the head, which implies that you are listening and understand what is being said.[1]

A similar message is conveyed by interjecting short words or phases such as 'yes', or 'I see', without interrupting the flow of the patient's narrative or following a pause saying, 'yes, I understand — please continue'.[1]

Confrontation

When the patient is not speaking freely, confrontation may be used. The therapist describes to the patient something obvious about his or her verbal or nonverbal behaviour.

This may includes comments such as: 'You seem sad', 'You sound upset or angry' or 'I notice that you have been rubbing the back of your neck'. Confrontation has to be used with tact and skill, and should reflect sympathetic interest in the patient.[1]

Questions

When the patient is asked a question, the therapist tends to take control of the consultation, and may end up directing it along the lines of his or her own opinion or hypothesis generation. If a patient is asked a question too early in the consultation, the amount of desirable information may be restricted and this may disrupt the true priorities of the patient's concerns.[1]

Support and Reassurance

The ability to be appropriately supportive and reassuring helps to create an atmosphere in which the patient is encouraged to communicate. Examples of supportive statements are 'I understand' or 'That must be very upsetting'. Reassurance should include words or actions which tend to restore the patient's sense of wellbeing, worthiness or confidence.[1]

Summarising

Summarising what the patient has said will keep the patient on track and also confirms the accuracy of the information by providing the patient with the opportunity to revise any misunderstandings.[1]

Factors Contributing to Poor Communication

Factors contributing to poor communication can be created unintentionally and patients will know if they are being listened to or ignored.

The Therapist–Client Interaction

There are factors that can influence the communication between the therapist and the patient:[1]

- Poor past relationships and experiences to unresolved interpersonal conflicts. This may include poor treatment outcome, indifferent compliance to a treatment or payment of accounts.
- Personal differences, openly expressed, may create subtle barriers including differences in age, sex, religion, culture, social status.
- The personal honesty and integrity of both parties in dealing with difficult messages.
- Familiarity between the patient and the therapist, e.g., friends and relatives.

The Environment

The physical environment in which the consultation is being done is important. The appearance, size and layout of the consultation room, waiting room and treatment room may affect communication, sometimes adversely, especially if privacy is threatened by, say, leaving a consultation room door open.[1]

Summary of Environmental Factors that can Adversely Influence Communication[1]

Waiting room	Poor physical layout Length of waiting time
Time pressure	Too busy Too noisy Sense of urgency
Physical factors	Desk — barriers Layout inappropriate Poor record system Substandard massage table
Privacy	Dressing/undressing Sound Interruptions — phone

Nonverbal Communication

Nonverbal communication or body language is one of the most important features of the communication process. Nonverbal cues comprise the majority of the impact of any communicated message.[1]

The ability to recognise nonverbal cues improves communication, rapport and understanding of the patient's fears and concerns. The interpretation of body language, which differs between cultures, is a special study in its own right but there are certain cues and gestures that can be readily interpreted.[1]

Having noted nonverbal communication, you must then know how to deal with it. This may require diplomatic confrontation. That is, bring these cues to the patient's attention and explore the associated feeling further. By recognising a patient's nonverbal cues, you can encourage communication and a better understanding of the patient.

A technique suggested by Pease is to watch television without sound for 15 minutes each day and check your interpretation each 5 minutes. By the end of three weeks, he suggests, you will have become a more skilled body language observer.[3]

Counselling Skills

The Macquarie Dictionary says that counselling is:

> *giving advice that is opinion or instruction given in directing the judgement or conduct of another.*[4]

In the clinical context counselling can be defined as:

> *The therapeutic process of helping a patient to explore the nature of his or her problem in such a way that he or she determines his or her decisions about what to do, without direct, advice or reassurance from the counsellor.*[1]

As an aromatherapist, you should provide a comfortable, safe and nurturing environment for your clients. This environment will facilitate your patient's level of trust in you. As your clients relax in this environment they will often disclose issues in their lives other than those you have been asked to treat — for example, difficulties in sexual relationship or sexual abuse.

Effective counselling requires clear communication. There are many facets to clients — these include their sex, their personalities, ways of dealing with the world, their belief systems, life experiences and cultural background.

To provide effective counselling, the therapist must first prepare for this role. The therapist must be prepared to acquire the knowledge and skills for basic counselling by reading, attending workshops and discussing cases with colleagues who are skilled in counselling. Interview techniques are essential, as is self-discipline to appropriate one's strengths and limitations.

Murtagh offers the following basic counselling hints:[1]

- listening and empathy are the beginning of counselling
- good communication is the basis of counselling
- the therapist must really care about the patient
- always be aware of the family context
- it is important for therapists to handle and monitor their own feelings and emotions
- maintain eye contact
- the therapist must tolerate and be comfortable with what the patient says
- confidentiality is essential
- counselling is easier if there is a good rapport with the patient, especially if a long-standing relationship exists
- counselling is difficult if a social relationship is present
- do not say to the patient 'I'm counselling you'.
- characteristics of an effective counsellor include a non-possessive warmth and accurate and empathic understanding
- use appropriate 'gentle' confrontation to allow self-examination
- help patients to explore their own situation and express emotions such as anxiety, guilt, fear, anger, hope, sadness, self-hate, hostility to others and hurt feelings
- explore possible feelings of insecurity and allow free expression of such feelings.

Murtagh says that one should also avoid:[1]

- telling patients what they must do or offering solutions
- giving advice based on your own personal experiences and beliefs
- bringing up problems that the patient does not produce voluntarily.

Murtagh also reminds us that:[1]

- we cannot solve patients' problems for them
- patients often have to change by only an inch in order to move a mile
- if a counselling relationship is no longer productive, then terminate and refer.

Clients Unlikely to Benefit from Counselling

The following groups of clients may not benefit from counselling:[1]

- Patients who have had an unrewarding experience with another therapist.
- People who are antagonistic to the notion of a psychosocial diagnosis.
- Patients who are dependent on contact with the therapist and are willing to do almost anything to maintain the relationship.
- Patients with a vested interest in remaining unwell who are therefore resistant to change — for example, patients with work-related disabilities or injuries who are awaiting legal settlement.
- Those in an intractable life situation who are unwilling to change.
- Patients who are unwilling to examine and work on painful or uncomfortable areas of their life.

The Diagnostic Phase

A detailed consultation form will ensure that you have all the necessary information to provide an accurate diagnosis and the correct treatment. The following is a guideline to developing your own consultation form.

A. Identification Data

Name, age, sex, marital status, occupation, religion, work address, home address, telephone number.

B. Main Complaint

The main complaint is a statement in the client's own words of their present condition. In order to analyse the condition, it must be fully described in all its dimensions. The following parameters might be used:

- time
- quantity
- location
- aggravating factors
- alleviating factors.

Other questions that should be asked include:

- What do you think is your problem?
- What do you want to do about it?
- What has been happening in your life recently?

C. Family History

Record the age and health (or death and cause of death where applicable) of parents, sibling and children. Is there a history of any of the following conditions in the family; diabetes, high blood pressure, stroke, heart problems, cancers, tumours, arthritis, gout, alcoholism, epilepsy, glaucoma, blindness, deafness, kidney problems, bladder problems, allergies, skin problems, stomach problems, bowel problems, gall bladder or liver problems, genetic or inherited diseases, other unusual diseases.

D. Past Medical History

- General health: Ask the client to rate their own health, e.g., excellent, good, fair or poor.
- Serious illnesses: Have they ever had chicken pox, measles, rheumatic fever, polio, herpes, pneumonia, diverticulitis, hernia, haemorrhoids, tension/anxiety problems, depression.
- Injuries: Have they ever had broken bones, lacerations or other injuries.
- Operations: List surgical procedures they have undergone.
- Medications: What medications (including nutritional or naturopathic supplements).

E. Diet

Brief breakdown of daily meals, special diets, alcoholic beverages, coffee, teas, bowel movement.

F. Review of Symptoms

The main symptoms referable to each system are reviewed. Information that belongs with the present illness will frequently be obtained and should be recorded here. Repetitions are to be avoided by referring to the previous sections that contain the same information.

- Skin: Texture, colour, sweating pattern, bleeding, bruising, eruptions, pimples, eczema, cracked skin, boils or itching.
- Lymph nodes: enlargement, pain, sinuses, drainage.
- Respiratory: asthma, oppressed breathing, acute or chronic bronchitis, cough, expectoration, hayfever, sinus, allergies, smoking.
- Cardiovascular: Amount and type of exercise, angina, chronic heart diseases, sluggish circulation, palpitations, oedema, hypertension, varicose veins.
- Gastrointestinal: Appetite, nausea, vomiting, constipation, diarrhoea, unusual stool colour of consistency, abdominal pain, food intolerances.
- Endocrine: impotence, sterility, menstrual history (age at onset, cycle, duration, amount, dysmenorrhoea, amenorrhoea, menorrhagia, date of last period, premenstrual syndrome, number of pregnancies, obstetric complications, age of menopause, hot flushes, post-menopausal bleeding).
- Urinary: Passing of urine, frequency, pain, colour, foul smelling.
- Musculoskeletal: Pain, swelling, stiffness, limitation of motion of joints, fractures, serious sprains.
- Nervous: Headaches, convulsions and seizures, loss of consciousness, paralysis, weakness.
- Emotions/Moods: anxiety, depression, sleep pattern, memory, thought content, attitude (towards friends, associates, family, disease).

G. Social History

Record nativity, occupation, marital status, clients' emotional relationship to parents throughout life. Marital history should contain age, health, occupation, education of partner and number of children. Describe the extended family group. Who do they live with at home? Learn exactly what they do in their occupation with particular attention to the degree of emotional tension or health hazard. Are there any debts or economic problems that may influence convalescence? How much do they participate in civic, social, religious or political activities of their particular economic and social group? Find out how they spend their day — what hobbies, how they relax, how the family responds to an illness.

Management Phase

The management phase involves immediate care, prevention and long-term care. A holistic approach implies that the therapist will listen to the patient's views, offer an explanation where necessary and adopt an educative approach to encourage the patient to actively participate in the management of the condition.

The treatment and education combine to alleviate the condition. In some simple situations the treatment alone is sufficient; in others, the condition may be redressed solely by the remedial actions of the client. Generally, the treatment and remedial measures carried out by the client are required to achieve lasting improvement.

This is especially true of chronic conditions. Unless clients are given a clear understanding of the origins of illness, and are shown what remedial procedures to adopt, the condition may drag on indefinitely, even though it is partly relieved by the treatment. Therefore the appropriate actions of clients to help themselves can greatly reduce their suffering and their need for treatment.

Client Education

There are two main aspects of client education.

- The first is concerned with the identification of the originating factors of the illness, and then with prescribing the appropriate remedial measures to these factors.
- The second is concerned with helping clients at a more personal level. To help people to help themselves it is first necessary to help them understand themselves, then accept themselves, and yet also to determine to change themselves.

Many origins of disease are not physical factors, but disharmonious patterns of thoughts and emotion. Changing these ingrained patterns of disharmony is the most important and the most difficult part of client education, since people are often reluctant to change. The regulation of these deeply embedded patterns of feeling and belief is core to client education.

Since some individuals may have difficulty in changing, progress must be gradual and only at a rate within the capacity of the client. The three main components for change are:

- understanding
- motivation
- discipline.

Understanding

Clients must first understand, as thoroughly as it is appropriate, the pattern of their disharmony in the context of the pattern of their lives. They need to know which aspect of their behaviour or constitution became the originating factors of their illness. In this way they can understand which of their patterns of thought, emotion and behaviour need to be modified, and thus which preventative and remedial measures are appropriate.

Motivation

Understanding alone is not enough. There must be the motivation to put the understanding into practice. This can only be done with motivation from within the client. The therapist may act as a catalyst, but cannot supply motivation to a person who altogether lacks it.

Discipline

Momentary enthusiasm, temporary motivation, is useless. Changing ingrained patterns of thought and emotion is the work of a lifetime. Discipline is the steady application of understanding and motivation over long periods of time, despite setbacks and discouragements. This is the only way that lasting change can be effective. Discipline does not mean sudden, harsh bursts of self-punishment and deprivations; it is the slow, steady, gentle implementation of change.

Case History

The purpose of writing a case history is to present:

- a client assessment.
- a description and details of the treatment programme including the client's responses to the treatment.
- an evaluation of the treatment programme.
- any future recommendations for further treatments.

The case history may include the standard consultation sheet used in the clinic. However, the consultation sheet alone — without description, assessment and evaluation — does not constitute a case history.

1. Client Assessment

Sex, age, occupation, body type, marital status, sleeping patterns, diet, activities, medical history, presenting conditions, skin texture, tone and colour, medications, indicators of stress.

2. The Treatment Programme

Type of massage treatment to be performed. Reasons for using this treatment.

1. Outline any other aromatherapy treatment prescribed.
2. List of essential oils used (base oils and essential oils)

3. Formulae: Drops of oil per mL of base oil; % of each oil in the formulae, % of the total blend.
   - Reasons for choosing the essential oils used.
   - Reasons for the percentage of oils used in the blend.
   - Any essential oils that are contra-indicated for this client.
   - As treatment progresses, all changes to the formulae must be noted and the reasons for such changes given.
4. Client's response to the treatment.
   - Note responses during and immediately after the treatment.
   - Note responses between treatments.
5. Home recommendations: Details of oils recommended and formulae used.
   - Frequency and method of usage by the client.
   - Nutritional supplements, homoeopathic remedies, exercises, changes to diet, etc., should all be noted if used.

3. Evaluation of the Treatment Programme

1. Response of client during and immediately after the treatment.
2. Response of the client between treatments. Any improvement, adverse reactions, or changes by the client which may/or may not directly relate to the condition being treated.
3. Evaluate changes to the programme: Have you had to adjust your treatment in any of the following areas?
   - Massage treatment
   - Oils and formulae
   - Home treatment programme
4. Evaluation of the treatment: Has there been significant improvement? Why/why not?
5. Has the client cooperated with the home treatment programme?
6. Your overall evaluation of this programme.

4. Future Recommendations

These are based upon your evaluation of the treatment programme:

1. Is further treatment required?
2. Is referral to another professional appropriate?

Patient Referral

The decision to refer a patient to another therapist is a very important skill. A referral may be considered when there is a risk of a serious, chronic or life-threatening condition. In this case the referral should be made to a general practitioner. A referral may also be necessary when the treatment strategy requires the skills of another health professional such as a nutritionist, homoeopath, acupuncturist, herbalist etc.

References

1. Murtagh J. *General practice*. The McGraw-Hill Companies Inc, Australia, 1998.
2. Mitchell A, Cormack M. *The therapeutic relationship in complementary health care*. Churchill Livingstone, Great Britain, 1999.
3. Pease A. *Body language*. Camel Publishing. London, 1985.
4. Delbridge A et al. eds. *Macquarie dictionary*. 3rd edn, Macquarie Library Pty Ltd, Australia, 1997.

A Holistic Approach to Prescribing Essential Oils

Objectives

After careful study of this chapter, you should be able to:

- outline a holistic approach to prescribing essential oils
- define the role of case history taking
- develop a treatment framework
- develop a patient management strategy
- develop a framework for selecting essential oils
- define the individual prescription
- determine the duration and dosage of essential oils.

Introduction

A holistic approach to prescribing essential oils in aromatherapy needs to include the following skills and knowledge:

- case history taking
- developing a treatment framework
- developing a patient management strategy
- the treatment.

All of these factors will influence the therapeutic effect and outcome, and the aim of the aromatherapist is to find the right combination of prescribing factors for each individual patient.

As with anything, experience will prove to be the best teacher, and these guidelines should not be seen as hard and fast rules. From a theoretical and practical perspective, it is usually impossible to take all factors into account.

Case History Taking

The aim of case history taking is to obtain the information needed to arrive at a treatment framework. This is achieved by conducting a consultation. The procedure for a consultation is described in *Chapter 17.*

A holistic approach should adopt a patient-centred consultation, which means that the focus is not only just on the condition but also takes into account the following:

- the patient as a person
- emotional reaction to the condition
- the effect on relationships
- work and leisure
- lifestyle
- the environment.

Therefore, particular emphasis should be given to:

- the historical factors behind the development of the presenting complaint
- factors which modify the presenting complaint
- current and previous medication
- information about the patient's constitution and current condition which can come from alternative methods of diagnosis and/or orthodox methods of diagnosis, e.g., blood tests
- diet
- social history
- past serious health problems and disorders related to the presenting complaint, as these can lead to information about the underlying causes of the complaint.[1]

Developing a Treatment Framework

The treatment framework sets out the aims of treatment. Information used to arrive at the treatment framework for a particular disorder is drawn from the following sources:

- the traditional holistic understanding of the condition
- the clinical experiences of the therapist in the treatment of the disorder
- a knowledge of scientific and clinical studies that have defined the underlying pathological process for that particular disorder
- a clinical understanding of the causes involved in the particular disorder
- the individual case history. The individual case history acts as a filter for all the above information
- the need for symptomatic treatment — this will depend on the individual case history.[1]

The knowledge required to develop a treatment framework based on a traditional holistic understanding of the condition, an understanding of the pathological processes and a clinical understanding of the condition is described in *Unit V: Clinical Index.*

We need take into account the physiological conditions and the psychological, emotional and spiritual aspects of our client. Once all these parameters have been clearly identified, the essential oils can be selected according to their properties and their nature.

Management Strategy

The objectives in developing a management strategy are to:

- involve the patient as much as possible in the management of his or her own condition
- educate the patient about the illness
- promote rational prescribing
- achieve compliance with therapy
- provide appropriate reassurance
- encourage continuity of ongoing care.[1]

Murtagh suggests a 10-point plan managing a treatment strategy. These guidelines will not always need to be applied in their entirety, and may be staged over a number of consultations.[1]

1. Explain the treatment strategy to the patient.
2. Establish the patient's knowledge of the condition.

3. Establish the patient's attitude to the condition. There may be a conflicting relationship with the patient without knowing why.
4. Educate the patient about the treatment strategy. This includes correcting any incorrect health beliefs recognised in point 2 and supplementing the patient's existing knowledge to a level appropriate to the needs of the patient and the therapist.
5. Develop a therapeutic strategy for the presenting problem: immediate, long-term and preventive.
6. Explore other preventive opportunities. This may include exercises, dietary modifications, advice about smoking and alcohol problems, just to name a few.
7. Reinforce the information. Encourage the patient to participate in decision making and in accepting some degree of responsibility for his or her own management.
8. Provide takeaway information.
9. Evaluate the consultation. The therapist should encourage feedback regarding the patient's reaction to the way the treatment was conducted, and establish whether the objectives have been met and the patient is happy with the outcome.
10. Arrange a follow-up. Follow-up sessions allow the therapist to reinforce and clarify preventive measures and information given.

The Treatment

The aromatherapy treatment should be energetically and constitutionally matched to the patient. The following guidelines are not hard and fast rules; in any event, experience proves to be the best teacher in prescribing:

- decide on the treatment goals based on the treatment strategy
- ensure the goals are individualised to the requirements of the individual case
- decide on the immediate priorities of the treatment
- choose reliable essential oils that have these actions
- if a particular action needs to be reinforced, do this by choosing more than one essential oil
- make sure that the choice of essential oils matches the energetic and the physiological state of the patient
- support the treatment with appropriate lifestyle management advice and preventive measures.

In acute conditions the dosage and timing of the administration of the essential oils are most likely to be critical, whereas in chronic conditions, the use of the right blend may well be the foremost consideration.

The nature of any treatment depends considerably on the extent to which the pathogen has penetrated the system. A passing cough, cold, headache or dyspepsia can be treated very simply and usually safely with home remedies, such as might be discussed at a symptomatic level of the average aromatherapy book. These treatments often combine reasonable efficacy with a lack of interference in vital processes.

Mills says that most of these problems would be self-limiting anyway; they would pass on whether they were treated or not. However, a condition that has persisted for a long period of time, either persistently or recurrently, is seen in traditional thought to have penetrated superficial defence measures. It will require increasingly substantial and carefully directed treatments and a greater practical expertise.[9]

Generally at the early, acute or superficial stages of disease the body will defend itself. This defence may often be uncomfortable or distressing and is often thought of as the illness. Symptoms may include vomiting and diarrhoea, coughing, fever, inflammations and skin eruptions. These mechanisms are caused by the body ridding itself of the pathogens causing the symptoms. It may be unwise to unduly suppress these symptoms. One may reduce the ferocity of the symptoms by making a cough more productive, managing a fever or by reducing inflammation by stimulating extra blood flow to the area. However, the priority should be management rather than suppression, as these symptoms should be seen as a sign of healthy resistance rather than an illness.[9]

However, if the symptoms have persisted for too long, or seem to have arisen out of another more substantial problem, then they should not be treated in quite the same way. Repeated bouts of bronchitis, sore throats, or rheumatic pains, even if these happen only every year or so, are more likely to be deep-seated rather than superficial problems. In chronic conditions there is a tendency for other vital signs to be subdued, for eliminatory functions like those of the bowels and urinary system to be diminished. Respiratory passages tend to dryness and sensitivity rather than the initial production of excessive catarrh.[9]

Selecting Essential Oils

The essential oils should be selected using the following guidelines:

- select the essential oils according to their therapeutic properties
- select the essential oils according to the constitution of your patient.

Classification of Essential Oils

Since there are so many essential oils to choose from, we need a practical and functional system that classifies the essential oils and makes it simple for us to decide which ones to select. There are several systems that can be used to classify the actions of essential oils.

The way in which medicinal plant substances have been organised and classified has always varied throughout the ages. The purpose of classification is to make plant remedies more readily accessible mentally and in written texts and hence easier to use in therapy. This can be done by using a system that is based on a botanical, pharmacological or a therapeutic classification of the essential oils. Each method has its advantages and disadvantages.

Botanical

Many important herbal compilations are organised according to plant families. An alternative botanical system sometimes used is classifying the essential oil's properties according to the part of the plant used.

Modern Pharmacological

This is a more analytical approach whereby plants are classified according to the purported main 'active principle', in other words according to the main biochemical substance thought to be responsible for their effects. The system used in aromatherapy classifies the essential oils according to their constituents' functional groups.

Topological

According to Holmes the aim of this system was to classify the therapeutic substances according to the part of the body in which they had the most influence. However, by the late 1600s, this system fused with the therapeutic classification, producing classifications such as hepatics (relating to the liver), cephalics (relating to the head), digestives (relating to the digestive system) and so on.[2]

Therapeutic

This is the most common system used by most therapists who have had training in western plant-based therapies. This system is based on anatomical-clinical medicine and pharmacological studies. The essential oils are organised according to their therapeutic properties. Holmes is very critical of this system:

> *The pharmacopoeia itself is now reduced to a state where each herb is individually ticketed with a little string of qualifiers such as sudorific, cathartic, hepatic — worn out labels meaningless to the modern practitioner untrained in Galenic medicine and oblivious to the meaning of its treatment strategies.*[2]

Holmes proposes a system that is 'energetically based'.

Energetics

Holmes says that there is no doubt that essential oils are successfully being used today in a variety of energy-based systems, such as acupuncture, reiki or chakra balancing.[3] In addition to their measurable scientific properties essential oils also work in subtle energetic ways beyond scientific analysis and terminology.

A holistic model should classify the essential oils according to an energetic based system. Such a system might incorporate the principles of Traditional Chinese Medicine or Ayurveda.[3]

Constitution of the Client

Classifying a person's personality to each essential oil has been done throughout most cultures and time. Typically, this is based on the aroma of the essential oil. The Chinese use the Yin/Yang and Five Element System, the Indians use Ayurvedic medicine, which recognises the three personalities and energy types of *Vata, Pitta* and *Kapha*, while the traditional Greek system used the four 'humours'.

According to Worwood, C.G. Jung adopted these four humours of air, fire, water, and earth into the concepts of the four aspects of a human being: thinking (air), intuition (fire), feeling (water), and sensation (earth).[4]

Galen, the ancient Greek, used the categories of *sanguine* (fire) — optimistic and happy; *melancholic* (earth) — depressed and anxious; *choleretic* (air) — irritable and impulsive; and *phlegmatic* (water) — listless and not easily moved. The different combinations of the four humours in any one individual constitutes his or her 'complexion' or 'temperament'. The ideal is to have equal proportions of all four.[4]

For example, Ayurvedic medicine can be used to diagnose a client in terms of the three doshas — *Vata, Pitta* and *Kapha*, which he or she will aim to bring into harmony with Ayurvedic medicines, diet, massage, meditation, yoga or essential oils. For example, vata dosha types are described as enthusiastic and lovers of new experiences but when out of balance they become anxious, exhausted and depressed, while pitta dosha types have a fiery temperament and are ambitious, perhaps overbearing and demanding.

The Individual Prescription

If an individual is drawn towards a particular essential oil, then is that essential oil defined as having the same personality characteristics? The answer to this is yes and no. There are two interrelated dynamics to take into consideration:

- **The signature scent** — i.e., the essential oil corresponds to the physical, emotional, and mental characteristics of the user.
- **The regulating scent** — i.e., the essential oil is needed to balance what is absent in the health or personality of the user.

As an example, Fischer-Rizzi discusses the nature of ylang ylang, emphasising the need to not only treat the symptoms but the role that the clients play in their own disharmony:

> *The spirit of ylang ylang usually fits that person who is naturally drawn to the oil. She is much like the title character, Carmen, from Georges Bizet's opera — fiery, temperamental, passionate and erotic. Although her emotions are deeply felt, she never loses her balance. Aware of her own fascinating radiance, she is capable of casting magical spells. Her wardrobe is bright and colourful and she loves to wear jewellery.*[5]

However, when ylang ylang is used for its regulatory scent it is more suitable for:

> *… this second woman often does not allow herself to live, who hides her femininity, dresses drably, and does not trust her intuitive powers. Extremely frustrated, she appears nervous, depressed and tense. Hormone imbalances, such as irregular, skipped or painful periods, or inflammation of the ovaries, may underlie certain illnesses.*[5]

Ylang ylang may be mistakenly classified as a feminine fragrance. Perfumers may have made a mistake in assuming (in a gender-biased way) that floral scents are for women and wood scents are for men.

The very nature of ylang ylang may also be utilised to help dominating masculine men bring out their more feminine side, awakening their intuition.

Duration of Treatment

The length of time in hours, days, weeks or months for which treatments should be administered can vary a great deal. The main considerations are to:

- treat the constitution of the individual
- rebalance the condition of disharmony
- relieve symptoms.

If the essential oils are used as preventive measures for the individual, extended or regular treatments are necessary. If the treatment is for symptom relief (not suppression), short-term use is enough. If the condition is chronic or degenerative such as multiple sclerosis or rheumatoid arthritis, the treatment might be ongoing and permanent. With acute conditions, short-term treatments may be sufficient. Please note that the imbalance that occurs from acute symptoms often needs further attention and longer-term treatments. Systemic conditions, such as those usually underlying skin eruptions, for example, are more likely to take longer to treat than purely local conditions such as injury or local infection.

What Dosage is Used?

One of the aspects that makes aromatherapy so intriguing is the range of principles involved. At one end of the spectrum the essential oils are being used for their pharmacological action, similar to allopathic medicine, yet under the assumption that the whole natural extract is best suited to induce true healing. At the other end of the spectrum is the psychotherapeutic use of the essential oils, where the scent is considered the most important agent to bring about healing.

According to Schnaubelt, the effects caused by olfactory triggering mechanisms in aromatherapy work in the same concentration ranges as homoeopathic preparations.[6]

The question of how much essential oil is needed to achieve the desired effect is important in aromatherapy. The size of most essential oil constituents, in conjunction with their volatile and lipophilic natures, means that the essential oils have the ability to penetrate human skin.

Many natural substances have been found to have a certain effect at one concentration and the opposite effect at another concentration. Tisserand, for example, states that:

> *… patchouli oil seems to be one of those oils that is either stimulating in small doses, and is sedative at larger doses. Its yang effect is most pronounced on the nervous system; it seems to be a very strong nerve stimulant, reminiscent of ginseng … The effect of sedation or stimulation not only depends on the dose but also on the state of the individual.*[7]

Holmes says that lavender can exert a cooling or a warming effect on the body. This would depend on the dosage of lavender used and the type of condition being treated. A person with a hot and acute condition — typified by congestion, inflammation or fever, dilutions of one percent or less are recommended. This will have a cooling, anti-inflammatory effect.[8]

On the other hand someone with a cold and chronic condition, characterised by chills, fatigue, cold extremities — a higher dose of lavender may be used to generate warmth and activity.[8]

Therefore lavender can cool and sedate or warm up and stimulate, depending on the dosage used.

This supports the assumption that increasing the dosage does not necessarily increase the effect; to the contrary, it may diminish it. It is usually advisable to use essential oils in small dosages. Test this yourself by using half the amount of essential oil you are currently using for a certain problem. I am sure you will be surprised to find that the observed effectiveness of the essential oils will not be diminished.

References

1. Murtagh J. *General practice*. The McGraw-Hill Companies Inc., Australia, 1998.
2. Holmes P. *The energetics of western herbs*. Artemis Press, USA, 1989.
3. Holmes P. *Energy medicine*. The International Journal of Aromatherapy 1999; 9(2): 53–56.
4. Worwood V. *The fragrant mind*. Doubleday, Great Britain, 1995.
5. Fisher-Rizzi S. *Complete aromatherapy handbook*. Sterling Publishing Company, USA, 1990.
6. Schnaubelt K. *Less is more*. The International Journal of Aromatherapy 1988; 1(3): 4.
7. Tisserand R. *The art of aromatherapy*. The C.W. Daniel Company Limited, Great Britain, 1977.
8. Holmes P. *Lavender oil*. The International Journal of Aromatherapy 1992; 4(2): 20–22.
9. Mills S. *The essential book of herbal medicine*. Penguin Books, 1991, England.

The Art of Blending

Objectives

After careful study of this chapter, you should be able to:

- explain the principles of blending
- define the term synergy, as it relates to aromatherapy blends
- create a therapeutic blend
- discuss the psychological impact of a blend
- utilise a range of blending principles to create a blend
- examine a range of aromatherapy formulae.

Introduction

There is a plethora of books on aromatherapy. Many of them are often laced with wonderful and intriguing recipes and blends; however, very few of them address the skills required to blend the oils. The art of blending essential oils is still shrouded in mystery. While there are some basic guidelines to assist you in blending, they will not help you to create a perfect synergy.

Many aromatherapists consider blending of essential oils as the fun, playful aspect of aromatherapy. In fact, Lavabre says that blending is one of the most enjoyable aspects of aromatherapy. It can become a very enjoyable hobby.[1]

However, it must be emphasised that while blending allows you to express your creative outlet, it plays a very important role in creating a powerful synergy of essential oils that will enhance the effectiveness of your treatment.

Lavabre says that blending is an art, but like any art it requires a balance of practice, skills and intuition.[1]

Principles of Blending

Creating a synergy is the most important part of blending. It requires a deep understanding of essential oils, a fair amount of experience and a lot of intuition. Intuition and experience are very important, because synergies are rather context-dependent. A given combination of oils might be an excellent synergy for one patient, but totally inappropriate for another.

To create a good synergy, you need to take into account not only the symptoms that you want to treat, but also the underlying causes of the disorder, the biological terrain and the psychological or emotional factors involved.

While the aesthetic appeal of a blend is often critical, I agree with Lavabre, who says:

> *When creating a blend, first look at the purpose of the blend. A blend to fight an infection will be very different from one to soothe emotional wounds or to relieve stress. An infection-fighting blend will be built like a small commando of very efficient no-nonsense soldiers. You want to get the job done as quickly and cleanly as possible. Your main concern is that the purpose be clear and that all oils used work in a very disciplined way towards the same goal. Fragrance is totally secondary.*
>
> *For emotional problems on the other hand, fragrance is of utmost importance, and you will need to carefully and skilfully build your blend to produce a pleasant one.*[1]

For example, the aesthetic appeal of a blend for a client with an arthritic condition is often of little consequence. It is necessary to find out more about the client's condition. If it is rheumatoid arthritis, it will be more appropriate to choose anti-inflammatory essential oils such as German chamomile and everlasting; however, ginger and cajeput are more appropriate for treating osteoarthritis, as these oils have excellent analgesic properties.

The goal of a holistic approach must also balance the body chemistry. Toxins must be eliminated and new accumulations of toxins must be prevented. Therefore, detoxifying essential oils such as juniper berry, carrot seed, sweet fennel or lemon are recommended.

The aesthetics of the blend becomes far more important when it is necessary to address the psychological and emotional factors of a condition. This is often the case with eczema and psoriasis, where it might be appropriate to select essential oils with anti-inflammatory properties such as German chamomile and everlasting. However, when stress is involved it is more appropriate to use essential oils that will help the patient cope better with stress.

In some circumstances, knowledge of the chemical constituents can be quite beneficial in creating a blend. For example, when a person has a chronic respiratory tract infection, the approach would be to bombard the person with essential oils rich in phenols as they have potent antimicrobial properties. However if the individual has a cough and there is excessive mucus, it is necessary to liquefy the mucous by using essential oils rich in ketones that are mucolytic. It will also be beneficial to use essential oils rich in oxides, as they are excellent expectorants and will assist in the elimination of excess mucus.

The throat may be red, sore and inflamed, so essential oils such as sandalwood and cedarwood that are rich in sesquiterpenes are beneficial because of their anti-inflammatory and soothing qualities.

The immune system can be supported by utilising monoterpenes in the blend. Therefore our blend might look like this:

Essential Oil	Principal Constituents	Property
20% thyme, red	phenols	antimicrobial
20% *Eucalyptus dives*	ketones	mucolytic
10% sandalwood	sesquiterpenes	anti-inflammatory
30% *E. polybractea*	oxides	expectorant
20% lemon	monoterpenes	immuno-stimulant

A different blend achieving a similar therapeutic outcome could be as follows:

Essential Oil	Principal Constituents	Property
20% cedarwood, Virginian	sesquiterpenes	anti-inflammatory
10% aniseed	ketones	mucolytic
30% bay, laurel	phenols, oxides	antimicrobial & expectorant
40% ravensara	oxides, monoterpenes	expectorant, immuno-stimulant

It may also be tempting to treat a patient with many symptoms and conditions with the one blend. This, according to Lavabre, is:

> *... the best recipe for failure and represents a misunderstanding of the concept of synergy. Essential oils can be used in many ways and applied to many areas of the body. Do not try to treat the lungs and the kidneys with the same blend. Instead, create a blend for each area that you want to address.*[1]

Lavabre suggests that one should not blend essential oils with opposite effects (e.g., a calming oil and a stimulating oil).[1] While this advice is correct in principle, it does not apply to all situations.

For example, lavender and rosemary would not be compatible for a person who is having problems sleeping and suffering from muscular aches and pain. However, if this person did not have sleeping problems the blend would be perfectly fine to use, as long as there was no hypertension and you were aware of other potential contra-indications associated with rosemary.

The Psychological Impact of a Blend

When blending essential oils it is necessary to be aware of the strong association between scent and memory.

The mute language of fragrance may summon up an elusive deja vu sensation — 'It reminds me of something, but I just can't think what'. It may often be more precise, reminding you of first love or a childhood visit to a well-loved grandmother who smelled of lavender.

The ability to build picture-bridges, to associate images and feelings with fragrances, can assist us in understanding the constitution of our client. For example:

- patchouli = oriental market
- sandalwood = spiritual and meditative
- jasmine = sensuous and erotic.

We need not have smelled a particular fragrance before for it to have an amazing influence. Generally speaking, pleasant odours will evoke happy and pleasant feelings, unless we have learned to associate particular 'pleasant' fragrance with an unpleasant experience, whereas unpleasant odours generally make us feel uneasy.

Make sure that the patients are comfortable with the aroma. If they associate a smell with an unpleasant experience, the smell will make them go through all the emotions associated with that unpleasant experience.

The concept of character/personality profiling of essential oils can be difficult to understand. This may be explained by imagining you are in a room, blindfolded, and someone wearing an essential oil as a perfume walks into the room. What does this tell you about her — her personality, what kind of interests she might have and what type of clothes she might wear?

In holistic aromatherapy, including an essential oil to match the character of your client may be essential for an effective blend.

Blending Techniques

While there are no hard and fast rules in blending essential oils for aromatherapy, the following hints may be helpful:

- Until you gain considerable experience, do not blend more than three or four oils at a time.
- It is important that the odour of the blend is pleasant to your patient.
- Ensure that your patient does not have any allergies to the essential oils that you have selected.
- Ensure that your patient does not have unpleasant memory associations with the essential oils that you have selected.

Perhaps John Steele gives us the best advice. At a workshop on blending that I once attended, he emphasised the importance of *learning to listen through your nose*. He also suggested that the person blending should be *empty and receptive*, as one would be during meditation.[2]

However, how do we go about creating a balanced and aesthetically pleasing blend? It must be emphasised that blending is highly subjective. A number of systems exist that will provide you with a basic framework for blending. They are as follows.

Top Notes	Middle Notes	Base Notes
Bergamot	German chamomile	Carrot seed
Clove	Cardamom	Cedarwood
Cinnamon	Geranium	Cistus
Grapefruit	Ginger	Clary sage
Lemon	Lavender	Frankincense
Lemongrass	Sweet marjoram	Myrrh
Lime	Palmarosa	Patchouli
Mandarin	Pine	Peru Balsam
Neroli	Rosemary	Sandalwood
Petitgrain	Rosewood	Spikenard
Sweet orange	Ylang ylang	Vetiver
Peppermint		
Thyme		

Top, middle and base note classification of essential oils commonly used in aromatherapy.

Top, Middle and Base Notes

Many aromatherapists resort to the traditional concept of top, middle and base notes for aromatherapy blending. This concept is extremely important in perfumery. A good blend should be a balanced synergy of top, middle and base notes. However, I believe that it has been overemphasised when blending essential oils for aromatherapy purposes.

In the first edition of *The Complete Guide to Aromatherapy* I cited work by Carles, a perfumer who suggests a ratio of 15–25% for top note, 30–40% for middle note and 45–55% for base note. While this ratio may be suitable for a perfume composition, I don't think it needs to apply to aromatherapy.

However, I agree with Lavabre, who suggests the following ratios:[1]

top notes:	20–30%
middle notes:	40–80%
base notes:	10–25%

What your sense of smell first experiences in a blend is known as the *top note*, or the *initial impact*. Then, after a few minutes, comes the *bouquet*, the *heart*, or the *middle note*, which gradually blends into the *back note*, also known as the *base note* or *fond* in French. The essential oils are placed in order from the very light (very volatile) oils to the heavy (least volatile) oils.

Top Notes

The top note is usually a fresh citrus and light, volatile green note and fruity ester notes. These form the blend's initial impression, giving brightness and clarity to it. They are usually refreshing and uplifting. Typical top notes are citrus essential oils such as bergamot, neroli, lemon, lime, sweet orange and essential oils such as peppermint, thyme, cinnamon and clove.

While most citrus top notes can be used liberally in a blend, the spice oils should be used in very small amounts.

Middle Notes

The middle or heart notes last longer, imparting the warmth and fullness of the blend. They give body to blends. Middle notes are mostly found in essential oils distilled from leaves and herbs. Essential oils such as geranium, lavender, marjoram, rosewood and rosemary are middle notes and they primarily influence digestion and the general metabolism of the body.

Base Notes

Then there is the heavy smelling, deeply resonating base note which has a profound influence on the blend as a whole. This includes essential oils such as frankincense, myrrh, patchouli, vetiver and sandalwood, which have a long-lasting scent and act as fixatives. This means they slow down the volatility rate of top and middle notes, thus improving the tenacity of the blend as a whole.

Base notes have a strong influence on the mental, emotional and spiritual plane. They have a sedative and relaxing effect.

Practical Tips

An essential oil blend should not break up into three stages, each of which smells differently, leaving the others behind. If the blend is well balanced, the top note will contain some middle note, the base note retains some of the middle note, and changes during the evaporation process will be as imperceptible as the movements of the hands of a watch. An essential oil blend that falls apart is badly formulated.

Bergamot, for example, though highly volatile itself, tempers the evaporation rate of the even flightier lemon or grapefruit, while neroli has the same action on bergamot. A good bridging essential oil has the ability to awaken the more receptive elements of the heavier aromas. The deeply resonating scent of vetiver can be elevated by using lime; patchouli, by using lavender; and ylang ylang, by using sweet orange.

If you have composed a blend that smells to garish, with the top note being too far removed from the middle note, you can bring the formula into harmony by adding an essential oil with a softer quality that at the same time vibrates from the middle towards the top, such as neroli, rose otto or clary sage.

If, on the other hand, the base note has become too pronounced, having no connection to the middle, you will have to lift the blend by adding an essential oil that smells a little brighter, resonating from the middle to the base, such as lavender, geranium, ylang ylang or rosewood.

If the blend is principally composed of top notes, consider using a small amount of rosewood or sandalwood. However, keep in mind that if the blend is composed of only top notes, do not expect the fragrance to be anything more than a brief encounter.

While the top, middle and base note classification certainly gives you some advice, Lavabre's classification of essential oils according to equalisers, modifiers and enhancers provides some excellent advice for anyone wishing to create a perfect synergy.

Blend Equalisers

Blend equalisers are those essential oils that will smooth out the sharp edges in a blend. They will balance the blend and allow it to flow harmoniously.[1] Lavabre says that essential oils such as fir, rosewood, Spanish marjoram, sweet orange, pine and tangerine are examples of equalisers. Fir and pine needle are ideal to use with the cineole-rich essential oils.[1]

The main purpose of the blend equaliser is to hold the blend together but it has little effect on the blend's distinctive personality. Blend equalisers can be used in large quantities — up to 50%, especially if you are also using blend modifiers.[1]

Blend Modifiers

Blend modifiers will give the blend a lift and contribute to its distinctive personality. If the blend is rather flat and uninteresting, adding a drop of a modifier may improve it. Blend modifiers include essential oils such as clove, cinnamon, peppermint, German chamomile, cistus and vetiver. They should be used sparingly (usually never more than 3%) as they have the ability to influence the overall fragrance of the blend even when used in very small amounts.[1]

Blend Enhancers

These essential oils have a pleasant fragrance and slightly modify the blend without overpowering it. Blend enhancers include essential oils such as bergamot, cedarwood, geranium, clary sage, lavender, lemon, lime, may chang, palmarosa, sandalwood, spruce, jasmine, neroli, rose otto and myrrh. Blend enhancers can be used up to 50%.[1]

Natural Extenders

Essential oils such as jasmine, rose and neroli are quite expensive. When you use these oils in a blend you wish to take full advantage of their exquisite aroma. Lavabre recommends using natural extenders that are compatible with expensive essential oils to make the blend more affordable.[1]

The formula below is an excellent use of natural extenders. This blend maintains its exquisite rosy aroma, by adding two affordable essential oils with a delightful floral and rosy odour — palmarosa and rosewood. The sweet, rich, earthy odour of patchouli is perfect as a base note.

palmarosa	10%
rose absolute	20%
rosewood	60%
patchouli	10%

Odour Intensity

Perfumers have developed analytical techniques for determining the odour intensity of essential oils. The odour intensities presented below were developed by Appell and are rated on a scale from 1 to 10. The odour intensity may be used as guide to blending. The key to balance is achieving olfactory equilibrium, which occurs when two or more essential oils are in a mixture and no single essential oil dominates the odour of the blend.

For example, if you are making a blend with everlasting and lavender, the respective odour intensities are 7 and 5. This means that the odour of everlasting is stronger than that of lavender. As a result, mixing one drop of everlasting and one drop of lavender will not produce a fragrance representing both essential oils. Everlasting would dominate. To create a balanced blend it may be necessary to mix one drop of everlasting to three drops of lavender. While the figures given for the odour intensity do not give an exact mixing ratio, they do make it easier to find the right proportions.

Essential Oil	Odour Intensity	Essential Oil	Odour Intensity	Essential Oil	Odour Intensity
Angelica root	9	Frankincense	7	Patchouli	7
Aniseed	7	Ginger	7	Pepper, black	7
Basil	7	Juniper	5	Peppermint	7
Bergamot	5	Lavender	5	Petitgrain	5
Cedarwood	6	Lavender, spike	6	Pine	5
Cinnamon	7	Lemon	5	Rose absolute	8
Citronella	6	Lemongrass	6	Rose otto	7
Clary sage	5	Mandarin	5	Rosemary	6
Clove bud	8	Myrrh	7	Rosewood	5
Eucalyptus	8	Neroli	5	Sage, Dalmatian	6
Everlasting	7	Nutmeg	7	Sandalwood	7
Fennel	6	Sweet orange	5	Thyme, red	7

The odour intensity of commonly used essential oils according to Appell.[3]

Odour Types

Blending can also be done according to odour types. For example, lavender has a floral herbaceous scent, so it will blend well with floral scents as well as herbaceous scents. This classification is considered quite subjective. However, it can provide some useful guidance.

Floral notes are usually expensive and the amount that will be used depends on the budget. Floral oils blend well with woody, fruity, sweet and musty notes and to some herbaceous notes. They are wasted with camphoraceous notes.[1]

Fruity notes are inexpensive and easy to blend. They do not blend very well with woods and poorly with camphoraceous.[1]

Green notes will blend well with any essential oil, if used in small amounts.[1]

Herbaceous notes blend well with camphoraceous and wood notes. Use with caution when using with florals.[1]

Camphoraceous notes give a medicinal feel to any blend. Will ruin floral notes and do not blend well with fruit notes. Best used with herbaceous and woody notes.[1]

Spicy notes should be used in very small amounts (0.5 to 5%). They can add an interesting note to any blend and, as Lavabre says, they can make or break a blend.[1]

Woody notes blend well with any oils. They create warmth and give the blend its heart.[1]

Earthy notes give depth and grounds any blend. Do not overuse, usually 3 to 10% is sufficient.[1]

Aromatherapy Blends

The following blends have been provided as a guide to illustrate the blending techniques discussed.

Detoxification Blend

This is an excellent detoxifying blend which can be used to support the lymphatic system, the liver and kidneys.

Carrot seed has a peculiar dry-woody, earthy scent — it has been used sparingly, or else it would easily dominate the blend. Grapefruit has been liberally used to tone down the medicinal odour of sweet fennel and juniper berry, while the herbaceous scent of rosemary gives this blend body.

grapefruit	35%
sweet fennel	20%
juniper berry	30%
carrot seed	5%
rosemary	10%

Arthritis Blend — Rheumatoid

The role of this blend is to reduce inflammation and pain. German chamomile and everlasting complement each other and are an ideal choice for their anti-inflammatory properties. However, they both have a high odour intensity so they have been used sparingly.

German chamomile	10%
everlasting	10%
cajeput	25%
spike lavender	35%
juniper berry	20%

Study Blend

This is a wonderful refreshing and stimulating blend, the rich herbaceous scents of basil, peppermint and rosemary have been beautifully complemented by liberal amounts of the zesty citrus scent of lemon. As basil and peppermint are both blend modifiers and have a high odour intensity they have been used sparingly.

basil	10%
lemon	50%
peppermint	10%
rosemary	30%

Sensitive Skin Blend

This wonderful synergy of woody, herbaceous and floral scents is soothing, harmonising and gentle. German chamomile has been used sparingly, so that it does not overwhelm the scent of the blend.

German chamomile	10%
lavender	40%
neroli	10%
sandalwood	40%

Insomnia Blend

Sweet orange and lavender are two delightful oils to blend. They form a perfect synergy, which has been complemented by the gentle woody aroma of sandalwood and the highly diffusive, sweet, herbaceous scent of Roman chamomile, which is important to this blend, but used sparingly.

lavender	30%
sweet orange	35%
Roman chamomile	10%
sandalwood	25%

Nervous Tension Blend

A very simple blend utilising the most effective therapeutic essential oils to deal with nervous tension. The essential oils chosen in this blend smell great. Neroli has been complemented with the floral scent of lavender and ylang ylang. Geranium has a powerful diffusive green, leafy and rosy scent so it is used sparingly.

lavender	35%
geranium	15%
neroli	20%
ylang ylang	30%

Colds and Flu Blend

This blend contains essential oils that will really pack a punch. It is a delightful citrus, camphoraceous and herbaceous blend which will fight off the symptoms of any cold or flu.

Eucalyptus polybractea	35%
E. citriodora	35%
ginger	5%
tea tree	20%
red thyme	5%

Sinus Blend

A simple therapeutic blend in which all the essential oils have been used in very similar quantities. Less peppermint is used because it has a high odour intensity, which would dominate the blend.

E. polybractea	30%
spike lavender	25%
pinus sylvestris	30%
peppermint	15%

Uplifting Blend

This blend makes use of some wonderful essential oils with antidepressant properties. It is a delicate combination of floral, citrus and woody scents.

bergamot	30%
neroli	15%
rose otto	15%
rosewood	40%

Heart Chakra Blend

The heart chakra is concerned with forgiveness, compassion and unconditional love. It is not difficult to see why the following essential oils have been chosen. This blend utilises expensive essential oils, but they have been used sparingly, yet they have a pronounced impact on the overall odour of the blend.

bergamot	20%
lavender	40%
melissa	3%
neroli	5%
rose absolute	2%
ylang ylang	30%

Third Eye Chakra

The third eye chakra offers us the ability to see and understand all things. Bergamot has been used as a blend equaliser and clary sage, a blend modifier, has been used sparingly. Myrtle and rosemary are camphoraceous and herbaceous, and liberal amounts of bergamot have been used as a blend enhancer to create a harmonious synergy.

bergamot	35%
clary sage	5%
lavender	30%
myrtle	10%
rosemary	20%

References

1. Lavabre M. *Aromatherapy workbook.* Healing Art Press, USA, 1997.
2. Steele J. *Blending workshop at AROMA'93 Conference*, England, 1993.
3. Appell L. *Cosmetics, fragrances and flavours: Their formulation and preparation.* Novox Inc, USA, 1982.

Methods of Administration

Objectives

After careful study of this chapter, you should be able to:

- describe methods of using essential oils
- outline the benefits of the various methods of using essential oils
- examine the internal use of essential oils.

Introduction

One of the advantages of aromatherapy is the ease in which essential oils can be administered in so many different ways:

- methods of percutaneous absorption such as massage; baths; foot, hand and sitz baths; compresses; skin care preparations and ointments; and neat application
- inhalation
- internal use.

Applying essential oils correctly is important if the full benefits of their properties are to be utilised.

Percutaneous Techniques

This means techniques that involve the application of the essential oil to the skin. Some of the commonly used methods are:

- massage
- bath
- compress
- topical application by the use of ointments, gels and creams.

Massage

Massage with essential oils is by far the most common method of using essential oils in holistic aromatherapy. Many studies have confirmed the importance of touch in the development of healthy human beings. Touch has been described as a basic human behavioural need and its importance for mental and physical health has been well researched.[1]

Therapeutic Benefits of Massage

The massage therapist may learn a variety of techniques that are designed to have a multitude of beneficial effects. The beneficial effects of massage include:

- inducing deep relaxation, relieving mental and physical fatigue
- releasing chronic neck and shoulder tension and backache
- improving circulation to muscles, reducing inflammation and pain
- relieving neuralgic, arthritic and rheumatic conditions
- helping sprains, fractures, breaks and dislocations heal more readily
- promoting correct posture and helping improve mobility
- improving, directly or indirectly, the function of every internal organ
- improving digestion, assimilation and elimination
- increasing the ability of the kidneys to function efficiently
- stimulating the lymphatic system to eliminate toxins
- helping to disperse many types of headache
- helping to release suppressed feelings, which can be shared in a safe setting.[1]

Aromatherapy Massage

Aromatherapy massage uses gentle, relaxing techniques and utilises the various energy systems of the body. The percussive techniques of Swedish massage or deep tissue massage work are generally not suitable for aromatherapy massage because they are too intense and stimulating when used with essential oils.

Aromatherapists may utilise a range of massage techniques. This obviously depends on their training and background, and partly on their personal outlook and preference.

Davis says that it does not matter too much which technique is used, provided that the therapist has been thoroughly trained in his or her chosen system and uses it with care and a nurturing attitude towards the client. It is far more important that the massage physically encompasses the whole body and that the therapist takes into account the whole person — body, mind and spirit.[2]

I have been privileged to train with Madame Micheline Arcier. This aromatherapy massage technique is described in *Chapter 22*.

How to Use Essential Oils in Massage

For massage purposes, essential oils are usually diluted in a carrier oil. The standard carrier oil used is a vegetable oil. There is no preferred vegetable oil. The selection of the base used is dependent on the benefits of the carrier oil and the cost of the carrier oil.

For example, someone with dry skin would benefit from cold-pressed avocado oil, someone with mature skin would benefit from cold-pressed rosehip oil and wheatgerm oil, while someone with sensitive skin would benefit from jojoba and evening primrose being used as a base oil.

The recommended dilution rate used is a 1% to 3% dilution of the appropriate essential oil to the carrier oil.

A general rule of thumb is that 1 mL of essential oil is approximately 20 drops. This is only an estimate as it will obviously depend on the size of the eye dropper or dripulator and the specific gravity of the essential oil.

If you are preparing a 3% dilution massage blend:

- to 100 mL of carrier oil, you add 3 mL of essential oil, or 60 drops
- to 50 mL of carrier oil, you add 1.5 mL of essential oil, or 30 drops.

If you are using more than one essential oil to make your massage oil, it must be emphasised that the dilution refers to the total combination of essential oils.

When working with babies, children, pregnant women, elderly and persons with sensitive skin you should use only 0.5% to 1.0% dilution.

If you are preparing a 1% dilution massage blend:

- to 100 mL of carrier oil, you add 1 mL of essential oil, or 20 drops
- to 50 mL of carrier oil, you add 0.5 mL of essential oil, or 10 drops.

Conditions that respond to massage include circulatory problems, digestive problems, fluid retention, headaches, insomnia, menstrual problems, musculoskeletal disorders and nervous tension.

Contra-indications for Massage

The aromatherapist must know when massage is recommended and when it should be avoided. The following conditions are generally contra-indicated for massage:[3]

Abnormal body temperature: Massage is contra-indicated when the client has a fever.

Acute infectious disease: Do not give a massage to an individual who is coming down with an acute viral infection such as a cold and flu. The massage will intensify the illness and also expose the therapist to the virus.

Inflammation: Where there is acute inflammation in a particular area of the body, massage is not advisable because it could further irritate the area or intensify the inflammation.

Osteoporosis: This condition leads to deterioration of bone. In advanced stages bones become brittle, sometimes to the point that they are easily broken. Osteoporosis is usually prevalent in the elderly.

Varicose veins: Varicose veins are a condition in which the valves in the veins break down because of back pressure in the circulatory system. The veins bulge and may rupture, usually in the legs. The development of varicose veins is often the result of gravity or other obstructed venous flow, as the result of crossing the legs or other sitting postures that inhibit circulation to or from the legs.

However, essential oils such as cypress, lemon and geranium can be blended with calendula-infused oil to effectively treat varicose veins. Special care is needed in the execution of the massage, and only gentle, almost superficial, upward effleurage strokes should be used.

Oedema: Oedema is a circulatory problem that generally appears as puffiness in the extremities, but it can be more widespread. Specific massage techniques such as lymphatic drainage are considered beneficial for the treatment of oedema.

High blood pressure: Massage is often contra-indicated for persons with high blood pressure. However, an aromatherapy massage that incorporates essential oils known to lower blood pressure, such as lavender, ylang ylang, sweet marjoram and may chang, will be beneficial.

Intoxication: Never massage a client who is intoxicated.

Other Topical Applications

These can be very useful mediums for the topical application of essential oils when a vegetable oil base is not suitable.

Ointments

Ointments are semisolid non-aqueous preparations that are not absorbed easily into the skin and are therefore used to provide a protective or remedial film over the skin. Being immiscible with water or skin secretions, ointments effectively form an occlusive layer over the skin, preventing evaporation.

The result is similar to an occlusive dressing. The skin becomes waterlogged (hydrated), permitting easier absorption of the essential oils in the ointment.

Ointments have topical protective, healing, soothing, moistening and cooling properties and provide a long-term effect when continuously applied. Some examples of the application of ointments are:

- For the treatment of boils, sores, infected cuts and fungal skin conditions a soothing and antiseptic ointment can be made using tea tree oil and calendul-infused oil.
- The rubefacient and analgesic properties of arnica-infused oil, black pepper, ginger, hypericum-infused oil, cinnamon and peppermint can be used in an ointment to treat arthritis and sports injuries. Use before an event to keep the muscles warm and prevent injuries.
- To moisten, soothe and protect dry, irritated skin conditions such as eczema, dry, chapped

skin or lips use calendula-infused oil, lavender, myrrh and German chamomile in an ointment.

Many recipes use lanolin, a wool fat, or petroleum jelly as a base. I prefer to use a vegetable-derived ointment such as the formula outlined below:[4]

20 to 15 g	beeswax or cocoa butter
80 to 85 mL	vegetable oil.

Alternatively, shea butter makes an excellent ointment base.[4]

While the recommended dilution for essential oils in a massage oil or lotion can be up to 3% dilution, in an ointment the amount of essential oil used can be much higher. This obviously depends on the condition being treated. For example, an ointment for wound care which incorporates essential oils such as lavender, everlasting and German chamomile could contain 20% or more essential oils. It is not uncommon to have an ointment for muscular aches and pains or arthritis to be made with 40% or more essential oils. These ointments would be used on localised areas of the body and usually for a short period.

Emulsions

Creams and lotions are examples of emulsions. They may be used to treat most skin conditions or any condition where a massage oil is considered.

An emulsion is a stable system of two or more immiscible liquids in which the droplets of one liquid are held in suspension in the other by emulsifiers.[5]

To create an emulsion, oil, water and an emulsifier must be mixed in a way to finely disperse the oil in water (or vice versa). Two types of emulsions can be made:

- oil in water emulsions
- water in oil emulsions.

The first disperses oil droplets in water and the second disperses water droplets in oil. If you are not to sure what kind of emulsion your favourite cream or lotion is made of, put some on your finger and let water run over it. If it washes off easily it is an oil in water product, if not, it is a water in oil emulsion. Sometimes it may be necessary to make a cream with more resistance to water e.g., when making a sunscreen or for environmental and occupational protection.

An emulsifier is a chemical compound that is used to join oil and water to form a stable mixture called an emulsion. Each emulsifier molecule has the unique property of being able to attract both water and oil at the same time at different sites of its molecular structure.[6]

The basic ingredients needed to make emulsions include:

- emulsifying waxes (emulsifier)
- water
- emollients such as vegetable oils
- active ingredients such as essential oils or herbal extracts
- preservatives.

A simple recipe for making a cream is as follows:[4]

Oil phase:

10 g	emulsifying wax
30 mL	sweet almond oil.

Water phase:

5 mL	vegetable glycerin
90 mL	purified water
2 mL	citrus seed extract.

In one bowl, melt the wax in a bain-marie and stir in the vegetable oil. Bring the water and glycerin to the same temperature in a separate bowl. Remove both bowls from the heat and slowly stir the water phase into the oil phase. Continue beating until the mixture cools, add the citrus seed extract and then add 1–3% essential oil to the preparation and store in a jar.

Gels

Gels are used to hydrate, soothe and cool the skin. Gels make an excellent base for essential oils when a vegetable oil base is not desired. Gels can be made from plants such as linseed, pectin from citrus peel, guar gum or xanthan gum.[4] Gels can be used as:

- moisturisers
- masks
- treatments for skin problems such as acne and blemished skin.

A simple recipe for making a gel base is as follows:[4]

2–5 g	powdered gum
100 mL	purified water.

Sprinkle the pectin, guar or xanthan gum slowly into purified water that has been heated to 35–40°C. Use a whisk or electric hand mixer to ensure the powdered gum is evenly dispersed throughout the water. Strain the gel, and add more water if a thinner consistency is desired. Add up to 1% essential oil.

Inhalations

When essential oils are diffused into a room they have a multitude of effects. There is the obvious olfactory pleasure that is gained. Unpleasant odours can be replaced by the natural aromas of essential oils, thus stimulating our senses and imagination by the memories that they evoke.

Essential oils have specific therapeutic properties on the wellbeing of those who breathe them in. They have long been known for their airborne antiseptic properties, allowing them to disinfect and purify the air in the event of bacterial contamination. For example, Valnet says:

> *The essence of lemon is second to none in its antiseptic and bactericidal properties. The work of Morel and Rochaix has demonstrated that the vapours of lemon essence neutralize the meningococcus in 15 minutes, the typhus bacillus in less than an hour, pneumococcus in 1–3 hours and staphylococcus aureus in 2 hours.*[7]

The use of essential oils as an inhalation for the treatment of respiratory conditions such as nasal congestion, coughs, colds and sore throat is a common and effective practice. Essential oils such as *Eucalyptus polybractea* or *Ravenara aromatica* act as mucolytics and pulmonary decongestants.

Inhalation of essential oils works predominantly on the mind via the olfactory/limbic/hormonal/emotional response. Inhalations may therefore be effective in overcoming problems such as stress, depression or tiredness and any other emotional dilemma that may be encountered.

Buchbauer believes that the only effective way of administering essential oils is via inhalation:

> *Aromatherapy applied in the correct way by inhalation only (where the resultant plasma concentration of aroma compounds is 100 to 10,000 smaller) leads to the desired effect.*[8]

Maury describes the effect of fragrance on the psyche and mental state of the individual:

> *Powers of perception become clearer and more acute, and there is a feeling of having, to a certain extent, outstripped events. They are seen more objectively and therefore in truer perspective.*[9]

The use of essential oils as an inhalation for the treatment of respiratory conditions such as a congested nose, headache, sore throat and coughs is a common and effective practice. Valnet cites Bardeau who found that essential oils that were vaporised were able to kill 90% of airborne microbes within three hours. The oils that were most effective when vaporised included clove, lavender, lemon, marjoram, mint, niaouli, pine, rosemary and thyme.[7]

One of the simplest methods to inhale essential oils is to place about 10 drops on a paper towel or handkerchief and regularly inhale. Another possibility is to place 10 drops of essential oil into boiling water and inhale the vapours emitted. The most effective method of using the essential oils as inhalations is by using an oil burner or vaporiser.

Conditions that respond to inhalations include nervous tension, headaches, respiratory problems, colds, sore throat, blocked sinuses and coughs.

Methods of Inhalation

Direct Inhalation

Apply 1–2 drops of neat essential oil to a tissue or handkerchief, hold this near the nose for a few moments and inhale the vapours.

One of the simplest methods to inhale an essential oil is to add 3–4 drops of essential oil to a handkerchief and regularly inhale. Another possibility is to add 5–10 drops of essential oil to a bowl of steaming water and breathe the vapours emitted.

Vaporisers/Diffusers

The most effective method of using the essential oils as inhalations is by using an oil burner or vaporiser.

To use a candle vaporiser place a small quantity of water in the small dish on top of the oil burner, then add 5–10 drops of essential oil. Light the candle and keep alight for approximately 15 to 30 minutes.

Remember, never leave a burning object unattended and never allow the oil and water in the oil burner to dry out. Keep the bowl clean by wiping it with a damp towel. To use the electric burners simply place 10 or more drops on the top of the vaporiser and plug in. Remember to follow the instructions provided by the manufacturer as each vaporiser is different.

Goeb says that micro-diffusers are the best apparatus for diffusing essential oils. This consists of an air pump, an injector and a glass container with an opening for filling. It is recommended that the glass container is designed to allow the finest particle of essential oils to be diffused into the air. This not only ensures maximum dispersion into the air, but also enhances absorption within the lungs.[10]

Steam Inhalation

Add 5–10 drops of essential oil to a bowl of steaming water. Then place a towel over your head and the bowl and inhale the vapours for a few minutes.

The eyes should be kept shut during inhalation. Steam inhalations are a traditional home remedy to ease congestion in the respiratory passage caused by colds, coughs and catarrh.

Benefits of Inhalations

Conditions that respond to inhalations are nervous tension and stress, mental and physical fatigue, headaches, respiratory problems, asthma, colds, sore throats, blocked sinuses and coughs.

Baths

An enjoyable method of using the essential oils is in a bath. This is a very effective method because the oil can act in two ways: by absorption into the skin and by inhalation. Baths can be an excellent way of using essential oils for client who cannot be massaged.

The main concern is that some aromatherapy books recommend adding the drops of essential oil directly to the water and then swishing it around to disperse the oil. Essential oils are not soluble in water so I fail to understand how a swish is going to help disperse the essential oil. The main concern is that undiluted essential oils may come into contact with the skin and cause irritation to the skin.

Aromatherapy baths are generally safe, provided that the essential oils are properly dispersed into the water. It is therefore recommended to use a dispersant whenever using essential oils in a bath.

Ensure that the dispersant is vegetable oil-derived, as this will have an emollient effect on the skin. The warmth of the water aids absorption of the essential oil through the skin and also causes the essential oil to vaporise, hence there is also the benefit via olfaction.

Essential oils can also be added to sea salt or magnesium sulphate. Bath salts can be used to promote detoxification, especially if essential oils such as grapefruit, juniper berry and geranium are used. Magnesium sulphate also helps to relieve tired sore muscles. Aromatherapy bath salts can be made by adding up to 1 mL of essential oils to every 100 g of salt.

Foot and Hand Baths

For foot and hand baths, place five drops of an essential oil into a teaspoon of dispersant and add to a bowl of lukewarm water. After soaking the hands or feet for 10 to 15 minutes, wrap them in a dry towel.

Conditions that respond to hand and foot baths are arthritis, oedema, circulatory problems, dermatitis, rheumatism, varicose veins and dry skin.

Full Bath

For a full bath it is advisable to use a dispersant. Conditions that respond to a full bath include circulatory problems, fluid retention, headache, insomnia, menstrual problems, muscular disorders and nervous tension.

Be cautious when using citrus oils such as peppermint, lemon or sweet orange and spice oils such as clove or cinnamon because they can easily irritate the skin when used in a bath. A prickly sensation may be felt and a rash may occur. If this happens the bath should be vacated immediately, the oil washed off and a vegetable oil such as jojoba should be applied to soothe the irritated skin.

Sitz Bath

Sitz baths are also known as a hip bath. A bowl or normal bath may be used, filled with enough water to cover the hips up to the waist only. Add 5 drops of essential oil to a dispersant and add to the bath water. Sitz baths are very effective for treating urinary, genital and lower digestive conditions.

A hot hip bath is generally taken for 3 to 10 minutes at 40–46°C. It will stimulate, relax, warm and relieve pain and is typically used for gynaecological conditions such as delayed or painful periods, for lumbar pain, urinary ailments, gout, haemorrhoids and constipation.[11]

A neutral sitz bath is more appropriate for situations of acute inflammation, such as cystitis and pruritus of the anus or vulva. It is generally taken for 15 minutes at 33–35°C.[11]

A cold hip bath should only last for one to three minutes at a temperature of 13–24°C. It is stimulating, decongesting and is ideal for treating blood congestion. Cold hip baths are great for treating copious menstrual or inter-menstrual bleeding and may also be used to prevent colds, flu and promote sound sleep.[11]

Douches

A douche is a vaginal wash using essential oils diluted in water. This method can be beneficial in the treatment of catarrhal or infectious conditions of the urinary tract, such as pruritus, cystitis or thrush.

Add five to ten drops of essential oil to one litre of warm water and shake the mixture well. Add one tablespoon of cider vinegar to help maintain the pH balance. This mixture can be used in a sitz bath, bidet or in an enema or douche pot, which can be brought from some chemists.[12]

The best position for applying a douche is lying on the back (to avoid spreading infection to the womb), and the douche should be retained for 10–20 minutes. Douches should be applied every day for up to a week when the symptoms are acute and once a month for maintenance.[12]

It should be kept in mind that douching should not be done on a regular basis as it disrupts the normal, healthy bacterial balance.[2,12]

Compresses

Compresses are generally recommended when the affected area or condition is too painful to massage.

Compresses are a very effective way of using essential oils to relieve pain and swelling and reduce inflammation. Hot compresses are often used to reduce pain of a chronic nature, to draw out boils or splinters and to relieve menstrual cramps. Cold compresses may be used to relieve tiredness due to overwork or stress, to alleviate acute pain and as a first aid for injuries such as sprains.

When preparing a compress you should use a clean cloth, a face flannel or a clean handkerchief for a very small compress and a folded hand towel for a larger one.

A hot compress should be replaced with a fresh one as soon as it has cooled to body heat.

To make a cold compress use some ice cubes. Davis says that a very large cold compress can be used to reduce a client's fever if it is dangerously high, but she says that this should only be done by therapists who are well trained in handling acute illness, and should never be applied to babies or elderly people, as their body heat control mechanisms are less efficient than those of adults and older children.[2]

Alternating warm and cold compresses may be used to help speed healing in pulled muscles, sprained ligaments and bruises.

The normal dilution of essential oils in a compress solution is 4 to 5 drops in 200 mL of water. Dip the cloth into the solution and wring it out so that it does not drip. Then cover the area being treated with the compress. Place a plastic wrap over the compress and then a towel or blanket on top. Leave the compress on for two to four hours. A cold compress should always be kept moist and renewed frequently to maintain the primary cold effect.

Internal Use

Oral

The use of essential oils internally is the most controversial issue in aromatherapy today. We need to remember that internal use of essential oils is common practice in France. Dr Lapraz, a French doctor who uses essential oils, says:

> *Our position with regards to the internal use of aromatherapy is very clear. As essential oils are extremely active agents having some demonstrable effects on the different organs of the body, they need to be administered under medical supervision.*[13]

Pénoël suggests that in the case of serious infections, the only way that aromatherapy can help is an internal, massive and repetitive aromatic treatment involving strong antimicrobial essential oils taken by oral ingestion every 20 minutes! He suggests that within three days such an infection can be completely eliminated by such a treatment.[14]

However, as Pénoël points out, the French patient in a stressful situation cannot easily make an appointment to receive an aromatherapy treatment 'in the English way', which he claims to be a delightful and highly efficacious treatment. The French doctor trained in aromatherapy is also not likely to include lifestyle changes which are necessary as part of a holistic aromatherapy treatment.[14]

Many professional aromatherapy associations do not endorse the internal ingestion of essential oils, unless the aromatherapist has suitable training. The International Federation of Aromatherapists Australia Code of Ethics states that:

> *No aromatherapist shall use essential oils for internal ingestion or internal application nor shall any aromatherapist advocate or promote such use of essential oils unless the practising aromatherapist has medical, naturopathic, herbalist or similar qualifications and holds an insurance policy which specifically covers the internal application of essential oils.*[15]

Oral ingestion of essential oils should only be recommended by suitably trained individuals such as doctors or medical herbalists who have an understanding of the pharmacological interaction of the essential oils, have an in-depth understanding of human physiology and pathology and who have extensive training in the French model of aromatherapy.

Oral administration does have a number of disadvantages:

- possibility of nausea and vomiting
- irritation of the gastrointestinal tract
- much of the essential oil will be metabolised by the liver
- destruction of the essential oil constituents by stomach acidity or enzymes in the intestines.[16]

Rectal

Suppositories are a common method of essential oil administration by French medical doctors. The advantages of using suppositories are:[17]

- The essential oils can be administered in higher doses than oral administration for the treatment of acute infectious conditions, especially lower respiratory tract conditions.
- There is the absence of the interaction between the essential oil and the gastrointestinal tract or the liver which possibly breaks down the essential oil.
- There is more rapid absorption of essential oil into the body.

- They reduce the possible hazardous effects on the liver, especially essential oils containing phenols. In order to excrete phenols the liver has to convert them into sulphonates which may cause damage to the liver by overworking it.
- Suppositories are easier to administer than oral ingestion.

It needs to be stressed that similar safety issues to those of oral administration need to be considered. Being lined with mucous membrane, the rectum is highly sensitive to irritation and there may be a risk of occasional irritation.

Benefits of Internal Use

Schnaubelt suggests that to successfully deliver essential oils to the stomach and/or the intestines to treat conditions associated with the digestive system the essential oils are best used internally.[18]

For essential oils to be successfully absorbed they must be used in an appropriate carrier or be emulsified in a liquid. Schnaubelt suggests that one or two drops will deliver the full pharmacological effect that can be gained from any given oil. Only a very small amount of essential oil may make it to the intestines as most of the ingested essential oil will be metabolised by the liver. He therefore recommends the use of suppositories.[18]

References

1. Price S, Price L. *Aromatherapy for health professionals.* 2nd edn, Churchill Livingstone, UK, 1999.
2. Davis P. *Aromatherapy A–Z.* 2nd edn, The C.W. Daniel Company Limited, Great Britain, 1999.
3. Beck M. *Milady's theory and practice of therapeutic massage.* Milady Publishing Company, USA, 1994.
4. Stubbin S. *Do it yourself pure plant skin care.* The International Centre of Holistic Aromatherapy, Australia, 1999.
5. Cowper A. *Manufacturing handbook for herbal medicines.* Allegro Printing Services, Australia, 1996.
6. Smeh N. *Creating your own cosmetics — Naturally.* Alliance Publishing Company, USA, 1995.
7. Valnet J. *The practice of aromatherapy.* The C.W. Daniel Company Limited, Great Britain, 1980.
8. Buchbauer G. *Molecular interactions.* International Journal of Aromatherapy 1993; 5(1): 11.
9. Maury M. *Marguerite Maury's guide to aromatherapy.* The C.W. Daniel Company Limited, Great Britain, 1994.
10. Goeb P. *Atmospheric diffusion of essential oils.* Aromatherapy Records 1996; 2: 96–100.
11. Pizzorno J, Murray M. eds. *Textbook of natural medicine.* 2nd edn, Churchill Livingstone, UK, 1999.
12. Worwood V. *The fragrant pharmacy.* Bantam Books, Great Britain, 1991.
13. Lapraz J. *In profile.* International Journal of Aromatherapy 1991; 3(4): 12–14.
14. Pénoël D. *This is also aromatherapy.* The International Journal of Aromatherapy, 1991; 3(3): 14–16.
15. *IFA code of ethics.* Simply Essential, No. 11 December 1993.
16. Tisserand R, Balacs T. *Essential oil safety.* Churchill Livingstone, UK, 1995.
17. Azemar J. *Galenic forms for aromatherapy — Suppositories.* Aromatherapy Records 1995; 1: 86–89.
18. Schnaubelt K., *Medical Aromatherapy.* Frog Ltd, USA, 1999.

The Aromatherapy Massage

Objectives

After careful study of this chapter, you should be able to:

- explain the benefits of aromatherapy massage
- list aromatherapy massage contra-indications
- describe the aromatherapy massage sequence and techniques.

Introduction

Massage is considered one of the most important methods of applying essential oils. Research indicates that massage can have the following benefits:

- reduction in anxiety levels
- emotional stress relief
- relief of muscular tension and fatigue
- improved local and distant lymphatic circulation
- better local blood circulation, leading to a feeling of warmth
- pain relief due to the release of endorphins, leading to relaxation.[1]

The benefits of a massage are enhanced by adding essential oils to the massage oil. However, simply using a massage oil with essential oils does not constitute an aromatherapy massage. What differentiates an aromatherapy massage from other forms of massage?

There are many different forms of aromatherapy massage. Davis suggests that it does not matter too much which aromatherapy massage technique is used, provided that the therapist has been thoroughly trained in his or her chosen system.[2]

The aromatherapy massage described in this chapter was developed by Madame Micheline Arcier, with whom I have had the privilege of being trained. This massage has a profound influence on a person's wellbeing because it utilises so many massage techniques that regulate the autonomic nervous system, stimulates the lymphatic system, eases muscular tension, promotes circulation, promotes the flow of *Qi* and balances the electromagnetic energy field of the body.

The aromatherapy massage utilises techniques such as Swedish massage, neuromuscular massage, lymphatic massage, reflexology, acupressure and polarity therapy.

Before describing the aromatherapy massage technique, let us examine some of the massage techniques incorporated in the aromatherapy massage.

Acupressure

Acupressure is based on the Chinese medical system of acupuncture. It is based on the principle that the energy of the body, known as *Qi*, circulates from the internal organs to the periphery of the body and returns again through the channels known as meridians.[3] There are six channels of yin energy and six channels of yang energy.[3]

Along these channels the *Qi* may surface to the exterior of the body at specific points. By applying pressure at these points the *Qi* may be stimulated or sedated according to the body's needs.

Lymphatic Massage

Lymphatic problems can be relieved by using specific lymphatic drainage massage techniques. Aromatherapy massage techniques developed by Maury and Arcier incorporate many lymphatic drainage movements.

Lymphatic massage was developed by Dr Emil Vodder. It is a sequence of movements that drains the lymph nodes.

Lymphatic massage should not be done on anyone who has active cancer, heart problems, thrombosis, phlebitis, high blood pressure, varicose veins, pregnancy, any acute inflammation or infection, or any other severe medical problem. Do not use lymphatic massage drainage techniques on anyone who has recently undergone chemotherapy, since the toxins filtered by the liver for elimination will be released into the bloodstream and make the person feel very ill.[1]

Neuromuscular Massage

Neuromuscular techniques are the backbone of the aromatherapy massage technique. Neuromuscular techniques evolved from the original work of Stanley Leif.[4] As a chiropractor and osteopath, he studied the work of a practitioner of Hindu manipulation, Dewanchand Varma. Varma, who practised a system called pranotherapy, stated:

> *We have discovered that circulation of the nervous currents slows down occasionally because of the obstruction caused by adhesions; the muscle fibres harden and the nervous currents can no longer pass through them.*[5]

Leif found the techniques of Varma useful and developed his own soft tissue method, which was called neuromuscular therapy.[4] The overall effect of this massage is the restoration of the balance of the autonomic nervous system.

The body constantly endures stress from trauma, improper body mechanics or of a psychological or emotional nature. Regardless of the nature of stress, the body will compensate by producing neuromuscular changes. These changes often result in reduced mobility, pain, fatigue or depression. Neuromuscular dysfunctions become apparent as contractures, hypersensitive areas and tissue restriction.[3]

The benefits of neuromuscular therapy include:

- it restores muscular balance and tone
- it restores normal tone in muscular and connective tissues
- it improves blood and lymph drainage

- it affects reflexively the related organs and viscera and to tonifies them naturally.[4]

Neuromuscular lesions are always hypersensitive to pressure and are often associated with trigger points. Besides trigger points, neuromuscular therapy utilises acupressure points, and neurolymphatic reflexes and neurovascular reflex points.

Neurolymphatic Reflex Points

The neurolymphatic reflexes are also referred to as Chapman's reflexes. Massaging these reflexes will provide additional localised lymphatic drainage.[4]

John Thie, author of *Touch for Health*, says that the neurolymphatic points regulate the energy of the lymph system. These points are mainly primarily located on the chest and back.[5] He describes how they work:

> *These reflex points act like circuit breakers or switches that get turned off when the system is overloaded. The location of the reflex points does not seem to correspond to the positions of the lymph gland. The neuro-lymphatic points vary in size from a little pellet to a small bean, and they occur either alone or in groups, sometimes scattered over the entire muscle. Some are palpable, can be felt, and others are not. They are usually greater in the front of the body than the back. The reflexes or areas which are found to be sore seem to be the ones in greatest need of massage.*[5]

Thie suggests kneading the point with the fingers, using deep massage and maintaining the pressure for 20–30 seconds. He says that the amount of tenderness can be an indication of the extent of the problem. As tenderness decreases, he says that the blockage in the energy of the lymph flow to the organ and muscles will be relieved.[5]

Neurovascular Reflex Points

These are also referred to as Bennett's Reflex Points.[4] They are primarily located on the head. When the scalp massage is performed and the massage technique is performed on the forehead, the neurovascular holding points are stimulated. Neurovascular reflex points are used for diagnostic and therapeutic use. Chaitow says that light pressure should be used. This may be accompanied by slight stretching of the skin. Generally, a pulsation can be felt.[4] Thie explains this pulsation:

> *A few seconds after contact is made, a slight pulse can be felt at a steady rate of 70–74 beats per minute. This pulse is not related to the heartbeat, but it is believed to be the primitive pulsation of the microscopic capillary bed in the skin. After a pulse has been felt on both sides and it has become syncronised, the neuro-vascular points may be held for about 20 seconds or up to 10 minutes depending on the severity of the problem.*[5]

Polarity Therapy

Some of the aromatherapy techniques use polarity therapy based on Dr Randolph Stone's work. The human body is a living being, emitting an electromagnetic energy field of many different frequencies, which must be in balance to maintain good health. Each part of the body has either a positive or negative charge, and polarity therapy utilises the therapist's own electromagnetic field to rebalance that of the client.

Reflexology

Originally referred to as zone therapy, reflexology is based on the principles that reflex points on the hands and feet are related to organs in the body, and that applying pressure to a reflex point will affect the associated organ.[3] Placed side by side, the soles of our feet reflect a map of our whole body.

Through the feet, the autonomic nervous system, the lymphatic system, the circulatory system and the energy meridians are all affected. This makes reflexology a holistic therapy that can be combined with aromatherapy.

Superficial Reflex Techniques

The aromatherapy massage incorporates a range of superficial reflex techniques. These massage techniques include static contact, superficial stroking and fine vibrations. They affect the levels of arousal, autonomic balance and the perception of pain. Static contact is used to enhance the flow of interventions, to achieve therapist rapport with the client and to reduce anxiety and induce sedation at the beginning and the end of the massage interventions that incorporate other techniques.[6] Some guidelines for performing static contact techniques include:[6]

- Hands are relaxed and in full contact with the client's body in a position that allows them to conform evenly to the contours of the client's body.
- Hands are usually placed on the client's body in a symmetrical position.
- You do not apply force or do not physically manipulate the client's tissue in anyway. The partial weight of your hands may rest on the client's body.
- Hands make and break contact with the surface of the client's body gradually and gently. It is the manner in which contact is made and broken that establishes relaxation; however making and breaking contact frequently may decrease the sedative effect of this technique.
- You hold your hands steady while they are in contact with the client's body. The hands

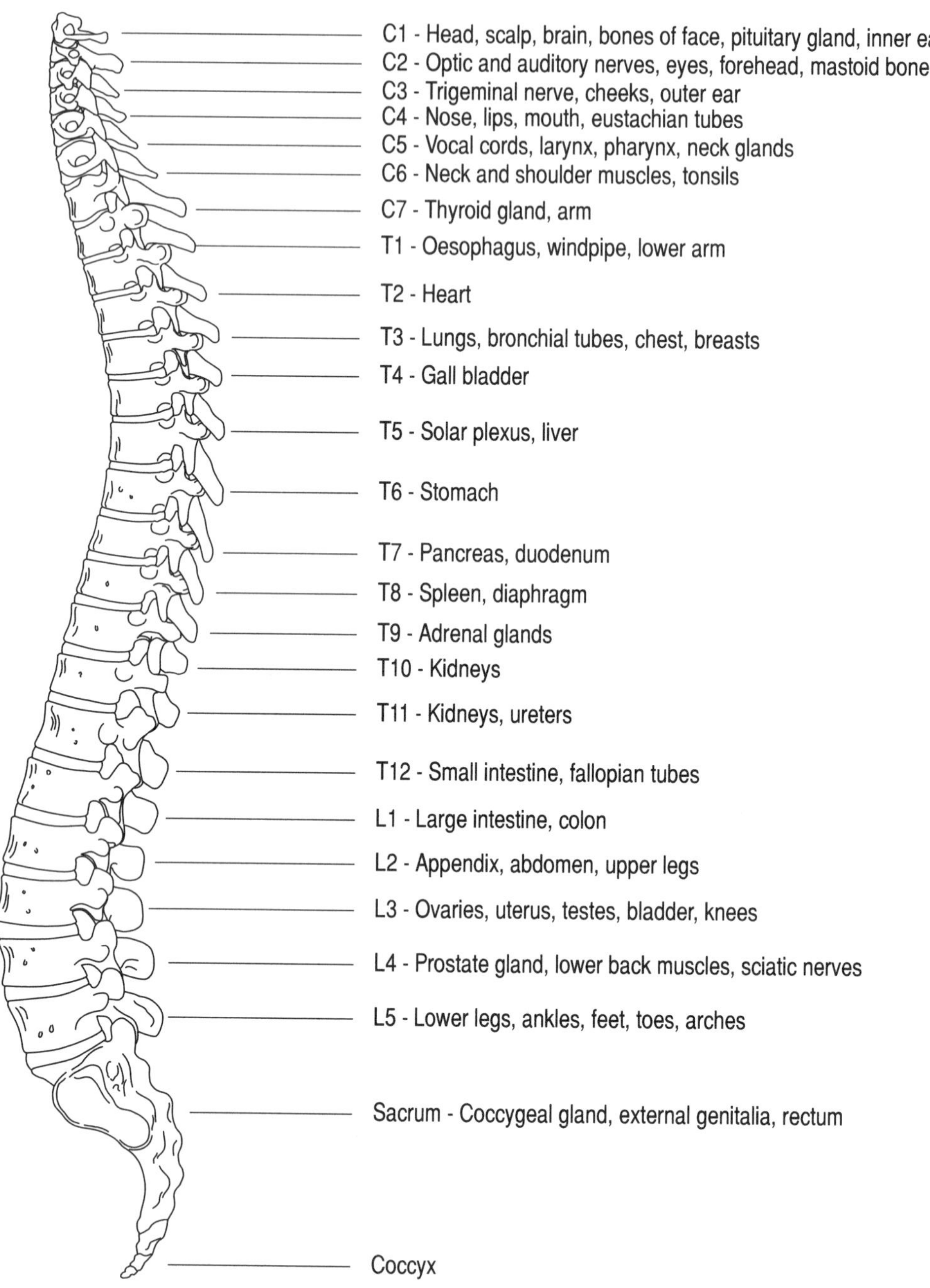

Reflex zones used in aromatherapy massage.

should not shake from fatigue, even during prolonged application.

Andrade and Clifford say that you are more likely to achieve a deep state of relaxation when applying static contact for 5 minutes or longer at the mid-sacrum, the occiput, the hands and the feet. They suggest that this is possibly due to the higher density of nervous innervation in these areas.[6]

Swedish Massage

Swedish massage was developed in the nineteenth century by Professor Ling of Sweden. He made a detailed study of massage, laying down the foundation of what is now taught and practised as 'Swedish massage'.[3]

Swedish massage employs remedial manipulative techniques such as effleurage, petrissage, vibration, friction and tapoment. The techniques used in the aromatherapy massage are effleurage, petrissage, vibration and friction. It usually starts with long, slow, gentle strokes, referred to as effleurage, over the back and body. The smooth flowing effleurage techniques of Swedish massage are used extensively in all aromatherapy massage techniques.

Petrissage is considered somewhat more aggressive. The thumbs and fingers work together to lift and 'milk' the underlying fascia and muscles in a kneading type of motion. Petrissage movements increase venous and lymphatic drainage and break up adhesions that may be present in the fascia.[7]

Friction techniques involve moving more superficial layers of the flesh against the deeper tissues. Whereas kneading involves lifting and pulling the flesh, friction presses one layer of tissue against another layer.[3] Friction is often used to separate the tissues and to break down adhesions and fibrosis, especially in muscle tissue and fascia.[3]

Vibrations are the continuous shaking or trembling movement that is transmitted from the hands of the therapist to a fixed point, or part of the body.[3]

Trigger Points

It is very interesting that many points along the back that are stimulated when you perform Stimulation of the nerve ganglia along the spine correspond to acupuncture points. These points can be sensitive to pressure and are valuable to you as a diagnostic technique. Chaitow cites Serizawe's nerve-reflex theory which states that when an abnormal condition occurs in the internal organ, alterations take place in the skin and the muscles related to that organ by means of the nervous system. This alteration is called a reflex action.[5]

Chaitow says that whether we classify these points as trigger points, acupuncture alarm points, neurolymphatic points or neurovascular points, it is merely a matter of convenience and it is simply a way of making sense out of the vast amount of information available to us.[4]

Generally tenderness elicited on palpitation of the acupressure back points may indicate dysfunction of the organ related to that point. In Traditional Chinese medicine if sensitivity is noted on light pressure, there is a *qi* deficiency. If heavy pressure is required, then the condition relates to a *qi* excess.

Preparation for Massage

It is important that you are physically and mentally prepared to perform an aromatherapy massage. You must have the appropriate equipment and treatment materials, such as tables, essential oils, carrier oils, infused oils bottles, labels and linen. During the treatment, you must ensure that the client is appropriately positioned and draped prior to and during the massage. You must also ensure that you use correct body mechanics during the treatment.

Psychological Preparation

It is important for you to ensure that you have allocated enough time to perform the treatment. Ensure that you also allow enough time before the treatment to review the client's files, to check any reference material and to think about each client. Andrade and Clifford recommend that you leave some time for gentle stretching, to facilitate your psychological preparation. They suggest conscious diaphragmatic breathing, correct body mechanics and the use of controlled repetitive movement during the performance of massage techniques can actually deepen your level of relaxation.[6]

Ensure that you practice some routine of calming the mind throughout the day, especially before each treatment. I agree with Andrade and Clifford who says that 'burnout' is very common in service-oriented professions such as massage because of the isolation often encountered. It is therefore wise to include opportunities for interactions with colleagues, such as continuing education courses and professional meetings. Service to others must not come at the expense of taking care of oneself.[6]

Preparation of Equipment

The massage table is an essential tool in the practice of the aromatherapy massage. The table should be solid, stable, easy to clean and at least 0.72 × 1.8 m, and adjustable for height, so that it can accommodate different clients and different types of treatments. The table should be padded with a high density foam on the to and sides. It should have a face cradle or head support.

For the therapist who travels frequently a well-built portable table is recommended. Stationary tables are referable for the clinic as they are usually very strong and stable. A hydraulic or electric height-adjustable table will provide quick adjustment to the different heights that may be required for the most effective application of different techniques.

Preparation of the Client

Once you have established a treatment strategy and discussed your treatment with your client, you need to identify the articles of clothing and jewellery to be removed and explain the rationale for doing so. You must also give the client clear instructions on how to position themselves on the table and how to arrange the draping.

Draping

Draping ensures that the client is safe, warm, modest and in a comfortable position to receive a massage. Draping also ensures that appropriate client-therapist boundaries are maintained. Andrade and Clifford recommend that therapists use the following draping guidelines:[6]

- only one part of the body is undraped at a time
- only the area that are to be treated are undraped
- the gluteal cleft, perineum, genitals and female breast are not undraped.

Therapist's Posture During the Treatment

The outcome and the characteristic feel of a 'good' massage depends very much on your posture. Andrade and Clifford recommend the following general principles of body mechanics when performing massage techniques:[6]

- Posture is aligned and is upright, except during controlled transfer of body weight.
- Both feet remain in contact with the floor.
- Reduce the vertical distance between yourself and the client by bending your knees, rather than bending over at the lumbosacral articulation
- Increases in pressure are achieved through the controlled use of body weight, rather than through muscle strength.

The Autonomic Nervous System

To understand the full benefits of the aromatherapy massage an understanding of the autonomic nervous system that regulates the activity of the smooth muscles, cardiac muscles and the glands is necessary.

The autonomic pathways consist of two neurons. One extends from the central nervous system to the ganglion. The other extends directly from the ganglion to the effector (muscle or gland). The ganglions are known as the cervical ganglia, thoracic ganglia, lumbar ganglia and the sacral ganglia. From these ganglia pass nerve fibres, which group themselves to form plexuses. From these plexuses, nerves radiate to supply the different organs in the thoracic, abdominal and pelvic cavities. These are responsible for controlling the processes that take place within the body but not under conscious control.

During the aromatherapy massage you will be using techniques to stimulate the nerve ganglia. This has a profound effect on the body. Most people who experience an aromatherapy massage comment on the gentleness of the aromatherapy massage technique, but are amazed at the way that they feel energised if they are suffering from lethargy or, if they are stressed, how relaxed they feel and how well they sleep. These responses are due to the effect that the aromatherapy massage has on the autonomic nervous system.

It is interesting to note that there is a similarity between the location of the ganglia and the position of the Chinese acupuncture points found along the bladder channel which run bilaterally to the spine. The acupuncture points along the back are referred to as 'back shu' points or 'associated' points. Each associated point can be used to identify a disharmony in its associated meridian and in its associated organ or function. These points are similar to the location of the chain of ganglia situated on either side of the vertebral column from the base of the skull to the coccyx.

Aromatherapy Massage Guidelines

Before performing an aromatherapy massage please follow the guidelines listed below:

- Ensure that your nails are short.
- Try not to break contact unnecessarily from your client's body. A break in contact can feel disconcerting to the client. Of course, breaks when you have reached a natural pause in the sequence are okay.
- Slow movements calm while brisk movements stimulate.

- Work with your whole body, rather than just your hands and arms. For example, when applying pressure, lean into the stroke, using your body weight rather than overworking your arms and wrists.
- If you forget the next sequence, use simple effleurage techniques until you remember. It is far better to improvise than to stop mid-flow.
- Be totally relaxed and confident, otherwise your client will sense your nervousness.
- The duration of the aromatherapy massage is approximately 45 minutes to one hour.

Contra-indications

There are a few situations when aromatherapy massage is not advisable or should be used with caution.

- **Post-operative states:** Always seek permission from your client's general practitioner or surgeon before massaging following any form of recent major surgery.
- **Heart conditions:** If the client has a history of heart attack, angina or stroke use only gentle massage which will assist the circulation.
- **Varicose veins:** Treat varicose veins with care and massage with extremely light pressure using upward strokes only. Massage above the area first.
- **Infectious diseases:** Do not massage any topical infectious disease, but instead use essential oil compresses, which are useful for the treatment of broken skin, wounds, inflammations and bedsores, etc. For respiratory infections such as sore throat or chest infections, chest massages may be very useful.
- **Cancer:** Aromatherapy massage may be beneficial in alleviating many of the symptoms and side-effects associated with chemotherapy or radiation therapy. However, any therapist who decides to use massage should have a very good understanding of both massage and cancer.
- **Inflamed joints:** With conditions such as gout or rheumatoid arthritis, massaging directly over the area will be extremely painful therefore compresses or baths are recommended. Massaging the joint above the affected area can be very beneficial to improve circulation.
- **Fractures and large areas of scar tissue:** Do not massage a recent fracture or large area of scar tissue for at least two months. Use only gentle massage techniques to apply the aromatherapy blend to aid scar healing and minimise scarring.

The Aromatherapy Massage Technique

The technique I will be describing is referred to as the 'Micheline Arcier Aromatherapy Massage'. I have not altered her sequence and have found it best to follow the exact sequence without alteration.

The actual massage should take about 45 minutes. Extending the duration of the massage is not recommended, as too much stimulation may neutralise the results. These are the main massage movements used. Unless otherwise specified the massage movements are repeated five times.

1. Attunement

This technique relaxes your client and establishes contact. It is done with dry hands. Cup your left hand around the base of the occipital bone and keep it there as you do the following:

- Right hand flat on the 5th thoracic for 20 seconds, then lift hand.
- Right hand flat on the 10th thoracic for 20 seconds, then lift hand.
- Right hand flat on the 2rd and 3rd lumbar for 20 seconds, then lift hand.
- Right hand on iliac crest pushing gently towards feet, right side first, then repeat on the left side, lift hand.
- Leave left hand on the occipital bone for 20 seconds, then slowly release.

2. Massaging the base of the cranium

- With dry hands start to massage the base of the cranium and the back of the neck.
- Hold the right side of the head with the left hand and with the right thumb start to apply pressure on the left side of the cranium under the occipital bone. When the centre part is reached, invert the position, but this time using the middle finger to apply pressure on the right side of the cranium. This alleviates muscle contraction and fluid infiltrations.

Repeat these movements five times, more if there is tension. Due to tension and congestion some people are very tender in this area, so gently at first, increasing the pressure if your client can tolerate it.

- Slide your fingers up along the cranium and then sweep your fingers over the top of the head and through the hair starting at the base of the skull. Carry the motion all the way to the ends of the hair, giving your hand a little flick at the end of each sweep. This stimulates the cranial nerves, releases the energy flow from the body and neutralises negative electrical charges from the body.

3. Applying the oil

Apply the aromatherapy massage oil blend all over the back with sweeping effleurage movements. Repeat until the oil is well spread and the client starts to relax. Effleurage can be done throughout the treatment between steps to give continuity to the treatment.

4. Stimulation of the nerve ganglia along the spine

- The two thumbs are used, alternating pressing, releasing and sliding. Each side of the spine must be done alternately five times, starting at the level of the coccygeal and working all the way up the spine to the neck. Do not press on the spinal bone.
- Follow by a similar, deep sliding movement.

These movements stimulate the chain of ganglia that make up the sympathetic nervous system.

5. Decongesting the back tissue

The tissue on the back often becomes tight and congested with tension and fatigue. This tension can be relieved by lifting the skin between your hands.

- Begin just above the buttocks and continue all over the back up to the neck and top of the shoulders. Scoop up the skin as if you were scooping up water. Your fingers should roll together and touch, as you turn your hands inward.

This movement will promote blood and lymph flow.

6. Liberation of the nerve influx

- Beginning at the base of the client's spine poise finger tips of both hands at the edge of the spinal column pointing towards the table, and sliding them over the back and down the massage table.

This movement should be continued up the back to the shoulder, then repeated on the left side. You should be standing on the left side, so you will find that your thumbs now move over the body and down the table before the fingers. Repeat on both sides of the back, from the bottom to top, five times.

7. Massaging the hips and buttocks

These movements can relieve problems associated with the uterus, bladder and sexual organs. When working on women this area often feels tender, and these techniques should break up much of the congestion. People with sciatica will also benefit.

- Effleurage hip and buttocks area.
- Circular movement with thumbs from coccygeal to the hip bone.
- Deep thumb sliding movement along the ganglia from the coccygeal to iliac crest, repeat fanning out over the buttock area.

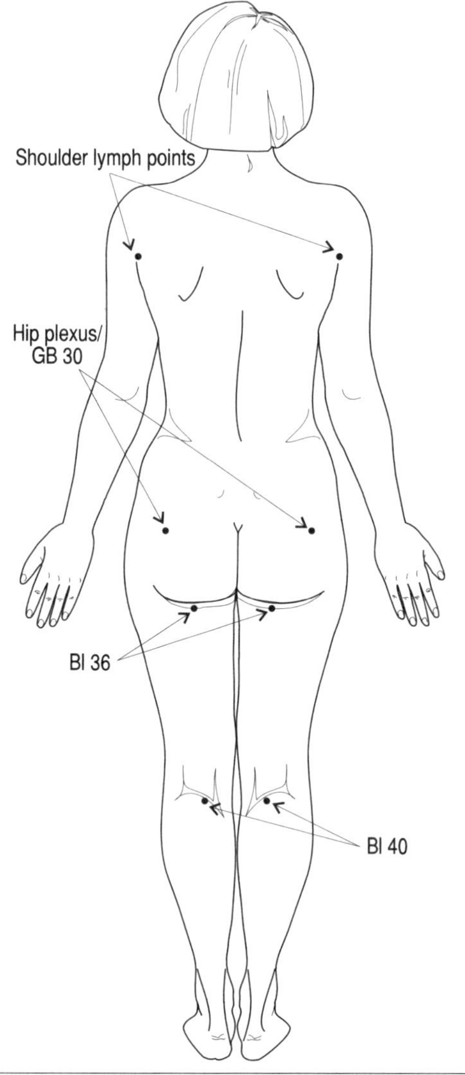

Location of pressure points used in aromatherapy massage.

- Apply pressure with the middle finger to the hip plexus for a count of four, and then rest flat of hand over the area to soothe. The hip plexus is collocated with the acupressure point GB 30, and is located posterior and inferior to the head of the greater trochanter, in the major gluteal depression. The depression is very obvious when the buttocks are tensed. This point will help relieve pain in the lower hip region, pain and weakness in the lower extremities and will help the energy circulate around the body.

These movements increase circulation and improve lymphatic drainage and relieve any congestive state.

8. Massaging the kidney area

Effleurage over the kidney areas.

9. Arms and hands

If your client's arms are not lying straight out, lift them onto the couch, palms up.

- Sliding movement from the coccygeal lumbar area to shoulder lymph points, just above the crease of the arm. Apply pressure with thumbs.
- Slide down arms, apply pressure on the inner centre fold at the elbow, slide down to the inner centre of the wrist; then apply pressure in the centre of the palm before sliding off from the finger tips.

These acupressure points affect the lymph circulation, metabolism and lung and heart function.

10. Relaxing tension in the neck and shoulder area

Massage shoulders and neck; finish by sliding along the cranium to the top of the head.

11. Massaging the back of the legs

- Apply the oil using effleurage movements.
- Standing at the end of the table, place your entire hand on the sole of each foot, your left hand on the left foot, your right hand on the right foot. Hold your hands on your client's feet for at least ten seconds.

This movement uses polarity therapy, which utilises the magnetic field of the person. In this position you are charging the body with two poles of the same polarity. By using the flat of your hands the effect is calming and energising.

- Curve your hands around your client's ankles and hold for two seconds.
- Then run your flat hands up to the back of the knees. The pressure should be firm, unless there is fluid retention. In this case always press lightly. Pause with the hands on the popliteal crease and apply pressure to acupressure point Bl 40 for two seconds.
- Now continue to run your hands up the legs and then sliding back down the lateral aspect of the thighs from the trochanter to just above the knee, applying firm pressure.
- Circular and sliding movements with the thumbs on the sole of the feet. Slide up to the ankles, circular movements around the ankles, slide up and rest the hands on the popliteal crease for two seconds. Now slide your hands up to just below the buttocks and press the lymphatic points that are collocated with acupressure point Bladder 36, at the midpoint of the gluteal fold between the femoral biceps and the semitendinosus muscles and is used for the treatment of pain in the lumbar, sacral, gluteal and femoral regions.

Repeat leg movements three times and finish by resting hands on the soles of the feet.

12. Front

Assist the client to turn over, ensuring the body remains covered. You should now wash your hands.

13. Pressing the head with your thumbs

- With dry hands, begin pressing midline of the forehead with your thumbs. Place one thumb on the top of the other to enhance the pressure, and press at 1 cm intervals, starting from the centre of the top of the forehead, then moving over the top of the head to the back of the head.

This movement affects the Governor Vessel meridian and stimulates the endocrine system because of its stimulating effect on the pituitary gland.

14. Stimulating the scalp

- With your fingers spread, firmly massage the scalp all over. Actually move the scalp, do not let your fingers slide around on the hair.

This loosens the scalp, increases blood flow to the hair follicles and stimulates the nerve endings that will alleviate tension to the head.

15. Magnetic cleansing

- Rake your fingers through the hair, starting at the scalp. Pull through to the very tips of the hair, giving your hands a flick as you reach the ends.

This action draws out negative magnetic charges from the head and the hair. Repeat six times.

16. Applying oil to the face and upper body

Apply a small amount of face oil into the palm of your hand, and apply it to the face, working both hands in unison on each side of the face, over the nose and chin, and carefully around the eyes.

17. Massaging the forehead

- With your thumbs facing each other, start above the eyebrows in the centre of the forehead and press in a straight line out to the hairline on the side of the head, pressing at 2 cm intervals, and moving up until you reach the hairline at the forehead. Pressure is decreased when on the temples.
- Deep pressure is applied to the corrugator muscle, which is a small muscle on each side of the root of the nose, sliding up to the hairline. This will help to release tension and soothes the frowning muscle.
- Complete the forehead massage sequence by a soothing almost hypnotic movement, sliding the hands alternately over the forehead. The centre of your palm should make the most contact with the head.

This soothing massage technique can be done between all movements performed on the face.

18. Circling the eyes

- With either your second or middle fingers, circle the eyes, starting from the inside corner of the eyebrows and moving out and around below the eyes. Exert more pressure over the brow, and very light pressure over the eyelid.

Do not drag the skin when performing this technique. This movement calms and revives the eyes and improves blood circulation.

19. Pinching the eyebrows

The corrugator muscle is lifted and pressure applied inside the bone near the eye. This relieves eye strain and sinus problems.

20. Decongesting the nose

- Using the fingers of both hands, make circles on each side of the base of the nose, working up the bridge. Then slide your fingers over the forehead to the hairline.

Be sure that you don't press too hard on the side of the nose as this may obstruct the breathing. This technique decongests the nose.

21. Sinus drainage

- Spread your fingers over the cheeks on each side of the nose. With firm pressure 'rake' over the cheeks towards the ear. This helps to drain the sinuses and benefits the lymph capillaries that run horizontally across the face into the submaxillary lymph glands in the jawbone under the ear.
- Just under the cheekbone at the nostrils where the acupuncture point Co 20 is located, press firmly, holding for ten seconds, then complete by sweeping the fingers out towards the ear.
- With two hands over the cheeks, vibrate your hands. This stimulates the muscles and helps their toxicity.

22. Liberating the lymph in the lower face

- Spreading the fingers of each hand over the upper lip and chin, rake outwards to the ear.
- With your hands over the cheeks, gently vibrate. This stimulates and tones the muscles.

This move encourages lymph flow into the nodes at the sides of the lower jaw, called the mandibular lymph nodes.

23. Stimulating the chin and jaw area

Massage contours of the face with fingers placed under the jaw bone, and thumbs working in a circular movement, from the chin to the end of the mandible.

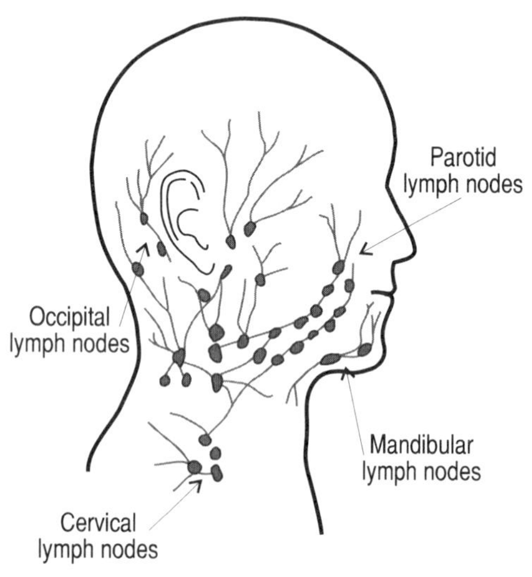

Lymph nodes of the face.

24. Toning the neck

- Holding your left hand under the neck, slide your right hand around the front of the neck, working from left to right.
- Now change hands, placing the right hand underneath the neck, and sliding with the left.

You should use a flat hand and make sure you are using enough oil so that you don't pull the skin. This improves the skin tone of the neck.

25. Stimulating the neurolymphatic reflex points

- Begin this movement by sliding your hands to the base of the neck over the clavicle down to just above the breasts; hold your hands about four inches apart. Hold for two seconds.
- Sweep your hands over the top of the shoulders and press them down, holding for ten seconds.
- Run your hands all the way up the sides of the neck and out through the hair.

As you move down the chest you are passing over lymph nodes, lymph vessels and nerves that affect the heart, liver, thyroid and lungs. If your client objects to oil in the hair, you can discontinue the movement at the hairline. Repeat the entire process three times.

26. Massaging the shoulders

- Slip your hands under your client's shoulder and massage with circular movements of the fingers, on the trapezius muscles in the shoulder area, to help relieve tension in the upper back and shoulders.
- A deep petrissage movement on the shoulders helps to relax muscles and release tension.
- Cup your fingers against the occipital bone and slightly stretch the neck. Do not lift the head from the massage table, repeat three times.
- Hand cupped under the back of the neck, lift and vibrate. Do not lift the head from the massage table, repeat three times.

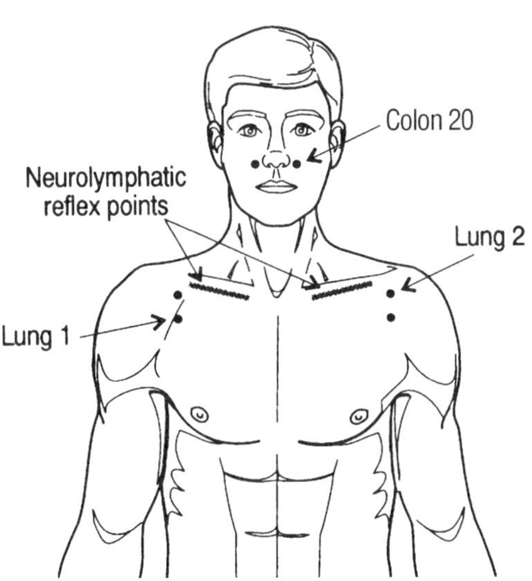

Location of neurolymphatic reflex and acupressure points on the chest.

27. Stimulating the neurolymphatic reflex point below the clavicle

- Sliding from the neck down to the midpoints under the clavicle, press with your first two fingers for two seconds, using both hands.
- Massage below the clavicle working your way out to the shoulders, up the side of the neck and head and off through the hair.

You are stimulating the lung acupuncture points as well as the neurolymphatic reflex point in the area.

28. Calming and reviving the diaphragm

- Apply oil to the abdomen.
- Keeping your left hand on the client's arm inscribe a counterclockwise movement with the flat of your hand around the solar plexus, make the circular movements at least six times, moving slowly and concentrating on putting your body energy into the treatment.
- Then liberate the diaphragm by sliding hands down the ribs. If the client complains of deep pain, stop the movement. If there is a lot of tension ask the client to do a few abdominal breathing exercises.

29. Massaging the feet

- Apply oil to the feet and legs using effleurage movements.
- Then with the wrists tilted inwards, grasp the tops of the feet with your finger tips, the thumbs on the heels.
- Now slide up the feet with your thumbs from the heel to the big toe. Repeat this movement, working towards the centre of the heel.
- When you cannot go any further in this position, move the hands to the outside of the feet and, grasping the tops of the feet with the fingers, work the thumbs up the heel to the little toe. Repeat this movement working towards the centre of the feet.

30. Stimulating the lymph in the feet

- Hold the soles of the feet with your fingers. At the same time, stroke between the toes in the direction of the ankle with your thumbs.

This encourages the lymph that flows down to the toes to start its upward journey to the nodes in the knees.

31. Massaging the legs

- Sliding your hands from the feet to the ankles, massage them with a circular motion.
- Then slide your hands up to the knee and rest them for two seconds. The popliteal lymph nodes that drain the bottom of the legs are located in the front of the knees, so by sliding up the leg and resting your warm hands on the knees you are encouraging lymph to travel into these nodes.
- From the knees slide up towards the groin and press in with your thumbs to stimulate the inguinal lymph nodes there. These nodes are located in the inguinal groove, level with the upper border of the symphysis pubis. This movement should be done with great care as the area is often tender and sensitive.

32. End of the treatment

End the aromatherapy treatment by placing the flats of your hands on the soles of your client's feet. Hold this position for a count of 20 seconds then slowly withdraw your hands and cover the legs with the sheet or towel.

This is always done at the end of the treatment to rebalance the flow of energy. Remember to wash your hands when the treatment is completed and shake them to release any negative magnetism.

References

1. Rankin-Box D. ed, *The nurses' handbook of complementary therapies*. Churchill Livingstone, United Kingdom, 1995.
2. Davis P. *Aromatherapy: An A–Z*. 2nd edn, The C.W. Daniel Company Limited, Great Britain, 1999.
3. Beck M. *Milady's theory and practice of therapeutic massage*. Milady Publishing Company, USA, 1994.
4. Chaitow L. *Soft-tissue manipulation*. 2nd edn, Thorsons Publishing Group, Engand, 1988.
5. Thie J. *Touch for Health*. De Vorss and Company, Australia, 1979.
6. Andrade C, Clifford P. *Outcome-based massage*. Lippincott Williams & Wilkins, USA, 2001.
7. Micozzi M. ed, *Fundamentals of complementary and alternative medicine*. 2nd edn, Churchill Livingstone, USA, 2001.

Bibliography

Arcier M. *Aromatherapy*. The Hamlyn Publishing Group, England, 1990.

Arcier M. *Aromatherapy training notes*.

Jackson J. *Aromatherapy*. Greenhouse Publications, Australia, 1987.

Aromatherapy for Health Professionals

Objectives

After careful study of this chapter, you should be able to:

- explain the benefits of aromatherapy in a primary health care environment
- develop guidelines for developing protocols for the practice of aromatherapy within a primary health care environment
- explain the role and benefits of aromatherapy for aged care, palliative care, cancer, persons with learning difficulties, midwifery and surgery and intensive care.

Aromatherapy in a Primary Health Care Environment

Primary health care is defined as the first level of contact that individuals and families in the community have with the National Health System. Aromatherapy is a very popular complementary therapy, which is becoming an integral part of primary health care.[1]

Price says that primary health care includes practice nurses, those working within a health centre or GP clinic, midwives and community nurses. There is a great potential in the community for aromatherapists/nurses to help patients and many have already added this skill to their caring.[1]

According to Stevenson, aromatherapy has the following therapeutic benefits in nursing for the treatment and management of:

- headaches, migraines, stress, anxiety and depression
- insomnia and restlessness
- acute asthma attacks and other respiratory problems
- common colds and influenza
- digestive disorders and constipation
- arthritis, muscular and neuralgic pain
- menstrual irregularities
- burns, eczema, psoriasis and a variety of other skin conditions
- wounds and scars
- pregnancy and labour.[2]

Holder says that in these days of rising costs of health care it may be prudent to introduce different modalities such as aromatherapy, because it is efficient and cost-effective.[3]

Gravett, a haematologist, investigated the use of essential oils for the treatment of chemotherapy-induced side-effects in a group of patients undergoing high dose chemotherapy, with stem cell rescue for breast cancer. He found that essential oils were just as effective as conventional symptomatic treatment and that essential oils were significantly less expensive.[4]

Holder warns us that it is imperative for nurses using essential oils to do so in an informed way. This means undertaking a recognised course of study. She says that some nurses believe that aromatherapy can be easily incorporated into their practice with very little formal training. This is a concern for both the patient and the therapist.[3]

Guidelines for Developing Protocols

When preparing for the introduction of complementary therapies into nursing practice, Holder, a qualified nurse and aromatherapist, provides us with the following advice:[3]

- Gather as much information and knowledge as possible about essential oils and massage.
- Seek other interested members of the team. Organise a meeting to discuss how to implement aromatherapy into practice.
- Seek specialist help and advice from a reputable practitioner. Visit centres that use complementary therapists in practice. Attend study days.
- Discuss with nurse managers and educators. Seek their support. Discuss with other members of a multidisciplinary team, and inform them of your intention to introduce essential oils and therapeutic massage.
- Make a strategy for introducing aromatherapy into the practice. Discuss the cost of the oils. Seek help from other agencies. Nominate a person to order the oils, find a reputable supplier.
- Write guidelines for the use of essential oils — discuss accountability/safety measures. Consult nurse management.
- Inform patients and relatives of availability of therapists — produce an information leaflet.
- Do not be over-ambitious. Introduce in a small way. As knowledge increases, extend repertoire and use of oils.
- Always discuss with patient before using oils.
- Plan an evaluation — share your knowledge with other people.

Price says that the ever-increasing interest by the nursing profession in complementary therapies, especially aromatherapy, has raised a number of important issues. They are as follows:

- the need for training
- identifying the knowledge and skills required for aromatherapy training
- the level of professionalism required for an aromatherapist
- the role of professional associations
- development of clear guidelines and policy for the practice of aromatherapy within a primary health care environment
- clearly defining the role of aromatherapy.[1]

McVey says that to date there have been few national guidelines to determine the practice of complementary therapies. However, she cites the UKCC Standards for the Administration of Medicines, which states that the practice of complementary therapies should be based upon sound principles, available knowledge and skill.[5]

Horrigan asks us to consider the following ethical issues:[6]

- Should patients have a choice of therapies or care elements and who should decide which is the most appropriate for them at the time?
- Should patients be able to choose a nurse or other health care professional with additional skills such as aromatherapy?
- Is it necessary to obtain written consent prior to treating patients with aromatherapy?
- How is accountability addressed when aromatherapy is used within patient care?
- Does a trained aromatherapist need the doctor's consent to treat a patient?

When introducing aromatherapy into a specific area of patient care, Horrigan says that it may be necessary to:

- give a demonstration to the ward or department staff
- offer to treat the manager or consultant
- treat a patient who usually has aromatherapy and ask him or her to talk to other staff.[6]

Funding is always an issue. However, there are many ways of obtaining funding. Horrigan suggests:[6]

- Utilising relatives and patients who often make donations to a ward — request that some of the money be used to establish an aromatherapy service.
- Organise fundraising activities.
- Use patient's own oils — provided you are happy to do so.
- Offer your own oils as a voluntary contribution.
- Some hospital pharmacies will purchase the essential oils of your choice — make an enquiry in your area of work.

Aromatherapy and Aged Care

Care of the elderly has usually been seen as the least glamorous side of nursing. However, it can also be the most rewarding.[1]

Price says that it was Helen Passant, who was one of the first nurses to introduce massage into a hospital.[1] She introduced massage to what was then called the geriatric ward at Churchill Hospital, Oxford, in the 1980s. It soon became apparent to her that with massage the patient's skin became stronger and more resistant to bruising and tissue damage. Passant also found that essential oils enabled the levels of conventional sedative drugs to be reduced.

Aromatherapy can play a crucial role in re-establishing the mind-body relationship, which is an intrinsic part of true and deep healing.[7] Bensouilah says that the sensuous, enveloping scent of ylang ylang, jasmine and geranium are superb at reawakening a long-forgotten sense of beauty, self-worth and grace — so often lost when an elderly person suffers isolation and lacks caring.[7]

Stankovic and Cook outline the normal aging process. This includes:

- degenerative changes that affect the structure and function of the body
- reduced respiratory and circulatory rates
- muscle tone and strength reduced
- bone tissue changes affecting posture and postural muscles
- rate of healing slows down.[8]

They state that abnormal processes that can occur include:

- osteoarthritis
- rheumatism
- pneumonia
- cardiac failure
- diseased arteries
- arteriosclerosis producing sluggish circulation
- loss of mobility through stiffness and aching joints
- inadequate temperature control
- decreased metabolism
- pain and direct discomfort due to arthritic conditions
- incontinence
- immobilisation, which can in turn cause additional health issues such as thrombosis, oedema, muscle atrophy, joint stiffness, osteoarthritis and reduced respiration.[8]

They also list emotional issues that can arise during the aging process including:

- fear due to failing physical health
- loss of status
- loss of independence
- loss of companionship

- bereavement and widowhood
- loss of emotional control
- depression
- poor self-image
- loss of femininity
- feelings of worthlessness.[8]

Stankovic and Cook suggest that the aim of an aromatherapy treatment should be to release physical and emotional stress; release feelings of fear, insecurity, loneliness and bereavement; promote relaxation and stimulate mental function. They also say that aromatherapy can be used to increase the rate of circulation, assist in the removal of toxins and inflammation, increase delivery of oxygen to cells, increase flow of lymph fluids assisting detoxification, reduce heart rate and blood pressure, reduce swelling and stimulate metabolic function.[8]

Aromatherapy can also be used for relaxing muscles, reducing tension, relieving pain, easing joint stiffness, cramps and spasms. Aromatherapy can assist in the removal of secretions from the lungs, decongest and stimulate expectoration, tone respiratory musculature and induce relaxed breathing. The skin will also benefit greatly with an increase in circulation to the skin, tone skin tissue, maintain skin elasticity, increase in sensory stimuli and improve healing rate. Aromatherapy can be used for reducing pain, reducing the amount of medication required, increasing awareness and improving memory.

Dosage and Dilutions

Price recommends that with older people whose bodily systems have begun to slow down, only half the normal concentration of essential oils should be used. This means that instead of the standard 2.5% dilution, a 1.25% dilution should be used: e.g., 25 drops per 100 mL of base or carrier oil.[1]

Bensouilah says that it is prudent to work with low dilutions, as older skin tends to be thin, dry and very absorptive. She says that substances are metabolised more slowly, especially if taking long-term medication.[7]

Circulatory Problems

Aromatherapy foot baths and foot massages can be very useful for treating poor circulation.

Dementia

The incidence of dementia increases with age, affecting approximately 1 person in 10 over 65 and 1 in 5 over 80 years. The causes of dementia are:

- degenerative cerebral diseases including Alzheimer's disease (60%)
- vascular (15%)
- alcohol excess.[9]

The characteristic features are impairment of memory, abstract thinking, judgement, verbal fluency and the ability to perform complex tasks. Personality may change, impulse control may be lost and personal care deteriorate. Murtagh cites the DSM-III-R criteria for dementia:[9]

a) memory impairment
b) at least one of the following:
    1. abstract thinking impairment
    2. impaired judgement
    3. disturbed higher cortical function:
        - language = aphasia
        - motor actions = apraxia
        - recognition = agnoxia
        - constructional difficulties
c) personality change
d) disturbance significantly interfering with work, social interaction or relationships
e) not due to delirium or others, e.g., major depression.

Murtagh says that the many guises of dementia can be considered in terms of four major symptom groups:[9]

1. Deficit presentations: due to loss of cognitive abilities, including:
    - forgetfulness
    - confusion and restlessness
    - apathy (usually a late change)
    - self-neglect with no insight
    - poor powers of reasoning and understanding
2. Unsociable presentations: based on personality change, including:
    - uninhibited behaviour
    - risk taking and impulsive behaviour
    - suspicious manner
    - withdrawn behaviour
3. Dysphoric presentations: based on disturbed mood and personal distress, including:
    - depression
    - irritability with emotional outbursts
    - lack of cooperation
    - insecurity

4. Disruptive presentations: causing distress and disturbances to others, including:
    - aggressive, sometimes violent behaviour
    - agitation with restlessness.

Murtagh says that there is no cure for dementia — the best thing that can be offered to the patient is tender loving care. Education, support and advice should be given to the patient and family. Multidisciplinary evaluation and assistance are needed. Regular home visits by caring sympathetic people are important. Sufferers tend to manage much better in the familiar surroundings of their own home and this assists in preventing behaviour disturbances.[9]

Price says that essential oils may have the ability to act as some kind of trigger and help patients remember some of their past experiences. She recommends essential oils such as rosemary and peppermint, because they are known to stimulate the mind and memory.[1]

Aromatherapy can offer versatile treatments for alleviating the symptoms of dementia including forgetfulness, anger, aggression, mood swings and confusion.

Digestive Disorders

Price suggests using essential oils for digestive conditions such as constipation, diarrhoea and diverticulitis. The oils can be:

- administered internally by suitably qualified therapists
- applied to the abdomen in a carrier oil
- massaged in a clockwise direction into the abdomen.[1]

Many elderly people suffer from constipation as a result of their medication or from a poor or over-refined diet. Essential oils are effective for constipation with massage of the abdomen and/or the reflex points on the feet. The most effective essential oils for treating constipation are: bitter orange, rosemary, basil, black pepper and ginger.

In cases where the diarrhoea is of a nervous origin, the relaxing effects of sweet marjoram and sweet orange are very effective. Price recommends using peppermint, clove bud, aniseed, nutmeg and geranium.[1]

For diverticulitis, Price recommends that the diet be changed to one rich in fibre, and massage with anti-inflammatory essential oils that act on the digestive system such as myrrh, German chamomile and neroli.[1]

Insomnia

The most commonly used essential oil for treating sleep disorders is lavender. Often a few drops on the pillow have helped to induce a relaxed sleep in many patients.

Price says that some of the sedative and calming essential oils such as sandalwood, ylang ylang and lemon have sleep-inducing properties.[1] The essential oils can be vaporised, used on a tissue, put in the bath or applied in massage.

Ulcers and Pressure Sores

An ulcer is a localised area of necrosis on the surface of the skin or mucous membrane. Ulcers are common on the legs and feet, areas exposed to the sun, and on pressure areas such as the sacrum in older people.

The most common causes of lower limb ulceration are venous disease, arterial disease and diabetes. Venous ulceration accounts for the majority of leg ulcers. Chronic venous insufficiency is one of the most common problems in the elderly. Clinical features of venous ulcers include:

- more common medial than lateral
- notoriously slow to heal
- generally not tender but can be painful
- associated pain is usually relieved by raising the leg.[9]

Murtagh suggests the following practices in the management of venous leg ulcers:[9]

- Promote clean granulation tissue to permit healing.
- Meticulous cleansing and dressing.
- Preventing and control of infection.
- Firm elastic compression bandage — use a minimal stretch bandage from base toes to just below the knee. The degree of compression depends on the blood flow and is proportional to it.
- Bed rest with elevation (if severe, 45–60 minutes twice a day and at night): ensure legs are elevated higher than the heart).
- Appropriate modification of lifestyle including weight reduction.
- Good nutrition including a healthy balanced diet with ample protein and complex carbohydrates.

Pressure sores tend to occur in elderly immobile patients, especially those who are unconscious, paralysed or debilitated. The cause is skin ischaemia from sustained pressure over bony areas, particularly the heels, sacrum, hips and buttocks. Poor general health, including anaemia, is a predisposed factor. Clinical features of pressure sores include:

- preliminary area of fixed erythema at pressure site
- relative sudden onset of necrosis and ulceration
- ulcer undermined at edges
- possible rapid extension of ulcers
- necrotic slough in base.[9]

Murtagh suggests the following practices to prevent pressure sores from developing:

- good nursing practice, including turning patient every two hours
- regular skin examinations by the nursing and medical staff. [Pressure points should be checked for erythema — red skin due to vasodilation in the dermis]
- special care of pressure areas, including gentle handling
- special beds, mattresses (e.g., air-filled ripple) and sheep skins to relieve pressure sores
- good nutrition and hygiene
- avoid the donut cushion.[9]

Barker recommends having clean, frequent changes of bed clothes, soft sheets to minimise irritations and suggests that physiotherapy involving passive/active exercises and hydrotherapy is very helpful.[10]

Baker has found lemon and niaouli the best essential oils to use, especially if there is a large amount of pus and debridement. He recommends applying the oil neat, either singly or blended into the debridement. Once the pus and debridement have been removed he recommends blending the essential oils of lemon and niaouli in a 1.5% dilution in distilled water, and using in a fine spray bottle over the whole area of the ulcer at frequent intervals.[10]

Baker also recommends honey.[10] This should be applied for up to a maximum of three days. This helps with the healing of the granular layer. He recommends adding niaouli, lemon and thyme. This honey poultice routine can be repeated at regular intervals if needed, given a period of 10 days between applications. The honey poultice is contra-indicated in diabetic patients.[10]

Price recommends calendula oil, which is known for its cicatrisant effect on wounds and persistent ulcers. Other essential oils recommended include frankincense, German chamomile, true lavender and geranium.[1]

Respiratory Problems

Elderly people suffering from catarrhal problems, such as chronic bronchitis or asthma, can benefit from a daily application of essential oils. Price recommends using the following essential oils because of their anticatarrhal, expectorant and mucolytic properties: frankincense — also antitussive, Atlas cedarwood, *Eucalyptus smithii,* hyssop, niaouli, peppermint, sweet marjoram, aniseed, scotch pine and *Salvia officinalis.*[1]

Rheumatism and Arthritis

There are many essential oils that are indicated for the treatment of rheumatism and arthritis. Essential oils should be used for their analgesic and anti-inflammatory properties. Price recommends black pepper, ginger, rosemary, clove, nutmeg and cajeput for their analgesic property.[1] Juniper berry essential oil should also be used to reduce any fluid around the joints. Price recommends applying the essential oils in a massage blend directly over the affected area or with a compress.[1]

Case Studies and Research

A number of case studies and clinical trials confirm the benefits and efficacy of using aromatherapy in aged care.

Aromatherapy's effectiveness in managing disorders associated with dementia was examined in a crossover clinical trial.[11] Six criteria were chosen to reflect functional disabilities and behavioural difficulties experienced by patients. These were:

- communication — appropriateness and coherence of verbal and nonverbal communication
- independence — level of self-care required
- functioning — feeding, toileting
- resistance — non-cooperative behaviour, abusiveness
- wandering — purposeless roaming
- restlessness — agitation, especially during the night.[11]

Lavender and melissa were chosen for the clinical trial. The method of application was as follows:

- morning — six drops of lavender to the patient's bath or wash basin
- midday — a 3% blend of melissa in a carrier oil dabbed onto the patient's chin as a cologne
- evening — three drops of lavender to the patient's pillow.[11]

The results of the trial identified that there was an improvement in communication, independence and functioning during the aromatherapy treatment. However, resistance and restlessness increased markedly during the treatment. This came as a surprise to researchers, as the oils used — lavender and melissa — are generally regarded as sedatives. It was suggested that the increased wandering represented improved mobility and that the patients did not wander aimlessly, but recreationally, as if to exercise and their wandering did not disturb other subjects, as normally occurs.[11]

Bowles, the primary researcher of the Aromatherapy Research Group in Australia, investigated the effects of essential oils and touch on resistance to nursing care procedures and dementia-related behaviours in a residential care facility.[12]

Essential oils of lavender, sweet marjoram, patchouli and vetiver were blended at 3.0% into a aqueous cream and 5 g was gently massaged five times per day onto the bodies and limbs of 56 aged care residents with moderate to severe dementia. The participants were divided into two groups and following a baseline period in which there was first no massage followed by massage with cream only, the groups received 4 weeks of massage with cream and essential oils or 4 weeks of massage with cream alone, and then there was a crossover period of 4 weeks.[12]

This trial highlighted some of the complex issues in using essential oils to manage dementia. For example, Bowles noted that in both groups, some participants showed extremes of behaviour during the period of essential oil treatment. It was suggested that it might be helpful for the trial to be repeated with a larger number of patients to establish how commonly such behaviour occurs.[12]

Bowles stated that people with less severe dementia as indicated by the MSSE (Mini Mental State Examination) may experience an increase in cognitive functioning as a result of gentle touching with essential oils. This needs further investigation, but may show a promising role for aromatherapy in helping people with early symptoms of Alzheimer's disease and other forms of dementia.[12]

Aromatherapy and Palliative Care

Palliative care is defined as caring for someone who may not get better, but who is nevertheless not at death's door, and may live for many years. Palliative care alleviates pain and gives temporary relief for people with chronic but not necessarily life-threatening conditions.[1]

People who need palliative care are often cared for in their own homes by a home carer, while others are cared for in hospices. Price says that hospices were the first health care establishments in Britain to embrace the benefits of aromatherapy. The primary aim of palliative and terminal care is to bring about an improvement in the quality of life of the patient.[1]

Essential oils can have a profound effect by alleviating stress, raising one's spirits, strengthening and revitalising the mind and providing comfort to the body by easing some of the distressing effects of the illness.

Living with a Serious Disease

Lynn and Harrold say that living with a serious illness can open up an unexpected variety of new possibilities. An individual may feel free to do those things that had been previously put off. It may open people up to the love and care of those around them. They suggest that serious illness can be a time of growth, meaning and healing. It should be an opportunity to heal relationships that were torn apart long ago. It may not necessarily be comfortable or rewarding, but coming to terms with the limits of life is a task that every thinking person undertakes. Some people may find new insights and make a commitment to live the rest of their life a little differently.[13]

Many people will die of chronic diseases such as heart disease, cancer, stroke or dementia. Many people, however, will live with these diseases for years before dying of them.[13] Often the condition can be managed with medications and complementary therapies, and the individual feels mostly well. Therefore, it is important for people to see themselves as *living with* rather than *dying of*.[13]

However, many people have a tough time coming to grips with the concept of dying, especially if there is some small chance of living. In general, people do not want to say someone is dying until they are almost 100% certain of death within days or weeks. To do so sounds like giving up on someone we love. People may feel guilty if they have given up on someone and the person gets better.[13] Lynn and Harrold recommend the following activities for individuals whose time may be short:

- spend time with people who are important to you
- create a legacy for those who care about you — letters, a tape recording, or a video can be a special gift
- call or visit an old friend and tell your story to those who will live on
- accept some compliments and gratitude (don't make people wait until the funeral)
- forgive yourself, and seek to make things right within
- right old wrongs

- take a 'last trip' or two
- make time for spiritual issues and struggles
- be at peace with the end to come, and the uncertainty of when you will die
- choose someone to make decisions for you when you are too sick to make them yourself
- write a will and help pass along obligations for your job and finances.[13]

Aromatherapy and Massage

Price says that aromatherapy with massage is particularly suitable for use in palliative care. Massage can provide warmth, comfort, pleasure and security. The essential oils may be added to relieve some of the anxiety, depression and promote a deeper, more relaxed sleep.[1]

With a bedridden patient, a full body massage may not be possible, therefore any massage should be modified to suit the needs of each individual patient. Price says that often the essential oils may bring hidden emotions to the surface. Carers should be aware of and prepare for this, using counselling skills they may have or referring the patient on if they feel they cannot deal with the situation themselves.[1]

Vale says that massage has a special place in caring for a person who is dying. She suggests that it is necessary to obtain permission from a medical practitioner and from the patient. It might also be necessary to have the family's consent to practise aromatherapy.[14]

Massage can encourage communication. It gives opportunities for the patient to talk about fears and anxieties. It may not be appropriate to do a full body massages; however, gentle hand or foot massage, which can be easy to deliver and simple to teach those closest to the patient, are recommended.[14]

Vale recommends using lavender for its relaxing effects or frankincense for its spiritual 'moving on' qualities. She also recommends a blend of ylang ylang and lemongrass to be used in a diffuser to encourage a peaceful atmosphere and dispel odours from wounds, colostomy sites or incontinence.[14]

A few drops of essential oil added to a bowl of water for the daily wash can again affect the atmosphere of the room, thus helping the patient. Lavender and geranium can be used for their uplifting and skin-rejuvenating properties. Patients often find essential oils such as grapefruit, lemongrass or may chang very refreshing and uplifting.

Aromatherapy and Cancer

Casey describes cancer as a group of neoplastic diseases, in which there is new growth of abnormal cells. The cells invade or replace normal tissue. This malignant process can occur within any of the body's structures.[15] There are two main 'groups' of cancers:

- cancers that originate in solid tissue structures of the body such as bone, brain, and liver
- cancers that never form a solid structure and are maintained within the blood and lymph systems within the body e.g., leukaemia and lymphomas.[15]

Cancers are commonly named according to the tissues and organs that they primarily arise from. All sarcomas arise from mesenchymal tissue including muscles and bone. Cancer of the bone is called osteosarcoma. All carcinomas arise from epithelial tissue. Basal cell carcinoma arises in the skin and is the most frequently diagnosed skin cancer and accounts for 75–80% of all skin cancers.[15]

Casey stresses that it is important for aromatherapists to know the type of cancer that the patient has as this will help to understand the physiological consequence of the disease and therefore the implications for aromatherapy treatment.[15] The following are terms used to describe the progression of cancer:[15]

- Remission — refers to the diminution or abatement of the symptoms of the disease. This is what the treatment strives for.
- Relapse — refers to the recurrence of cancer after a period of apparent cessation.
- Metastasis — refers to the spread of cancer from the primary tumour site to a distant location, where a secondary tumour subsequently develops.

The Australian Institute of Health and Welfare (AIHW) estimates that 30% of cancers can be attributed to active smoking, 30% to dietary influences, 2% to radiation exposure, 5–15% to infectious agents and the remainder to other miscellaneous risk factors. Some of these risk factors can be modified through lifestyle changes and others are inherited. While some risk factors are unavoidable, risks of particular cancers may be reduced through clinical monitoring of people and their risk factors and treating newly diagnosed cases early in their development.[16]

Approximately 345,000 new cancer cases are diagnosed in Australia each year. Approximately 270,000 are non-melanocytic skin cancers, which, if treated early, are far less life-threatening than most other cancers. According to the AIHW cancer currently accounts for 29% of male deaths and 25% of female deaths.[16]

Orthodox Treatment Methods

Buckle states that despite many years of research, cancer has not been eradicated and affects approximately one person in three. Some cancers are easier to treat than others, but the side effects of many conventional treatments for cancer can be very difficult to tolerate.[17]

Conventional or orthodox treatment for cancer falls into three main categories — chemotherapy, radiation therapy and surgical excision. Patients may be offered a single treatment modality or a combination of modalities.

Chemotherapy

Cancer cells tend to divide more rapidly than normal cells. This fundamental principle is the basis for cytotoxic chemotherapy. Chemotherapy is given to the patient orally or intravenously. The aim is to destroy the rapidly dividing cells of the tumour. However, chemotherapy is a systemic therapy and any body tissue that has a high rate of proliferation is also destroyed. This includes mucosal lining, bone marrow, hair follicles and ovarian and testicular tissues. This gives rise to complications of mucositis, anaemia (low haemoglobin), thrombocytopenia (low platelets), immunosuppression, alopecia and infertility.[15]

Chemotherapy is given in administration cycles. These cycles consist of a period of drug administration, followed by a period of recovery where the normal cell regeneration occurs. This occurs faster than the cancer cell replication. When normal cells have recovered then the cycle starts again, reducing the cancer cell load. A majority of adult solid tumours are relatively slow growing so they do not respond well to chemotherapy.[15]

Radiation

Radiation therapy uses an external beam or an internal device to deliver radiation to the tumour that consequently damages the cell's DNA, preventing it from replicating. Unlike the effects of chemotherapy, the effects of radiation are usually limited to the area directly around the tumour site. Patients have their skin marked to indicate the target site. It is important that the area, once marked, be kept free from all soap, lotions and oils as these can enhance local reaction burns within the tissues.[15]

Surgery

Casey says that surgery is undertaken for two reasons. The first is to gain an exact histological diagnosis which is an important source of information in regards to the treatment and the prognosis. The second is to remove all or part of the tumour. This may also involve taking surrounding tissue including lymph glands. Surgery may be done in conjunction with chemotherapy and/or radiation.[15]

Aromatherapy Considerations

Today a diagnosis of cancer does not necessarily mean an early and untimely death. People are now learning to 'live with' rather than 'die from' cancer. However, patients still may have to contend with the symptoms of their disease and the side effects of the therapies that are helping them survive.[18]

If the cancer is diagnosed early, it can be helped. Many natural therapies and holistic approaches can be instrumental in reducing anxiety and encouraging a positive outlook. For this, Denyer recommends modalities such as relaxation techniques, creative visualisation, mediation, massage and aromatherapy.[19]

Denyer stresses that this often leads to a new self-assessment and personal growth in the patient. This spiritual dimension plays an important role in supporting the immune system.[19]

Aromatherapy can help patients and carers. Many factors such as feelings of wellbeing affect a patient's quality of life and these are often related to symptom control and the patient's perceived levels of independence. Combining orthodox and complementary therapies can offer powerful control of distressing symptoms such as vomiting and pain.

Horrigan says that nurses are ideally placed to initiate methods of symptom control including the use of touch and aromatherapy. There are no clear guidelines concerning the use of aromatherapy for cancer, and normally there are no specific essential oils recommended.[18] Patients vary in their need for aromatherapy, depending on:

- the amount of pain suffered
- the site and extent of the tumours
- the frequency of radiotherapy if being treated
- the rate of circulation
- the ability to sleep
- the condition of the skin
- the medication being taken
- whether or not they are on chemotherapy
- the state of their morale.[18]

According to Price the benefits of those who elect to receive aromatherapy treatment are:

- reduction of anxiety, stress and tension

- gaining a sense of wellbeing, which reduces the inability to cope, strengthening self-belief
- relief of constipation, headaches, muscular aches and pains, insomnia, infections
- improvement in the circulation of blood and lymph, helping to eliminate unwanted toxins more efficiently
- stimulation of the immune system. There is ample evidence of the overall increase in immune functioning when relaxation is achieved by massage.[1]

Denyer says that gentle massage with essential oils can help the patient relax, which eases the physical pain. Patients tend to open up and say what they are feeling and what their fears are. This in turn allows the therapist to counsel the patients far more easily and deal with the psychological pain, as well as the physical pain.[19]

Millar says that there are nine main aims for the use of aromatherapy in the management of people with cancer:[20]

1. Improve the quality of life.
2. Give the patient something to live for.
3. Aid relaxation.
4. Help relieve stress, tension and anxiety.
5. Help relieve symptoms of the disease and its treatment, both holistically and clinically.
6. Provide security and comfort through touch.
7. Give empathy and time which is not hurried.
8. Use a holistic approach whenever possible to evaluate each patient's needs.
9. Provide a one to one environment, where patients can talk freely and in confidence.

There are some points to consider when using massage and aromatherapy with patients who have cancer. Horrigan says that aromatherapists and nurses have a duty to confer with any other practitioners to ensure that the patient receives the optimum combination of therapies. The patient and the carer should also be given enough information to enable them to make decisions based on knowledge and trust. They should be given time to discuss the benefits, costs and daily routines.[18]

There are differing opinions on whether or not massage and aromatherapy should be carried out in the early and middle stages of cancer. Evidence indicates that at all stages, massage and aromatherapy have produced beneficial results as long as the following guidelines are followed:

- During massage use only effleurage, not deep movements of petrissage, tapotement, cupping or hacking. Chemotherapy and radiotherapy can cause thrombocytopaenia (low platelet count) and patients who have undergone these therapies are at risk of bruising.
- Do not massage over solid tumours or over connecting lymph nodes. This may cause pain or discomfort, and unless the therapist is trained in lymphatic drainage techniques for lymphoedema this could cause inappropriate lymph drainage.
- Do not massage areas that are currently receiving radiotherapy. These areas must be kept free of contaminants as they may interfere with the radiation used and patients will have been forbidden to use oils, lotions or products that contain perfumes. Also the overlying skin will be delicate and may be sensitive to touch; massage may cause discomfort or breakdown of the tissue. The massage and essential oils should be adjusted accordingly; use very diluted essential oils.
- Aromatherapy should not be used while the patient is experiencing nausea or vomiting caused by chemotherapy. These unpleasant side effects may be triggered by the use of essential oils. Horrigan says that it could be possible for the olfactory memory to be triggered, bringing a return of the nausea and vomiting associated with the previous chemotherapy and aromatherapy combination.[18]
- Any health professional who decides to use massage should have a very good understanding of the massage techniques and cancer.
- Patients who are undergoing intensive therapy for their cancer often experience fatigue. Some patients will not be able to tolerate massage treatments longer than 1 hour. Ensure that the duration of the treatment is modified to suit the individual.[15]
- Patients undergoing chemotherapy often experience a heightened sense of smell. It would therefore be important for you assist clients in choosing an appropriate blend that they are comfortable with. Casey says that a patient will enjoy blends that are made using a dilution of around 1–1.5%.[15]

Casey says that aromatherapists should always seek the permission of a medical person when treating a patient who has cancer. She suggests the following considerations when assessing the suitability of the patient to a particular method of treatment:[15]

- Low platelet count — Platelets are responsible for helping our blood clot. A low count causes the patient to bruise easily. Therefore, it is advisable to avoid massaging these patients, so use inhalation and vaporisation.

- Patients who are febrile — Fever in patients who are undergoing treatment for cancer may indicate infection. The treatment should therefore be aimed at reducing the fever.
- Patients with a low albumin level — Patients with a low albumin level will have a higher concentration of essential oils in their bloodstream. Therefore, it is advisable to reduce the dose of essential oils.

There are certain myths about massage which need to be corrected. Massage will not:

- **Make the cancer grow due to increased blood supply.** While the blood circulation is increased following a massage, this will not stimulate cancer growth. The tumour growth is dependent on many other factors than blood supply.
- **Make the cancer spread.** If the cancer is the type which has the tendency to spread (metastasise) then it will do so of its own accord. Massage will not increase or decrease metastasis.
- **Interfere with the chemotherapy and radiation therapy**. Both these treatments are far too powerful to be over-ridden by any effects of massage.

Aromatherapy Treatments

Aches and Pains

Aches and pains in the limbs and joints may be caused by patients having to stay in bed for prolonged periods or because they have reduced mobility. Essential oils such as ginger, rosemary and lavender are recommended in a base oil and used as a massage oil to alleviate such aches and pains.

Alopecia

Horrigan says that some chemotherapy treatments and radiation therapy can cause total loss of hair. While this can be initially distressful to some patients, most patients will cope very well. The follicles need time to recover and the patient can be assured of regrowth, sometimes better than the original and sometimes a different colour and type.[21]

Provided that the quality of the skin is good, essential oils may be used to encourage regrowth, and for stimulating the scalp capillaries with massage. Horrigan recommends preparing a massage oil for the scalp using cedarwood and rosemary in a carrier oil at 1% dilution.[21]

Anorexia

Anorexia can be caused by fear and anxiety, the disease process, unpleasant sights or smell, pain, or as a result of chemotherapy or radiation therapy. Loss of weight may be rapid and irreversible leading to the atrophy associated with the terminal stages of cancer. Horrigan says that if this can be delayed, patients' quality of life may be increased as they will be able to maintain their strength for a little longer.[21]

When the patient is not feeling nauseated try one or two drops of lime, geranium, lemongrass or cardamom on a tissue. Allow the patient to choose the oil and remove the tissue from the room immediately if the nausea returns.

Anxiety and Fear

For many people with cancer, the side effects of chemotherapy or radiation start before the treatment has begun. The anticipation and anxiety of long-term drug therapy or the long-term stay in hospital are often amplified by the fact that the side-effects of cancer treatments are wellknown for their severity. Horrigan recommends using neroli oil for its gentle hypnotic effect. It may be used alone or blended with melissa or bergamot.[21]

Constipation

Horrigan recommends using juniper berry oil as it is reputed to stimulate peristalsis. It may be used in a massage oil and massaged in a clockwise direction over the abdomen. She also recommends a blend of sweet orange and rose.[21] Millar recommends rosemary, black pepper, Roman chamomile or sweet marjoram to be incorporated in an abdominal massage to stimulate peristalsis.[20]

Cystitis

Horrigan says that cystitis may be due to catheterisation, to neutropenia (low white blood cell count) or reaction to a specific regime of chemotherapy. She says that because of the risk of an overwhelming infection, cystitis must be treated with a high fluid intake and antibiotic therapy. She recommends using essential oils to soothe and relax an inflamed bladder.[21]

Depression

Horrigan recommends that the aromatherapy blend should be refreshing, yet with some relaxing and seductive richness. The patients need to be pampered, so she recommends offering them essential oils such as bergamot, neroli, jasmine or ylang ylang.[21]

Other essential oils recommended include frankincense, which is a useful addition for those with sleeping difficulties due to depression. She also recommends using rosewood, petitgrain and frankincense in equal parts in a base oil. As the condition improves, the oils can be lightened to include oils such as grapefruit, orange and lemon. Horrigan warns us not to use them too soon as the patients may still need time to work through their depression.[21] Casey has found the uplifting effects of bergamot to be invaluable. She recommends it is applied as a hand massage or a few drops on a tissue.[15]

Dry Skin

Dry skin will lead to itchiness and this can be very distressing. The causes are many and include drying from radiation therapy and allergic reaction to medication. Essential oils such as German or Roman chamomile, rose absolute or otto, neroli and lavender are recommended in a base oil or blended in an aqueous cream base with calendula-infused oil.

Horrigan recommends obtaining permission from the doctor prior to using anything on post-radiation therapy skin.[22] Geranium, lavender and sandalwood are recommended because they have a balancing effect on the production of sebum. Millar also recommends using sweet almond oil, avocado oil and calendula-infused oils as the base.[20]

Fatigue

Fatigue is caused by a combination of emotional, mental and disease process factors. Horrigan recommends sandalwood oil for physical exhaustion with a little bergamot or lavender. She says that this will encourage refreshing sleep. When the patient feels rested and wishes to resume intellectual activities, rosemary and lemon essential oils may be used to stimulate and aid memory.[22]

Grief

Horrigan says that anticipatory grief is when the patient accepts that he or she may have a short time to live and is grieving for a lost body image. She recommends uplifting and euphoric essential oils such as neroli, petitgrain, melissa, jasmine or rose.[22]

Headaches

This may have a pathological cause, especially if the patient has a brain tumor. It may be due to chemotherapy or radiation therapy or simply nervousness and tension. Horrigan recommends essential oils such as lavender or rosemary to be used in a cool compress or in massage.[22]

Casey suggests gentle massage around the neck, shoulders and scalp with essential oils such as Roman chamomile and mandarin to relieve headaches due to tension and stress.[15]

Indigestion

Horrigan says that indigestion may be due to the tumour spreading in the thorax or sluggish digestion. She recommends essential oils such as sweet orange, sweet marjoram and rose, which are known to stimulate peristalsis.[22]

Nausea

Buckle says that one-third of patients with cancer experience nausea and vomiting. Nausea is common during radiation or chemotherapy. She says that up to 75% of patients develop anticipatory nausea and vomiting during the course of repeated chemotherapy. Patients become very sensitive to smells, often smelling something which they had not noticed before, or feeling great distaste of a smell which had not previously bothered them.[17]

Buckle recommends peppermint, ginger and cardamom to alleviate nausea. Just a few drops of essential oil on a tissue can alleviate nausea. Buckle also recommends sipping a ginger herbal tea prepared with freshly grated ginger root.[17]

Neuralgia

In cancer patients, neuralgia may be caused by the infiltration of the nerves by tumours. Horrigan suggests that orthodox therapies and medication are of paramount importance to control this type of pain.[23] Hypericum-infused oil as base oil and essential oils such as rosemary, cajeput and spike lavender should also be considered as part of the aromatherapy treatment.

Oral Mucositis

Gravett says that usually 100% of patients undergoing high-dose chemotherapy suffer chemotherapy-induced damage to the lining of the mouth. This ranges from mild soreness to total mucosal loss with ulceration, haemorrhage and secondary infection. The conventional treatment consists of mouthwashes with proprietary antiseptic preparations, often with analgesics. He says that most patients don't like the mouthwashes as they provoke a burning sensation and possibly add chemical damage to the fragile mucosa which is already compromised by the chemotherapy.[4]

In a clinical trial conducted by Gravett, a mouthwash was made by using 1 drop of tea tree, 1 drop of bergamot and 1 drop of geranium in a tumbler of boiled warm water, taken 5 times daily.[4]

Tea tree was selected because it is a good all-purpose antiseptic, antifungal and antibacterial agent with very little recorded sensitivity or toxic reactions. Bergamot is also a good antiseptic and healing agent for wounds and ulcers and is traditionally used for infections of the mouth, skin, respiratory and urinary systems. Geranium is a traditional remedy for wounds, tumours and ulcers and has been used to treat stomatitis, glossitis and enteritis.

The results of this clinical trial indicated that there was no significant difference between aromatherapy and the control group. (The control group received conventional treatment with Corsodyl or Difflamm as well as analgesia such as paracetamol or continuous diamorphine infusion with patient-controlled administration).[4]

However, those patients who had previously received conventional mouthwashes universally preferred the aromatherapy preparation since it did not cause the same level of burning discomfort. Gravett was also impressed with the substantial difference in the cost of the treatment. The essential oil treatment cost an average of 11 pence per day whereas the conventional treatment cost 210 pence per day.[4]

Palliative and Terminal Care

Horrigan says that palliative care begins when the patient is no longer receiving treatment aimed at controlling or curing the cancer. It is designed so that the patient may continue to lead a comfortable and reasonably active life and the therapeutic intervention is designed to focus on symptom control. While aromatherapy can help patients in many ways during active treatment, the benefits are most notable once palliative care commences.[18]

Lymphoedema

Lymphoedema often occurs following a mastectomy, but is also common following lumpectomy if there is any removal of lymph glands under the arms. Buckle says that lymphatic drainage needs to be conducted regularly. She says that normal massage may be contra-indicated under such circumstances as it is important that movement is only one way. The pressure of normal massage can cause spasm in the lymph vessels, temporarily suspending the lymphatic flow. She also recommends using an essential oil such as juniper, as it can reduce inflammation by encouraging lymph flow back into the system.[17]

Radiation Burns

Price cites work done by Peneol who says that essential oils should be used prior to the treatment on the area to be irradiated, to reduce deep burning and scarring. Peneol suggests using any of the Melaleuca oils — *Melaleuca viridoflora, alternifolia* or *cajeputi*. He recommends applying the oil neat before the radiation session, and after the session a blend of 50% *M. viridoflora* in *Hypericum perforatum* or 50% *M. iridoflora* in *Rosa rubiginosa*.[1]

Casey found a combination of lavender and German chamomile very effective for radiation burns. She suggests applying it as a compress with the aid of a dispersant and then in a non-mineral oil cream base. Treatment should begin the day after the completion of the full radiation treatment.[15]

Millar recommends a blend of Roman chamomile, German chamomile, tagetes and yarrow for 2 to 3 weeks before the radiotherapy begins to prevent radiation burns.[20]

Respiratory Problems

Dyspnoea is associated with the terminal stages of many cancers, especially those which have invaded the lungs. Horrigan says that the main treatment for controlling this symptom is diamorphine. This drug assists by making the patient less aware of their respiratory effort, and any feeling of suffocation.[23]

Essential oils must be chosen to enhance these effects. The aim is to ensure comfortable breathing and enhancement of the euphoria produced by diamorphine.[23]

The positioning of the patient is important. Massage and inhalations will probably be most comfortable in an upright position which allows for full expansion of the compromised lungs. Horrigan recommends using relaxing and euphoric essential oils such as neroli, petitgrain or rosewood. Often patients with dyspnoea may feel nauseated by heavy-smelling oils or very sharp smelling oils.[23]

A dry cough may be suppressed with massage using essential oils such as cypress, whereas a productive cough may be assisted by the expectorant properties of essential oils such as frankincense, myrrh, cedarwood, myrtle, cajeput and ravensara.

Case Studies

A number of published case studies and clinical trials confirm the benefits and efficacy of using aromatherapy in promoting wellbeing and the management of cancer. The effects of massage and aromatherapy on the wellbeing of cancer patients was examined by Corner.[25]

The clinical trial evaluated the effects of massage with essential oils on the patient's perception of their:

- quality of life
- symptom distress
- levels of anxiety and depression.[25]

Fifty-two patients were recruited: 24 had breast cancer, 10 had gynaecological malignancy, 8 had haematological malignancy and the rest had sarcomas, cancers of the head and neck, or lungs.[25]

Twenty-two patients were being treated for a primary tumour and 21 either had local recurrence or metastatic disease. Nine patients were either disease-free or were described as being in remission. Ten of the patients had advanced disease which confined them to bed for more than 50% of the time. Thus the sample represented a broad range of patients with cancer.[25]

Just over half of the patients in the study were receiving chemotherapy, radiotherapy or surgery during the eight weeks of the trial. The intervention was standardised to a 30-minute massage, once a week for 8 weeks. The procedure was as follows:

- 5–10 minutes talking and preparation
- 20-minute back massage in sitting or lying position
- rest, talk, glass of water.[25]

Three groups were tested:

- group 1: massage with essential oils
- group 2: massage without essential oils
- group 3: no intervention.[25]

Each of the participants had to complete a regular evaluation form:

- immediately after the treatment
- hours after the treatment
- and one week after the treatment before the next treatment.[25]

A standard blend using lavender, rosewood, lemon, rose and valerian was used. The observations were:

- the effects were variable
- the positive effects ranged from one day to a week
- the duration of the effects were shorter in those undergoing chemotherapy and radiotherapy
- cumulative effects were reported.[25]

The results of her 8-week clinical trial were overwhelmingly positive. Some of the conclusions included:

- significant levels of reduction in anxiety and symptom reduction
- patients who had massage with essential oils had a greater improvement in anxiety reduction
- feelings of peace and calm, letting go, being pampered and feeling cared for.[25]

Corner made the following suggestions in regards to nursing:[25]

- A minority of patients were anxious about being massaged for the first time. This was not a deterrent for them, but it needed to be handled with sensitivity.
- That the massage was very important and that twice a week would have been more beneficial than once a week.
- Massage sessions were cumulative and peak effect for anxiety reduction was not reached until four sessions.
- Massage provoked emotional release and crying in some patients which required sensitive and skilled handling.
- Patients also used the massage session to talk and therefore the therapist needs to be skilled in communication/counselling skills.
- Massage and aromatherapy is a skilled and time-consuming activity if it is to have an optimum effect. It therefore needs adequate investment of time and space by the nurses.

Aromatherapy and Learning Difficulties

Aromatherapy has had some surprising successes in one of the least responsive therapeutic areas — the treatment of people with learning difficulties. Occupational therapists (OTs) are at the forefront of this development, and an introduction to aromatherapy is now included in some OT training courses in the UK.

It has been encouraging to see the many changes in the support offered to people with learning difficulties. The term 'mental handicap' has been replaced with the preferred term 'learning difficulties'. There is now a move to resettle people in the community rather than encouraging long, even permanent, hospital stays.[27]

The concept of treating people with learning difficulties as patients with a long term illness has been replaced by supporting them to make their own choices, speak for themselves and form relationships.[27]

This has been achieved within a supportive structure made up of a multidisciplinary team including physiotherapists, speech therapists, nurses and social workers. Within such a network the different roles blend together with a common goal of supporting people to achieve a lifestyle of high quality.[27]

Sanderson says that within Health and Social Services, quality of life issues involve five key areas of choice: community, participation, respect, relationships and competence. She says that each of these areas needs to be addressed when choosing any activity which involves aromatherapy.[26]

This framework should apply to all people with learning difficulties, even those who are severely disabled, or those with severe or profound learning disabilities. Often people with learning difficulties have had the majority of choices made for them and have been touched only when it is necessary to care for their personal care needs such as toileting, dressing and washing. It is therefore important to give people as much choice as possible when introducing them to aromatherapy: choice of oils, choice of which part of the body to massage, choice of when and where to receive the massage.[26]

Often people with severe learning difficulties have very limited mobility and are unable to care for themselves and may have virtually no language. These problems are compounded by deafness and/or blindness. The OT's role involves a holistic approach that helps people with learning difficulties to develop communication skills and an awareness of themselves and their environment.[26]

Touch is central to working with people who have severe learning difficulties, yet the issues that it raises are rarely addressed and clarified. A professional or supportive role involves much functional touching, taking people to the toilet, washing them, moving them in and out of wheel chairs. Yet many struggle with issues around the 'appropriateness' of hugging an adult with learning difficulties.[27]

Price says that children and adults need to feel loved and to be completely accepted, including the acceptance of any particular physical impairment or negative emotional behaviour.[1]

Touch

Sanderson says that for people who have severe learning difficulties, there is an even greater need because of their sensory deprivation in other areas. She cites Montagu, author of *Touching — the human significance of the skin*, who says that when people do not receive the touch that they need, their behaviour will become 'abnormal'. She suggests that being deprived of touch could result in 'challenging behaviours' such as rocking or self-injury.[26]

Therefore massage and aromatherapy can provide us with an opportunity to give affirming, valued and appropriate touch to people who are usually denied close physical contact.

Smell

Sanderson says that the sense of smell is 10,000 times more sensitive than that of taste and yet it is not generally considered to be clinically important. If people with severe learning difficulties are not encouraged to use this neglected sense then they will lack another avenue from which to gain pleasure and information from the environment.[26]

Multisensory Massage

Aromatherapy is being used to enhance sensory awareness through 'Multisensory Massage' and to improve communication with the use of 'Interactive Massage'.[27]

Multisensory massage incorporates various textures and essential oils into the treatment in order to stimulate different senses. It is often used with children to improve their awareness of the environment and their ability to respond to it.[27]

Up to 80% of people with severe learning difficulties have visual or hearing impairments, therefore the information received from the other senses is vital to learning and development.[27]

Sanderson explains that as we grow as children we are able to recognise and explore different objects and interpret and assimilate information about them — for example, what does grass look like, feel like, what happens when you touch it, even its taste.[26]

Sanderson says that people with severe learning difficulties need help to do this and may not have had the same opportunities or even inclination to find out and explore. Once people understand what things are like, then it is possible to learn about what things do and, more importantly, what the individual can do.[26]

Sanderson explains that the first step is for the therapist and individual with learning difficulties to form a relationship, and aromatherapy provides an ideal basis for this. One of the main goals is to help the individual to comprehend that 'When I do this — something happens'. Multisensory massage can be used to provide experiences in both these areas.[26]

'What are things like?' and 'When I do this something happens' can introduce people to different surfaces, human touch, vibration and smell.

A typical session might begin by helping the individual to choose two or three refreshing and invigorating essential oils. Uplifting and refreshing oils are usually used because the session is about learning and experiencing rather than relaxation. Sanderson says that people with severe learning difficulties cannot speak, but when you know them well you can often tell by their face or body movements whether they like the smell or not. Once an essential oil has been chosen, it is then made up into a massage oil and stroked onto the skin. The hands, legs, arms or feet are generally chosen, and a wooden massage tool and then perhaps an electric massager are used for short periods, perhaps just 5 to 10 minutes, on the back of the hands and arms or feet and lower legs.[26]

The session always ends with a 10 minute foot spa (vibrating warm water with an invigorating fragrance of peppermint), followed by drying the feet with a soft, fluffy towel and then gently rubbing the feet with different textured materials such as velvet, soft bristles, hessian or fake fur. The feet are subsequently massaged with diluted essential oils, the patient is encouraged to choose the fragrance from a range which the therapist feels will be beneficial.[26]

Interactive Massage

In addition to using essential oils to encourage sensory awareness, many OTs use interactive massage to help develop communication, interaction, responsiveness and active participation. It involves a series of responses, known as the interactive sequence, through which the person with severe learning difficulties is supported and guided by the OT.[26]

The sequence is made up of the following steps:

- resistance
- tolerance
- passive cooperation
- enjoyment
- cooperation
- leading
- imitation
- initiation.[26]

Sanderson says that interactive massage involves supporting people with severe learning difficulties to work through this sequence. Initially when massage is introduced to them, they may be resistant and hide their hands. From this stage of resistance, they will be able to tolerate the massage for short periods, fleeting initially, progressing to a number of minutes, until they co-operate passively with the massage and later begin to show signs of enjoyment.[26]

In the fifth stage, which is 'responds cooperatively', they will cease to be just passive recipients but will begin to respond cooperatively offering their hands and selecting creams and oils. From this stage they may begin to lead the session, anticipating the sequence and direction of the activity.[26]

The next stage involves beginning to imitate the carer's movements either on the back of their own hands or beginning to rub the carer's hand. At the final stage they will initiate the session independently, finding the massage oil or indicating that a massage is wanted.[26]

Aromatherapy and Communications

Durell, a community learning disability nurse and aromatherapist, documented the results of an aromatherapy service provided to people with learning difficulties.[28] The survey found that the aromatherapy service was rated very highly:

> *An estimated 40–50% of adults with learning disabilities have communication difficulties. This means reduced/no ability to communicate needs, wants, emotion, pain.*
>
> *Speech and language therapists strive to facilitate communication by whatever means possible, focusing on a combination of formal communication systems (verbal language, signing) and non-formal systems (objects of reference, eye pointing and touch). Once a communication system has been established, it allows the service user to achieve five accomplishments of normalisation:*
>
> - *relationships*
> - *choice*
> - *respect and dignity*
> - *community presence*
> - *personal development*
>
> *Having a means of communication allows a person to develop their identity.*[28]

A lack of a means of communicating leads to high levels of anxiety. It has now been identified that challenging behaviour has been linked to the inability to communicate. High levels of stress and anxiety will affect:

- motivation to communicate
- ability to understand — verbal/nonverbal and environment
- ability to listen
- ability to reason
- muscle tension.[28]

Aromatherapy is useful for each of the above issues. It has been suggested that because aromatherapy uses very little language, it is less cognitively demanding for the patients, therefore they respond in a more relaxed state. By relaxing more, communication can appear to be a less daunting task.

Aromatherapy and Midwifery

Pregnancy is a time of joy for most women and for the middle 4 or 5 months of a healthy pregnancy the mother has a look about her of glowing good health and usually feels well and happy. During the early and late months of many pregnancies, however, and sometimes during the middle months also, a number of conditions related to the pregnancy can arise which cause the mother varying degrees of discomfort or even distress. The judicious use of essential oils together with appropriate forms of massage by a skilled therapist can help ease the discomforts of pregnancy and provide a sense of nurturing that will comfort the mother at times when she is likely to be feeling rather fragile. Aromatherapy is even more appropriate when the heightened sense of smell during pregnancy is taken into consideration.

Waters says that the main cause of infant death is premature birth and that the number one cause of premature birth is stress.[29] There appears to be an epidemic of stress in much of the world today and it affects pregnant women at least as much as it does the rest of the population and possibly more. Caring use of aromatherapy treatments should help to reduce the stress felt by pregnant women and thereby possibly play a valuable role in reducing premature births caused by stress and the resulting prenatal deaths associated with it.

It is suggested that if a pregnant woman is not accustomed to regular massage that prenatal massage does not commence until she is three months pregnant. Reasons for this are:

- that many miscarriages occur during the first trimester and the woman may associate such a misfortune with the massage, and
- if she is suffering from severe nausea, massage might add to her discomfort.[30]

The pregnant woman's doctor must be contacted, if she is suffering from any serious health problem, for an opinion as to whether it is safe for her to have aromatherapy treatment during the pregnancy. If at any time during the pregnancy any condition arises which is outside the therapist's range of skills, the woman should be advised to contact her doctor. Should the therapist find that the woman is experiencing a sudden onset of pain, swelling, heat or redness of the calf or thigh muscles, a deep vein thrombosis may be suspected and the woman should be urged to contact her doctor immediately.

In positioning the client for massage, avoid lying her flat on her back (she should recline at an angle of about 45°) because the growing uterus presses on the inferior vena cava in this position and can cause an alarming drop in blood pressure.

Where massage is not possible (for example, if she has deep vein thrombosis), the pregnant woman may still be able to experience the benefits of aromatherapy. The therapist can make appropriate blends for bath or footbath, inhalation, oil burner or compress.

Aromatherapy blends during pregnancy should not exceed a strength of 2%. Suggestions are listed below for the relief of some of the discomforts of pregnancy.

Clinical Trials and Case Studies

A clinical trial investigated the benefits of lavender in a bath for minimising perineal discomfort. The researchers found that as many as 85% of women surveyed felt that lavender was beneficial.[31]

The study examined the practice of adding six drops of pure lavender oil to bath water daily for 10 days following childbirth to reduce perineal discomfort. 635 women participated in the clinical trial.[31]

They were divided into three groups, each using one of the following bath additives:[31]

- Group A: pure lavender oil
- Group B: synthetic lavender oil
- Group C: A placebo which consisted of distilled water containing a GRAS additive (generally regarded as safe compound).

The mothers randomly selected a bottle number so that neither the mothers nor the midwives were aware of the contents of the bottles that they had to use. All groups were given identical instructions:[31]

To use six drops of their additive to the bath on postnatal day one and every day until day 10. Half and hour after each bath the mother completed a Visual Analogue Scale (VAS) which graded her discomfort and mood scores.[31]

The results of the trial provided no statistical evidence to support the practice of using lavender to reduce perineal discomfort. However, mothers using the oil found it pleasant to use, and no unpleasant side effects were experienced. Comparison of mood scores showed little statistical difference. The pattern of discomfort scores showed no statistical differences between the groups. However, those using lavender oil experienced a lower mean discomfort score between days 3 and 5. This is usually the time when the mother finds herself discharged from hospital and perineal discomfort is usually high. It was suggested that further studies should examine other methods of applying the essential oils and the dosage of essential oil used.[31]

Aromatherapy for Surgery and Intensive Care

Many factors need to be considered when utilising aromatherapy for patients in intensive care. Price says that this includes minimising the risk of invasive infections and reducing stress and anxiety often experienced by the patient and relatives.[1]

Price says that often patients view the intensive care unit as a 'hostile environment', in which they are surrounded by a bewildering array of monitoring and support equipment and have been subjected to a variety of invasive therapeutic techniques.[1]

Aromatherapy can be most useful for alleviating anxiety and reducing recovery time for persons who have just had surgery.

Clinical Trials and Case Studies

Aromatherapy has been found to be extremely valuable in the care of post-operative coronary heart disease patients. Stevenson, a qualified nurse and aromatherapist, found that neroli reduced discomfort and side effects of patients who have undergone cardiac surgery. Neroli was chosen because of its abilities in calming the nervous system, alleviating insomnia, relieving anxiety, reducing palpitations and being a cordial or heart tonic.[32]

References

1. Price S, Price L. *Aromatherapy for health professionals*. 2nd edn, Churchill Livingstone, UK, 1999.
2. Rankin-Box D. *The nurse's handbook of complementary therapies*. Churchill Livingstone, UK, 1995.
3. Holder R. *Aromatherapy in hospitals — A study in acceptance*. The Aromatherapist 1995; 2(2): 11–19.
4. Gravett P. *An investigation of the use of essential oils for the treatment of chemotherapy-induced side-effects in a group of patients undergoing high dose chemotherapy with stem cell rescue for breast cancer*. AROMA'95 Conference proceedings, Aromatherapy Publications, England, 1995.
5. McVey M. *Policy development*. from *The nurses' handbook of complementary therapies*, edited by Denise Rankin-Box. Churchill Livingstone, UK, 1995.
6. Horrigan C. *Aromatherapy in patient care*. AROMA'93 Conference Proceedings, Aromatherapy Publications, UK, 1994.
7. Bensouilah J. *Aromatherapy of the elderly*. Aromatherapy Quarterly 1998; 56: 9–11.
8. Stankovic S, Cook S. *Aromatherapy in aged care: A gift to the senses*. Simply Essential 2000; 35: 26–27.
9. Murtagh J. *General practice*. 2nd edn, McGraw Hill, Australia, 1998.
10. Barker A. *Pressure sores*. Aromatherapy Quarterly 1994; 41: 5–7.
11. Mitchell S. *Dementia*. The International Journal of Aromatherapy 1993; 5(2): 20–23.
12. Bowles J. et al. *Effects of essential oils and touch on resistance to nursing care procedures and other dementia-related behaviours in a residential care facility*. The International Journal of Aromatherapy 2002; 12(1): 16–21.
13. Lynn J, Harrold J. *Handbook for mortals*. Oxford University Press, USA, 1999.
15. Casey M. *Caring for cancer patients*. Aromatherapy Today, 1999; 12: 10–13.
16. Australian Institute of Health & Welfare, *Australia's Health: 1998*. Commonwealth of Australia, 1998.
17. Buckle J. *Cancer and clinical aromatherapy*. Aromatherapy Today, 2000; 14: 32–35.
18. Horrigan C. *Complementary cancer care*. The International Journal of Aromatherapy 1991; 3(4): 15–17.
19. Denyer J. *Cancer — The gentle approach*. The International Journal of Aromatherapy 1988; 1(2): 9.
20. Millar R. *The use of aromatherapy in hospitals for patients with cancer*. The Aromatherapist 1996; 3(2):14–28.
21. Horrigan C. *Complementary cancer care II*. The International Journal of Aromatherapy 1992; 4(1):18–19.
22. Horrigan C. *Complementary cancer care III*. The International Journal of Aromatherapy, 1992; 4(2): 28–29.
23. Horrigan C. *Complementary cancer care IV*. The International Journal of Aromatherapy 1992; 4(3): 34–36.
24. Gravett P. *Aromatherapy treatment of severe oral mucositis following high dose chemotherapy*. The International Journal of Aromatherapy 2000; 10(1/2); 52–53.
25. Corner J. *An evaluation of the use of massage*. AROMA'95 Conference Proceedings, Aromatherapy Publications, England, 1995.
26. Sanderson H. *Learning difficulties*. AROMA'93 Conference Proceedings, Aromatherapy Publications, UK, 1994.
27. Sanderson H, Harrison J, Price S. *Aromatherapy and massage for people who have learning difficulties*. Birmingham University Press, UK, 1991.
28. Durrell S. *An Aromatherapy service for people with a learning disability*. The International Journal of Aromatherapy, 12(3): 145–151.
29. Waters B. *Massage during pregnancy*. Research Triangle Publishing Inc, USA, 1995.
30. Guenier J. *Essential obstetrics*. The International Journal of Aromatherapy 1992; 4(1): 6–8.
31. Cornwell S, Dale S. *Modern midwife*. March 1995; 31–33.
32. Stevenson C. *Orange blossom evaluation*. The International Journal of Aromatherapy 1992; 4(3): 22–24.

Unit V

Clinical Index

Unit V provides you with the knowledge and skills for the treatment of a wide range of conditions. Each condition is listed with a description of:

- The cause and symptoms.
- The recommended treatment, including:
  - The appropriate essential oils and their application.
  - Suggestions regarding diet, herbs, acupressure and additional complementary therapies.

Unit V includes the following chapters:

The Cardiovascular System

Objectives

After careful study of this chapter, you should be able to:

- identify the factors that contribute to cardiovascular disease
- identify, list and describe common pathophysiologies of the cardiovascular system
- explain the aromatherapy treatment for specific conditions and disorders of the cardiovascular system
- explain the role of other holistic strategies for specific conditions and disorders of the cardiovascular system.

Introduction

The cardiovascular system is made up of the heart, arteries, arterioles, capillaries, veins, venules and the blood. The basic function of the cardiovascular system is to ensure that blood reaches all parts of the body. Every cell must receive nourishment that is provided by the blood. The cardiovascular system also ensures that waste products of the cells (carbon dioxide, urea, lactic acid, etc.) are carried to the kidneys, intestines, lungs and skin where they are excreted.

Statistics from the Australian Institute of Health and Welfare indicated that cardiovascular disease accounted for 41.9% of all deaths among Australians in 1996. Coronary heart disease was the major cardiovascular cause of death, accounting for 23% of all deaths. Strokes accounted for 9%, heart failure for 2.3% and peripheral vascular disease for 1.6% of all deaths.[1]

Many cardiovascular diseases require medical diagnosis and treatment. However, aromatherapy, as with other forms of natural therapy, can play a vital role in the prevention of cardiovascular disease. Its main forms are coronary heat disease, stroke and peripheral vascular disease, which are caused by damaged blood supply to the heart, brain and legs. The main underlying problem in cardiovascular disease is a process known as atherosclerosis that clogs blood-supply vessels. It is most serious when it affects the blood supply to the heart, causing angina or a heart attack, or to the brain, which leads to a stroke.[1]

Much evidence shows that lifestyle is a contributing factor to the disease process. Risk factors such as cigarette smoking, excess intake of salt, saturated fats and refined processed foods, alcohol, lack of exercise can all potentiate disease processes.

Biochemical risk factors such as high cholesterol and triglycerides, reduced high density lipoproteins (HDL) levels, decreased levels of plasma copper, high blood sugar, increased blood viscosity and high blood pressure can also significantly influence circulatory problems.

General Considerations

Although there may not be complete agreement on any set of rules for preventing or delaying the onset of heart disease, many authorities concur that the following factors apply to cardiovascular diseases:

- exercise
- diet
- smoking
- stress.

Diet

Proper nutrition, including the basic food elements, will help to maintain all tissues in optimum condition. The most important dietary factors that will reduce the risk of heart disease are:

- reduce the consumption of dietary fats
- increase the consumption of fish oils or cold-pressed polyunsaturated oils
- reduce the intake of salt to less than 2 to 3 g per day
- avoid tea, coffee, cocoa and excessive sugar
- increase dietary fibre by eating raw fruit and vegetables
- reduce alcohol intake
- reduce weight if necessary
- eat more garlic, onion and ginger.

Exercise

Appropriate exercise is an important part of prevention as well as the treatment of heart disease. Regular exercise programs, with gradual increases in the length and difficulty of activity, have been found to be very helpful. To begin with, simple walking may be the most effective, followed by activities such as swimming, bicycling and jogging. Even a minimal amount of regular exercise, such as walking 30 minutes three times a week, has been shown to be of major benefit.

Smoking

People who smoke are at a greater risk of developing coronary heart disease, stroke and peripheral vascular disease and other chronic conditions from smoking tobacco products.[1] In addition to heart disease, it is estimated that 30% of cancers are attributed to active smoking.

Stress

There is a correlation between stress and diseases of the circulatory system. It would be more appropriate to consider the individual's ability to deal with stress in his/her lifestyle.

'Type A' personalities are generally considered competitive, ambitious and over-conscientious, while type B are more relaxed and easygoing. With coronary heart disease it is predominantly type A who experience myocardial infarction.[2]

Massage and aromatherapy can be very important in allowing Type A personalities to experience how it feels to be relaxed. This re-experience of relaxation is what massage treatment aims to achieve.[2]

Aromatherapy Considerations

Many circulatory and most cardiac problems require professional diagnosis and treatment, but aromatherapy in combination with simple preventative recommendations can prevent the deterioration of the circulatory and cardiovascular system.

Aromatherapy has been found to be extremely valuable in the care of post-operative coronary heart disease patients. Stevenson, a qualified nurse and aromatherapist, found that neroli reduced discomfort and side-effects of patients who have undergone cardiac surgery.[3] Neroli was chosen because of its ability to calm the nervous system, alleviate insomnia, relieve anxiety, reduce palpitations and because it is a heart tonic.[3]

When someone has had a heart attack — whether it be mild or severe — the experience can lead to the patient remaining in a state of great anxiety and tension. The worry of having subsequent heart attacks may actually cause another heart attack.[4]

It is therefore vital for the therapist to provide the right kind of support. This means not to pander to or encourage an attention-seeking, self-pitying attitude in the patient, as this does very little to aid recovery. The best course of action is for the therapist to restore an attitude of equilibrium, which can be achieved by using aromatherapy.[4]

The following list of properties indicates how essential oils may be used to help prevent and treat some of the more common problems associated with the cardiovascular system.

Nervines

Anxiety and stress can lead to cardiovascular problems. The use of relaxing nervines such as bergamot, Roman chamomile, lavender, clary sage, geranium, neroli, sandalwood and ylang ylang should be considered to reduce stress and anxiety.

Circulatory Tonics

Essential oils such as cypress, geranium, yarrow and lemon are useful for treating swellings, inflammations and varicose veins.

Hypotensives

Essential oils such as lavender, sweet marjoram, may chang and ylang ylang have been found to reduce blood pressure.

Hypertensives

Hypertensives may be used for poor circulation, chilblains, listlessness and low blood pressure. Essential oils such as rosemary and thyme have been found to increase blood pressure.

Rubefacients

Essential oils such as black pepper, ginger, clove bud, rosemary and thyme stimulate circulation locally to the area where they are applied. Rubefacient oils cause the capillaries to dilate, increasing the blood flow, which speeds up the healing process.

Associated Conditions

Bruises

Useful Oils

• arnica-infused oil • black pepper • everlasting
• German chamomile • hyssop • sweet fennel
• spike lavender • lemon • sweet marjoram
• rosemary

Clinical Features

The skin is not broken when bruised, but the underlying tissue is injured, resulting in pain, swelling and black and blue marks due to blood that has collected under the skin.

Aetiology

Although body parts become bruised after contact with hard objects, there are several factors that predispose one to bruising. Anaemia, overweight, malnutrition, leukaemia and excessive use of anti-clotting drugs can lead to vessel rupture, resulting in bruising.

Aromatherapy Treatment

Essential oils such as fennel, hyssop, rosemary or spike lavender are effective if applied to the area as soon as possible after bruising has occurred, preferably in an ice-cold compress. Arnica-infused oil is a classic remedy for bruising and it can be applied neat to unbroken skin.

In case of severe bruising such as that resulting from accident, oils which stimulate the spleen such as black pepper, German chamomile and lavender will be helpful.[5]

Other Treatments

Balch and Balch suggest the following for the treatment of bruises:[6]

- 3,000 to 10,000 mg of vitamin C with bioflavonoids taken in divided doses during the day.
- Avoid aspirin or other nonsteroidal anti-inflammatory drugs.
- If bruising is frequent seek medical advice.
- The diet should include an abundance of dark green leafy vegetables and fresh fruit which are rich in vitamin C.
- Apply a comfrey ointment on a daily basis.

Chilblains

Useful Oils
• black pepper • cinnamon bark or leaf • clove bud • ginger • lavender • lemon • nutmeg • rosemary • sweet marjoram • red thyme

Clinical Features

Chilblains are reddish blue discolourations of the skin, accompanied by swelling, which affects parts of the body that are exposed to cold, particularly toes, fingers, and the backs of legs. Children are particularly prone to chilblains on their feet in winter.

Aetiology

Poor circulation of the blood is a contributory factor.

Therapeutic Strategy

- Stop smoking.[6]
- Follow the basic recommendations for a healthy diet.[6]
- Get regular exercise to promote blood flow.

Aromatherapy Treatment

Essential oils that are rubefacients will stimulate the local circulation. The most effective essential oils are black pepper, cinnamon bark, clove bud, lemon, ginger, nutmeg, rosemary and red thyme.

Massage the affected area with a massage oil containing a 3% dilution of any of these oils. This will reduce pain and itching and help to disperse the chilblains.

Other Treatments

- Boost circulation by dry skin brushing.[6]
- The diet should include garlic and foods containing high levels of vitamin C and E that will improve circulation.[6]

Hypertension

Useful Oils
• bergamot • Roman chamomile • lavender • lemon • sweet marjoram • may chang • neroli • melissa • ylang ylang

Definition

Hypertension is the clinical term for high blood pressure. The definition is blood pressure persistently elevated above 140 mm Hg systolic and/or 90 mm Hg diastolic.[7]

Clinical Features

It is perfectly normal for the systolic blood pressure to increase on exertion or during emotional stress, but in a healthy body it will return to normal quite quickly. Blood pressure is a parameter that reflects the circulating blood volume, peripheral vascular resistance, efficiency of the heart as a pump, the viscosity of the blood and the elasticity of the arterial walls. Thus a change in any of these parameters will result in blood pressure changes.

The blood pressure reaches its highest point during systole and its lowest point during diastole. The blood pressure of a healthy young adult is approximately 120 mm Hg (column of mercury) during systole and 80 mm Hg in diastole. By convention, this is expressed as 120/80.[8]

Hypertension is divided into several levels:[9]

- borderline (120–160/90–94)
- mild (140–160/95–104)
- moderate (140–180/105–114)
- severe (160+/115+).

Hypertension is an important preventable cause of cardiovascular disease. Studies have shown that without treatment, hypertension greatly increases the incidence of cardiac failure, coronary heart diseases with angina pectoris and myocardial infarction, and renal failure.[6]

Arteriosclerosis and atherosclerosis are common precursors of hypertension. Because the arteries become obstructed with cholesterol plaque, circulation of blood through the vessels becomes difficult. When the arteries become hardened and constricted, the blood is forced through narrower passageways. As a result the blood pressure becomes elevated. Advanced warning signs include persistent morning headaches, sweating, rapid pulse, shortness of breath, swollen ankles and fingers, recurrent nose bleeds, dizziness and vision disturbances.[6,10.]

Aetiology

High blood pressure can be divided into two categories:

- Cause is of a known origin (renal, adrenal tumour types), referred to as secondary hypertension.
- Cause is of unknown origin, referred to as essential hypertension.

About 95% of all diagnosed hypertension is essential hypertension.[7] Cigarette smoking, stress, obesity, excessive use of stimulants such as coffee and tea, drug abuse and high sodium intake have all been identified as risk factors.[6]

Secondary hypertension is due to kidney diseases. The kidneys secrete a large amount of a hormone called renin. The function of renin is to constrict the arterial walls, and in doing so, raise the pressure of the vessels. Many kidney diseases such as pyelitis, nephritis or polycystic kidneys increase the possibility of hypertension.[6]

Therapeutic Strategy

Hypertension is closely associated with lifestyle and dietary factors. Diet, exercise and relaxation therapies have all proven to be very effective in managing borderline to mild hypertension.[9]

Aromatherapy Treatment

While it will be necessary to make changes to the diet and lifestyle, aromatherapy can help to lower and stabilise blood pressure. Clinical research shows that regular massage effectively reduces high blood pressure.

Essential oils will alleviate hypertension by their:

- hypotensive effect
- sedating and calming effects
- detoxifying effect.

The three most important essential oils are lavender, sweet marjoram and ylang ylang.[5]

While these essential oils may be used to lower high blood pressure, a selection of sedative, antidepressant and uplifting oils are also recommended. Roman chamomile, bergamot, neroli and frankincense may be used. Detoxifying essential oils such as juniper berry and lemon oil are also recommended.

Precautions

There is certainly an amount of controversy regarding hypertensive essential oils. It has been traditionally believed that essential oils such as rosemary, sage, hyssop and thyme are hypertensives, therefore they should not be used by anyone suffering from high blood pressure.[5,11] However, Tisserand and Balacs state that it is very unlikely that any essential oils can exacerbate hypertension.[12]

Other Treatments

Nutrition

- Avoid all alcohol, caffeine and tobacco.[6]
- A high fibre diet and supplemental fibre are recommended. Oat bran is a good source of fibre. Eat plenty of fruit and vegetables.[6,10]
- A salt-free diet is essential in lowering blood pressure. Lowering salt intake is not good enough; eliminate all salt from the diet. Excessive consumption of dietary sodium chloride, coupled with diminished dietary potassium, induces an increase in extracellular fluid volume and an impairment of the blood pressure regulating mechanisms. This results in hypertension in susceptible individuals.[6,9,10]
- Increasing the amount of cold-pressed polyunsaturated vegetable oils which are an excellent source of linoleic acid has a profound hypotensive action. This is due to the normalisation of the E series prostaglandins which are known to be decreased in hypertensive patients.[9]
- Increase intake of calcium-rich foods. Calcium deficiency has been linked to high blood pressure.[10]
- Reduce the intake of animal proteins — lean towards a vegetarian diet.[6,9,10]
- Garlic, onions and ginger should be used in cooking. Garlic has been shown to decrease the systolic pressure by 20–30 mm Hg and the diastolic by 10–20 mm Hg.[10]

Herbs

- Hawthorn berries have long been used in Europe as a cardiovascular tonic.[9]

General Advice

- Check blood cholesterol and blood sugar as these are usually elevated in hypertension. If elevated treat accordingly.[10]
- Stress reduction techniques have been shown to be beneficial in lowering blood pressure.[9]
- Keep body weight down. Regular moderate exercise is important to maintain proper circulation.[6,9]

Palpitations

Useful Oils

• lavender • may chang • melissa • neroli • rose otto • ylang ylang

Definition

Palpitations are referred to as an individual's awareness of the beating of the heart. By definition it does not always imply 'racing' of the heart but any sensation in the chest such as 'pounding', 'flopping', 'skipping', 'jumping', 'thumping' or 'fluttering' of the heart.[10]

Tachycardia is defined as an abnormal increase in the heart rate above the normal resting range — 60 to 100 beats a minute.[14]

Aetiology

Although palpitations commonly occur in structurally diseased hearts, palpitations are usually quite normal after exercise, or when stressed and frightened, or when stimulants such as caffeine or nicotine have been taken.

When palpitations are associated with chest pain, oedema or loss of consciousness, a pulse that is slower than 50 beats per minute or faster than 120 beats per minute, the client should be referred to a medical practitioner. Symptoms such as these are likely to indicate a more serious cardiovascular disease for which medical attention is required.

Aromatherapy

In the case where palpitations have not been linked to structural heart disease, and particularly where there may be a psychological reason for their occurrence, aromatherapy will be effective in treating palpitations.

An emergency procedure is to simply inhale essential oils such as neroli, lavender, rose otto or ylang ylang directly from the bottle. A person who is subject to frequent palpitations would benefit from regular massage with any one of the above essential oils.

Other Treatments

- Avoid coffee, tea, cola and caffeine drinks, chocolate, alcohol and smoking.[10]
- During an 'attack', dip the hands and arms up to the elbow in cold water for at least 10 seconds.[10]
- Acupressure points Heart 7 and Pericardium 6 can be used to relieve anxiety, nervous tension and palpitations.[13]
- Reduce anxiety state through meditation or relaxation techniques.[10]
- Stop smoking.[10]
- Increase the intake of essential fatty acids.[10]
- Increase consumption of potassium, magnesium and calcium-rich foods.[10]

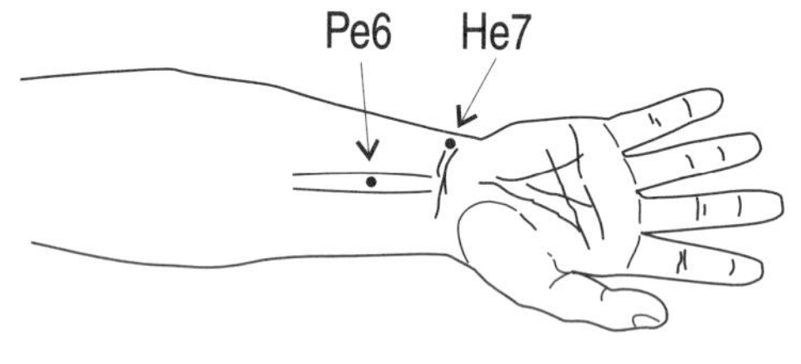

Location of acupressure points used to treat palpitations.

Oedema

Useful Oils

• carrot seed • cypress • sweet fennel • grapefruit • juniper berry • geranium • mandarin • sweet orange • rosemary • tangerine • sage

Definition

Oedema is an excessive accumulation of fluid in tissue spaces. It may be generalised or localised.[14]

Clinical Features

Fluid retention usually causes swelling of the feet and ankles and is made worse by standing and hot weather. Being stationary for a long time, such as a prolonged journey, may produce ankle swelling. More generalised fluid retention may result in swelling of the fingers, with tightness of rings on the fingers and puffiness of the upper and lower eyelids and face.[15]

Aetiology

There are many possible causes, the most serious one being some form of kidney disease. Pregnancy, oral contraceptives, premenstrual tension, allergic reaction, standing or sitting for too long and injury to the body can all cause the body to retain fluid.

Treatment Strategy

- Treat the cause where known.
- Restrict sodium chloride intake.
- Use diuretic and detoxifying essential oils in massages and baths.

Aromatherapy Treatment

Massage is useful for reducing fluid retention of the legs and ankles that has occurred after prolonged standing. Massage the legs with long, upward strokes, always moving away from the ankle.

Any essential oil that has diuretic properties may be used in a massage oil. This includes carrot seed, sweet fennel, juniper berry, grapefruit, lemon, cold-pressed lime, tangerine, mandarin and sweet orange. These oils may also be used in a bath.

Fluid retention is often caused by an accumulation of toxic wastes in the body, as in the case of cellulite. Detoxifying oils such as carrot seed, sweet fennel, juniper berry and lemon can be useful in such cases.

Other Treatments

- Reduce salt intake; salt helps retain fluid in the body.[15]
- Reduce refined carbohydrates, such as sucrose-containing foods, honey and glucose. All these foods require a considerable amount of water to be metabolised. Often just cutting these foods out will increase urine output.[15]
- Food allergies produce significant fluid retention. Wheat, other grains and milk are common culprits.[15]

- Persistent fluid retention can be caused by heart problems which will require medical treatment.[15]
- The following herbs may be beneficial for the treatment of fluid retention— dandelion root or leaf, juniper berry, celery seed, parsley and burdock root. These herbs have diuretic properties.[15]

Varicose Veins

Useful Oils
• calendula-infused oil • cypress • lemon
• geranium • juniper berry • rosemary
• wheatgerm cold-pressed oil

Definition

Varicose veins are abnormally enlarged swollen veins that usually occur in the legs. They are the result of weakness of the valves inside the veins that allow the blood to flow back to the heart. If the valves do not work properly, blood accumulates in the veins, stretching them and causing varicosities.

Clinical Features

The prominent blue bulging veins are often accompanied by dull, nagging aches and pains. Swellings, sore legs, leg cramps and feelings of heaviness in the legs are also characteristic of varicose veins.[6]

Generally, varicose veins are not considered harmful if the involved vein is near the surface. However, these veins are often cosmetically unappealing. Although significant symptoms are not common, the legs may feel heavy, tight and tired.[6,9]

A more serious form of varicose vein involves obstruction and valve defects of the deeper veins of the leg. This type of varicose vein can lead to problems such as thrombophlebitis, pulmonary embolism, myocardial infarction and stroke.[9]

Aetiology

- Genetic weakness of the veins or venous valves.[9]
- Excessive venous pressure due to a low fibre-induced increase in straining during defecation.[9]
- Lack of exercise, obesity, pregnancy and anything that reduces the circulation in the legs.[9]
- Poor posture such as sitting cross-legged or standing upright all day long.[9]

Constipation, phlebitis, heart failures, liver disease and abdominal tumours can all play a role in the formation of varicose veins.[6]

Therapeutic Strategy

- Modifying dietary factors.
- Increasing bulking agents.
- Physical activity.
- Use of herbs and essential oils to tonify the veins.
- Avoid standing in one place for long periods.

Aromatherapy Treatment

Essential oils can assist in the treatment of varicose veins because of the following properties:

- venous decongestants
- circulatory stimulants
- astringent action.

Holmes says that cypress oil is a true venous blood decongestant as well as an astringent and recommends its use for the treatment of venous blood stagnation such as varicose veins, haemorrhoids and phlebitis. It should be used in a massage oil.[16]

Special care needs to be taken with the massage techniques used. Only gentle, upward, almost superficial effleurage strokes should be used. Work up the legs from the feet towards the heart. It may take months to produce any improvement in the varicose veins, and as in any chronic condition, prolonged treatment is required.

It is important to vary the essential oils used from time to time. Alternate cypress and lemon with lavender, juniper, geranium or rosemary. Daily application is needed. These essential oils may also be used in a bath or blended in a clay lotion compress.

Mailhebiau recommends using sage with cypress for treating venous problems such as varicose veins.[17]

Other Treatments

Nutrition

- Vitamin C aids circulation and reduces the tendency of blood clots. Up to 3,000 mg daily is recommended.[6]
- The diet should be low in fat and refined carbohydrates and contain plenty of fresh fruit and vegetables. Avoid processed and refined foods.[6]
- Flavonoid-rich berries, such as hawthorn berries, cherries, blueberries and blackberries are beneficial in the prevention and treatment of varicose veins since they increase the integrity of the walls of the veins. Consumption of these berries or their extracts is indicated for individuals with varicose veins.[9,10]
- Ensure that the diet contains adequate fibre to avoid constipation. A high fibre diet is the most important component in the treatment and prevention of varicose veins and haemorrhoids. A diet rich in vegetables, fruit, legumes and grains promotes peristalsis. Fibre will attract

water, forming a gelatinous mass which keeps the faeces soft, bulky and easy to pass. The effect of a high fibre diet is less straining during defecation.[9]

- Individuals with varicose veins have a decreased ability to break down fibrin. The result is that fibrin is deposited in the tissues near the varicose veins. The skin becomes hard and lumpy due to the presence of fibrin and fat. Cayenne, ginger, garlic and onions all increase fibrin breakdown. Liberal consumption of these spices in foods is recommended for individuals with varicose veins and other disorders of the cardiovascular system.[9]

Herbs

Duke recommends the following botanicals:[18]

- Violet flowers contain rutin which helps to maintain the strength and integrity of the capillary walls. He says that 20 to 100 mg of rutin a day can significantly strengthen the capillaries. According to his calculations, he estimates that you would need only a few tablespoons of violet flowers to obtain 100 mg of rutin. They are quite safe to eat and suggests adding them to salads.
- Witch hazel comes in both a water extract and alcoholic extract. Both preparations are soothingly astringent and are excellent as an external treatment for various conditions from bruising to varicose veins.
- Lemon contains flavonoids, including rutin, that reduce the permeability of the blood vessels, especially the capillaries.
- Onions are one of the best sources of quercetin. Like rutin, quercetin reportedly decreases capillary fragility.
- Bilberry helps circulation by stimulating new capillary formation, strengthening capillary walls and increasing the overall health of the circulatory system.
- Ginkgo biloba is well known for its ability to increase circulation and has been used for treating varicose veins.

General Advice

- Gentle exercise such as yoga and swimming is beneficial. Walking and gentle exercises are suitable, but jogging, skipping, aerobic and other exercises which involve repeated impact can do more harm than good.[6,10]
- Wear loose clothing that does not restrict blood flow.[6]
- Do not sit cross-legged as the blood flow will be inhibited.[6]
- Avoid standing as much as possible and lie with the feet higher than the heart.[6]

References

1. Australian Institute of Health & Welfare, *Australia's Health: 1998*. Commonwealth of Australia, 1998.
2. Anderson L. *The heart of massage*. The International Journal of Aromatherapy 1992; 4(3): 20–21.
3. Stevenson C. *Orange blossom evaluation*. The International Journal of Aromatherapy 1992; 4(3): 22–4.
4. Barker A. *Aromatherapy and heart attack*. Aromatherapy Quarterly 1996; 48: 13–18.
5. Davis P. *Aromatherapy: An A–Z*. The C.W. Daniel Company Limited, Great Britain, 1988.
6. Balch J, Balch P. *Prescription for nutritional healing*. Avery Publishing Group, USA, 1997.
7. Werner R. *A massage therapist's guide to pathology*. Lippincott Williams & Wilkins, USA, 1998.
8. Cohen BJ, Wood DL. *Memmler's the human body in health and disease*. 9th edn, J.B. Lippincott Company, USA, 2000.
9. Pizzorno J, Murray M. *A text book of natural medicine*. 2nd edn, Churchill Livingstone, UK, 1999.
10. Osiecki H. *The physician's handbook of clinical nutrition*. Bioconcepts Publishing, Australia, 1990.
11. Lawless J. *The encyclopaedia of essential oils*. Element Books Limited, Great Britain, 1992.
12. Tisserand R, Balacs T. *Essential oil safety*. Churchill Livingstone, UK, 1995.
13. Reed Gach M. *Acupressure's potent points*. Bantam Books, USA, 1990.
14. Murtagh J. *General practice*. The McGraw-Hill Companies Inc, Australia, 1998.
15. Davies S, Stewart A. *Nutritional medicine*. Pan Books, Great Britain, 1987.
16. Holmes P. *The energetics of western herbs Vol.1*. Artemis Press, USA, 1986.
17. Mailhebiau P. *Portraits in oils*. The C.W. Daniel Company Limited, Great Britain, 1995.
18. Duke J. *The green pharmacy*. Rodale Press, USA, 1997.

The Respiratory System

Objectives

After careful study of this chapter, you should be able to:

- outline a general treatment strategy for conditions associated with the respiratory system
- identify, list and describe common pathophysiologies of the respiratory system
- explain the aromatherapy treatment for specific conditions and disorders of the respiratory system
- explain the role of other holistic strategies for specific conditions and disorders of the respiratory system.

Introduction

Human life depends on the ability to utilise oxygen and to eliminate carbon dioxide. Respiration is defined as the exchange of oxygen and carbon dioxide between the atmosphere and the cells in the body. The respiratory system consists of:

- **the upper respiratory tract** — the nose, pharynx, larynx, trachea, bronchi and bronchioles
- **the lower respiratory tract** — the lungs, alveoli, pleura and diaphragm.

Mills describes the lungs as an extremely efficient unit in allowing gas exchange between air and fluid:

> *In creating the lungs the maker faced several intriguing engineering problems. Exchanging oxygen and carbon dioxide in a fluid environment, initially by simple diffusion through cell walls, and then through specialised gill structures, is a relatively uncomplicated business. Air breathing is much harder. Because gas exchange is less efficient between air and fluid, a relatively much larger surface area of body fluids has to be exposed for aeration. A way of passing large quantities of air over these fluids has also to be devised.*
>
> *The resulting design is the lungs, vast networks of fine blood capillaries surrounded by air whose movement is powered by an efficient bellows unit, the diaphragm. It works extremely well.*[1]

However, what happens when we inhale air that is contaminated with dust, smoke and other pollutants?

Fortunately, a number of ingenious systems ensure that the air we breathe is cleaned. Mills explains the ingenious role of the mucociliary escalator and the coughing reflex:

> *... However there remains a problem. Air is likely to be contaminated with dust, smoke and other pollutants. Sucking all this into a closed moist sponge inevitably means that a lot of rubbish will get trapped inside. ... As air is inhaled, the anatomy of the airways sets it spiralling in a vortex down the bronchial tubes. Centrifugal forces thus ensure that most particles in the air get thrown to the bronchial walls. Here a sticky mucus secretion traps the particles like flypaper. This film is supported on a bed of cilia, contactile filaments projecting from the surface of the epithelium.*
>
> *They are involved in a phased series of contractions, always upwards, to give the effect of repeated waves rising up the airways, carrying the impregnated mucus with them. This emerges at the top, at the throat, as phlegm or sputum usually to be swallowed unconsciously, to be destroyed in the sterilising vat of the stomach. The whole upward elimination is attractively referred to as the 'mucociliary escalator'.*[1]

So, by the time the air reaches the fine alveoli in the lungs, where it meets the capillaries, it is usually clean. This is just as well, as there are no cilia or mucus secretions at this level. Any impurity that has made its way to the lungs can only be removed by wandering phagocytes, or possibly by powerful upheavals of the diaphragm, exercise or coughing. The cough is the backup to the mucociliary escalator. It is clearly an attempt at removal. Unfortunately coughing is often seen as a hindrance that is better suppressed.

To understand the various respiratory disorders it is important to understand the principles of the mucociliary escalator. The mucociliary escalator can fail if there is:

- insufficient mucus, or
- too much mucus.[1]

The first case is common with allergic and asthmatic conditions and in dry irritating coughs, the mucus is too tacky to flow adequately. If the problem is prolonged, congestion may occur and a secondary bronchitis can result.[1]

The second case is more common in cooler and damp climates, when excessive mucus, otherwise known as catarrh, can overload the ciliary mechanism and a primary congestion can occur. Opportunistic infection can easily supervene and bronchitis and other lung infections are the common result.[1]

With this in mind it is possible to develop a holistic approach to the treatment of respiratory problems.

General Considerations

Many respiratory problems such as the common cold are self-limiting and the person would get better irrespective of any treatment. However, this assumes that the person has sufficient energy to combat the infection and that nothing is done to deplete the body's natural defence mechanisms. When someone is feeling fatigued or stressed then it is more difficult to fight a cold.

It is not wise to sedate the cough reflex because this is the means by which the air passageway is cleared of excess tenacious mucous or foreign matter. However, when the constant coughing causes exhaustion, sleeplessness and irritation, an antitussive is called for.[1]

Smoking has a devastating effect not only on the lungs and respiratory system, but on the overall health of the individual and the unfortunate people who happen to be next to the smoker.

Treatment Strategy

In the treatment of respiratory conditions, diet and lifestyle are of paramount importance. Aromatherapy may assist by accelerating the healing process, by toning debilitating tissues, encouraging proper elimination of toxins and by relieving symptoms until the underlying causes have been dealt with.

The following dietary and lifestyle measures should be considered essential for long-term cure:

- restructuring the diet, including the acid/alkaline balance of the diet in favour of alkaline-forming foods
- reduction or elimination of refined sugars and refined wheat products
- reduction or elimination of salt, sugar, tea, coffee and alcohol
- reduction or elimination of suspected allergens (for example, yeast, gluten, artificial food additives and dairy products; make sure that there is a corresponding supplementation of foods high in calcium)
- a high intake of foods rich in vitamin C
- regular exercise, fresh air and correct breathing
- no smoking.

Aromatherapy Considerations

Extensive research and clinical trials have proven that essential oils are very effective for treating respiratory problems. The best method of using the essential oils for the treatment of respiratory tract infections is by inhalations, chest and back massages, compresses, diffusers and oil burners.

Many essential oils used in treating respiratory problems come from the trees — leaves, resins and woods. One school of thought suggests using the leaf oils for acute and short-term respiratory problems and the wood and resin oils for more chronic conditions. Generally the wood and resin oils tend to be more drying and soothing, while the leaf oils are more stimulating and active in fighting pulmonary bacteria. Gumbel says that the leaves of the plant have a direct affinity to the function of the lungs, since they are the respiratory organs for the plants, and indirectly for the earth itself.[2]

The therapeutic properties of essential oils that have a particular affinity to the respiratory system are:

Antimicrobial Properties

The antimicrobial properties of essential oils are well documented and their use for the treatment of respiratory tract infections is well known.[3,4]

Many essential oils have antimicrobial activity. Essential oils such as cajeput, cinnamon, clove bud, lavender, lemon, lemon scented eucalyptus, manuka, niaouli, pine, rosemary, tea tree and thyme are of particular value for the treatment of flu, colds, sore throats, tonsillitis and other infections.

Antispasmodics

These essential oils relax the bronchioles of the lungs and may be used for the treatment of asthma, dry cough and whooping cough.

Essential oils that are classified as having an antispasmodic effect on the respiratory system include angelica root, aniseed, basil, bay laurel, Virginian cedarwood, cajeput, cypress, clary sage, eucalyptus, sweet fennel and thyme.

Antitussives

Antitussives are remedies that prevent coughing. Some work by soothing irritability (respiratory demulcents), and others remove congestive mucus (expectorants).[5]

Essential oils such as aniseed, cypress, *Hyssop var. decumbens,* eucalyptus, peppermint and thyme are incorporated in sugar-based lozenges to suppress coughs. Cough lozenges with essential oils apparently function by stimulating the formation and secretion of saliva, which produces more frequent swallowing and thereby tends to suppress the cough reflex.[6]

Demulcents

Demulcents soothe and relieve irritated or inflamed mucous membranes. In herbal medicine the herbs with mucilaginous properties such as flaxseed, liquorice, marshmallow leaf and mullein are valuable as demulcents.[6]

Sandalwood is an effective demulcent essential oil as it soothes and relieves irritated and inflamed mucous membranes. It is recommended for dry, irritable and ticklish coughs.[8] Holmes recommends gargles and syrups for throat infections, itchiness or hoarseness, and chest compresses for dry bronchial disorders.[8]

Expectorants

An expectorant promotes the expulsion of phlegm by coughing or spitting.[5] An expectorant may be defined as a substance which increases the output of demulcent respiratory tract fluid.[5] Expectorants are also used to alleviate coughing by:

- assisting the removal of a substance causing the cough reflex
- providing a more demulcent respiratory tract fluid.

Mills says that there are three categories of expectorants:

- stimulating and warming expectorants
- relaxing expectorants
- antitussives.[5]

Stimulating and warming expectorants are essential oils that also have circulatory stimulant properties. Their principal effect on the lungs is to provoke an expectoration of congested phlegm in the airways and to dry up excessive catarrhal production. Essential oils such as angelica root, aniseed, everlasting, sweet fennel and ginger are warming expectorants.

Bone and Mills say that relaxing expectorants are high in mucilage and occasionally volatile oils. They generally act to reduce spasm and improve deficient mucus secretion in the airway.[5]

Tyler classifies expectorants according to their mode of action:

- nausea-expectorants
- local irritants
- surface tension modifiers.[6]

However, he states that the classification is imprecise because the functions of many botanicals are not understood and have multiple actions. Of interest in aromatherapy are the local irritant expectorants, including essential oils such as aniseed, sweet fennel and thyme.

Balacs says that menthol, camphor, eucalyptus oil and 1,8-cineole appear to have the effect of reducing surface tension between water and air in the lungs, a property which can enhance the effect of the lung's own surfactants.[9]

Essential oils such as Atlas cedarwood, cajeput, frankincense, *Hyssop var. decumbens,* spike lavender, myrrh, myrtle, pine, sandalwood and thyme are also expectorants.

Immunostimulants

Essential oils can support and strengthen the immune response in two ways; by directly inhibiting the threatening micro-organisms or by stimulating the immune system.[7] Essential oils such as cajeput, eucalyptus, lavender, lemon, niaouli, rosemary, tea tree and thyme act against a wide variety of bacteria and viruses whilst at the same time increasing the immune response.

Associated Conditions

Asthma

Useful Oils

• aniseed • Atlas cedarwood • cajeput • clary sage
• Roman chamomile • cypress • sweet fennel
• frankincense • everlasting • *Eucalyptus radiata*
• *Hyssop var. decumbens* • lavender • spike lavender
• pine • lemon • mandarin • myrtle • niaouli
• peppermint • petitgrain • pine • rosemary

Definition

Asthma is defined as the reversible narrowing of the bronchioles, by inflammation of the mucus membranes or contraction of the muscular walls of the diaphragm. Difficulty in breathing, tightness in the chest, prolonged expiration phase, wheezing and coughing caused by excessive mucus are common symptoms.[10]

Clinical Features

Asthma is typically divided into two categories; extrinsic and intrinsic. Extrinsic or atopic asthma is generally considered an immunologically mediated condition with a characteristic increase in serum IgE. This is closely linked with the presence of eczema, hay fever, urticaria and migraine in the patient, or in his or her close relatives. People with this kind of family history are called atopic.[11,12]

Childhood asthma is often preceded for several months or years by episodic coughing that develops into a wheezy bronchitis and eventually into asthma. Such children often have a history of slow recovery from upper respiratory tract viral infections.

Intrinsic or nonatopic asthma is associated with a bronchial reaction that is not due to antigen-antibody stimulation, but rather to such factors as chemicals, cold air, exercise, infection, agents that activate the complementary pathway and emotional upset.[9,10]

The classic symptoms of asthma are wheezing, coughing (especially at night), tightness in the chest and breathlessness.[13]

Asthma should be suspected in children with recurrent nocturnal cough and in people with intermittent dyspnoea or chest tightness, especially after exercising.[13]

A series of stages has been characterised for describing the severity of an acute asthma attack:

- **Mild:** mild breathlessness
- **Moderate:** respiratory distress and wheezing at rest
- **Severe:** marked respiratory distress
- **Respiratory failure:** severe respiratory distress (life threatening).[14]

Aetiology

No single cause for asthma has been found, but a variety of factors may trigger an attack. These include specific factors such as viruses and allergens (inhaled allergens — house dust mite, animal dander, cigarette smoke; ingested allergens — foods, drugs, food additives, yeasts and moulds on food) and non-specific factors such as emotional stress, weather changes and exercise.[13,15]

Allergy is an integral part of most patients with asthma which presents first in childhood. It is not, as many people believe, an integral part of all asthma.

Therapeutic Strategy

Pizzorno suggests the following therapeutic approach:

- determine and rectify the underlying defect that allows the development of sensitisation
- determine and balance the underlying metabolic defect that causes an excessive inflammatory response
- find the allergens and develop a lifestyle, diet and environment that allows the allergens to be avoided
- modulate the inflammatory process to limit the severity of the response
- prepare an effective treatment for the bronchoconstriction of the acute attack.[11]

General advice in the management of asthma should also include:[10]

- Patients with asthma should not smoke.
- Atopic patients should avoid exposure to furred or domestic animals if they have a problem.
- About 90% of children with atopic symptoms and asthma demonstrate positive skin-prick responses to dust mite extract. Total eradication of house dust mite from the home is difficult.
- The asthmatic's emotional life may also need regulating. The lungs are linked to the emotions in an obvious way (for example, think about laughter or crying). If a person with asthma has difficulty in expressing feelings, it is worth exploring why this is so.
- Deep breathing can strengthen our connection to our feelings and can help improve asthma if practised regularly. Other regular exercise such as walking, swimming, yoga, Tai Chi, or other relaxation classes can also help to deepen and relax breathing and provide emotional balance.

Aromatherapy Treatment

The selection of essential oils is dependent upon:

- the presence of an infection
- the emotional factors involved
- the allergic response involved.

Asthma precipitated by infection (cold, flu, bronchitis etc.) with loose, copious mucus secretions is best treated with oils such as cajeput, eucalyptus, myrtle, lemon and spike lavender.

Asthma with viscid, tenacious mucus is best treated using essential oils with expectorant properties such as aniseed, fennel, *Hyssop var. decumbens,* rosemary and peppermint.

While Hoffman is referring to herbal preparations, the following advice is excellent when prescribing essential oils for asthma sufferers:

> *Most successful are the antispasmodic and bronchodilator plants, but they will do little for short-term relief of attacks. When used over a period of time, however, especially in conjunction with pulmonary tonics that strengthen the lungs, they can reduce both the frequency and severity of attacks. Expectorant remedies will be essential to ensure minimum build up of sputum in the lungs. However, as stimulant expectorants can potentially aggravate breathing difficulties, only the relaxing expectorants should be used. Antimicrobial support will guard against secondary infection. Anticatarrhals will help the body to deal with any over production of sputum in the lungs or sinuses. Nervines can help either where stress is a primary trigger or where the asthma itself becomes a source of stress that in turns triggers attacks.*[14]

Hoffman and Davis both recommend the inhalation of essential oils with antispasmodic properties for the treatment during an acute asthma. Inhale the oil directly from the oil bottle, or from drops placed on a tissue.[14,16] Steam inhalations may aggravate the condition, as the heat will increase inflammation of the mucus membranes and make congestion worse.

Asthma is sometimes representative of the psychosomatic illnesses present in industrial Western societies. The psychosomatic effect was observed with asthma patients who suffered allergies to cats. It was in many cases sufficient only to show the afflicted person a photograph of a cat in order to precipitate a crisis.[17] Usually asthma patients are people who convey messages asking for love and attention. The typical personality of an asthma sufferer demonstrates extreme sensitivity with poor self-esteem. Typically, asthma sufferers have difficulty creating boundaries between themselves and others.

For asthma sufferers with allergies, essential oils such as everlasting, lavender and Roman chamomile are recommended. Another oil that has been found to be beneficial is frankincense.[16] It is an expectorant and is known to relax, slow down and deepen the breathing. This may be useful as a preventive measure in asthma.

Other Treatments

Nutrition

- Check for food sensitivities and avoid foods found to precipitate an asthma attack. Double-blind food challenges in children have shown that immediate onset sensitivities are usually due to eggs, fish, shellfish, nuts and peanuts. Delayed onset is triggered by milk, chocolate, wheat, citrus fruit and food colourings, particularly tartrazine.[11,15]

- Include garlic and onions in the diet. These foods contain quercetin and mustard oils, which have been shown to inhibit an enzyme that aids in releasing inflammatory chemicals.[10,11]
- Vitamin C inhibits experimentally induced bronchial constriction in normal and asthmatic subjects. It appears that vitamin C has a wide variety of pharmacological effects that appear important for treating asthma.[11]
- Vitamin B12 appears to be especially effective in sulphite-sensitive individuals.[10,11]
- Supplement the diet with essential fatty acids (GLA, EPA) or take linseed oil, one tablespoon per day and cod liver oil, one teaspoon per day.[11,15]
- Improve immunity by supplementing with antioxidant nutrients, zinc and vitamin B6.[15]

Herbs

- Duke recommends anise and fennel seeds. He suggests that they will be beneficial to loosen bronchial secretions. Both of these herbs can be used as essential oils and are rich in ketones, which are known for their mucolytic properties.[15]
- Ginkgo biloba has been found to be beneficial for the treatment of asthma. This is because ginkgo biloba blocks the action of the platelet-activating factor, a chemical mediator in asthma, allergies and inflammation.[11,13]
- Liquorice root contains glycyrrhizin, which shows steroid-like activity and has a long history of use as an anti-inflammatory and anti-allergenic agent. Liquorice root is also an expectorant, a useful action to help alleviate asthma.[11,18]

General Advice

- Keep the ambient temperature in the bedroom at a comfortable level of warmth to try to prevent airway cooling during the night. Avoid wide open windows in winter as warm humid conditions have been clearly shown to prevent asthma provoked by airway cooling.[15]
- Avoid drinking cold fluids.[15]
- Reduce exposure to cigarette smoke, pollutants, cold winds and air-conditioning ducts.[15]
- Practise allergen avoidance as efficiently as possible, i.e., keeping bedding/bedroom as dust free as possible, avoiding feather pillows, eiderdown quilts etc. Wash linen in 1% tannic acid solution.[15]
- Relaxation and breathing exercises should be performed every day.[15]
- Acupressure is particularly helpful in cases of acute asthmatic attack. It probably won't make the symptoms disappear but it will alleviate them. Use acupressure points Lu 1 and Ki 27 to relieve chest congestion and asthma.[19]
- According to Louise Hay, asthma is caused by 'smothered love' and an inability to breathe for one's self. She states that an asthmatic feels as though he/she doesn't have the right to breathe. The asthmatic takes on guilt feelings for whatever seems wrong in his/her environment.[20]

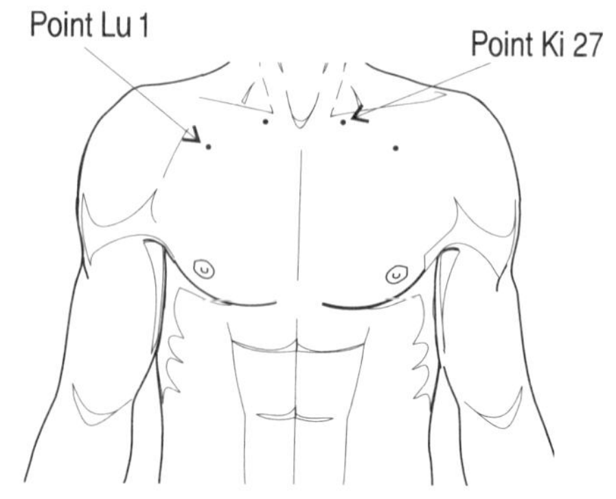

Location of acupressure points used to treat asthma.

Bronchitis

Useful Oils

• aniseed • Alas cedarwood • basil • bay • cajeput
• cypress • sweet fennel • everlasting
• *Eucalyptus radiata* • frankincense
• *Hyssop var. decumbens* • spike lavender • myrrh
• myrtle • niaouli • peppermint • ravensara • rosemary
• sandalwood • thyme

Definition

Bronchitis is the inflammation of the bronchi due to infection or irritation that may occur as a primary disorder or as part of another pulmonary disease such as tuberculosis, bronchiectasis or emphysema. Bronchitis can be acute or chronic.

Clinical Features

The clinical features of acute bronchitis are:

- cough and phlegm (main symptoms)
- wheezing and dyspnoea.[13]

Chronic bronchitis is characterised by a chronic productive cough for at least 3 successive months in 2 successive years. The clinical features of chronic bronchitis include:

- wheezing and progressive dyspnoea

- recurrent exacerbations with acute bronchitis
- occurs mainly in smokers.[13]

Aetiology

Acute Bronchitis

Acute bronchitis is usually caused by an infection and is generally self-limited.[10] Acute bronchitis is rarely serious in adults; however, in infants, small children, in debilitated clients and in clients with chronic pulmonary disease, it may be severe and life threatening.

Acute bronchitis is most prevalent in winter as part of an acute upper respiratory tract infection. It may develop following the common cold or other viral infection. Exposure to air pollutants, possible chilling, fatigue and malnutrition are often predisposing factors.[10]

Other predisposing factors include poor diet, improper treatment of the common cold, or flu, lowered resistance, chest weakness, frequent colds, smoking, allergies and poor digestive function.

Chronic Bronchitis

Chronic bronchitis involves significant, irreversible, generalised obstructed airways associated with varying degrees of chronic bronchitis, abnormalities in small airways and emphysema.[5]

Chronic bronchitis is characterised by a productive cough of long duration without a clear predisposition to acute upper respiratory infection. Cigarette smoking appears to be a common causal factor.[10]

The possibility that the 'bronchitis' is secondary to some serious underlying condition must always be kept in mind. Sources of possible chronic irritation should be avoided (for example, smoking, allergenic agents, fumes). A change of climate to a dry, temperate area may sometimes be required.[10]

Therapeutic Strategy

The following therapeutic strategy should be considered:[10]

- Bed rest is highly advisable, especially if fever is present. Once the fever subsides, alternating periods of rest and periods of moderate activity to prevent secretions from settling in the lungs.
- Drink plenty of fluids such as pure water and herbal teas.
- Add moisture to the air. Use a humidifier and steam inhalations to relieve bronchial inflammation.
- Cough suppression may be used if the cough is troublesome and interferes with sleep, but care should be used if the patient also has chronic obstructive lung disease.
- Smoking is a big no-no. If the client has chronic bronchitis, little improvement can be expected unless smoking is stopped.
- Apply a warm, moist compress, or a hot water bottle over the chest and back before bedtime to aid in sleeping and reducing inflammation.

Aromatherapy Treatment

The aromatherapy treatment for bronchial infections should be as follows:

- combat the infection with antibacterial and immunostimulant essential oils
- soothe and heal the inflamed bronchial mucosa
- facilitate the removal of sputum from the bronchi and trachea by using expectorants
- relax bronchial spasm.

Aromatherapy combats the infection, reducing the fever, easing the cough and expelling the mucus. In the first stages when coughing is dry and painful, steam inhalations with essential oils such as *Eucalyptus radiata*, spike lavender, cedarwood, cypress, myrtle, pine, ravensara or frankincense will provide relief. These essential oils are used for their antispasmodic and expectorant properties. In the later stages of acute bronchitis, it is very important to clear all the mucus from the lungs and any essential oil such as aniseed, basil, cajeput, eucalyptus, *Hyssop var. decumbens,* spike lavender, rosemary, myrrh or thyme may be used.

A person suffering from acute bronchitis needs to be kept warm and rested, preferably in bed. It is important to avoid anything that may aggravate the cough such as smoke and very dry air. Make sure that there is sufficient humidity in the room, by using a humidifier or by simply using a large bowl of hot water and adding 10 drops of eucalyptus oil.

Parsley seed and bay laurel essential oils are beneficial for maintaining the tissue structure integrity of the lungs.[21]

Davis suggests using ginger essential oil, as it is ideal for any condition where the body is not coping effectively with moisture, whether internal or external.[16]

Most adults recover from bronchitis without complications, given the above care and treatment. However, the elderly and frail, babies and young children and people with heart conditions or a history of lung infections are at a much greater risk and must always be treated under properly qualified supervision.

Other Treatments

Nutrition

- Include garlic and onions in your diet. These foods contain quercetin which has been found to inhibit lipooxygenase, an enzyme that aids in releasing an anti-inflammatory chemical in the body. Garlic is also a natural antibiotic.[10]
- Balch suggests a daily dosage of 3,000–10,000 mg of vitamin C plus bioflavonoids.[10]
- Avoid mucus-forming foods such as dairy products, processed foods, sugar, sweet fruits, and white flour.[10]

Herbs

- Fenugreek tea is good for reducing the flow of mucus.[10]
- Goldenseal has antimicrobial properties and is effective for treating inflammation of the mucous membrane of the bronchial tubes, throat, nasal passages and sinuses.[10]
- Garlic, mullein, stinging nettle, couch grass, plantain, horehound and marshmallow are all beneficial for the treatment of bronchitis.[13]
- Marshmallow root is a demulcent and also has an anti-inflammatory effect. It is beneficial for treating bronchitis, colds, coughs and sore throat.[13]

Catarrh

Useful Oils

• aniseed • cajeput • Atlas and Virginian cedarwood
• German chamomile • eucalyptus • everlasting
• sweet fennel • frankincense • ginger
• *Hyssop var. decumbens* • lavender • lemon
• sweet marjoram • myrtle • niaouli • peppermint
• pine • ravensara • rosemary • sandalwood
• thyme • tea tree

Definition

Catarrh is the excess production of mucus in the lungs. It is common to many respiratory problems. Catarrh is seen in holistic medicine as being a vicarious elimination mechanism.[1]

Clinical Features

Catarrh as a medical condition does not really exist, the term is used extensively to explain the thick mucus that is expelled from the nose or coughed up from the throat.

There is either faulty elimination by the usual organs responsible for detoxification, or an excessive intake of environmental and dietary toxins. The body will seek to restore its internal harmony by using the mucous membranes to expel these waste products.

Aetiology

The most common causes are asthma, colds, flu, hay fever, bronchitis, sinusitis and rhinitis. Many of these conditions are dealt with under separate headings.

Therapeutic Strategy

In addition to general dietary and lifestyle factors, long-term treatment of catarrhal problems will involve the use of depurative or detoxifying essential oils, particularly those that encourage drainage of the lymphatics, those that promote elimination of acid metabolites — diuretics, and those that stimulate the immune system.

Aromatherapy Treatment

Many essential oils are decongestants and expectorants — helping to clear out the chest and lungs — helping to alleviate catarrh. For immediate relief of congestion, a steam inhalation with any of the following essential oils is recommended: aniseed, cajeput, Atlas and Virginian cedarwood, eucalyptus, fennel, frankincense, ginger, *Hyssop var. decumbens,* lavender, myrtle, peppermint, pine, rosemary, thyme or tea tree. A massage oil for the upper back, chest and shoulders using any of the above essential oils will also be of assistance.

For catarrh caused by pollens and other irritants, anti-allergenic essential oils such as everlasting, lavender or German chamomile are recommended.[20]

Massage of the face, with particular attention to the sinus area around the nose, will help to drain away excessive mucus.

Other Treatments

- Diet plays an important role in the management of catarrhal conditions. Dairy products and wheat are known to provoke catarrh in many people, and they should be avoided for a period by anybody who suffers catarrh frequently.
- See *Asthma, Bronchitis, Hay Fever* or *Sinusitis.*

Hay Fever

Useful Oils

• cajeput • German chamomile • *Eucalyptus radiata*
• lavender • spike lavender • myrtle • peppermint
• petitgrain • pine • ravensara • rosemary • thyme
• tea tree

Definition

Hay fever is the common term for allergic rhinitis due to the seasonal spread of pollens, but the condition is not necessarily seasonal and may result from exposure to antigens other than pollens.[10]

Allergic rhinitis is characterised by sneezing, runny nose, swelling of the nasal mucosa, itching of the eyes and tearing.[13]

Clinical Features

The symptoms of hay fever include sneezing, runny nose, swelling of nasal mucosa, itching of the eyes, watery eyes, reduced sense of smell, hypersecretion of mucus and headaches. These symptoms may be secondary to acute colds or flu, or hay fever.[13]

Aetiology

Common allergens that precipitate symptoms are house dust, animal dander, some foods (cow's milk, eggs, peanuts, peanut butter), fungus spores, feathers, powders, insecticides and many grass pollens (from trees in spring and grass in summer). A history of allergies aids in distinguishing allergic rhinitis (hay fever) from upper respiratory tract infections.[15]

Sinusitis may also develop in these individuals due to bacterial infection that becomes associated with impaired drainage of the nasal mucosa.[15]

People who suffer from hay fever may also suffer from other so-called atopic disorders such as asthma and dermatitis. People prone to allergies are usually aware of the time of the year and the conditions under which they are most sensitive. For a definitive diagnosis, the radioallergosorbent test (RAST) is easily done and gives reliable results.[10] Factors that aggravate rhinitis include:

- emotional upsets
- fatigue
- alcohol
- chilly, damp weather
- air conditioning
- sudden changes in temperature and humidity.[13]

Therapeutic Strategy

The following therapeutic strategy should be considered:

- avoid or reduce exposure to the offending antigen
- reduce sensitivity by building integrity of mucosa and reducing inflammatory response
- improve immunity
- dietary changes including low acid diet and reduction of dairy products.[13]

Aromatherapy Treatment

Essential oils that assist in the treatment of hay fever have expectorant, anti-inflammatory, astringent, antimicrobial and immunostimulant, restorative and tonic properties.

Davis suggests that any essential oil that will relieve the symptoms of the common cold will help to relieve the symptoms of hay fever.[16]

Essential oils such as eucalyptus, lavender, spike lavender, ravensara and myrtle can be used in inhalations to reduce sneezing and a runny nose. German chamomile may be beneficial if allergies are present due to its anti-allergenic properties.

Some people may find that steam inhalations aggravate them. If so, simply place the essential oil on a tissue and inhale it whenever needed during the day.[16]

Other Treatments

General Advice

Advice to the client should include the following:

- Keep healthy, eat a well-balanced diet, avoid 'junk food' and live sensibly with balanced exercise, rest and recreation.[13]
- Avoid using decongestant nose drops and sprays. Although they may relieve symptoms at first, a worse effect occurs on the rebound.[13]
- Avoidance therapy: avoid the allergen, if you know what it is.[13]
- Sources of the house mite are bedding, upholstered furniture, fluffy toys and carpets. Seek advice about keeping your house dust free, especially if you have perennial rhinitis.[13]
- Pets, especially cats and dogs, should be kept outside.[10,13]
- Avoid chemical irritants such as aspirin, smoke, cosmetics, paints and sprays.[13]

Herbs

- Drink two cups of fenugreek tea a day.[15]
- Ginger's anti-inflammatory property may be beneficial for treating hay fever.[15]
- Stinging nettle is an excellent blood purifier. Several cases of hay fever have been successfully treated by drinking stinging nettle tea every day for several months before the pollen season commences.[10,22,23]

Nutrition

- A diet rich in raw vegetables and fresh fruit which contains vitamin C is recommended. Vitamin C is an immunostimulant, anti-inflammatory and also has antihistamine activity.[10]
- Increase consumption of fish oils, e.g., GLA/EFA and cod liver oil.[15]

- Introduce beeswax into your diet. This may decrease sensitisation to pollens by orally stimulating the blocking antigens.[15]
- Test for milk and dairy product sensitivity. These encourage the formation of catarrh and mucus in the alimentary tract.[15]
- Eat yoghurt or any soured products three times a week.[10]
- Use garlic and horseradish in your cooking.[15]
- Researchers have found that three bananas contain enough magnesium — 180 mg is recommended — to quell a hay fever attack. Other foods rich in magnesium are kidney beans, soyabeans, almonds, lima beans, whole wheat flour, brown rice, molasses and peas.[10]

Upper Respiratory Tract Infections

Useful Oils

• aniseed • Atlas and Virginian cedarwood • cajeput • cedarwood • clary sage • cypress • fennel • frankincense • everlasting • *Eucalyptus radiata* • *Hyssop var. decumbens* • lavender • spike lavender • lemon • sweet marjoram • myrtle • peppermint • pine • ravensara • rosemary • tea tree • thyme

Definition

The upper respiratory tract comprises the nose and nasal sinuses, the mouth, the pharynx and larynx.[13] Because of its exposure to all noxious physical, chemical, allergic and infective agents it is not surprising that upper respiratory tract infections constitute the most frequent minor illnesses of humanity.

Any infection that is confined to the nose, throat, larynx or trachea is called an upper respiratory tract infection (URTI). The respiratory tract may become infected as the organisms travel along the lining membrane. The disorder is named according to the part involved, e.g., pharyngitis, laryngitis, bronchitis and so on.

Clinical Features

The patient complains of malaise, feverishness and headache. Nasal discomfort and discharge and sneezing are followed by mucoid to purulent discharge and nasal obstruction. The runny nose, an unpleasant symptom of the common cold, is an attempt on the part of nature to wash away the pathogens and thus protect against further infection. The pattern of each infection varies depending on where it starts and how it spreads. Common symptoms include sore eyes, sore throat, headaches, limb pain, nasal obstruction, mouth ulcers and earache.

Often the lower respiratory tract becomes involved so that bronchitis with cough, sputum and possibly wheezing are part of the clinical picture.

Aetiology

Infections are caused by an extremely wide range of viruses. Among the infections transmitted through the respiratory tract are the common cold, diphtheria, chickenpox, measles, influenza, pneumonia and tuberculosis.[10]

Therapeutic Strategy

General measures should include bed rest, consume plenty of fluids to prevent dehydration, limit sugar consumption and a balanced diet.[11,13]

Congestion, cough and/or a sore throat are signs of a cold, but if these symptoms occur together with a fever or fatigue you may have the flu.

Aromatherapy Treatment

An aromatherapy treatment should aim to:

- Treat the infection with antimicrobial essential oils such as tea tree, cajeput, lemon and red thyme.
- Support the immune system by using immunostimulants such as eucalyptus, lavender, lemon, and tea tree.
- Eliminate excess catarrh and mucus by using mucolytics and expectorants such as aniseed, eucalyptus, everlasting, fennel seed, angelica root and hyssop.
- Soothe the inflamed mucous membranes by using sandalwood.

For immediate relief of congestion a steam inhalation with essential oils is very effective. Hoffman recommends very hot steam — as hot as can be tolerated without burning the nose and throat. This itself is a hostile environment for viruses. The steam inhalation in combination with the essential oils will ease congestion and help to combat the infection that has caused it.[14]

For a sore throat add three drops of tea tee oil to warm water and gargle. Repeat this up to three times a day.

Other Treatments

Nutrition

- To prevent and treat colds, include garlic in the diet and take 1–3 g of vitamin C with bioflavonoids daily.
- Diet plays an important part when catarrh is involved. Dairy and wheat products are known to promote excessive catarrh and should be excluded for a period of time by anyone who suffers catarrh frequently, to see whether any

improvement is noticed. If so, these catarrh-forming foods should be excluded permanently from the diet, or included in very small amounts only.[5,10]

Herbs

- Diaphoretic herbs such as catmint, elderflowers, ginger, lime flowers, peppermint, thyme and yarrow tea will help to manage and improve febrile response.[5,18]
- Echinacea is one of the most important immune enhancing and supporting herbs. It also has a direct antiviral activity to prevent the infection.[5,6,10,11,18]
- Garlic has immune potentiating properties and has broad spectrum antimicrobial properties.[11,15]
- Herbal tea made from fresh ginger rhizomes is recommended at the onset of an upper respiratory tract infection.[5,10]
- For a sore throat mix one tablespoon of slippery elm powder with one part boiling water and half a cup of honey for cough and sore throat.[10]
- Make an infusion of sage and add a few clove buds and a teaspoon of glycerine if the throat is dry. Use this as a gargle.[23]

Sinusitis

Useful Oils

• cajeput • everlasting • *Eucalyptus radiata*
• *E. dives* • ginger • *Hyssop var. decumbens*
• spike lavender • lemon • myrtle • niaouli
• peppermint • pine • ravensara • thyme • tea tree

Definition

The sinuses are located close to the nasal cavities and near the ear. Infection may travel quite easily into the sinuses from the mouth, the nose and the throat along the mucous membrane lining; the resulting inflammation is called sinusitis.

Clinical Features

Symptoms of acute sinusitis include headache, earache, toothache, purulent post-nasal drip, nasal obstruction, facial pain, cranial pressure, loss of sense of smell, tenderness over the forehead and cheekbones and occasionally a high fever. Sometimes sinusitis produces a swollen face followed by a stuffy nose and thick discharge of mucus.[10,13]

If the mucus is clear after a week you probably do not have an infection. If the mucus is greenish or yellowish, you do. If the mucus is clear without a cold, you probably have allergies.[10]

Long-standing, or chronic, sinus infection may cause changes in the epithelial cells, resulting in tumour formation. Some of these growths have a grape-like appearance and cause obstruction of the air pathway; these tumours are called polyps.

Clinical features of chronic sinusitis include vague facial pain, offensive post-nasal drip, nasal obstruction, toothache, malaise and halitosis.[13]

Aetiology

More than 50% of all cases of sinusitis are caused by bacteria.[10] The sinuses affected by this infection include those above the eyes, inside each cheekbone, behind the bridge of the nose and in the upper nose.

Factors involved in chronic sinusitis include pollution, occupational dust exposure, tobacco smoke, adenoids, allergies, rhinitis, cold and damp weather, dental problems, trauma and flying.[5]

Structural problems such as a deviated septum or growth of nasal polyps can obstruct the flow of mucus out of the sinuses. This is not an infectious condition to begin with but since the mucus is obstructed, this creates a perfect environment for bacteria to create an infection.[12]

Therapeutic Strategy

The treatment strategies for acute and chronic sinusitis are similar:

- support the immune system
- use mucolytics, anticatarrhals and decongestants
- use steam inhalations containing antimicrobial and anti-inflammatory essential oils
- chronic sinusitis may represent a vicarious elimination; this needs to be treated with depuratives and lymphatics
- reduce exposure to harmful environments
- a dairy-free, low salt diet should be followed for at least 3 months.[5]

Aromatherapy Treatment

Steam inhalations using essential oil will be the most effective treatment for effectively promoting drainage and easing the pain. Add a few drops of any of the following essential oils (cajeput, eucalyptus, spike lavender, lavender, lemon, myrtle, ravensara, peppermint, pine, thyme, tea tree). These oils have been chosen for their antiseptic, antimicrobial, analgesic and decongestant properties).

While massage techniques to drain the sinuses are often recommended, sufferers of acute sinusitis may find the techniques painful and it would be best to avoid facial massage over the sinuses until the massage was tolerable.

Massage may be introduced after a day or two, or whenever a steam inhalation has reduced the congestion enough for massage to be tolerable.

Other Treatments

General Advice

- Apply a hot compress over the sinus area.[10,15]
- Check for inhalant or food intolerances.[15]
- Acupuncture and acupressure are very effective therapies for sinusitis and can be used alongside aromatherapy. The acupressure points commonly suggested for the treatment of sinuses are LI 4, St 3 and Bl 2. Bl 2 is located at the bridge of the nose and is helpful for frontal headaches and sinus conditions, while LI 20, located next to the edge of the nose, is the best point for dealing with the maxillary sinuses located in the cheek area.[20]
- Harrison suggests that sinusitis is linked to poor bowel function and that constipation of the bowel reflects mental constipation, mostly in inflexible individuals, and often indicates a reluctance to cry.[24]

Herbs

- Drink 2 cups of fenugreek tea per day.[15]
- Support the immune system in its fight against the bacteria with immune-enhancing herbs such as echinacea.[5]
- Goldenseal is effective in combating sinusitis.[5,10] Its benefits are enhanced by combining it with 250 to 500 mg of bromelain, an enzyme present in fresh pineapple. Goldenseal can be taken as a tea, or the tea can be used as an intranasal douche.[10]
- Ginger root can be crushed and applied as a poultice to the forehead and nose to stimulate circulation and relieve congestion.[10]
- Mucolytic herbs such as garlic and horseradish will clear congestion.[5,10]

Nutrition

- Increase intake of garlic, onion and ginger or poultice of onions and garlic applied to sinus.[18]
- Eliminate sugar from your diet. Reduce salt intake.[10]
- Do not eat dairy foods, except for low-fat soured products such as yoghurt and cottage cheese. Dairy products increase mucus formation.[5,10]
- Duke recommends the following 'sinusoup'. Begin with a vegetarian minestrone and add helpings of garlic, plus horseradish, hot peppers and ginger. He says that on a cold winter day, it warms the soul as it opens the sinuses.[18]
- A diet of 75% raw foods is recommended.[10]
- Vitamin C increases immunity against infection and reduces mucus.[10]
- Vitamin A increases the health of epithelial tissue lining of the sinuses.[10]

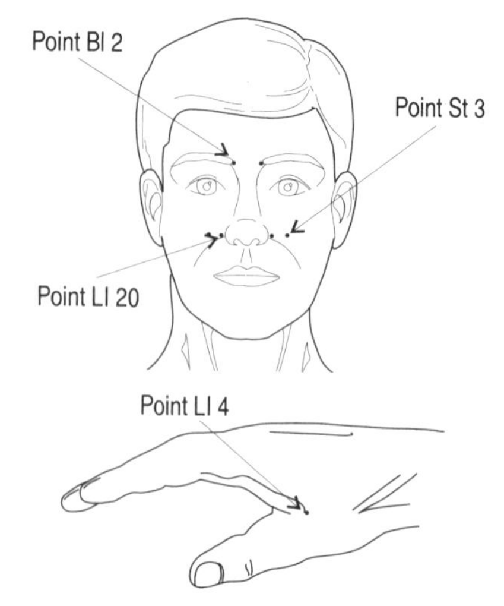

Acupressure points used to treat sinus problems.

Sore Throat

Useful Oils

• cajeput • Atlas and Virginian cedarwood • *Eucalyptus radiata* • frankincense • lavender • lemon • ravensara • sandalwood • tea tree • thyme

Definition

A sore throat can be caused by anything that irritates the sensitive mucous membranes at the back of the throat.

Clinical Features

Typically, a sore throat is an extension of the common cold, tonsillitis, sinusitis or a viral infection.[10] An acute sore throat should run its course within a few weeks.

Aetiology

Some irritants include viral and bacterial infections, allergic reactions, dust, smoke, fumes, extremely hot foods and drinks, tooth or gum infections and abrasions. Chronic coughing and excessively loud talking also irritate the throat.[10]

Therapeutic Strategy

The therapeutic strategy for the treatment of sore throats includes:[5]

- Immune enhancement.
- The use of lymphatics and depuratives.
- A dairy-free diet rich in fruit and vegetables.
- Use of lozenges which contain herbs such as echinacea, propolis, sage, liquorice root, marshmallow and myrrh.

Aromatherapy Treatment

Steam inhalations using essential oils such as lavender, tea tree, cajeput and ravensara will ease discomfort. A gentle massage to the throat and chest area with a massage oil blend containing frankincense, lavender and sandalwood can be used. These essential oils should also be used in a vaporiser, especially if using at night before going to bed.

Add three drops of tea tree oil to a glass of warm water, mix well and gargle. Repeat two or three times a day. Continue until the condition has cleared up.

Other Treatments

Nutrition

- Vitamin C and bioflavonoids can be used to improve immunity and vitamin A can be used to increase the resistance of epithelial tissue.[10,11]
- Ginger, honey and lemon juice is good for alleviating sore throats.[18]

Herbs

- To stimulate immunity and phagocytosis use echinacea and goldenseal.[10,11]
- Liquorice root combined with honey has demulcent and expectorant properties.[10,18]
- Marshmallow tea will soothe a sore throat.[10,18]

Tonsillitis

Useful Oils

• eucalyptus • lemon • tea tree • thyme

Definition

Tonsillitis is an inflammation of the tonsils, the glands of the lymph tissue located on either side of the entrance to the throat.

Clinical Features

Symptoms of tonsillitis include soreness, redness, pain and inflammation of the tonsils, difficulty in swallowing, hoarseness and coughing.[3,10] Other symptoms include headaches, earache, fever and chills, nausea and vomiting, nasal obstruction and discharge, and enlarged lymph nodes throughout the body. The disorder is common in children but people of any age can be afflicted with inflammation of the tonsils.[10]

Aetiology

The inflammation is typically caused by viruses and other bacteria, often streptococcal organisms, which are present when the body's resistance is lowered. Tonsillitis can be caused by improper diet which is high in carbohydrates and low in protein and other nutrients. Repeated bouts of tonsillitis indicate a weak state of resistance, making it difficult to cure.[10]

Treatment Strategy

The treatment strategies for tonsillitis and sore throat are similar.

Aromatherapy Treatment

Steam inhalations at frequent intervals will relieve the pain and help combat infection. Essential oils such as thyme, lavender, lemon, tea tree and eucalyptus should be chosen for their antiseptic and anaesthetic properties.

Other Treatments

- Chamomile, echinacea, garlic, sage and thyme are excellent herbs to use for the treatment of tonsillitis.[10,18]
- Use a warm salt-water gargle.[10,11]
- Fortunately, the practice of removing the tonsils, particularly during childhood, is now far less common than it was 20 or 30 years ago.

References

1. Mills S. *The essential book of herbal medicine.* Penguin Books, England, 1991.
2. Gumbel D. *Principles of holistic skin therapy with herbal essences.* Karl F. Haug Publishers, Germany, 1986.
3. Valnet J. *The practice of aromatherapy.* The C.W. Daniel Company Limited, Great Britain, 1980.
4. Williams L. *Ranking antimicrobial activity.* The International Journal of Aromatherapy 1996; 7(4): 32–35.
5. Bone K, Mills S. *Principles and practice of phytotherapy.* Churchill Livingstone, UK, 2000.
6. Tyler V. *The honest herbal.* Haworth Press, USA, 1993.
7. Schnaubelt K. *Medical aromatherapy.* Frog Ltd., USA, 1999.

8. Holmes P. *Sandalwood — The wisdom of being*. The International Journal of Aromatherapy 1994/5; 6(4): 14–17.
9. Balacs T. *Cineole-rich eucalyptus*. The International Journal of Aromatherapy 1997; 8(2): 15–21.
10. Balch J, Balch P. *Prescription for nutritional healing*. Avery Publishing Group, USA, 1997.
11. Murray M, Pizzorno J. *A text book of natural medicine Vol 2*. 2nd edn, Churchill Livingstone, UK, 2000.
12. Werner R. *A massage therapist's guide to pathology*. Lippincott Williams & Wilkins, USA, 1998.
13. Murtagh J. *General practice*. 2nd edn, The McGraw-Hill Companies Inc., Australia, 1998.
14. Hoffman D. *An elders' herbal*. Healing Art Press, USA, 1993.
15. Osiecki H. *The physician's handbook of clinical nutrition*. Bioconcepts Publishing, Australia, 1990.
16. Davis P. *Aromatherapy: An A–Z*. 2nd edn, The C.W. Daniel Company Limited, Great Britain, 1999.
17. Haas M, Schnaubelt K. *Breathing space*. The International Journal of Aromatherapy 1992; 4(4): 13–15.
18. Duke J. *The green pharmacy*. Rodale Press, USA, 1997.
19. Hay L. *You can heal your life*. Specialist Publications, Australia, 1987.
20. Reed Gach M. *Acupressure's potent points*. Bantam Books, USA, 1990.
21. Goeb P. *Broncho-pulmonary pathologies*. Les Cahiers de L'Aromatherapies, No. 1 September, 1995.
22. Lininger S. et al. eds, *The natural pharmacy*. Prima Health, USA, 1999.
23. Beckman N. *The family library guide to natural therapies*. Family Library, Australia, 1992.
24. Harrison J. *Love your disease: It's keeping you healthy*. Angus & Robertson Publishers, Australia, 1984.

The Musculoskeletal System

Objectives

After careful study of this chapter, you should be able to:

- identify, list and describe common pathophysiologies of the musculoskeletal system
- explain the aromatherapy treatment for specific conditions and disorders of the musculoskeletal system
- explain the role of other holistic strategies for specific conditions and disorders of the musculoskeletal system.

Introduction

Our skeleton, the connective tissue, our muscles and our joints hold us together, enable us to stand, to move and give us form. The musculoskeletal system is used and misused; it often becomes the site of much physical wear and tear. Some of the diseases of the musculoskeletal system such as arthritis can be extremely disabling, having a major adverse impact on normal living and work.

If problems are due to muscular injury or structural misalignments, a great deal can be done to realign the body with the help of remedial massage techniques, osteopathy, chiropractic techniques and psychophysical adjustments like rolfing, Alexander technique or Feldenkrais.

Aromatherapy Considerations

Aromatherapy is very effective in treating musculoskeletal problems. Essential oils used in massage and baths have an almost immediate effect on muscle tissue, which is heightened by the effects of the massage. Some essential oils bring warmth to the body and can provide a considerable amount of pain relief. Such oils can also relieve local inflammation by setting free mediators in the body which in turn cause the blood vessels to expand, so the body is able to move more quickly and the swelling is reduced.

To treat problems that manifest in the bones and muscles effectively, digestion and assimilation have to function correctly, as do the various aspects of elimination. The particular therapeutic properties of essential oils which have a particular affinity for the musculoskeletal system are:

Analgesics

Many of the essential oils with anti-inflammatory or rubefacient properties also have analgesic effects. Some of these essential oils include German chamomile, eucalyptus, cajeput, lavender, sweet marjoram, peppermint, rosemary and thyme.

Anti-inflammatory

For swellings, inflammations, arthritis use German chamomile, everlasting and yarrow essential oils. These essential oils are non-irritating to the skin. Essential oils such as thyme, clove bud and cinnamon are also anti-inflammatory; however, they are well known for their skin irritant properties.

Antirheumatics

Some essential oils can relieve rheumatic problems. Antirheumatics are selected according to the specific action on the body such as detoxifying, anti-inflammatory, rubefacient and diuretic.

Essential oils with antirheumatic properties include black pepper, cajeput, German chamomile, eucalyptus, ginger, juniper berry, lemon, sweet marjoram, pine, rosemary and thyme.

Detoxifiers

Detoxifiers, also known as depuratives, cleanse and purify the bloodstream and restore healthier functioning. The main clinical use of depuratives is in the treatment of chronic inflammatory disease, especially of the joints and connective tissues.

Essential oils that are detoxifiers include juniper berry, carrot seed, lemon, and sweet fennel.

Rubefacients

Rubefacients are used to promote circulation to the muscle tissue and skin. The result promotes not only circulation to the muscle tissue and skin but also brings an agreeable feeling of warmth and relief from pain and an anti-inflammatory effect.

Essential oils that are rubefacient include black pepper, cajeput, clove bud, ginger, juniper berry, spike lavender, rosemary, sweet marjoram and thyme.

Associated Conditions

Arthritis

Useful Oils

• black pepper • cajeput • carrot seed
• cinnamon bark • clove bud • German chamomile
• eucalyptus • ginger • juniper berry • lavender
• spike lavender • lemon • sweet marjoram • nutmeg
• pine • rosemary • thyme

Definition

The term 'arthritis' means inflammation of a joint. There are many different types of arthritis. Some are due to infection and others are due to wear and tear; for many the cause is obscure. The two most common forms of arthritis are rheumatoid arthritis and osteoarthritis. Conventional treatment often reduces pain, but there is little improvement in the arthritic process itself.

The accepted medical view is that arthritis is incurable and treatment is confined to the relief of pain with analgesic and anti-inflammatory drugs, often with undesirable side effects. Joint replacement surgery is often offered where there is serious degeneration of the joint, but this can only be done for the largest joints such as the hips and knees and involves major surgery.

Clinical Features

Osteoarthritis

Osteoarthritis is the most common type of arthritis, occurring in about 10% of the adult population and in 50% of those aged over 60. It is a degenerative disease of the cartilage and may be primary or secondary to causes such as trauma and mechanical problems.[1]

Primary osteoarthritis is usually symmetrical and can affect many joints. Unlike other inflammatory disease the pain is worse on initiating movement and loading the joint, and eased by rest. Osteoarthritis is usually associated with pronounced stiffness, especially after activity, in contrast to rheumatoid arthritis.[1] Other clinical features of osteoarthritis include:

- morning stiffness is often the first symptom
- pain is worse by the end of the day, aggravated by use, relieved by rest, worse in cold and damp
- variable disability

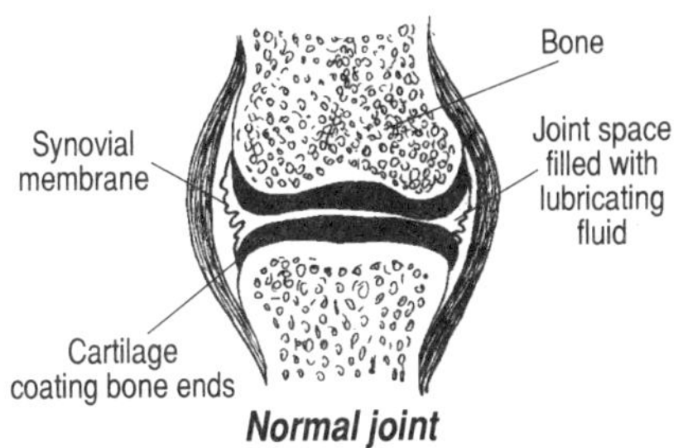

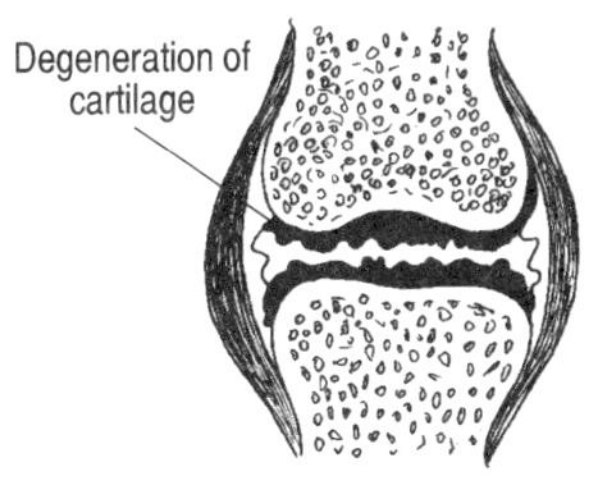

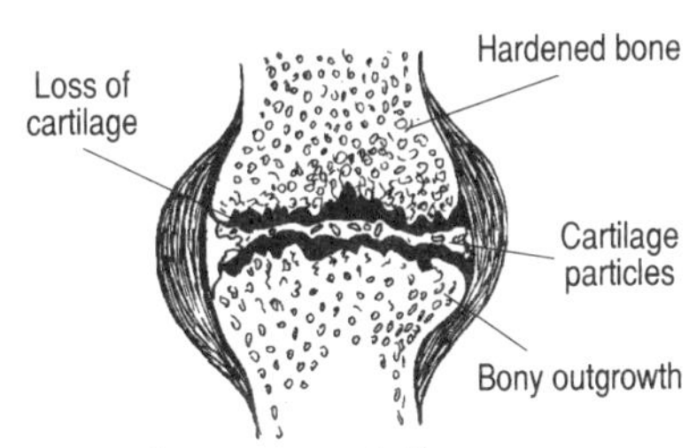

How osteoarthritis develops.

- hard and bony swelling, joint deformity
- signs of inflammation are mild.[1,2]

In the acute stage of osteoarthritis the joints will be hot, painful and swollen. In the subacute stage the joints will have milder pain and stiffness.

Rheumatoid Arthritis

The onset of rheumatoid arthritis is generally slow however it can be abrupt. Fatigue, low-grade fever, weakness, joint stiffness and vague joint pain may proceed the appearance of painful, swollen joints by several weeks. The joints will be quite warm, tender and swollen. As the disease progresses, deformities develop in the joint of the hands and feet.[2]

Typical characteristics of rheumatoid arthritis include:

- soft swelling
- warmth
- tenderness on pressure and movement
- limitation of movement
- muscle wasting
- later stages — deformity of joints.[1]

In the acute stage of rheumatoid arthritis, the affected joints are red hot, painful and stiff, although they improve considerably with moderate amounts of movement and stretching. The joints most often affected are the knuckles in the hands and toes. Rheumatoid arthritis can also appear in the ankles and wrists, generally the knees are less common.

Aetiology

Osteoarthritis

Osteoarthritis is divided into two categories: primary and secondary. In primary osteoarthritis, the degenerative 'wear and tear' process occurs after the 5th and 6th decade, with no apparent predisposing abnormalities.[2]

Secondary osteoarthritis is associated with some predisposing factor which is responsible for degenerative changes. Predisposing factors in secondary factors in secondary osteoarthritis include:

- trauma (obesity, fractures and injuries along joint surfaces, surgery)
- crystal deposits
- presence of abnormal cartilage
- previous inflammatory diseases of the joints.[2]

The cartilage lining of the joint tends to soften, fragment and ulcerate as the damage progresses. In an effort to overcome this, the body manufactures new bone around the joint margins. This tends to have the effect of altering the mechanics of the joint, increasing the rate of damage and producing greater inefficiency of the joint.

The primary chemical change observed is the loss of proteoglycan (a protein sugar or mucopolysaccharide). These 'proteoglycans' are responsible for cartilage resilience or bounce and their loss from cartilage results in a stiffer material that is more easily damaged by wear and tear. Proteoglycans account for 75–80% of normal cartilage. In osteoarthritis the percentage of proteoglycans is reduced to 35–40%.[3]

Rheumatoid Arthritis

Osiecki says that almost all definitions of rheumatoid arthritis emphasise its chronic and inflammatory nature. This is immediately evident from the examination of the red, swollen, tender joints of the affected individual. An inflammatory response is usually considered as the body's adaptation to protect itself from a hostile environment.[3] This response should be accomplished without significant injury to the body's own tissue. However, it appears that the inflammation in rheumatoid arthritis is an inappropriate response.[3]

While it is not clearly known how this occurs, there are a number of factors that predispose the joint to become inflamed. They are as follows:[3]

- Microtrauma resulting in microvascular injury — that is, blood supply to the joint capsule being either sluggish or impaired.
- Infection of the synovial membrane by virus or bacteria.
- Metabolic conditions being hostile to normal function of the joint — for example, synovial hypoxia and increased joint acidity.
- Excessive synovial antibody production due to cell hyperactivity stimulated by virus; unrestrained T helper/inducer cells and the removal of waste from tissue.
- Increased viscosity of blood resulting in poor nutrient and oxygen flow to the joint capsule.
- Increased synovial fluid resulting in a rise in intra-articular pressure and hence obstruction of capillary and venous circulation, which contributes to the formation of effusions and hypoxia.
- Precipitation of chemicals, toxins, metabolic waste products or allergic material in joint space resulting in inflammatory responses.

Therapeutic Strategy

While it can be difficult to differentiate between rheumatoid arthritis and osteoarthritis, the following clues may help: rheumatoid arthritis is not a result of joint wear and tear, it does not usually target the weight-bearing joints, it tends to act symmetrically on the body, rather than the joints that have been damaged through wear and tear.

Rheumatoid arthritis is a multifactorial condition that requires a comprehensive therapeutic strategy that focuses on reducing those factors that may be involved in the disease process. A holistic approach involves improving digestion, food allergies, increased gut permeability, increased circulating immune complexes and excessive inflammatory processes.[2]

Diet is strongly implicated in rheumatoid arthritis. The major focus should be:

- eliminate food allergies
- follow a vegetarian diet
- modify the intake of dietary fats and oils
- increase the intake of antioxidant nutrients.[2]

The therapeutic strategy for managing osteoarthritis is based on reducing joint stress and trauma, promoting collagen repair mechanisms, and eliminating foods and other factors that may inhibit normal collagen repair.

Whether the condition is rheumatoid arthritis or osteoarthritis many therapeutic principles are similar. In all cases the following points will need to be considered:

- control pain using appropriate essential oils
- suggest appropriate activity, exercise and physical therapy to preserve function and prevent deformity
- reduce factors that may lower the coping threshold such as stress, depression and anxiety
- reduction of inflammation of the joint
- restoring body chemistry to reduce the inflammatory process — that is, detoxification.

Aromatherapy Treatment

The aromatherapy treatments for rheumatoid and osteoarthritis are similar. As osteoarthritis is less likely to be inflammatory, essential oils that are predominantly analgesic and rubefacient should be used. On the other hand rheumatoid arthritis is likely to respond to anti-inflammatory essential oils as it is more of an inflammatory nature. The following essential oils should be considered:

analgesic: cajeput, clove bud, cinnamon leaf, ginger, spike lavender, marjoram (Spanish or sweet), rosemary, pine, thyme.

anti-inflammatory: German chamomile, clove bud, everlasting, ginger, nutmeg, yarrow.

circulatory stimulants: black pepper, cinnamon bark, clove bud, ginger, lemon, rosemary, pine, thyme.

eliminating toxins from the body: carrot seed, juniper berry, lemon.

These essential oils may be used in a bath, local massage or compress over the affected area. Whenever heat and warmth are applied to a stiff painful joint in the form of a bath, hot compress or warming massage, it is important to move the joint as much as possible afterwards, otherwise the heat can cause congestion which makes the symptoms worse rather than better.

If the inflamed joint is very tender and painful to touch, the essential oils should be used in a compress or in a bath.

Massage is contra-indicated in the acute phase of rheumatoid arthritis osteoarthritis; however, during the subacute phase, massage is recommended. It can help to improve mobility and the health of the soft tissues surrounding the joint.

Other Treatments

Nutrition

There is no single dietary treatment recommended for arthritis because there are a number of causes and predisposing factors. Arthritis sufferers should determine by trial and error which treatment will be of the most benefit to them.

- Lose weight. This is especially important for those who have osteoarthritis of the hips, knees and ankles. This will mean eating less refined carbohydrates and less animal fats.[4,5]
- Exclusion diets. Plants from the solanaceae family (such as tomatoes, eggplants, capsicums, paprika and potatoes) adversely affect some people and should be avoided for a period of one to two months. Avoid any foods such as wheat, milk, dairy foods and beef which are suspected to be the cause of allergies.[5]
- For those who are underweight, have a poor appetite or have a poorly balanced diet, supplements should be used before going on an elimination diet. Elimination of allergic foods has been shown to offer significant benefits to some individuals with rheumatoid arthritis.[5]
- Older people often do not respond well to an elimination diet. For these people it is best to make use of supplements such as zinc, evening primrose oil, fish oils and other nutrients such as vitamin C and B complex which are involved in the metabolism of essential fatty acids. Such supplements may have a general anti-inflammatory effect, but this may take several weeks or even months for their full effect to be felt.[5]
- Fresh ginger or powdered ginger used in cooking has been proven to be effective in reducing inflammation. Eat fish, plenty of green vegetables, salads, nuts, seeds, wholemeal bread and cereals.[2,5]
- Increase consumption of coldwater fish such as cod, tuna and mackerel.[2,3,4,5]
- Many people with arthritis seem to improve if digestion is improved. This can be done by taking digestive enzymes or apple cider vinegar with meals. Improving digestion and the acidity of the stomach ensures complete breakdown of any antigenic food protein that may exacerbate the condition.[5]
- Reduce the intake of red meats and avoid tea, coffee, alcohol and processed or refined foods.[2,3,4]
- An extract from the New Zealand green-lipped mussel has been used in rheumatoid arthritis and osteoarthritis with encouraging results.[5]
- Where allergens exist, avoid all nightshade foods or plants such as tomato, potato, eggplants and peppers. These foods are known to aggravate the arthritic condition in some patients.[2,3]
- For rheumatoid arthritis, evening primrose oil may be beneficial in doses of 2 × 500 mg capsules taken 4 times daily, together with a supplement providing vitamins C, B6, B3 and zinc.[5]

Herbs

The following herbs have been traditionally used for the treatment of arthritis, gout and rheumatism: celery seed, stinging nettle, elderflower, yarrow, meadowsweet, burdock, dandelion, ginger root, liquorice root, angelica, cayenne.[6]

Celery seed and nettle have an alkalising effect and help to eliminate excess acid in the body. Celery seed has a diuretic effect and nettle contains essential nutrients such as iron, minerals and vitamins. Elderflower, yarrow and meadowsweet have diaphoretic and anti-inflammatory properties. Burdock and dandelion are alteratives and will help purify the blood and rid the body of excess toxins. Angelica, ginger and cayenne pepper are warming remedies, helping to stimulate circulation and having an analgesic affect.[6] Ginger has anti-inflammatory effects by inhibiting prostaglandin synthesis.[7] Devil's claw has been reported to have anti-inflammatory and analgesic effects.[2]

General Advice

- Rest is necessary where practical for any acute flare-up of rheumatoid arthritis.[1]
- It is important to have regular exercise, especially walking and swimming.[1]
- Refer to a physiotherapist or occupational therapist for preparing an appropriate physical

therapy and advice on how to cope at home and work.[1]

- Each joint should be put daily through the full range of motion to keep it mobile and reduce stiffness.[1]
- According to Louise Hay, arthritis is a disease that comes from a constant pattern of criticism of self and criticism of other people.[8]
- For osteoarthritis, heat is generally used to help relieve stiffness and pain, relax muscles, and increase the range of motion. Moist heat such as moist packs and hot baths are more effective than dry heat.[1]

Backache

Useful Oils

- arnica-infused oil • black pepper • cajeput
- cinnamon bark • clove bud • German chamomile
- eucalyptus • ginger • juniper berry • lavender
- spike lavender • lemon • sweet marjoram • nutmeg
- peppermint • pine • rosemary • thyme

Clinical Features

At least 85% of adults are affected by back pain at some point in their lives. At least 50% of these people will recover within 2 weeks and 75% within 1 month, but recurrences are frequent and have been reported in 40–70% of patients.[1]

Aetiology

The most common cause of back pain is minor strain to muscles and/or ligaments. Most of these soft tissue problems resolve rapidly.[1]

The main cause of back pain is dysfunction of the intervertebral joints of the spine due to injury (this accounts for 70% of low back pain). Another common cause of back pain is spondylitis (synonymous with osteoarthritis and degenerative back disease, this accounts for about 10% of cases of low back pain).[1]

Other common causes of back pain include poor posture, improper footwear and walking habits, improper lifting, straining, calcium deficiency, slouching when sitting, and sleeping on a mattress that is too soft.[4]

Therapeutic Strategy

The therapeutic strategy for backaches should include:

Physical therapies: Massage can be a valuable way of re-educating tense muscles. Many people are not aware of the tension they are holding in some areas of the body, and relaxation can be achieved through massage.[1]

Rest: for acute painful back problems 2 days' strict rest lying on a firm surface is optimal treatment.[1]

Patient education: Appropriate education leads to a clearer insight into the causes and aggravation of the back disorder plus coping strategies.[1]

Exercises: An early graduated exercise program as soon as the back pain subsides has been shown to promote healing and prevent relapses. All forms of exercise (extension, flexion and isometric) appear to be effective.[1]

Analgesics and rubefacients: Essential oils with an analgesic effect should be used in massage.

Other effective treatments to consider in the management of backaches include hydrotherapy, transcutaneous electrical nerve stimulation (TENS), acupuncture and biofeedback.[1]

Aromatherapy Treatment

Aromatherapy massage is very effective treatment where the pain is due to muscular fatigue, spasm or tension. There are many essential oils that will help reduce pain in the short term and treat the muscular problem or injury in the longer term.

Spike lavender, sweet marjoram, rosemary, eucalyptus and cajeput are commonly used in combination with warming oils such as black pepper, nutmeg and ginger, where there is acute pain.

It is important to have a good knowledge of anatomy and decide whether to refer a patient to an osteopath or chiropractor for manipulation. When manipulation for any spinal displacement is required, aromatherapy massages before and after the manipulation can reduce pain and increase the effectiveness of the treatment.

Many back injuries arise because of poor muscle tone. The muscles are no longer capable of supporting the vertebrae, or the various joints associated with it. The best way of improving the condition of the back is to increase muscle tone, usually through exercise. However, the exercise has to be carefully chosen to improve the condition of the back without placing further strain on it. Osteopaths and physiotherapists will often provide the best advice on suitable exercise. If there is injury it is usually best to avoid exercise until the injury has been treated.

Baths using relaxing essential oils such as lavender and ylang ylang are a very useful form of self-help when backache is caused by tension.

The best form of treatment for backache is prevention. Regular massage with essential oils and baths will prevent pain by reducing stress, improving muscle tone, relaxing tight muscles and improving the general level of wellbeing.

Other Treatments

Balch and Balch recommend the following treatments for backache:[4]

- To relieve back muscle pain, soak in a very warm bath or apply a heating pad directly to the back.
- When carrying things on your shoulder, switch the weight to the other side from time to time. Carrying heavy shoulder bags may produce neck, back and shoulder pain.
- Learn to recognise and reduce stress. Relaxation techniques can be very helpful.

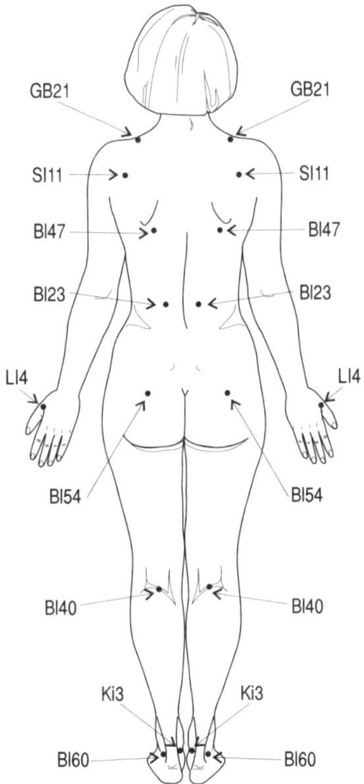

Acupressure points to relieve backache.

- Always push large objects, never pull them.
- Wear comfortable, well-made shoes. The higher the heel of the shoes, the greater the risk of backache.
- Move around. Do not sit in the same position for long periods of time.
- Never lean forward without bending your knees. Lift with your legs, arms, and abdomen — not with the muscles of the small of your back.
- Do not sleep on your stomach with your head raised on a pillow. Instead, rest your back by lying on your side with your legs bent, so that your knees are slightly higher than your hips. Sleep on a firm mattress with your head supported by a pillow.
- Maintain a healthy weight and get regular moderate exercise. A lack of exercise can cause back pain.
- The following acupressure points will tonify the lower back. Bl 40, located in the centre of the back of the popliteal crease, is a special tripper point for alleviating lower back pain. Bl 23, located on the lower back between the second and third lumbar, two finger widths away from the spine at waist level, also tonifies a weak back. If this point is tender, stationary light touch, instead of deep pressure, can be quite healing. Bl 54, located 1 to 2 finger widths outside the sacrum and the base of the buttocks lateral to the midline of the lower third of the sacrum, is used to relieve lower back aches, sciatica, pelvic tension, hip pain and tension.[7]

Bunions

Useful Oils

• German chamomile • lavender • lemon
• sweet marjoram • peppermint • rosemary

Definition

This condition is also known as *hallux valgus*, which means 'laterally deviated big toe.' The proximal phalanx of the great toe is laterally deviated, the joint capsule is stretched and a callus grows over the protrusion.[9]

Clinical Features

Bunions are a very painful inflammation of the joint between the big toe and foot which can lead to a deformity of the joint of the big toes.[9]

Aetiology

In a majority of cases, bunions are the result of shoes that do not fit properly — too narrow, too tight or too high. Children and young people should always wear shoes that are the correct size and width, as their bones are more easily deformed than those of adults.

Therapeutic Strategy

The first step in treating bunions is to remove the factors that are causing it, or making it worse. This often means changing footwear.[9]

Massage can help to reduce adhesions and inflammation. However, it must be remembered that massage will not make bunions go away.[9]

Aromatherapy Treatment

Essential oils can be used to relieve the pain, and sometimes reduce the amount of tender swelling around the joint, but they will be useless unless other physical measures are also included.

If the joint is inflamed, very gentle massage with essential oils such as German chamomile, lavender, rosemary, and peppermint may be used for their analgesic and anti-inflammatory properties.

Other Treatments

- Wear comfortable shoes that support the feet.
- In hot weather, do not forget that your feet swell, therefore shoes that are not too tight are best. Go barefoot whenever possible.
- Severe cases should be treated by a podiatrist.

Bursitis

Useful Oils

• cajeput • eucalyptus • ginger • juniper berry • rosemary

Definition

Bursitis is an inflammation of the bursa. The bursae are small sacs containing lubricating fluid which is situated between moving joints. It often affects shoulders, but it is well known for its appearance in elbows and knees (tennis elbow and housemaid's knee).[4,9]

Clinical Features

Bursitis can affect anyone. However, older people and athletes are more likely to get them. It can be difficult to differentiate between bursitis and tendinitis, the inflammation of a tendon. Bursitis is characterised by a dull persistent pain that increases with movement, whereas tendinitis typically causes sharp pain on movement.[4]

The symptoms of bursitis include pain on any kind of movement, passive or active, along with heat, oedema and extremely limited range of motion.[9]

Aetiology

The bursa can become inflamed through injury, infection, repetitive stress and unusual pressure when the liquid content increases, causing pain and limited movement.

Aromatherapy Treatment

Essential oils such as rosemary, cajeput, juniper berry or eucalyptus blended in a massage oil and gently rubbed into the inflamed area will assist in reducing the inflammation and relieve pain. A warm moist compress is also recommended.

Other Treatments

Avoid using the joint until the inflammation has diminished.[4]

Cramps

Useful Oils

• black pepper • Roman chamomile • clary sage • cypress • geranium • lavender • sweet marjoram • thyme

Clinical Features

A cramp is the sudden involuntary contraction of a muscle or group of muscles which causes acute pain.[9] Many people suffer from cramps in the legs or feet during sleep. While the smooth muscles of the body may also be prone to cramps, this section specifically relates to the skeletal muscles.

Aetiology

Muscle cramping in different parts of the body is commonly caused by mineral deficiencies, particularly calcium and magnesium.[9]

Heat cramps are primarily due to salt depletion. The use of diuretic drugs for high blood pressure or heart disorders may also be the cause of muscle cramping. If someone is taking these drugs be sure to include potassium in the diet.[10]

Poor circulation contributes to leg cramps. Cramps during the day while active may be a sign of impaired circulation.

Aromatherapy Treatment

Massaging the legs vigorously using black pepper, sweet marjoram, geranium, lavender, cypress and thyme in a massage oil will relieve cramps.

Other Treatments

- Cramps in the legs can be relieved by bending the knee as far as it will go, or contracting the opposite muscle to that in contraction. If cramps are experienced while reclining, the flow of blood to the legs will be increased if you stand up.
- Sodium chloride, 1 g every 30–60 minutes with large amounts of water or a saline solution usually relieves heat cramps promptly.[10]
- Hot foot baths using mineral salts are beneficial.[4]
- Daily walking and regular exercise help to increase circulation, reducing the incidence of cramps.[4]

Gout

Useful Oils
• carrot seed • juniper berry • lemon • pine • rosemary

Definition

Gout is a common type of arthritis that occurs when there is too much uric acid in the blood, tissues and urine. The uric acid crystallises in the joints, acting as an abrasive causing swelling and pain.[4]

Clinical Features

Gout has been called the rich man's disease, since it is associated with too much rich food and alcohol. 90% of sufferers are men, usually over 30 years of age.[3,4]

The metatarsophalangeal joint of the great toe is the most susceptible joint, although others, especially those of the feet, ankles and knees are commonly affected. Gout is characterised by sudden acute attack — the pain is usually intense. The involved joints are swollen and extremely tender and the overlying skin is tense, warm and dusky red. Fever, headache, malaise and tachycardia are common.[4]

Subsequent attacks are common, with the majority having another attack within one year. This may lead to gouty arthritis in the long-term, with progressive functional loss and disability. Hypertension, renal stones and renal failure may also be associated with gouty arthritis.

Aetiology

High uric acid levels may be attributed to:

- Increased uric acid synthesis from purine metabolism.[2,3]
- Reduced ability to excrete uric acid. Drugs such as diuretics and aspirin may contribute to this. Alcohol decreases excretion from the kidney and increases synthesis of uric acid.[2,3]

Uric acid is a by-product of certain foods, so this condition is closely associated with diet. It can be brought on by stress. Obesity and an improper diet increase the tendency for gout.

Therapeutic Strategy

The therapeutic strategy should include:

- a low purine diet is important
- aromatherapy treatment that aims at detoxifying the body, thus reducing the high levels of uric acid which cause gout.

Aromatherapy Treatment

Massage is often not appropriate for the treatment of gout due to the inflammatory nature of the condition. Foot baths and compresses are suitable treatment methods. Place several drops of carrot seed, pine, rosemary or juniper berry oil in a warm foot bath and keep the feet in the bath for 10 minutes.

Other Treatments

Nutrition

- Lose weight if overweight.[2,3,4]
- Avoid alcohol.[2,3,4]
- No meat.[4]
- Eat only raw fruits and vegetables for 2 weeks.
- Cherries, blue berries and strawberries are excellent as they help neutralise uric acid.[2,3,4]
- Drink celery juice diluted with purified water.[2,3,4]
- Avoid purine rich foods such as anchovies, asparagus, herring, mushrooms, mussels, all organ meats, sardines and sweetbreads.[2,3,4]
- Take vitamin C to increase the loss of uric acid via the kidneys.[4]

Herbs

- Antirheumatic and detoxifying herbs such as celery seed, burdock and juniper berry will be beneficial.[4]

Sciatica

Useful Oils
• black pepper • cajeput • cinnamon bark
• clove bud • German chamomile • eucalyptus
• ginger • juniper berry • lavender • spike lavender
• sweet marjoram • nutmeg • peppermint • rosemary
• thyme

Definition

Sciatica is defined as pain in the distribution of the sciatic nerve or its branches (L4, L5, S1, S2, S3) that is caused by nerve pressure or irritation. Most problems are due to entrapment neuropathy of a nerve root, in either the spinal canal or the invertebrate foramen.[1]

Clinical Features

Sciatica is often accompanied by or precedes lumbago, and may be the first warning of a prolapsed or slipped vertebral disc. It is also caused by lifting heavy objects incorrectly or bending awkwardly.

Therapeutic Strategy

It is important to realise that the pain of sciatica is a symptom, and that treating the pain alone is not an effective treatment. The cause must be found and treated. The therapeutic strategy should include:

- back care education
- bed rest (2 days is considered optimal)

- analgesic and anti-inflammatory essential oils
- basic exercise program, including swimming.[1]

Aromatherapy Treatment

When the sciatic pain is so intense that massage is contra-indicated, use these oils by applying a cold compress to reduce the pain and inflammation. The most useful essential oils for sciatica are peppermint, ginger, nutmeg, spike lavender, rosemary and cajeput. Gentle massage with any of these oils at times when there is less or no pain can be very beneficial, and baths can also be helpful.

Other Treatments

- Exercises which gently stretch and strengthen the sciatic nerve are beneficial. Lie on the back with one knee placed over the other and pull the top knee gently towards you using your hands. You will feel your lower back stretching. Change over knees to stretch the other side.
- The following acupressure points stimulate he lower back and relieve sciatica. Bl 40, the point behind the knee, is a special point for alleviating lower back pain and sciatica. Bl 23 and Bl 47 relieve lower back aches and sciatica and strengthen the back. Bl 54, located on the buttocks, is an effective lower back point and sciatica point. These points can be used separately or together in a sequence for relieving sciatica.[8]

Sports Injuries

Natural remedies go hand in hand with the standard methods of treating sporting injuries and maintaining the wellbeing of the body which is pushed by sport to the limits of endurance, stamina and skill.

Management of Soft Tissue Injuries

RICE

'Rest, ice, compression and elevation' are words so often repeated by physiotherapists and sport therapists that they have been shortened to form the acronym 'RICE' which is drummed into anyone with an injury that needs care.

Rest: Resting an injury is extremely important to ensure that no further damage takes place.[11]

Ice: Applying ice to all sorts of injuries, as long as it is done correctly, can stop internal bleeding, bruising, and inflammation. In doing so, it reduces the healing time.[12]

Ice can be placed in a bowl or bucket into which you immerse the toes, feet, fingers, hands or elbows or any other parts of the body that are affected. An ice compress may be used. Put ice or a bag of frozen vegetables in a plastic bag, place between two towels and then wrap around the affected area.[11]

Ice packs should be applied for 15 minutes every 2 hours for 24 hours, then 15 minutes every 4 hours for 24 hours.[11]

Compression: Compressions can be made with a bandage or piece of material which is folded to form a pad. This should be wrapped firmly over the area to prevent swelling. Compresses can be hot or cold. Compresses are needed to reduce the level of blood flowing to the area but should never be so tight that they impede circulation and cause the injured person to experience pain, numbness or the skin turning blue.[12]

Elevation: By raising the injured limb higher than the heart, swelling and pain can often be prevented or reduced by reducing the volume and pressure of blood flow through the injured limb. It also promotes the return of blood away from the injured part and back to the heart.[12]

Strains

Useful Oils

• arnica-infused oil • black pepper • cajeput
• cinnamon bark • clove bud • ginger • spike lavender
• sweet marjoram • nutmeg • rosemary • thyme

Definition

A strain refers to an injury to the muscle–tendon unit.[10,12]

Clinical Features

Symptoms include mild or intense local pain, stiffness and pain on resisted movement or stretching. Unless it is a bad strain, there is no heat and swelling present. Pain is exacerbated by stretching.[10]

Treatment

- RICE treatment.
- Massage will help reduce adhesions, oedema and re-establish range of motion.
- Use of rubefacient essential oils such as black pepper, clove bud, ginger, spike lavender, nutmeg and rosemary to promote healing of injured muscle tissue.

Achilles Tendinitis

Useful Oils

• clove bud • German chamomile • ginger
• juniper berry • spike lavender • lavender
• sweet marjoram • nutmeg

Definition

Inflammation of the Achilles tendon. This restricts movement and the area may be hot and painful.

Clinical Features

Achilles tendinitis is common in runners who change routine, or are unaccustomed to running or long walks. Symptoms include aching pain on using tendon, tendons feel stiff, especially on rising and there may be swelling and bruising.[1]

Treatment

- RICE
- Use essential oils which are anti-inflammatory and analgesic. For the first 3 days use cold compresses to which you have added 3 drops each of German chamomile and lavender. Then use a hot compress to which you have added 3 drops of ginger and German chamomile. Also massage the area with a massage oil blend of spike lavender and German chamomile.

Sprains

Useful Oils

• arnica-infused oil • black pepper • clove bud
• German chamomile • ginger • juniper berry
• spike lavender • lemongrass • sweet marjoram
• nutmeg • peppermint • rosemary • thyme

Definition

Sprains are tears to ligaments, the connective tissue that joins bone to bone.[9]

Clinical Features

- Sprains are injured ligaments, not muscles or tendons.[9]
- Sprains are more serious than strains and tendinitis. Muscles and tendons are more elastic and less densely arranged than ligaments. Ligaments do not have the same rich blood supply that muscles have. This makes them slower to heal.[9]
- Inflammation is common.[9]
- The signs of an acute sprain are pain, redness, heat and inflammation.[9]

Treatment

- Use the RICE treatment for 48 hours.[1]
- If exercise is overdone, it will cause more tearing and scar tissue.[9]
- Commence gentle stretching and encourage full range of movement with isometric exercises as soon as possible.[1]
- Massage using analgesic and anti-inflammatory essential oils such as cajeput, ginger, nutmeg, peppermint and clove bud.
- Keep the ankle bandaged to prevent further damage. Use ice packs for three days (followed by massage), three times a day, and if the pain continues begin to apply alternate hot and cold flannels, to both of which you have added 4 drops of peppermint. Using steaming hot flannels and ice-cold ones, and apply them alternately several times. Do this three times a day.
- To prevent sprains, do stretching exercises before and after exercise. Massage with essential oils such as black pepper, ginger, clove bud, spike lavender, lemongrass and rosemary before massage.

References

1. Murtagh J. *General practice*. 2nd edn, The McGraw-Hill Companies Inc, Australia, 1998.
2. Pizzorno J, Murray M. *A text book of natural medicine*. 2nd edn, Churchill Livingstone, UK, 1999.
3. Osiecki H. *The physician's handbook of clinical nutrition*. Bioconcepts Publishing, Australia, 1990.
4. Balch J, Balch P. *Prescription for nutritional healing*. Avery Publishing Group, USA, 1997.
5. Davies S, Stewart A. *Nutritional medicine*. Pan Books, England, 1988.
6. Hoffman D. *The new holistic herbal*. Element Books Limited, USA, 1983.
7. Reed Gach M. *Acupressure's potent points*. Bantam Books, USA, 1990.
8. Hay L. *You can heal your life*. Specialist Publications, Australia, 1987.
9. Werner R. *A massage therapist's guide to pathology*. Lippincott Williams & Wilkins, USA, 1998.
10. Krupp M, Chatton M. *Current medical diagnosis and treatment 1980*. Lange Medical Publications, USA, 1980.
11. Australian Sports Medicine Federation, *The sports trainer: Care and prevention of sporting injuries*. The Jacaranda Press, Australia, 1986.
12. *St John Australian first aid manual*. 3rd edn, St John Ambulance of Australia, 1998.

The Reproductive System

Objectives

After careful study of this chapter, you should be able to:

- identify, list and describe common pathophysiologies of the reproductive system
- explain the aromatherapy treatment for specific conditions and disorders of the reproductive system
- explain the role of other holistic strategies for specific conditions and disorders of the reproductive system.

Introduction

The focus of this chapter is primarily the reproductive system of women. By the nature of human anatomy, there is not the same degree of complexity of structure and function in the male reproductive system.

The major female reproductive organs include the ovaries, which produce ova; the uterine (fallopian) tubes, which transport the ova to the uterus (womb); the vagina; and the external organs that constitute the vulva. The mammary glands are also considered part of the female reproductive system.[1]

The functions of the female reproductive system are to:

- produce ova
- secrete sex hormones
- receive the sperm from the male during coitus
- provide sites for fertilisation, implantation and development of pregnancy
- facilitate delivery of the baby
- provide nourishment for the baby through the secretion of milk from the mammary glands in the breasts.[2]

The pituitary secretes sex hormones in response to the secretion of hormones from the hypothalamus. The hypothalamus also has links to the higher centres of the brain and it is known that its function can be affected by thoughts, feelings and environmental stress. It is easy to see how emotional problems and stress can upset the hypothalamus and hence cause problems with menstruation and hormonal balances.[3]

Aromatherapy Considerations

Aromatherapy is considered one of the most effective methods of dealing with menstrual, pregnancy and menopausal problems. Many essential oils can help to regulate hormone production, relax or uplift, or are useful for reducing stress-related tension that often exacerbates symptoms.

Essential oils such as jasmine and rose have a general strengthening effect on the reproductive system and may be used to relieve specific complaints such as menstrual problems.

Some essential oil constituents have hormone-like behaviour because their structure is similar to hormones, so they interact with the receptors that identify hormones. Oestrogenic activity has been found in essential oils such as aniseed and sweet fennel. Anethole, a methyl ether of oestradiol, is responsible for the oestrogenic activity of these oils.[4]

There are no essential oils that have progesterone-like activity, nor are there any oils used in aromatherapy that have androgen-like activity. Essential oils with oestrogenic activities may influence the menstrual cycle, lactation and secondary sexual characteristics.

In treating conditions associated with the reproductive system the following properties are considered useful:

Antimicrobial

Essential oils with antiseptic and bactericidal properties may be used to treat leucorrhoea, vaginal pruritus and thrush. Essential oils that are antimicrobial include bergamot, German chamomile, eucalyptus, myrrh, rose, sandalwood and tea tree.

Antispasmodics

For menstrual cramps and labour pain, essential oils such as Roman chamomile, clary sage, lavender and sweet marjoram may be used.

Emmenagogues

Essential oil with emmenagogue properties have the ability to promote menstruation and are used to treat amenorrhoea and scanty periods. Essential oils that are emmenagogues include basil, carrot seed, German and Roman chamomile, sweet fennel, clary sage, juniper berry, lavender, sweet marjoram, myrrh, parsley seed, rose, rosemary, peppermint and tarragon.

Galactagogues

Galactagogues are remedies that are used to increase milk flow. Essential oils that are galactagogues include aniseed, dill, sweet fennel, jasmine and lemongrass.

Parturients

Essential oils with parturient properties help induce labour by stimulating contraction, helping to give a swift and relatively painless birth. Essential oils that are parturients include jasmine, rose and nutmeg.

Uterine Tonics

Uterine tonics have a toning and strengthening effect on the whole system, on the tissue of the organs and on their function. Essential oils that are uterine tonics include clary sage, jasmine, rose, myrrh and frankincense.

Associated Conditions

The conditions of the reproductive system are considered in four groups:

- those associated with pregnancy and childbirth
- those associated with the menstrual cycle
- those associated with menopause
- those associated with infections.

Pregnancy

Pregnancy is a time of joy for most women and for the middle four or five months of a healthy pregnancy the mother has a look about her of glowing good health and she usually feels well and happy. During the early and late months of many pregnancies, and sometimes during the middle months, a number of conditions related to the pregnancy can arise which cause the mother varying degrees of discomfort or even distress.

The judicious use of essential oils together with appropriate forms of massage by a skilled therapist can help ease the discomforts of pregnancy and provide a sense of nurturing that will comfort the mother at times when she is likely to be feeling rather fragile. Aromatherapy is even more appropriate when the heightened sense of smell during pregnancy is taken into consideration.[5]

The popularity of aromatherapy in the field of obstetrics has been mostly attributed to midwives willing to incorporate natural and safe techniques to assist the birth process.

The main cause of infant death is premature birth and the number one cause of premature birth is stress.[6] There appears to be an epidemic of stress in much of the world today and it affects pregnant women at least as much as it does the rest of the population and possibly more.[6]

Caring use of aromatherapy treatments should help to reduce the stress felt by pregnant women and thereby possibly play a valuable role in reducing premature births caused by stress and the resulting prenatal deaths associated with it.

If at any time during the pregnancy any condition arises which is outside the therapist's range of skills, the woman should be advised to contact her doctor. Should you find that the woman is experiencing pain of sudden onset, swelling, heat or redness of the calf or thigh muscles, a deep vein thrombosis may be suspected and the woman should be urged to contact her doctor immediately.[6]

In positioning the client for massage, avoid lying her flat on her back. She should recline at an angle of about 45 degrees, because the growing uterus presses on the inferior vena cava in this position and can cause an alarming drop in blood pressure.[6]

Where massage is not possible (for example, if she has deep vein thrombosis), the pregnant woman may still be able to experience the benefits of aromatherapy. The therapist can make appropriate blends for a bath or foot bath, inhalation, oil burner or compress.

Aromatherapy blends during pregnancy should not exceed a strength of 2%. The following is a description of some of the problems encountered during pregnancy, the aromatherapy remedies and the holistic advice that the pregnant woman can follow to overcome the problems.

Backache

Many women experience some lower back pain as their pregnancy advances, due not only to the increased weight of the baby, but also to the changing shape of their own body, and the way this increases the lumbar curvature of the spine.

To minimise back pain during pregnancy, the mother should not stay in one position for too long, should not wear high-heeled shoes and should not do any forward bending or strong upward stretching exercises.[7]

Yoga and specific natal exercises are beneficial. It is important to rest for at least 20 minutes each day, lying flat on the back, with the legs bent at the knees and supported on a chair. The thighs should be at right angles to the body, and the calves at right angles to the thighs. This position straightens out lumbar curve and relaxes the overworked muscles of the lower back.[7]

A massage blend with essential oils such as spike lavender, cajeput and lemon will provide relief from pain and help to tone the muscles which are supporting the increased weight.

When massaging a pregnant woman it is very important to ensure she is comfortable and relaxed. Finding comfortable positions in later pregnancy is often difficult. To facilitate back massage on a pregnant mother, she should sit forward over a straight backed chair leaning onto a cushion. For head, neck or foot massage use a bean bag or cushions with the arms and legs supported.

Constipation

Bowel sluggishness is common in pregnancy. It is due to the suppression of smooth muscle motility by increased steroid sex hormones and pressure upon displacement of the intestines by the enlarging uterus. Constipation should not be allowed to continue untreated as it frequently leads to haemorrhoids and aggravates diverticulitis.

The most effective aromatherapy treatment for constipation is massage of the abdomen, always in a clockwise direction. Essential oils to use for this massage are German chamomile, neroli, sweet orange, tangerine and black pepper. Refer to *Constipation* for further recommendations.

Fatigue and Insomnia

Fatigue can occur at any stage of the pregnancy. It can be one of the overwhelming symptoms, particularly in the first and second trimester if the pregnant woman is still working. The body is adjusting to the fluctuating hormone levels and is providing energy for foetal development and growth. Increased weight, a variety of physical discomforts and an element of anxiety towards the end of pregnancy may lead to fatigue and an inability to go to sleep or to sleep for long periods.[9]

Essential oils such as lavender, Roman chamomile, sweet orange and neroli are excellent oils to use in a bath, massage or vaporiser to help one overcome fatigue, feel more relaxed and to assist with sleep.

Flatulence

Keep a record of all the foods eaten in order to determine what foods or food combinations are causing the flatulence. Eat four to five small meals a day instead of three big meals. Walking a kilometre a day should assist the digestion and elimination.[7]

Essential oils to relieve flatulence during pregnancy include dill, ginger and spearmint. Prepare a 2% dilution of one of these oils and massage over the abdomen several times a day.

Haemorrhoids

Haemorrhoids are a related problem to varicose veins. The following advice and treatments are recommended:

- To obtain relief the mother needs to avoid constipation and drink at least eight glasses of water a day.[7]
- Increase the intake of roughage in the diet with foods such as raw vegetables, fruit, whole bran and whole grain breads. This often helps to soften the stools and makes elimination easier. Hard stools may be very painful and cause bleeding.[7]
- Use cold witch hazel compresses to help shrink the haemorrhoids.[7]
- Worwood suggests blending 15 drops of geranium and 5 drops of cypress essential oils into the contents of a small tube of KY jelly squeezed into a small glass jar. This should be mixed well and rubbed around the anal area when required. This treatment will not only alleviate the symptoms, it prevents haemorrhoids occurring in the first place.[8]

Heartburn

Heartburn can occur in later pregnancy due to compression of the stomach. Guenier suggests ginger, lavender, lemongrass and coriander seed essential oils for baths and vaporising and for massage of the abdomen and middle back.[5] Roman chamomile and tangerine could also be used. Other helpful hints include:

- Do not consume spicy or greasy foods, alcohol or coffee.[7]
- Drink one tablespoon of milk before eating to coat and soothe the stomach and eat four to six small meals a day.[7]
- Refrain from bending or lying flat for several hours after eating.[7]

Leg Cramps

Leg cramps in pregnancy are usually worse in the last months of pregnancy and can be caused by the position of the baby or due to the reduction in the level of diffusible serum calcium or increase in the serum phosphorus level (or both). To relieve cramps try the following formula in a foot bath:

geranium	5 drops
lavender	10 drops
cypress	2 drops

You may also try rubbing or kneading the contracted, painful muscle using a massage oil containing black pepper and ginger essential oil. Other helpful hints include:

- Increasing calcium and potassium intake by eating foods such as bananas, grapefruit, oranges, cottage cheese, yoghurt, salmon, sardines, soybeans, almonds and sesame seeds.[7]
- While sleeping or sitting, elevate the legs higher than the heart.[7]
- Do not stand in one place for too long.[7]
- Walk one kilometre a day to stimulate the flow of blood through the legs.[7]
- When experiencing a cramp, apply a hot water bottle or heating pad to the cramping area and apply pressure using your hands.[7]

Miscarriage

Some women cannot carry a baby to full term and experience a miscarriage or spontaneous abortion. There may be many reasons for this, including emotional stress, malnutrition, general malaise, illness such as infection and glandular disorder.[7]

A common contributing factor to miscarriage is an altered progesterone level. Progesterone is necessary for the maintenance of pregnancy. At about the third month of pregnancy the placenta takes over the major role of progesterone secretion from the corpus luteum. If the placenta fails to carry out this vital function, miscarriage will occur. The first symptom of miscarriage is bleeding, sometimes accompanied by cramping. Slight bleeding, although alarming, does not necessarily mean a miscarriage will occur. Some women may lose small amounts of blood regularly throughout their otherwise healthy pregnancy. However if the persistent or heavy bleeding occurs, urgent medical advice should be sought.[3]

The emotional trauma experienced after a miscarriage can be considerable, and the support of an experienced and caring practitioner can be a helpful addition to that of friends and family. Dr Bach's Rescue Remedy can have a very calming effect during this distressing time. Take a few drops as often as required.

The essential oils recommended for use after a miscarriage not only help the body back to its pre-pregnancy state, they also heal on an emotional and spiritual level. Any of the following essential oils should be used in a massage blend, bath or vaporiser — geranium, frankincense, jasmine, clary sage, neroli, rose otto, rosewood and sandalwood.

Morning Sickness

Morning sickness is a positive sign meaning that the placenta is sited.[5] It often occurs in the morning, but can occur at any time of the day. It is believed to affect about 50% of women during the first three or four months of pregnancy.[7]

Four to five drops of ginger, lavender or spearmint essential oil may be used as an inhalation or used as a compress over the stomach. Alternatively, a few drops of the same oils on the pillowcase at night or inhaled from a tissue are helpful. Other helpful hints include:

- Mothers suffering from morning sickness should eat small, frequent meals and snack on wholegrain crackers.[7]
- An infusion of freshly grated ginger helps to relieve nausea.[7]
- Red raspberry leaf and peppermint taken as a tea helps relieve nausea.[7]
- Avoid all fats, sugars, alcohols, caffeine, cigarette smoke and processed orange juice.[7]
- Vitamin B complex with additional vitamin B6 and magnesium during pregnancy helps control morning sickness. Foods rich in vitamin B6 and magnesium include brewer's yeast or torula yeast, sunflower seeds, soya seeds, brown rice, walnuts, bananas, salmon, tuna, chicken and wheatgerm.[7]

Oedema

A rise in oestrogen in the body causes swelling of the hands and feet. Some swelling is to be expected and is acceptable. Avoid all highly processed foods, while maintaining a well balanced diet. Wear loose, comfortable clothing. Be sure to wear properly fitting shoes, which may be larger than your normal size.[7]

A hand or foot bath containing a few drops of lime, sweet orange, tangerine, grapefruit or geranium should relieve fluid retention.

Skin Problems

Common skin problems during pregnancy include pimples, acne, red marks and mask of pregnancy (dark blotches on the skin and face). These skin changes will, however, disappear with the birth of the baby. 5 mg of folic acid before each meal may help the pregnancy mask to disappear.[7]

Studies have shown a correlation between pregnancy mask and adrenal gland depletion due to increased stress. Vitamin B complex and Vitamin C supplements are recommended. Avoid physical and emotional stresses.[7]

Stretch Marks

Stretch marks are wavy reddish stripes, that gradually turn white, appearing on the abdomen, buttocks, breasts and thighs. They are caused by excessive and rapid weight gain typically associated with pregnancy, and appear when the skin becomes over-stretched and the fibres in the deep layers tear. Unfortunately, once they appear they are permanent, even though they become less prominent with time.[7]

Stretch marks can be prevented by applying the following massage oil blend to the places in which they would commonly appear.

wheatgerm oil	10 mL
apricot kernel oil	10 mL
avocado oil	50 mL
neroli	5 drops
tangerine	20 drops
lavender	5 drops

Guenier suggests geranium, frankincense and lavender essential oils for stretch marks.[5]

Varicose Veins

Varicose veins are enlarged veins close to the surface of the skin. They usually disappear after the birth of the baby. The following guidelines will help alleviate varicose veins:

- Do not wear restrictive knee socks, garters, belts or high-heeled shoes.[7]
- Do not stand for long periods of time or sit cross-legged.[7]
- Walking one kilometre a day is beneficial.[7]

Varicose veins can be alleviated or prevented by using the following massage blend and gently massaging it to the legs. Massage should be in the direction from the ankles to thighs:

calendula-infused oil	20 mL
wheatgerm oil	10 mL
sweet almond oil	30 mL
geranium	15 drops
cypress	5 drops
lemon	10 drops

Preparing for Birth

In preparation for labour, the pregnant woman may be advised to prepare for delivery by self-massage of the perineum for five to ten minutes daily for the last six weeks of pregnancy. Guenier reports the results of a clinical trial of women having their first baby, which indicated that only 48% of the women using perineal massage needed an episiotomy or had a second degree tear compared with 77% of women in the control group.[5] She says:

> *The procedure is best carried out following a warm bath to increase circulation and soften tissues, and with an empty bladder. The woman should use a mirror so she can see she is applying the oils to the perineum and the posterior vaginal wall, special attention being given to any scar tissue from previous deliveries. The oil is made up using a base oil, wheatgerm oil, lavender and geranium. Two index fingers are inserted two inches into the vagina pressing down towards the rectum. The massage movement should be in a 'u'. The tissues relax and stretch very quickly. The vagina should be stretched open for 20 seconds to feel the tingling or burning process associated with the head crowning.*[5]

Aromatherapy can provide an enriching dimension to a woman's experience of pregnancy, ease her discomforts, nurture her, help reduce her stress and possibly reduce her risk of giving birth prematurely. It can also make her labour quicker and easier, with less need for drug use and other interventions, giving her more control over the birth.

From about the seventh month raspberry leaf tea is recommended in preparation for childbirth. Raspberry contains fragrine that relieves uterine pains by dilating the pelvic muscles. Use one teaspoon of raspberry leaf tea to one cup of boiling water.[7]

Aromatherapy can be of great help during childbirth. Some essential oils strengthen and deepen contractions, while also having an analgesic effect. In the labour ward an anxiety-free atmosphere can be created with the help of vaporised essential oils. Oils such as bergamot, grapefruit, tangerine, neroli, jasmine, rose and lavender prove to be the most useful.

Labour

Tiran stresses that the induction of labour should not be attempted by anyone other than a member of a conventional obstetric team.[9] Aromatherapy is now being used by an increasing number of health professionals involved in childbirth. Labour is divided into three stages:

- the first is the dilation of the cervix
- the second is the expulsion of the baby
- the third is the delivery of the placenta.

The average length of the first stage of labour with the first baby is about 12 hours and with subsequent children about 7 hours. However, this stage may take anywhere from 2 to 24 hours, or more, depending on the size of the baby, the baby's position, the size of the mother's pelvic area and the behaviour of the uterus. During this stage massage with oils such as clary sage, jasmine, neroli or rose to help the mother relax between contractions. Use a few drops of bergamot or lavender in a bowl of warm water to refresh and disinfect the atmosphere.

Burns and Blamey evaluated the benefits of essential oils in a labour ward. The essential oils used included lavender, clary sage, peppermint, eucalyptus, chamomile, frankincense, jasmine, rose, lemon and mandarin.[10] The results of the study were:

- lavender was the most commonly used oil. It was used to reduce maternal anxiety (174 times), for pain relief (38 times) and to lighten mood (12 times)
- peppermint was the oil most commonly selected to relieve nausea and vomiting (108 uses)
- clary sage was the oil most commonly used to increase contractions (77 times).[10]

The most common reasons for using the essential oils were to reduce anxiety (321 uses), relieve nausea (130 uses), increase contractions (111 uses) and for pain relief (88 uses).[10]

13% of the women who participated used no other form of pain relief and 67% of women were given essential oils first before any other analgesia.[10]

71% of women had a spontaneous vaginal delivery, 20% had an instrumental delivery, while 8% had a Caesarean section; 7% emergency and 1% elective. The last 1% of deliveries were not recorded.[10]

The most frequent comment was the relaxant effect of the essential oils, lavender, clary sage and chamomile being the most popular. Lavender was regarded as the best mood enhancer. It was found that lavender was most effective to calm down uterine contractions if the mother was exhausted and needed to sleep, while clary sage was given to encourage labour. Once in labour, lavender was once again used to minimise anxiety.[10]

Not all the uses were necessarily effective, for example:[10]

- 29 mothers found peppermint relieved nausea and 8 mothers stated that peppermint did not stop nausea.
- 24 midwives and 10 mothers found clary sage accelerated labour, while 17 midwives found that clary sage did not affect labour.

The results from the mothers' perception on the effectiveness of the essential oils was that:[10]

- 62% said that the essential oils were effective
- 12% found the essential oils were not effective
- 17% of women could not make a decision
- 9% of women did not record a decision.

It was suggested that aromatherapy softens the atmosphere in the delivery room, thus enabling a holistic approach in what would be a rather stressful environment where care can include a lot of technology. Mothers commented on the pleasant smelling delivery suite. Burns and Blamey say that a relaxed woman in labour is empowered to having greater control over what happens to her.[10]

Oils for the Delivery Room

Rose [8, 9, 10]	Uterine relaxant
	Natural antiseptic
	Slight analgesic effect
Neroli [8]	Facilitates easy breathing
	Calming
	Antiseptic
Lavender [8, 9, 16]	Circulatory stimulant
	Analgesic
	Calming
	Antiseptic
	Anti-inflammatory
	Promotes wound healing
	Relieves headaches
Clary sage [8, 9]	Uterine tonic
	Analgesic and antispasmodic
	Euphoric
Jasmine [8, 9, 16]	Euphoric
	Antidepressant
	Uterine tonic

Post-natal Care

Breast and nipple care is very important for the comfort of the mother and the wellbeing of the child. Cracked nipples are a common problem. They are not only painful but there is the possibility of infection. A good massage oil to prepare is:

almond oil	40 mL
calendula-infused oil	5 mL
wheatgerm oil	5 mL

Post-natal Depression

The uplifting properties of essential oils are excellent to use after childbirth. Some of the essential oils recommended include bergamot, rose, neroli, clary sage, geranium, grapefruit, frankincense, mandarin, patchouli, rosewood, tangerine, vetiver and ylang ylang.

Giving birth is not only the most profound chemical change that the human body undergoes in the space of several hours, but also the most profound social change for the mother. As well as the unrelenting demands of the baby, and the worry that the baby is healthy, there are the unremitting rounds of washing and cleaning, and of relatives and friends all offering conflicting advice. It is far better to be prepared for these changes and difficulties. Profound changes have taken place hormonally, psychologically and socially. Essential oils can help at all levels.

Menstrual Problems

Menstruation should not be considered as an illness although it is unusual to meet someone who does not suffer from at least a small amount of premenstrual syndrome, period cramping, some irregularities in the cycle or menopausal symptoms.

Premenstrual Syndrome

Useful Oils
• bergamot • German and Roman chamomile
• carrot seed • clary sage • sweet fennel • geranium
• juniper berry • lavender • sweet marjoram • neroli
• rose otto and rose absolute • rosemary
• ylang ylang

Definition

Premenstrual syndrome (PMS) is defined as a group of physical, psychological and behavioural changes that begin 2–14 days before menstruation and are relieved immediately when the menstrual flow begins.[11]

Clinical Features

PMS is estimated to affect 20 to 40% of menstruating women, with peak incidence occurring among women in their 30s and 40s.[12] In many cases, symptoms are relatively mild; However, in about 10% of women, symptoms can be severe.[12] PMS symptoms include: fluid retention, distended stomach, tender breasts, weight gain, constipation, insomnia, headaches and mood swings.

In an attempt to bring some order to the clinically and metabolically confusing picture of PMS. PMS has been subdivided into four distinct subgroups according to specific symptoms and hormonal patterns.

The four subgroups are detailed in the table below. Any woman may have a number of symptoms from each subgroup and not necessarily from one group only. The most common symptoms are depression 71%, tiredness 35%, headache 33%, bloatedness 31%, breast tenderness 21%, tension 19% and aggression/violence 13%. Other important symptoms include weight gain, lowered general performance, decreased libido and feeling out of control.[11]

Aetiology

The pathogenesis of PMS is still uncertain. Among the proposed causes are pyridoxine deficiency, excess prostaglandin production and increased aldosterone production in the luteal phase.[11] Cabot cites several theories as to the cause of PMS:

- Imbalances in the prostaglandins — this may increase various types of physical pains but it does not explain the mental symptoms of PMS.[3]
- Excessive levels of the hormone prolactin which comes from the pituitary gland. This may be a factor in PMS sufferers with very painful breasts and infrequent periods and this hormone should be checked out in these cases. It is not, however, a universal finding.[3]
- Psychological defect or personality disorder — undoubtedly the underlying personality and environment can influence the development of PMS. Personality factors may intensify PMS symptoms but they cannot be held responsible for causing them.[3]

PMS sufferers consume 62% more refined carbohydrates, 27% more refined sugar, 79% more dairy products, 78% more sodium, 53% less iron, 77% less manganese and 52% less zinc.[12]

Treatment Strategy

According to Cabot there are two essential prerequisites in the treatment of PMS:

- As PMS is a recurrent disorder, it is essential that any treatment be safe and free from side-effects that could accumulate on a long-term basis.[3]
- As PMS has many possible symptoms, any effective treatment must be broad-based and capable of treating all those symptoms.[3]

Cabot says that the two main aims in the holistic treatment of PMS are:

- To improve the women's own ovarian function by ensuring adequate nutrition, avoidance of stress and a healthy lifestyle.[3]
- To alleviate each individual symptom of PMS using physiological and natural substances. She refers to vitamins and minerals and herbal medicines as natural substances.[3]

Aromatherapy Treatment

Essential oils and aromatherapy techniques are beneficial in reducing the severity of PMS. The use of sweet fennel, juniper berry and geranium in a

Type	Description	Causes
PMS-A (anxiety)	Symptoms of nervous tension, anxiety, mood swings and irritability are characteristic of this group. Biochemically, this group shows a high oestrogen to progesterone ration in the luteal phase.	Could be related to excess milk and animal fats. Also nervous excitability.
PMS-Ç (craving)	This group shows increased appetite, sweet craving, headache, fatigue, dizziness or fainting and heart pounding.	Low blood sugar, low prostaglandins.
PMS-D (depression)	Depression, crying, forgetfulness, confusion and insomnia may characterise this group.	High progesterone, low oestrogen, high androgens. Also appears to be higher levels of lead in the body.
PMS-H (hyper-hydration)	Fluid retention, weight gain, swelling of extremities, breast tenderness and abdominal bloating characterise this group.	These symptoms are attributed to increased retention of sodium in the body.

The main classifications of PMS.[12]

massage oil in lymphatic drainage massage can minimise fluid retention.

Essential oils such as clary sage, sweet fennel, geranium and rose influence the production of hormones and are beneficial for the treatment of PMS. Bergamot, Roman chamomile and rose may be used to reduce depression and irritability.

For aromatherapy to be used successfully to manage PMS, it is necessary to use a daily massage blend made up of any of the above essential oils in a massage base of evening primrose oil.

Other Treatments

Nutrition

- Advise the patient to eat regularly and sensibly; eat small rather than large meals.[11, 13]
- Increase the amount of complex carbohydrates, whole grains, vegetables and fruit, leafy green vegetables and legumes.[11, 13]
- Decrease or avoid refined sugar, salt, alcohol, caffeine, tobacco and red meat.[11, 13]
- Vegetarian women have been shown to excrete two to three times more oestrogen in their faeces and have 50% lower levels of free oestrogen in their blood compared to women who eat meat. It appears that many of the effects that a vegetarian diet has on lowering circulating oestrogen levels are related to a higher intake of dietary fibre. The fibre promotes the excretion of oestrogen directly and indirectly.[12]
- Eating foods high in sugar increases insulin secretion and can be harmful to blood sugar control. Sugar, especially if combined with caffeine, has a detrimental effect on PMS and mood. A high intake of sugar also impairs oestrogen metabolism.[12,13]
- Caffeine must be avoided by patients with PMS, especially if anxiety, depression or breast tenderness are major symptoms.[12,15]
- Evening primrose oil contains GLA, a vital essential fatty acid for regulating menstruation. Evening primrose oil needs to be taken for 2 to 3 months, two 500 mg capsules three times a day which will decrease many PMS symptoms, particularly depression and irritability.[12] The results of scientific studies using evening primrose oil have been good, with more than 60% of women with PMS experiencing a reduction of depression, irritability, breast pain, bloating and headaches using evening primrose supplements.[12] The study did not include any vitamins, minerals, dietary or lifestyle recommendations. The response rate is likely to have been higher if these had been included.[12]
- Vitamin B6 (pyridoxine) has been shown in clinical trials to relieve headaches, depression, anxiety, irritability and fatigue in over 50% of PMS sufferers.[12] According to Cabot this is because B6 is essential for the production of mood-regulating brain chemicals, serotonin and noradrenaline.[3]

Herbs

- Cabot recommends uva ursi, parsley and juniper berry as diuretic herbs. These herbs will assist in reducing abdominal swelling, pelvic congestion and weight gain due to fluid retention.[3]
- If progesterone is high, then oestrogenic herbs such as alfalfa, red clover, sage, aniseed, sweet fennel and fenugreek are useful.[14]
- If PMS is characterised by low levels of progesterone then herbs such as false unicorn and wild yam should be considered.[14]
- Dong Quai has been found to relieve PMS symptoms.[7]
- Liquorice root is particularly useful in PMS as it is believed to lower oestrogen, while simultaneously raising progesterone levels.[12]
- *Vitex agnus-castus*, known as chaste berry, appears to be very beneficial in PMS associated with breast pain and infrequent periods.[12]
- Hoffman recommends an infusion of equal parts of skullcap and valerian. If there is associated cramping, cramp bark and passion flower might be used and if there is fluid retention, dandelion and juniper berries can be added to the herbal infusion.[13]

General Advice

- Gentle exercise such as swimming, yoga or just going for a walk when depression or irrational anger threaten can also be a big help.[7,11,12]
- Advise patients to plan activities that they find relaxing and enjoyable at the appropriate time. Consider stress reduction techniques including counselling.[11,12]

Amenorrhoea

Useful Oils

- carrot seed • German and Roman chamomile
- clary sage • sweet fennel • evening primrose oil
- geranium • juniper berry • lavender
- sweet marjoram • rose otto and rose absolute
- yarrow

Definition

The absence of menstrual bleeding is called amenorrhoea, and it is diagnosed when a woman who previously had regular cycles fails to menstruate for over three months. It is quite a common event and 20 to 30% of women will experience episodes of amenorrhoea at some time during their reproductive life.[3]

Clinical Features

Many women may miss one or two periods during the fertile phase of their lives, perhaps during times of emotional stress, and if periods then return to normality there is nothing to worry about. It is obvious that amenorrhoea occurs during pregnancy.

Primary amenorrhoea refers to the failure to begin menstruating by the age of 18.[11] A physical examination may be necessary just in case there is physical obstruction. If no physical obstruction is evident then a constitutional treatment of essential oils and herbs should be considered to stimulate the onset of menarche.

Secondary amenorrhoea refers to the disappearance of menstruation for more than 3 months after normal periods have been established, but before the onset of menopause.[11] Missing periods during the several months following menarche is very common — it may take some young women several months or even years to establish a regular cycle. This should be taken into account when secondary amenorrhoea is being considered, as should the possibility of pregnancy and the early onset of menopause.

Aetiology

The most common cause of amenorrhoea is hormonal imbalance. Another obvious cause of amenorrhoea is pregnancy. Hormonal imbalance can result from upsets in the sensitive hypothalamus-pituitary-ovarian communication link. Factors such as weight loss, excessive exercise, obesity or emotional stress may upset the hypothalamus and pituitary, resulting in failure to stimulate the ovaries with resultant failure of normal female hormonal production and menstruation.[3]

Aromatherapy Treatment

Any essential oil that is an emmenagogue such as Roman chamomile, German chamomile, carrot seed, clary sage, sweet fennel, lavender, sweet marjoram and sage can be used.[15, 16, 17]

Mailhebiau describes sage as the 'saving' herb. It is described as a typically feminine essential oil and its effect on the reproductive organs is remarkable, both physiologically and psychologically. He says that it brings rapid relief in cases of painful periods and, in amenorrhoea and dysmenorrhoea, its emmenagogue power is very active.[18]

Mailhebiau suggests blending sage with clary sage to regulate dysmenorrhoea, activate periods that have ceased, temper and regulate heavy, painful periods and clear up vaginal discharges (leucorrhoea) which are characteristic of adolescence.[18]

Other Treatments

Nutrition

If there is no underlying medical problem a good basic diet, and correction of any nutritional deficiencies with a broad spectrum nutritional program, should restore the menses to normal function within two to three months.

Herbs

Duke says that emmenagogue herbs might help amenorrhoea. These herbs include chaste berry, black cohosh and blue cohosh, carrot seed, celery seed and turmeric.[19]

Dysmenorrhoea

Useful Oils

- German and Roman chamomile • cypress
- clary sage • sweet fennel • geranium
- jasmine absolute • lavender • sweet marjoram
- peppermint • rosemary • rose otto

Description

Dysmenorrhoea is the term used to describe painful periods.

Clinical Features

Intermittent aching to cramp-like discomfort in the lower midline usually accompanies the onset of bleeding. Cabot says that the best way to determine the severity of dysmenorrhoea is to determine how much it interferes with a woman's normal daily activities. It is often the most common cause of women being unable to attend school or work.[3]

Aetiology

Primary Dysmenorrhoea

Primary dysmenorrhoea, pain that occurs with menstrual periods and for which no organic cause can be found,[11] accounts for about 80% of cases of painful menses. Although primary dysmenorrhoea is particularly common during adolescence, it may continue well into adult life.[20]

Secondary Dysmenorrhoea

Pain can occur as the result of some underlying cause other than strong muscular contractions of the uterus. The underlying cause will usually be associated with a disease of the female organs in the pelvic cavity. The diseases most commonly implicated are infection of the tubes, ovarian cysts, uterine fibroids and endometriosis.[17]

Therapeutic Strategy

The therapeutic strategy should include:

- regular exercise

- avoid smoking and excessive alcohol
- relaxation techniques such as yoga
- avoid exposure to extreme cold
- place a hot water bottle over the painful area.[11]

Aromatherapy Treatment

Essential oils that are antispasmodic, emmenagogues and analgesics will be beneficial in treating dysmenorrhoea. These include essential oils such as aniseed, Roman chamomile, clary sage, cypress, sweet fennel, jasmine absolute, juniper berry, sweet marjoram, peppermint, rose absolute or otto, rosemary.

The choice of essential oils depends on the type of pain. For congestive pain, oils such as Roman chamomile and cypress are more useful, whereas spasmodic pain is relieved by oils such as peppermint, lavender or clary sage.

Davis suggests that some women may get more relief from massage or compresses over the lower back, and for others both lower back and abdomen will need to be massaged to get the best possible relief.[15]

Beckman says many women will just want to lie down with a hot water bottle.[21] If this is the case, select essential oils which are of a warming nature such as sweet marjoram, aniseed, fennel or rosemary. Use these essential oils in a massage blend before using the hot water bottle.

Other Treatments

Nutrition

- Calcium and magnesium are most important for the control of muscular contractions. A deficiency of either of these is indicated if the spasms are eased by heat. If only magnesium is lacking, then further relief can be gained by pressure or massage. If only calcium is missing no amount of pressure will make a difference.[25]
- Dysmenorrhoea usually responds to evening primrose oil, magnesium, vitamin B6, niacin, rutin and vitamin E. The effectiveness of niacin (200 mg/day) is enhanced by the addition of rutin and vitamin C. Supplements must begin 7–10 days prior to menses to be of any effect.[25]

Herbs

- Hoffman recommends a mixture of black haw bark, cramp bark and passion flower. Other herbs like black cohosh, false unicorn root and wild yam should also be considered.[13]
- Ginger tea is highly recommended for alleviating menstrual cramps.[19]
- Black cohosh has been found to be effective for the treatment of dysmenorrhoea.[19, 22]

General Advice

- Cold sitz baths — one a day for a few minutes, at least a week before the periods.
- Yoga and relaxation techniques often help, but need to be done consistently. An appropriate and regular exercise programme is recommended.[11]
- Increase the level of exercise. Many sufferers of dysmenorrhoea have found their symptoms improved after regular walking, exercise or swimming.[11]
- Constipation may contribute to the general congestion, so avoid processed foods and have a high wholegrain and vegetable diet.

Menopause

Useful Essential Oils

• bergamot • German and Roman chamomile
• cypress • sweet fennel • geranium • jasmine
• neroli • rose otto and rose absolute • ylang ylang

Definition

The word menopause means the end of cyclical menstrual bleeding and this occurs on average at 50 years of age, however the normal range can vary from 45 to 55 years.[12] There is a slow downturn in ovarian activity with resultant hormonal imbalances for as long as five years before menstrual bleeding finally stops. During these premenopausal years one finds abnormalities of ovarian activity, interspersed with some normal cycles.

Aetiology

Menopause is believed to occur when there are no longer any eggs left in the ovaries.[12]

> *There is no way that the ovary can be brought back to life after its supply of eggs is exhausted. During their active life span, the ovaries have an amazing potential. Each ovary contains approximately 200,000 eggs at the time of puberty and each month some of these eggs are stimulated to grow. One of these eggs (usually only one) will develop into a small hormone factory called the corpus luteum which makes two female hormones, oestrogen and progesterone. The function of the ovaries is controlled by the pituitary gland. After menopause there are no eggs left to respond to the chemical messengers called FSH and LH and develop into hormone producing glands.*[3]

Clinical Features

The most common symptoms of menopause are:

- hot flushes
- headaches
- atrophic vaginitis

- frequent urinary tract infections
- cold hands and feet
- forgetfulness
- an inability to concentrate.[12]

The lack of female hormones causes a disruption in the control of body temperature and this results in hot flushes and sweating, especially at night, which in turn will cause disturbed sleep with resultant fatigue the next day.

The skin becomes dry, fragile and itchy, particularly in cold weather. The female hormones normally exert a slight anti-inflammatory effect, and when they disappear, there is often an increase in rheumatic aches and pains, backaches and headaches, and arthritis may flare up for the first time.

The sexual tissues of the pelvis such as the uterus, vagina and bladder become dry and shrink without hormonal support. This causes loss of elasticity and lubrication and can result in pain during sexual intercourse, vaginal infections and discharge, urinary frequency and burning, and prolapse of the bladder and uterus.

It is important to remember that menopause is not a disease. It is a natural process in a woman's life. How a woman views this time of her life can have a lot to do with how frequent and severe her symptoms are.[7] If menopause is viewed as the end of youth and sexuality, this time will be much more difficult than if it is viewed as the next, natural phase of life. With a proper diet, nutritional supplements and exercise, most of the unpleasant side-effects of menopause can be minimised, if not eliminated.[7]

Hormone Replacement Therapy

Hormone replacement therapy (HRT) is one option often considered by many women to help them through the symptoms of menopause. However, it is important to give careful consideration to the risks as well as the potential benefits of HRT.

The goal of HRT is to restore a woman's hormonal balance, primarily her oestrogen level, to something closer to her normal premenopausal state. In addition to relieving temporary premenopausal and menopausal symptoms, oestrogen replacement appears to be an effective prevention against osteoporosis and heart disease.[11, 12]

However, there is evidence that the use of oestrogen increases the risk of serious cardiovascular disease, especially blood clots. HRT is also linked to an increased risk of cancer of the breast and uterus.[7, 12, 23]

Therapeutic Strategy

Rather than use oestrogens to artificially counteract the symptoms of menopause, the natural approach focuses on improving physiology. This can be accomplished by diet, exercise, nutritional supplements and herbs with phytoestrogens.[12]

Aromatherapy Treatment

The aromatherapy massage is considered very nurturing. A range of essential oils for use in menopausal treatment includes:

- bergamot, Roman chamomile, clary sage, jasmine, neroli and ylang ylang for their calming and antidepressant effects[15]
- sweet fennel — contains natural phytoestrogens[15]
- geranium — traditionally known as a hormonal regulator and balancer[15]
- rose — helps to tone the uterus and regulate the menstrual cycle. Rose is also beneficial for women who feel that they have lost their femininity — it can help them feel feminine, nurtured and desirable.[15]

Other Treatments

Nutrition

- Eat a diet of 50% raw foods and take a protein supplement to help stabilise blood sugar. Add black strap molasses, broccoli, dandelion greens, kelp, salmon and white fish to the diet.[7]
- Avoid alcohol, caffeine, sugar, spicy foods and hot soups and drinks; they can trigger hot flushes, aggravate urinary incontinence and make mood swings worse. They also make the blood more acidic, which prompts the bones to release calcium to act as a buffering agent. This is an important factor in bone loss.[7]
- Follow a diet low in salt and fats and high in fibre and complex carbohydrates with adequate calcium to limit the risk of osteoporosis. During menopause a woman's calcium needs increase to 1,000–1,500 mg daily — the same requirement as needed during pregnancy and lactation. Fat-reduced dairy products are the easiest way to obtain sufficient calcium. Non-dairy sources of foods high in calcium are sardines, tuna with bones, whole sesame seeds, rhubarb and tofu.[3]
- The diet should avoid or severely limit fried foods and 'junk' foods and include plenty of fruit, vegetables, breads and cereals. Water intake should be increased to two litres daily to help combat hot flushes, to help ease dry skin and dry vagina and to speed up the elimination of wastes.[3]

- Eat foods high in phytoestrogens. These include fennel, celery, parsley, soy products, whole grains, apples and alfalfa.[12]
- Take evening primrose oil, 3,000 mg daily, to help control hot flushes, dry itchy skin and dry vagina.[3]
- Fish oil or linseed oil, four capsules daily, should be taken for muscle and joint aches and pains.[3]
- Antioxidants such as vitamin A, C and E are helpful for hot flushes, dry itchy skin and dry vagina, aging of the skin and thinning of the hair.[3]
- High-potency vitamin B complex tablets, one daily, are useful for fatigue, poor memory and reduced mental efficiency and for anxiety, irritability and insomnia.[3]

Herbs

Many of the symptoms of menopause may be relieved by a variety of herbs and herbal extracts.

- For anxiety, irritability and insomnia, sedative herbs such as hops, skullcap, passion flower and valerian may be used.[7]
- Ginkgo biloba and Siberian ginseng are useful for forgetfulness and reduced mental efficiency that seems to accompany menopause.[7,12]
- Dong Quai is known as 'the female ginseng' and is ideal for balancing hormones and relieving symptoms of hot flushes and night sweats, as well as for vaginal dryness.[12,19]
- Red clover contains 1–2.5% isoflavones, which are phytoestrogens similar to those found in soya products.[19]
- The oestrogen-like activity of liquorice root is beneficial.[12,19]

General Advice

- Smoking is associated with early menopause.[11,12]
- Many doctors recommend hormone replacement therapy (HRT) to control the severe symptoms caused by oestrogen deficiency in menopausal and postmenopausal women. Although hormone therapy appears to be effective, it may have possible serious risks which should be carefully considered.[11]
- Get regular moderate exercise.[7,11,12]
- Frequent sexual intercourse can help relieve vaginal dryness.[7]
- If sexual intercourse is painful, try using vitamin E oil or an aloe vera gel to lubricate the vagina.[7]
- For itching in the vaginal area, use vitamin E cream or use vitamin E capsules.[7]

Mercer says that often menopause coincides with other events that may be stressful in themselves. Children may be leaving home, there may be problems with teenagers, parents and in-laws are aging and it may be necessary for a woman to provide more help and care for them at the very time when she may start to feel that her own life is becoming more difficult.[24]

Often one's career may have reached a crossroad, or the pressure of work itself is an added burden. These extra problems added to the hormonal, physical and emotional changes that can occur during menopause often make this time of one's life very difficult to manage.[24]

It is important that any counselling or instruction covers a wide range of methods in dealing with this stress. Acceptance of these changes occurring is very important and help with attitudinal change in the way of counselling may be necessary. Instruction in relaxation and meditation techniques is often a much-needed part of this process.

Endometriosis

Useful Oils

- clary sage • Roman chamomile • cypress
- sweet fennel • geranium • nutmeg
- rose otto and rose absolute

Definition

Endometriosis is a common gynaecological disorder affecting at least 8% of women. It is a unique disease in which the lining of the uterus, called the endometrium, develops in other sites of the body. In a healthy woman, this lining gradually thickens between periods under the influence of oestrogen, in preparation for the fertilised egg. If the egg does not arrive, the blood-rich lining is sloughed off and travels out of the body as a menstrual period. Endometriosis occurs when stray fragments of the endometrium somehow escape into the pelvic cavity and become attached to different pelvic organs.

Clinical Features

The symptoms vary tremendously from none at all to painful menstruation, continual dull lower abdominal pain, backache, sciatica or irregular heavy periods. Pain during sexual intercourse can be very distressing and affects three out of every four women with endometriosis.

Another common sign of endometriosis is infertility and 40% of women with endometriosis have difficulty falling pregnant. The infertility results for a number of reasons. Scar tissue and endometrial implants sometimes block the fallopian tubes and, as the tubes are bound down by adhesions, they cannot move to hover over the ovary at the time of ovulation to draw in the released egg. The production of inflammatory prostaglandins from the implants can also reduce the movement of the fallopian tubes, preventing them from hovering over the ovary at the time of ovulation. Because intercourse is unpleasantly painful, it is often avoided, and this too reduces chances of conception.

Aetiology

Small pieces of the endometrial lining find their way out through the Fallopian tubes and into the abdomen, where they implant onto the outside of the uterus and tubes, the ovaries, bladder or bowel. In these abnormal sites, the endometrial implants respond to the influence of the cyclic production of oestrogen and progesterone from the ovaries, so that they grow and bleed each month, just as the uterine lining does.

However, there is nowhere for the blood to escape and it accumulates in the ovaries and on the pelvic organs, provoking scar tissue formation, eventually sticking all the pelvic organs together like cement.[3]

Psychologically, endometriosis can have devastating effects on a woman's sexuality and self-esteem. Dyspareunia (painful coitus) is a common symptom as lesions and implants behind the uterus can lock it in a retroverted position making sexual intercourse very painful. One third of endometriosis sufferers are infertile.

If endometriosis is suspected, the diagnosis is often confirmed through a hospital procedure called a laparoscopy. During a laparoscopy, a slender, telescope-like instrument is passed into the abdominal cavity either through a small puncture wound beneath the navel, or through the upper vagina. This telescope allows the size and number of stray fragments of the endometrium tissue to be estimated.[7]

Conventional Treatment

By creating a pseudomenopause, drug therapy can be effective, although lesions may recur when the therapy is discontinued. A commonly used drug is Danazol, a synthetic androgen thought to block the pituitary stimulation and production of luteinising hormone (LH) and follicle-stimulating hormone (FSH).[3]

Synthetic androgens produce male characteristics and 85% of patients experience side-effects such as a deepening of the voice, alopecia, hirsutism, reduced breast size, clitoris enlargement and acne. Other side-effects may include weight gain, high blood pressure and joint problems.[3]

Pregnancy was long thought to halt the progress of the disease and is still suggested as an alternative to drug therapy. However, pregnancy is not a panacea; some women report no change or even a worsening of their problems.[3]

Aromatherapy Treatment

It is recommended that professional aromatherapy treatments be carried out over a 3-month period, with two visits a week initially. Lymphatic drainage should be avoided in the early stages due to the remote possibility of the endometrial cells being spread to other parts of the body. Gentle stress reducing aromatherapy massage techniques have no significant effect. However, neuromuscular and deep tissue massage can be very beneficial. Many women with endometriosis have trigger points which contribute to the amount of pain they are experiencing.

Essential oils such as cypress, geranium and rose are recommended. Essential oils with analgesic and antispasmodic properties such as nutmeg, clary sage and Roman chamomile should be used in a massage oil over the abdomen and the hips.

Use of the essential oils in a bath is also recommended. Worwood recommends alternating hot and cold sitz or hip baths. Ideally the water should be waist deep. About 15 minutes should be spent in the hot sitz bath and 5 minutes in the cold sitz bath.[8]

Worwood recommends a blend of geranium, rose, cypress, nutmeg and clary sage to be added to the hot bath only. The entire treatment should be repeated two to four times, depending on the severity.[8]

Other Treatments

- Diet is very important. Avoid caffeine, salt, sugar, animal fats, dairy products, fried foods, red meats and junk foods.[7]
- The diet should include 50% raw vegetables and fruits. In addition, eat plenty of wholegrain products, raw nuts, seeds and fish. Eliminate shellfish from the diet.[7]
- There should be an emphasis on calcium-rich foods such as almonds, tahina, green leafy vegetables, sunflower seeds and hazel nuts. Calcium improves muscle tone and helps reduce menstrual cramps common in endometriosis sufferers.[7]
- Evening primrose oil is rich in GLA, necessary to keep the cardiovascular and nervous systems healthy. Endometriosis patients may find it helpful for dealing with depression and fatigue,

especially when there are side-effects from hormone therapy.[3]

- An infusion of freshly grated ginger eases menstrual pain due to the antispasmodic effects. An infusion of chamomile tea, lime flowers and passion flower is also effective for cramping. This may also assist in reducing tension and irritability.[3]

Vaginal Candidiasis

Useful Oils

• bergamot • German chamomile • lavender • myrrh • petitgrain • tea tree

Definition

Vaginal candidiasis, commonly known as thrush, is an infection with the fungus *Candida albicans*.

Clinical Features

Clinical features include intense vaginal and vulval pruritus, vulva soreness, vulvovaginal erythema, white curd-like discharge, discomfort with coitus and dysuria.[11]

Aetiology

Candida infections have been viewed for many years as minor infections that affect the mucous membranes such as the vagina passages and the mouth. However, *Candida albicans* is more than an opportunistic infection. It has now been associated with a range of conditions such as deranged immune system, food intolerance, gastric upsets and PMS.

Predisposing factors to candida overgrowth include decreased digestive secretions, dietary factors, impaired immunity, nutrient deficiency, drugs (especially antibiotics), impaired liver function, underlying liver function, underlying disease states and altered bowel flora.[12]

All persons on long-term antibiotics are at greater risk of severe forms of candida. Oral contraceptives or corticosteroids should not be taken until the condition improves as they can upset the balance of the *Candida albicans* organism.[7]

Therapeutic Strategy

The therapeutic strategy for treating candida is to:

- enhance immunity
- a number of dietary functions promote the overgrowth of candida
- manage food allergies
- promote detoxification
- recommend probiotics.[12]

Aromatherapy Treatment

The treatment consists of baths and local applications of essential oils. The oils chosen should have antiseptic, antifungal and immune-stimulant properties such as those found in German chamomile, geranium, lavender, petitgrain, myrrh and tea tree.

A sitz bath is also very effective for vaginal irritation. 2–3 drops of the essential oil should be added to a bidet or large bowl of warm water twice a day whilst symptoms persist.

Other Treatments

- Avoid all yeast-containing foods such as breads, mushrooms, Vegemite, Marmite, cheese, soya products, miso, beer, wine, and all preserved and pickled meats.[12, 25]
- Avoid all refined carbohydrates — sugars, soft drinks, pastries, canned fruits, chocolate, honey and dried fruits. Candida thrives in a sugary environment.[12, 25]
- Eliminate citrus and acid fruits (oranges, grapefruit, lemons, tomatoes, pineapples) from the diet for one month; then add back only twice weekly. These fruits are alkalising and candida thrives in an alkaline environment.[25]
- Garlic should be taken every day.[25]
- Supplement the diet with vitamin B12, B6, biotin and folic acid as they maintain the candida in the non-invasive form.[25]
- Eat yoghurt which contains acidophilus and will help to restore the natural balance of the bowel and vagina.[25]

Cystitis

Useful Oils

• bergamot • German chamomile • lavender • sandalwood • tea tree

Definition

Cystitis is an infection of the bladder, usually caused by some type of bacteria.[7]

Clinical Features

Nearly 85% of urinary tract infections are caused by *Escherichia coli*, a bacterium that is normally found in the intestines.[7]

In women, bacteria introduced by means of faecal contamination or from vaginal secretions can gain access to the bladder by travelling up through the urethra. Cystitis occurs more frequently in women than in men because of the proximity of the anus, vagina and urethra in females. This allows for relatively easy transmission of bacteria from the anus to the vagina and urethra, and thus to the bladder.[7]

The symptoms of cystitis include a frequent desire to pass urine, burning and pain during the passing of urine and a strong odour of the urine. There may be blood in the urine. The possibility of developing a bladder infection can be increased by many factors, such as sexual intercourse, the use of a diaphragm and pregnancy.[7]

Aetiology

Intense sexual activity can trigger signs and symptoms — hence the term 'honeymoon cystitis'. Urinating before and after intercourse and washing afterwards with cool water can help to prevent this. It can also occur during pregnancy when the foetus is pressing down on the bladder, preventing it from emptying.[7]

Often a yeast infection in the bowel is the culprit. Hyperacidity and stress can quickly bring on cystitis.[7]

Therapeutic Strategy

The therapeutic strategy for treating cystitis is to:

- enhance the flow of urine by achieving proper hydration
- promoting a pH which will inhibit the growth of the infectious organism
- enhance the immune system
- employ essential oils and botanical remedies with antimicrobial activity.[12]

Aromatherapy Treatment

The most beneficial oils in the treatment of cystitis are bergamot and tea tree, usually externally as a local wash and in the bath.[15] As with all use of essential oils on delicate mucous membranes, a very low dilution should be used.

A massage oil containing bergamot, lavender and German chamomile should be massaged over the lower abdomen.[15] Sandalwood oil has also been used as an urinary tract antiseptic.

If there is pus or blood in the urine, or a high temperature, it may be advisable to consult a medical doctor, because cystitis can quickly lead to more serious kidney infection.

Other Treatments

Nutrition

- Cranberry is considered one of the best herbal remedies for bladder infections. Balch says that a good quality cranberry juice produces hippuric acid in the urine, which acidifies the urine and inhibits bacterial growth. Other components in cranberry juice prevent bacteria from adhering to the lining of the bladder.[7] Research has found that 0.5 litres/day of cranberry juice is required to produce beneficial effects. Use pure, unsweetened juice.[7]
- Avoid citrus fruit because these produce alkaline urine that encourages bacterial growth. Increase acid content in the urine to inhibit bacterial growth.[7]
- It is important to drink lots of water every day, but avoid tea and coffee.[3]
- Drink raw vegetable and fruit juices, especially carrot, celery, cucumber, watermelon and parsley, every day.[3]
- Vitamin C, 1,000 mg three times daily, can act as a urinary antiseptic.[3]
- Include celery, parsley and watermelon in your diet. These foods act as natural diuretics and cleansers.[7]
- Avoid the consumption of excessive amounts of sugar as people with high blood sugar levels are more susceptible to recurrent infections.[3]
- Acidophilus will replace some of the 'friendly' bacteria, especially if antibiotics have been prescribed.[3]

Herbs

- Diuretics can help to cleanse the system. Dandelion tea acts as liver cleanser and diuretic. Bearberry and uva ursi act as mild diuretics and antiseptics.[7]
- Goldenseal is considered one of the most effective antimicrobial herbs.[7]
- Buchu is recommended for a bladder infection with a burning sensation upon urination.[7]
- Garlic should be taken every day.[3]
- Marshmallow root increases the acidity of urine, inhibiting bacterial growth.[7]

General Advice

- Increase urine flow by increasing the amount of liquids consumed. Ensure the liquids are pure water, herbal teas and fresh fruit and vegetable juices diluted with at least an equal amount of water.[12]
- Good hygiene — wipe the vulva from front to back to avoid wiping anal bacteria onto the urethra.[3]
- Use sanitary pads rather than tampons.[7]
- Avoid excessive consumption of analgesic drugs as they can irritate the urinary tract.[3]

References

1. Tortora G, Anagnostakos N. *Principles of anatomy and physiology*. 4th edn, Harper & Row Publishers, New York, 1984.

2. Van de Graaff K, Fox S. *Concepts of human anatomy & physiology*. 3rd edn, Wm.C. Publishers, USA, 1992.
3. Cabot S. *Women's health*. Pan Macmillam Publishers, Australia, 1987.
4. Balacs T. *Hormones and health*. The International Journal of Aromatherapy 1993; 5(1): 18–20.
5. Guenier J. *Essential obstetrics*. The International Journal of Aromatherapy 1992; 4(1): 6–8.
6. Waters B. *Massage during pregnancy*. Research Triangle Publishing Inc, USA, 1995.
7. Balch J, Balch P. *Prescription for nutritional healing*. Avery Publishing Group, USA, 1997.
8. Worwood V. *The fragrant pharmacy*. Macmillan London Limited, England, 1990.
9. Tiran D. *Clinical aromatherapy for pregnancy and childbirth*. 2nd edn, Churchill Livingstone, UK, 2000.
10. Burns E, Blamey C. *Soothing scents in childbirth*. The International Journal of Aromatherapy 1994; 6(1): 24–28.
11. Murtagh J. *General practice*. 2nd edn, The McGraw-Hill Companies Inc, Australia, 1998.
12. Pizzorno J, Murray M. *A text book of natural medicine*. 2nd edn, Churchill Livingstone, UK, 1999.
13. Hoffman D. *The new holistic herbal*. USA, Element Books Limited, 1983.
14. Mowrey D. *The scientific validation of herbal medicine*. Keats Publishing, USA, 1986.
15. Davis P. *Aromatherapy: An A–Z*. 2nd edn, The C.W. Daniel Company Limited, Great Britain, 1998.
16. Lavabre M. *Aromatherapy workbook*. 2nd edn, Healing Arts Press, USA, 1997.
17. Ryman D. *Aromatherapy*. Piatkus Press, England, 1991.
18. Mailhebiau P. *Portraits in oils*. The C.W. Daniel Company Limited, Great Britain, 1995.
19. Duke J. *The green pharmacy*. Rodale Press, USA, 1997.
20. Krupp M, Chatton M. *Current medical diagnosis & treatment*. Lange Medical Publications, USA, 1980.
21. Beckman N. *The family library guide to natural therapies*. Family Library, Australia, 1992.
22. Tyler V. *Herbs of choice*. Haworth Press, USA, 1993.
23. Kersley E. *Female menopause*. Australia, 1983.
24. Mercer B. *Menopausal relief without HRT*. The Perfect Potion Aromatherapy Newsletter, 1996; 4.
25. Osiecki H. *The physician's handbook of clinical nutrition*. Bioconcepts Publishing, Australia, 1990.

The Integumentary System

Objectives

After careful study of this chapter, you should be able to:

- describe a range of skin lesions
- discuss the procedure for examining the skin
- identify, list and describe common pathophysiologies of the integumentary system
- explain the aromatherapy treatment for specific conditions and disorders of the integumentary system
- explain the role of other holistic strategies for specific conditions and disorders of the integumentary system.

Structure of the Integumentary System

The integumentary system consists of the skin and the subcutaneous layer that contains structures extending from the skin. The skin itself consists of three main layers. These are the:

- epidermis, or the outermost layer, which is divided into strata or layers, and is made entirely of epithelial cells with no blood vessels
- dermis, or true skin, which has a framework of connective tissue and contains many blood vessels, nerve endings, and glands
- hypodermis, or the subcutaneous layer — consisting of loose connective tissue and fat.[1]

Functions of the Integumentary System

Although the integumentary system has many functions, the three that are most important are:

- protection of deeper tissues against drying and invasion of pathogenic organisms and their toxins through a mechanical barrier
- regulation of body temperature by dissipation of heat to the surrounding air
- receipt of information about the environment by means of nerve endings that are profusely distributed throughout the skin.[2]

The outermost layer of the skin, the stratum corneum, protects the body against invasion by pathogens and against drying. These dry, dead cells, composed of keratin, are found in a tight, interlocking pattern that is impervious to penetration by organisms and by water. The outermost cells are constantly being shed, causing the mechanical removal of pathogens.

The regulation of body temperature, the loss of excess heat as well as protection from cold, is a very important function of the skin. Indeed, most of the blood that flows through the skin is concerned with temperature regulation. The skin forms a large surface for radiating body heat into the air. When the blood vessels dilate, more blood is brought to the surface so that heat can be dissipated. The activation of the sweat glands and the evaporation of sweat from the surface of the body also helps cool the body. In cold conditions, the flow of blood in the veins deep in the subcutaneous tissue serves to heat the skin and protect deeper tissues from excess heat loss.

Observations of the Skin

The identification of skin problems depends on astute clinical skills based on a systemic history and examination and, of course, experience. If you are in doubt it is preferable to refer your client to a skilled co-operative therapist or medical practitioner who has experience in identifying the skin lesions.

Terminology of Skin Lesions

A lesion is a pathologic change of the tissues due to disease or injury. Lesions are described by their appearance, location, colour and size.

Abscess: a localised collection of pus in a cavity less than 1 cm in diameter formed by necrosis of tissue.[4]

Atrophy: thinning or loss of the epidermis and/or dermis with loss of normal skin markings. Atrophic skin is thin, translucent and wrinkled with easily visible blood vessels.[4]

Atrophic scar: settles below the skin surface.[3]

Blackhead: an open comedo.[3]

Bulla: a vesicle larger than 1 cm in diameter.[4]

Carbuncle: a cluster of boils discharging through several openings.[4]

Comedo: a plug of keratin and sebum in a dilated sebaceous gland.[4]

Crust: a superficial dried secretion (serum and exudate).[4]

Cyst: a nodule consisting of an epithelial-lined cavity filled with fluid or semisolid material.[4]

Erosion: a skin defect with complete or partial loss of the dermis; they heal without scarring.[4]

Fissure: a linear split in the epidermis and dermis.[3, 4]

Furuncle: a purulent infected hair follicle.[4]

Hypertropic scar: rises above the skin surface.[3]

Keloid: overgrowth of dense fibrous tissue extending beyond the original wound.[4]

Lichenification: thickening secondary to chronic scratching or rubbing (in dermatitis).[4]

Macule: a discoloured, flat skin lesion such as a freckle or flat mole that is less than 1 cm in diameter.[4]

Nodule: similar to a papule but larger than 0.5 cm in diameter.[4]

Papule: a small, solid, raised skin lesion that is less than 0.5 cm in diameter.[4]

Plaque: a solid raised lesion that is greater than 2 cm in diameter. Plaques are rarely more than 5 mm in height and can be considered as extended papules.[4]

Pustule: a visible collection of pus in a blister. Pustules may indicate infection, but not always, as pustules are seen in psoriasis which is not infected.[4]

Scale: a flaking or dry patch made up of an excess of dead epidermal cells. Scales usually indicate inflammatory change and thickening of the epidermis.[4]

Scar: a healed dermal lesion where normal structures are replaced by fibrous tissue.[4]

Ulcer: a circumscribed deep defect with loss of all the epidermis and part or all of the dermis; they usually heal with scarring.[4]

Vesicle: a fluid-filled blister less than 0.5 cm in diameter.[4]

Wheal: a smooth, slightly elevated, swollen area that is redder or paler than the surrounding skin that is usually accompanied by itching; for example, an insect bite or an allergic reaction.[4]

Whitehead: a closed comedo.[3]

Classifying Dermatological Conditions

Most of the common dermatological problems fall into one of the categories as follows:[3]

Common Dermatological Problems

Infections		
	Bacterial	• impetigo
	Viral	• warts
		• *Herpes simplex, H. zoster*
	Fungal	• tinea
		• candidiasis
Acne		
Psoriasis		
Atopic dermatitis (eczema)		
Urticaria		
	Acute and chronic	
	Papular	• pediculosis
		• scabies
		• insect bites
Sun-related skin cancer		
Drug-related eruptions		

Hoffman classifies skin conditions into the following causes:[5]

Internal causes, where the origins of a skin disease are the result of internal disharmonies, as in psoriasis or eczema.

External causes, where the skin problem is a direct result of external influences, as with wounds, bruises or sunburns.

Internal reaction to external factors, where the skin problems are due to the body's inability to cope with external factors, such as allergic eczema or skin infections due to bacteria or fungi.

Examining the Skin

Taking a History

There are three basic questions that need to be asked:[3]

1. Where is the rash and where did it start?
2. How long have you had the rash? Refer to the table below that will be of assistance with this question.
3. Is the rash itchy? If so, is it mild, moderate or severe? The nature of the itch is very helpful diagnostically.

How long has the rash been present?[3]

Acute (hours–days)	urticaria atopic dermatitis insect bites drugs
Acute — chronic (days–weeks)	atopic dermatitis impetigo scabies pediculosis drugs *Pityriasis rosea* psoriasis tinea candida
Chronic (weeks–months)	psoriasis tinea warts cancers

Further questions to ask include:[3]

- Do you or have you been in contact with a person with a similar eruption?
- What medicines are you taking or have you taken recently?
- Have you worn any new clothing recently?
- Have you been exposed to anything different recently?
- Do you have a past history of a similar rash or eczema or an allergic tendency — for example, asthma?
- Is there a family history of skin problems?

The Nature of the Itching

The characteristics of the itch can be a very useful tool in identifying the condition. While the following table is very helpful, nothing is absolute; for example, tinea and psoriasis are sometimes itchy and sometimes not.[3]

Is the rash itchy?[3]

Very itchy	urticaria atopic dermatitis insect bites chickenpox (adults)
Mild to moderate itchy	*P. rosea* psoriasis drugs tinea candida stress itching/ lichen simplex
Often not itchy	psoriasis, impetigo tinea warts cancers seborrhoeic dermatitis

General Considerations

In the treatment of skin diseases the following holistic approaches are essential:

- Attention to dietary and lifestyle factors is of paramount importance.
- Use holistic principles for restoring vitality and resistance, building health rather than killing a disease.
- Treat the obvious cause according to the properties of the essential oils and the pathology of the diseases — for example, use an antiseptic oil to treat an infection.
- Treat the underlying cause following philosophical or holistic principles applied to the observation of symptoms and what they reveal.
- Treat symptoms.

When treating skin problems, you need to have patience, as improvement is rarely dramatic and treatment needs to be continued for several months. Beckman says that the estimated time that it will take to treat certain skin conditions such as eczema and dermatitis is one month for every year suffered by the client.[6]

Aromatherapy Considerations

An extensive amount of research has been done on the use of essential oils for skin problems. German chamomile has been reported to have an anti-inflammatory property.[7] The effect of chamomile was tested on 14 patients following dermabrasion of tattoos. It was note that the healing and drying process was significantly increased.[8]

The effects of tea tree oil and benzyl peroxide in the treatment of acne were compared. Tea tree oil was found to reduce the number of inflamed and non-inflamed lesions more slowly, but fewer side effects were experienced by those treated with tea tree oil.[9]

From the above studies it can be seen that essential oils are particularly valuable because they are able to address skin conditions on a variety of levels. The therapeutic properties of essential oils which are beneficial for the integumentary system are:

Alterative

Skin diseases traditionally associated with toxaemia or septicaemia and many cases of eczema and urticaria can be managed by alteratives. An alterative's primary aim is to detoxify.[11] Essential oils such as carrot seed, everlasting and juniper berry are beneficial.

Antiseptic

The antiseptic property of essential oils is well known. For cuts, infections such as acne and boils, and insect bites, essential oils such as eucalyptus, tea tree, lavender and lemon can be used.

Anti-inflammatory

For the treatment of eczema, infected wounds and bruises, essential oils such as German and Roman chamomile, everlasting, lavender, sandalwood and yarrow are beneficial.

Antipruritic

An antipruritic will relieve the sensation of itching or prevent its occurrence. Essential oils such as German and Roman chamomile, lavender, peppermint and sandalwood can be used.

Astringent

Astringents are beneficial where the skin is broken and discharging. Astringent essential oils such as cypress and lemon can reduce discharge, sepsis and promote healing.

Cicatrisant and Cytophylactic

To encourage cell regeneration for the treatment of burns, cuts, scars and stretch marks, essential oils such as German chamomile, everlasting, frankincense, geranium, lavender, myrrh, rose and neroli and are recommended.

Demulcent

Demulcents are helpful in reducing itching and inflammatory pain due to skin diseases. Sandalwood is considered an excellent demulcent.

Fungicidal

For the treatment of fungal infections such as athlete's foot and candida, essential oils such as lavender, tea tree, myrrh and patchouli are recommended.

Vulnerary

A vulnerary is a remedy that promotes healing of wounds. Essential oils such as berg-amot, cajeput, German chamomile and Roman chamomile, frankincense, everlasting, geranium, lavender, myrrh, niaouli, rosemary, sage, tea tree, thyme and yarrow are recommended.

Associated Conditions

Acne

Useful Oils

• bergamot • cajeput • geranium • juniper berry • lavender • lemon • lime • mandarin • neroli • niaouli • palmarosa • petitgrain • rosemary • rose otto • sandalwood • tea tree

Definition

Acne is a chronic inflammation of the pilosebaceous units, producing comedones, papules, pustules, cysts and scars.[4]

Clinical Features

Acne is most common in adolescence. It is slightly less common in girls and worse around 14 with premenstrual exacerbations.[3] It affects regions of the skin containing large sebaceous glands — that is, the face, back and upper anterior chest. The lesion consists of closed (white) or open (black) comedones (blackheads), papules, pustules, nodules and abscesses.[3]

The lesion begins in the upper portion of the follicular canal, with hyperkeratinisation being the first microscopic change. This leads to blockage of the canal, resulting in dilation and thinning. Eventually a comedo is formed. The formation of open or closed comedones appears to be related to the degree of keratinisation and the level of blockage of the duct. Once exposed to the air the contents of the comedone oxidises and turns black, and a blackhead can be seen. However, if the top of the opening is closed, and oxidation cannot take place, it becomes a whitehead.[10]

Aetiology

Acne vulgaris is the most common of all skin problems.[3] The onset of *A. vulgaris* reflects an increase in pilosebaceous gland size and sebum secretion due to androgenic stimulation. The severity and progression are determined by a complex interaction between hormones, keratinisation, sebum and bacteria.[10]

Despite a large amount of purulent exudate in pustular and cystic lesions, the only bacteria commonly cultured are normal skin species: *Pripionibacterium acnes* and *Staphylococcus albus*. These microbes are believed to release lipases that hydrolyse sebum triglycerides into free fatty acid lipoperoxides, thus promoting an inflammatory cascade.[10]

Acne is considered to be an androgen-dependent condition. Androgens control the sebaceous gland secretion and exacerbate the development of abnormal keratinising follicular epithelium.[3,4,10,11]

Therapeutic Strategy

Acne is a multifactorial condition requiring an integrated therapeutic approach:

- unblock pores
- decrease bacteria in the sebum
- decrease sebaceous gland activity
- keep the affected area as free of oil as possible.[3,4]

Many adolescents will find acne very stressful as they are concerned about their appearance. Sympathetic care and reassurance is required.[3,4]

Aromatherapy Treatment

Essential oils can assist in the management of acne by:

- helping to clear the infection
- reducing the amount of sebum produced
- minimising the extent of scarring and to promote healing
- reducing inflammation
- reducing stress and anxiety
- helping the body to eliminate toxins.

The antiseptic property of tea tree is well known for the treatment of acne. Clinical trials using a 5% tea tree solution were found to demonstrate similar beneficial effects as 5% benzyl peroxide in acne, but with fewer side-effects.[4]

However, it has been suggested that a 5% tea tree solution is probably not strong enough for moderate to severe acne. Stronger solutions (up to 15%) may provide better results.[10]

Other essential oils known for their antiseptic properties that may be used in the treatment of acne include bergamot, lemon, niaouli and petitgrain.

Essential oils such as geranium and palmarosa balance sebum production.[12,13] Rose otto is beneficial because it is highly antiseptic and reduces stress.[13]

Many aromatherapists recommend the use of vegetable oils such as jojoba as a base for essential oils. Saunders recommends jojoba because of its fine texture, and it is the most suitable for oily skin. She also suggests using hazelnut oil, as it is slightly astringent and is suited for oily skin.[14]

Massage is useful as it stimulates the circulation and helps the body to eliminate toxins. Essential oils such as rosemary, geranium and juniper can be used in a body massage to stimulate the lymphatic system.[12,13] To minimise the possibility of scarring, use essential oils such as neroli, sandalwood and true lavender in wheatgerm.

Carrot-infused oil is beneficial for its high beta-carotene content, which helps heal scar tissue. Hypericum- and calendula-infused oil are recommended as they both enhance wound healing and have anti-inflammatory properties.

While vegetable and infused oils may be a useful carrier medium, be careful, as excessive use of base oils tends to clog the pores and will exacerbate acne. Many people with acne may shun the idea of using an oily preparation on skin which already is quite oily.

Compresses, facial saunas, water-based creams and lotions, plant-derived gel bases and the use of dispersants to make aqueous extracts of essential oils are the preferred methods of application.

Other Treatments

The following guidelines and recommendations may be beneficial in the management of acne.

General Advice

- Avoid oily or creamy cosmetics and all moisturisers. Use cosmetics sparingly.[3]
- Avoid picking and squeezing blackheads. To do so is to risk increasing the inflammation by causing breaks in the skin in which harmful bacteria can lodge. Do not touch the affected area unless your hands have been thoroughly cleaned.[3]
- Avoid stress as it can affect hormonal changes which in turn may cause acne flare-ups.
- Ultraviolet light such as sunlight may help improve acne. Many dermatologists recommend at least 15 minutes of sunshine each day.[3,15]
- Benzyl peroxide is an active ingredient found in many over-the-counter acne preparations. While it may be helpful, it is extremely drying on the skin and has been known to cause allergic reactions.

Nutrition

- While conventional medicine suggests that diet is not considered to be a contributing factor, Osiecki and Pizzorno recommend high-protein diets and low-carbohydrate diets.[10,11]
- Food high in iodine should be eliminated, and milk consumption should be limited.[10,11,15]
- Avoid all refined sugars, saturated fats and processed foods.[11]
- Improve digestion by taking digestive enzymes or apple cider vinegar with meals.[11]
- Increase the intake of foods rich in zinc and vitamin A. Retinols, including oral vitamin A, have been shown in many studies to reduce sebum production and hyperkeratosis of sebaceous follicles.[10,11]
- Zinc is important in the treatment of acne. It is involved in local hormone activation, retinol-binding protein formation, wound healing, immune system activity and tissue regeneration.[10,11,15]
- Menstrual-related acne responds to vitamin B6. This reflects its role in the normal metabolism of steroid hormones.[10,11]

Herbs

- Alfalfa, burdock root, dandelion root herbs will detoxify the body and echinacea will stimulate the immune system.[15]
- Beckman recommends burdock root, echinacea, evening primrose oil, fenugreek, lemongrass, red clover and sarsaparilla as the herbs that should be used internally and suggests using herbs such as calendula and goldenseal externally.[6]
- Saunders recommends lemon juice. Pure lemon juice can be used neat, or in a mix with water. It is beneficial for oily skin, has astringent, anti-inflammatory powers and also cleanses the pores.[14]

Boils and Carbuncles

Useful Oils

• bergamot • carrot seed • geranium • grapefruit • juniper berry • lavender • lemon • rosemary • tea tree • thyme

Definition

A boil is an inflamed, infected lump, on or under the skin, as a result of a staphylococcus infection. A carbuncle is a close collection of boils filled with pus.

Clinical Features

Boils often appear on the scalp, buttocks, face and underarms. They are tender, red, inflamed, painful and can appear suddenly. Within 24 hours they become red and filled with pus. Swelling of the nearest lymph glands often occurs and the glands become swollen and tender.[15]

Boils are contagious. The pus that drains when a boil opens can contaminate the skin, causing more boils, or it can enter the blood, causing septicaemia. If the boils are very large, medicinal assistance may be required.[15]

Aetiology

Boils may be caused by a bacterial infection, an airborne or food allergy, stress, poor hygiene, an illness, a lowered resistance, certain drugs, poor nutrition, an infected wound, a toxic bowel and bloodstream, or thyroid disorders. They may be caused when the deepest portion of the hair follicle becomes infected and the inflammation spreads, often with staphylococcus bacteria. Constipation is also a common underlying cause.

Therapeutic Strategy

The most effective treatment for a boil is a hot compress with essential oils. This will 'draw out' a boil and speed healing. It is also important to purify and detoxify the blood and enhance the immune system.

Aromatherapy Treatment

The most suitable essential oils to use in a hot compress are tea tree, bergamot and true lavender because of their antiseptic properties. The area around the boil should be washed several times a day with a 1–3% dilution of lavender or bergamot.

If numerous or recurring boils are evident, there is a need to reduce the level of toxicity in the body. Regular massages and baths using detoxifying oils such as juniper berry, carrot seed, geranium, grapefruit and rosemary are considered beneficial.

Other Treatments

Nutrition

- The diet should be especially high in fruit and vegetables.[10]
- 3,000 to 8,000 mg daily of vitamin C. Vitamin C is an anti-inflammatory and an immune system stimulant.[15]
- Garlic should be taken daily to detoxify the body and stimulate the immune system.[10]

Herbs

- Prepare a detoxifying blend of herbs such as burdock root, red clover and yellow dock daily.[15,16] Mix equal parts of each herb and place a teaspoon of the herbal blend into a cup of boiling water, allow it to steep for 10 minutes, and drink. Repeat this three times a day.
- Echinacea and goldenseal help to cleanse the lymph glands.[15]

General Advice

- It is important to never squeeze or pop a boil. This may cause the infection to go deeper into the body.[17]
- Poultices will bring the boil to a head much faster. Some poultices often used include:
    - Mix half a tablespoon of slippery elm with one tablespoon of linseed oil. Add a teaspoon of charcoal. Apply to the boil as a poultice.
    - Take a handful of comfrey roots, grind up in a pulp and apply to the boil as a poultice.
    - Onion poultice. Apply pieces of onion wrapped in a cloth.[17]
- If a compress does not drain the boil, a doctor may be required to lance the boil.[17]

Burns

Useful Oils

• bergamot • carrot seed • everlasting • frankincense • lavender • lemon • manuka • neroli • tea tree

Definition

The severity of the burn is determined by how deep it is and how much of the surface area it covers. There are three basic classifications of burns:

- **First degree** burns affect only the outer layer of the skin, causing redness and sensitivity to touch. Sunburn is usually a first degree burn.[17,18]
- **Second degree** burns involve all layers of the epidermis and possibly the dermis. The burn area is small and is characterised by redness, blistering and acute pain.[17,18]
- **Third degree** burns go right down to the bottom of the dermis, destroying hair shafts, sebaceous glands, sweat glands and nerve endings. The skin may be red, or it may be white or yellowish, or leathery and black. There is usually little or no pain because the nerves in the skin are severely damaged.[17,18]

Therapeutic Strategy

Follow standard first aid procedures for the management and treatment of burns. Cool a first or second degree burn at once to reduce pain and swelling. Immerse the burn in cool running water until the body has returned to normal temperature (up to 10 minutes).[17]

- After the burn has been cooled, apply an aloe vera gel to ease the pain and promote healing.
- Do not apply any vegetable oils, greasy ointments or butter on burns.[18]
- Do not break the blisters.[18]
- Cover the burn with a sterile, non-stick dressing.[18]

If you suspect a third degree burn seek urgent medical attention. The burn is deep (full thickness) — the skin may look white, or may be black and charred. Do not attempt to treat the burn or do not remove clothing that is stuck to the burned area. A third degree burn requires immediate medical treatment.

Aromatherapy Treatment

Lavender's reputation for the treatment of burns was possibly the catalyst for aromatherapy itself. If Gattefosse had not been accidentally burnt and used lavender to treat the burn, aromatherapy as we know it today would probably not exist. In his own words he describes the benefits of lavender:

> *The external application of small quantities of essences rapidly stops the spread of gangrenous sores. In my personal experience, after a laboratory explosion covered me with burning substances which I extinguished by rolling on a grassy lawn, both of my hands were covered with a rapidly developing gas gangrene. Just one rinse with lavender essence stopped 'the gasification of the tissue'. This treatment was followed by profuse sweating and healing began the next day.*[19]

Mailhebiau recommends using lavender with hypericum-infused oil for the treatment of burns. He also suggests adding carrot seed essential oil to help regenerate the skin for someone who has suffered even serious burns.[20]

Davis recommends pouring neat lavender onto a sterile gauze and applying this to the burn. The gauze should be renewed every few hours. She attributes lavender's remarkable properties for the treatment of burns because of its analgesic properties, its ability to promote rapid healing and its ability to reduce scarring.[12]

Tea tree oil is also highly recommended for the treatment of burns and may be used together with lavender oil.[12]

Other Treatments

- Aloe vera pulp, gel or liquid can be applied to the burn as needed to relieve pain and speed healing.[15,16]
- Drink plenty of water during the healing phase.[15]
- Keep the burn lightly covered to minimise the chance of a bacterial infection.[15]
- Balch recommends 10,000 mg of Vitamin C immediately after the burn and 2,000 mg three times a day thereafter until the burn has healed.[15]

Eczema and Dermatitis

Useful Oils

• bergamot • carrot seed
• Atlas and Virginian cedarwood
• German chamomile • everlasting • juniper berry
• lavender • myrrh • palmarosa • patchouli
• sandalwood • tea tree • yarrow

Definition

The terms dermatitis and eczema are often used synonymously. Dermatitis can be divided into exogenous causes (allergic contact and primary irritant) and endogenous, which implies all forms of dermatitis not directly related to external causative factors.[3] Eczema is a non-infectious inflammatory condition of the skin.[4] The dermatitis–eczema group of skin diseases includes the following:

- contact dermatitis, being either toxic or allergic in origin
- atopic dermatitis
- seborrhoeic dermatitis
- photodermatitis.[11]

Clinical Features and Aetiology

Contact Dermatitis

Contact dermatitis is an acute or chronic inflammation that results from direct contact with chemicals or other irritants.[11] Lesions are often on exposed parts of the body. The lesions consist of erythematous macules, papules and vesicles. Signs and symptoms often include itching, burning and stinging of the skin, the affected area is often red, hot and swollen with exudation, crusting and secondary infection.

Contact dermatitis is caused by an allergen that provokes an allergic reaction in some people. It is due to delayed hypersensitivity. The location will often suggest the cause: the scalp suggests hair tints or shampoos, the face suggests cosmetic products and the hands suggest cleaning substances or chemicals that may have been handled during work.

While the dermatitis is initially confined to the site of contact, the irritation or increased hypersensitivity may cause the dermatitis to spread to other parts of the body. Generally, dermatitis may be provoked by a few substances; however, the patient may eventually develop hypersensitivity to many substances.

Atopic Dermatitis or Eczema

The term 'atopic' refers to a hereditary background or tendency to develop one or more of a group of conditions such as allergic rhinitis, asthma, eczema, skin sensitivities and urticaria. Atopic eczema is a constitutional condition marked by papules, especially of the flexural surfaces of the knees and elbows, with itching. Itching is often extremely severe and prolonged, leading to emotional disturbances.[3,11]

There is a family history of allergic manifestations such as asthma, allergic rhinitis and eczema. It may begin in the first few months of life, remissions frequently recur during childhood, adolescence and adulthood.[3] Intolerance to primary irritants is common; emotional stress, environmental temperature or humidity changes, bacterial skin infections and wool garments also commonly cause exacerbations.[3]

Seborrhoeic Dermatitis

An inflammatory scaling condition of the scalp, face and occasionally other parts of the body.[4] Endogenous and genetic factors and an overgrowth of commensal yeast *Pityrosporum ovale* seem to be involved.[3,4] Infants within the first month of life may develop seborrheic dermatitis, with a thick, yellow, crusted scalp lesion (cradle cap), fissuring and yellow scaling behind the ear.

Photodermatitis

Photodermatitis is an acute or chronic inflammatory skin reaction due to overexposure or hypersensitivity to sunlight, other sources of electromagnetic rays or photosensitisation of the skin by certain essential oils or drugs.

Therapeutic Strategy

While the aetiology of dermatitis may vary, the holistic treatment principles do not differ in principle. In managing dermatitis it is important to consider the following factors:

- Lifestyle and dietary factors are of utmost importance. Check for allergies in the diet. In particular, be wary of dairy products, especially implicated in the onset of childhood eczema. The avoidance of common allergens such as cows' milk, eggs, cheese, foods with food additives and refined sugars should be undertaken.[11]
- Test for food or chemical hypersensitivity. Common contact sensitivities include cosmetics, hair dyes, shampoos, fragrances, insecticides, aerosol allergens such as polishes, nasal sprays, synthetic resins, toothpastes, salicylate-rich food, detergents, soaps and lanolin.[11]
- The use of alteratives to promote detoxification.
- The use of essential oils that are anti-inflammatory.

Aromatherapy Treatment

Essential oils and aromatherapy has proven to be beneficial for the management of eczema and dermatitis. Application of antipruritics such as German chamomile, true lavender and sandalwood will reduce the sensations of itching. This will also help to reduce the degree of physical trauma caused by the scratching.

Essential oils with anti-inflammatory and vulnerary properties such as German chamomile, everlasting and yarrow applied topically will enhance the healing of skin lesions.

An astringent essential oil such as juniper berry used topically will reduce any 'weeping' or oozing of fluids. If an infection is present it will be necessary to include essential oils with antimicrobial properties such as tea tree or true lavender. Eczema is often seen as an attempt by the body to eliminate accumulated toxins through the skin.[12] Detoxifying essential oils such as carrot seed, rosemary, everlasting and rock rose should be used in a blend if the treatment strategy is to assist in the elimination of toxins.

In many situations eczema and dermatitis are triggered by stress[3,11], therefore essential oils which will help one deal with the 'stressors' will be valuable. Essential oils which are relaxants, such as bergamot, Roman chamomile, Atlas or Virginian cedarwood, lavender, geranium, sandalwood and ylang ylang, will play an important role in reducing the level of stress.

It is important to treat the clinical type and stage of eczema appropriately. According to Weiss, the basic rule for treating acute weeping eczema is 'wet on wet'. This means using wet dressings that have been bathed in solutions containing essential oils. Apply for 30 minutes three or four times a day.[21]

Moist compresses are needed until the weeping stage and acute inflammation have passed. The compresses or dressings should be loose, moist, and allow plenty of evaporation. The most effective essential oils to use would be German chamomile, yarrow, everlasting, myrrh, lavender and juniper berry.

With chronic dry lesions the essential oils are best applied topically using ointments and emollient creams. Essential oils such as German chamomile, Indian or Australian sandalwood, true lavender, palmarosa and patchouli are beneficial and should be used in a 1% dilution.

Other Holistic Treatments

Nutrition

- A diet rich in omega-3 fatty acids is recommended. This can be achieved by either fish oil supplements or by eating cold-water fish such as mackerel, herring and salmon. This increases the eicosapentaenoic fatty acid level, which has been shown to reduce the incidence of eczema.[11]
- Include high-quality cold-pressed sunflower, safflower or linseed oil in the diet. Evening primrose oil normalises the essential fatty acid imbalances and reduces symptoms of eczema.[11,15]
- Avoid dairy products, sugar, refined and processed foods, fats and fried foods in your diet.[15]
- A gluten-free diet is often of therapeutic benefit in controlling dermatitis.[15]

Herbs

Hoffman recommends the alterative herbs as the internal treatment of eczema. He recommends the leafy alteratives such as nettle and red clover rather than the rooty alteratives which he says tend to be more active on the liver and are often too strong for eczema, aggravating rather than healing the problem.[5]

Tyler suggests the use of tannin-containing herbs such as witch hazel leaves, oak bark and English walnut leaves. He recommends using witch hazel extract topically to relieve local inflammation of the skin.[22]

General Advice

- Patients with phototoxic dermatitis should avoid exposure to light.[11]
- Avoid scratching the lesions.[11]

Herpes Simplex

Useful Oils

• bergamot • cajeput • geranium • lemon • melissa • niaouli • ravensara • rose otto • tea tree

Definition

Herpes simplex is a common infection caused by the *H. simplex* virus which can cause a vesicular rash anywhere on the skin or mucous membranes.[3]

Clinical Features

There are two major antigenic strains of herpes:

- Type I (*H. simplex* or *H. labialis*) is recognised by cold sores and skin eruptions. It can also cause an inflammation of the cornea of the eye. If the eye becomes infected, refer to a medical practitioner immediately.[3,15]
- Type II (genital herpes) is sexually transmitted and is the most prevalent herpes infection. This viral infection can range in severity from a silent infection to a serious inflammation of the liver with fever, severe brain damage and stillbirths. Babies can pick up the virus in the birth canal, risking brain damage, blindness and death.[3,15]

H. simplex is contagious. It is present in saliva and can be spread in a family by sharing of drinking and eating utensils and toothbrushes, or by kissing.[3] The virus then remains in the body, and repeated outbreaks may be triggered by fever, a cold, or other viral infection, exposure to the sun and wind, stress, or depression of the immune system.[3,15]

The first sign of a developing cold sore is local tenderness with a small bump. The bump turns into a blister and there is tenderness in the area. The adjacent lymph nodes may become swollen and tender. Recurrences may be precipitated by many factors such as:

- sunburn
- sexual activity
- menses
- stress
- food allergies
- drugs
- certain foods.[10]

Therapeutic Strategy

Enhancement of the immune system is the key to controlling the herpes infection.[13] In addition, it is important to control food allergies and to manage stress.

Aromatherapy Treatment

Essential oils have been successfully used for the treatment of herpes. The antiviral properties of melissa extracts have now been recognised and the immediate application of melissa and other essential oils often prevents the viruses from replicating.[19,23]

Wabner suggests three applications of undiluted melissa oil directly onto the blister, for one day. The herpes usually disappears within 24 hours.[23] Care must be taken to apply the oil only to the blister as melissa may cause irritation on the surrounding skin. For children, he suggests blending melissa with rose otto to reduce the risk of irritation.

Davis recommends using bergamot, tea tree and eucalyptus oil. She says that these oils should be applied very quickly at the first signs of eruption. Prepare these oils in an alcohol base. She recommends 6 drops of each of the above essential oils into 5 mL of alcohol. Dabbing this blend at first onset will often stop blisters from developing.[10]

Other Treatments

Nutrition

- 5,000 to 10,000 mg of vitamin C daily will prevent and inhibit the growth of the virus.[15]
- Oral supplements of zinc (50 mg/day) have been beneficial in clinical studies.[10,15]
- 300 to 1,200 mg daily of the amino acid lysine, together with a diet low in its contrasting amino acid arginine (avoid peanuts, chocolate, seeds and cereals), is beneficial because lysine inhibits the growth of *H. simplex* virus and arginine stimulates its growth.[10,15]
- Avoid alcohol, processed foods, colas, white flour products, sugar, refined carbohydrates, coffee and drugs to lessen the chance of an outbreak.[15]
- Do not consume citrus fruits and juices while the virus is active.[15]

Herbs

- Herbal treatment for herpes should include echinacea, goldenseal, myrrh and red clover.
- Melissa herbal extract and liquorice root have topical antiviral activity and inhibit the growth and cell-damaging effects of *H. simplex.*[10,15,24]

General Advice

- Get plenty of rest and reduce stress.[15]

Psoriasis

Useful Oils

- bergamot • cajeput • carrot seed
- German chamomile • evening primrose oil
- calendula-infused oil • everlasting • juniper berry
- lavender • sandalwood • yarrow

Definition

Psoriasis is a common benign, acute or chronic and recurrent inflammatory disease characterised by dry, well-circumscribed, silvery, scaling papules and plaques of various sizes.

Clinical Features

Psoriasis is a classic example of a hyperproliferative skin disorder. The rate of cellular division rate in psoriatic lesions is 1,000 times greater than normal skin.[10] The normal period from new skin cell to desquamation is 28 days, but for psoriasis sufferers this is reduced to 4 days. Psoriasis first appears on the body as small dull red patches covered with dry silvery scales.[10]

Areas usually affected are the elbows, knees, lower back, ears and scalp. There may be itching and the nails can be affected. Remission is common.

Psoriasis is occasionally eruptive, particularly during periods of stress. While general health is not usually affected, the psychological stress of an unsightly skin disease often compounds the problem.

Aetiology

Causes are difficult to determine but they are generally regarded as metabolic disturbances as psoriasis affects the entire body, not just the skin. Indications include:[10]

- Some lesions are closely associated with a deficiency of essential fatty acids.
- Incomplete protein digestion or poor intestinal absorption of protein breakdown products.
- A number of gut-derived toxins are implicated in the development of psoriasis.
- Psoriasis can be triggered by nervous tension and stress, illness, cuts, several viral and bacterial infections, sunburn or drugs such as lithium, chloroquine and beta blockers.

Therapeutic Strategy

Psoriasis is a stubborn and difficult problem to treat. It requires patience, diligence and long-term treatment to observe lasting benefits. In particular, it is also important to consider the following:

- Avoid stressful situations, fatigue and environmental changes (such as exposure to cold) and trauma to the skin, as these can initiate new skin lesions.[11]
- Identify and address food allergies.[10]
- Manage inflammatory response by the use of anti-inflammatory remedies.
- Use alteratives to promote detoxification.
- Use essential oils that are anti-inflammatory or antipruritic.

Aromatherapy Treatment

Essential oils are very effective in dealing with psoriasis. A large number of patients (39%) report a specific stressful event occurring within one month prior to their episode.[10]

Aromatherapy plays a very important role in reducing stress. Any of the essential oils which help to alleviate stress and anxiety, such as bergamot, sandalwood and lavender, are most suitable. These oils may be used as an inhalation, in a bath or prepared in a 0.5–1% massage blend.

When preparing a massage oil, use evening primrose oil as a carrier. Wheatgerm oil can be applied to patches of psoriasis on the face. Mix two to three drops of tea tree to every 10 mL of wheatgerm oil and apply to the skin morning and evening.

Any of the essential oils with anti-inflammatory properties should also be considered, such as German chamomile, yarrow or everlasting.

Essential oils such as carrot seed and everlasting may be used to correct abnormal liver function. The connection between the liver and psoriasis relates to one of the liver's basic tasks of filtering and detoxifying the blood. If the liver is overwhelmed by excessive levels of toxins in the blood, or if there is a decrease in the liver's detoxification ability, the toxicity level in the blood will increase and the psoriasis will worsen.

Other Treatments

Nutrition

- The involvement of arachidonic acid cascade to form the inflammatory intermediates of skin inflammation suggests that dietary manipulation of this pathway through essential fatty acids such as gamma-linolenic acid (GLA) and eicosapentaenoic acid (EPA) via ingestion and topical application would be reasonably effective.[10]
- Avoid saturated fats (milk, cream, butter, eggs), sugar, processed foods, white flour and citrus fruits. Avoid red meat and dairy products.[15]
- Take linseed oil (1–2 tablespoons per day) or supplement with GLA/EPA.[10,11]
- Improve digestion by supplementing with digestive enzymes with each meal.[11]
- Increase intake of dietary fibre.[10]
- Increase the intake of fish oils, particularly those rich in EPA — sardines, tuna, mackerel and salmon.[11,15]

Herbs

- St Mary's thistle herbal extract increases bile flow and protects the liver, which in turn helps to purify the blood.[10,15]
- Other herbal extracts known to be blood purifiers are red clover, burdock and sarsaparilla. These herbs are all recommended for treating psoriasis.[15,16,22]
- For symptomatic relief use chickweed as a lotion or a cream.[16]
- Liquorice root exerts an effect similar to that of topical hydrocortisone in the treatment of psoriasis.[10]
- Topical applications of aloe vera in a hydrophilic cream are highly effective.[10]

General Advice

- Many drugs can initiate or aggravate psoriasis in susceptible individuals. These are alpha interferon, cortisone, lithium, phenylbutazone, aspirin, progesterone, iodine, nystatin, indomethacin and beta blockers.[11]
- Topical applications of cold-pressed vegetable oils rich in essential fatty acids such as GLA/EPA.
- Sunlight is very beneficial in most cases. A standard medical treatment for psoriasis involves the use of the drug psoralen and exposure to UV light.[10]

Wound Management

Useful Oils

• German chamomile • calendula-infused oil
• everlasting • lavender • lemon • myrrh • niaouli
• sage • tea tree • yarrow

Definition

A wound can be described as any break in the continuity of the skin resulting from physical, mechanical or thermal damage.

Clinical Features

The process of wound healing depends on the extent and severity of the wound. Trauma to the epidermal layers stimulates an increased mitotic activity in the stratum basale, whereas injuries that extend to the dermis or subcutaneous tissue elicit activity throughout the body as well as within the wound itself. General body responses include a temporary elevation of temperature and pulse rate.

In an open wound blood vessels are broken and bleeding occurs. Through the action of blood platelets and protein molecules, called fibrinogen, a clot forms and soon blocks the flow of blood and entry of pathogens. A scab forms and covers and protects the damaged area. Mechanisms are activated to destroy bacteria, dispose of dead or injured cells and isolate the injured area. These responses collectively are referred to as inflammation and are characterised by redness, heat, oedema and pain. Inflammation is a response that confines the injury and promotes healing.[1]

The next step in healing is the differentiation of binding fibroblasts from connective tissue forming fibrin at wound margins. Together with new branches from surrounding blood vessels, granulation tissue is formed. Phagocytic cells migrate into the wound and ingest dead cells and foreign debris.

Eventually the damaged area is repaired and the protective scab is sloughed off.[1]

If the wound is severe, the granulation tissue may develop scar tissue. Scar tissue differs from normal skin in that its collagenous fibres are more dense and it has no stratified squamous epidermal layer. Scar tissue has fewer blood vessels and may lack hair, glands and sensory receptors. The closer the edges of a wound, the less granulation tissue develops and the less obvious the scar. This is one of the main reasons for suturing a large wound or break in the skin.[1]

Therapeutic Strategy

Irrespective of the type of wound being treated the main objective is to promote healing and prevent infection. Please refer to a first aid manual for the management of wounds. The first aid manual should have clear instructions on several types of wounds ranging from minor skin abrasions, open wounds, penetrating wounds through to foreign objects in wounds. If in doubt seek medical aid, as the wound may require suturing.

According to the St John first aid manual the aim in the management of an open wound is to:

- control bleeding
- clean the wound as well as possible
- apply a sterile or clean dressing
- seek medical aid.[18]

To minimise infection:

- wash your hands well before and after management
- avoid coughing, sneezing or talking while managing a wound
- handle the wound only when it is necessary to control severe bleeding
- use sterile or clean dressings.[18]

Dirty and penetrating wounds should be examined by a doctor, as tetanus or other serious infection may result.

Aromatherapy Treatment

While the use of botanically derived substances have been used throughout all cultures and in natural healing for their capability to speed wound healing and prevent infection, it is surprising that modern medical practice does not recognise the utilisation of these plant-based remedies.

Certainly the most inspiring text on the use of aromatherapy for wound healing is Gattefosse's Aromatherapy, originally published in French in 1937, and translated into English in 1993.

In this book, Gattefosse cities many case studies from various physicians such as Drs Sassard, Meurisse, Forgues and Malchand, all of whom worked with essential oils in treating a wide variety of wounds, burns and injuries with often amazing success. The following is a quote from Dr Forgues' observations:

> *Wound to the forehead and the temporal bone area resulting from an automobile accident. Wounds on the bruised, purplish, swollen lips. The skin had detached and the muscles were severed; a haematoma was forming and was lanced; the wound reached the top of the head and extended towards the nape of the neck. Treatment: washing with four litres of water containing 5/1,000 lavender essence, drying the wound, dry dressing. Same treatment for four days, after a time the underlying layers healed and the skin reattached. Stop washes, but application of 15/1,000 solution. Completely healed eight days later. Although the wound was not sutured and there was therefore a risk of infection, it nonetheless healed in twelve days.*[19]

Guba conducted a clinical trial to investigate the wound-healing effects of various essential oils often cited as being effective. The following essential oils and vegetable oils were found to be effective:

- true lavender
- mugwort and sage
- everlasting
- German chamomile
- calendula-infused and CO_2 extract oils
- calophyllum oil
- borage and flaxseed oils
- shea butter
- citrus seed extract.[25]

Essential oils such as mugwort and sage contain ketones which have been generally found to exhibit cicatrising properties. Everlasting oil contains a number of unusual diketonic hydrocarbons known as b-diones (15–20% italidones I, II and III). It has shown strong effects in topical use as an anti-coagulant (for bruising) and as a noted cicatrising agent in wound healing.[25]

Recent research indicates that topically applied oils containing essential fatty acids will speed the wound-healing process by assisting the formation of prostaglandins. Prostaglandins serve the wound-healing process by increasing local blood supply, mediating leucocyte emigration into the wound and assisting the synthesis of granulation tissue. Rosehip, evening primrose, borage and flaxseed oils are rich sources of polyunsaturated fatty acids, linoleic, alpha-linoleic and gamma-linoleic acid. These oils are highly susceptible to oxidation, therefore only fresh oils should be used.

Shea butter has been traditionally used for sprains, muscular pains and to help heal wounds and burns. It has an exceptionally high content of unsaponifiables that are particularly useful in wound healing. Some clinical trials suggest that shea butter increases the microcirculation in the skin-increasing tissue oxygenation.[25]

Weiss says that St John's wort oil is an old-established medicinal plant, which has excellent properties for the external treatment of wounds and burns.[21]

Other Skin Conditions

Pressure Sores

Pressure sores, also known as bed sores, are deep ulcers that form when pressure is exerted over bony areas of the body, restricting circulation and leading to necrosis in the overlying tissue.

Aetiology

Pressure sores tend to occur in elderly immobile patients, especially those who are unconscious, paralysed or debilitated.[3] The cause is skin ischemia from sustained pressure over a bony area, particularly the heels, sacrum, hips and buttocks. Poor general health, including anaemia, is a predisposing factor.[3]

Clinical Features

- preliminary area of fixed erythema at pressure site
- relatively sudden onset of necrosis and ulceration
- ulcer undermined at edges
- possible rapid extension of ulcers
- necrotic slough in base.[3]

Therapeutic Strategy

In managing bed sores it is important to consider the following:

- good nursing care including turning the patient every two hours
- regular skin examinations by nursing and medical staff
- special care of pressure areas, including gentle handling
- special beds, mattresses (for example, air-filled ripple) and sheepskin to relieve pressure areas
- good nutrition and hygiene
- control of urinary and faecal incontinence
- avoid the donut cushion.[3]

Aromatherapy Treatment

Guba outlines a trial using a wound-healing formula that he prepared in six nursing homes. The wound-healing formula was applied at least once a day for skin tears and twice a day for pressure ulcers and venous ulcers. The formula was applied to dry gauze and then taped over the wound. Normal wound management practices were carried out as usual such as cleaning with a normal saline solution.[26]

The essential oils used on the wound-healing formula include lavender, sage, German chamomile and calendula-infused oil blended in a base of borage seed, flaxseed, *Calophyllum inophyllum* and shea butter.[26]

The results of this formula have been favourable. Guba cites Ellershaw, who says:

> *The standard treatment for pressure areas, such as alginate dressings, generally slough off the necrotic tissue producing a cavity. However, when using the wound healing formula, we find the necrotic tissue only slowly flakes off opening up to healthy granulation tissue with only a small cavity or no cavity at all developing. We find the wound healing formula works without exception on pressure sores.*[26]

Price recommends the use of cicatrisant oils together with those that are strongly antiseptic. They should be used in a spray with water when the sores are suppurating — 10 mL drops in 100 mL of water, shaking well each time before spraying the area.[27]

If it can be touched, gently apply the essential oils in a calendula-infused oil base. Price also recommends compresses, but it is important to ensure that the dressing used is non-stick. Essential oils recommended include frankincense, German chamomile, lavender and geranium.[27]

Nappy Rash

Nappy rash (or diaper dermatitis) is an inflammatory contact dermatitis occurring in the napkin area and can be a common presentation of mild or moderate underlying skin disease. It is found in children up to 2 years old and has a peak incidence from 9 to 12 months.[3]

Aetiology

The main predisposing factor in all types is dampness due to urine and faeces. Other aggravating or causative factors are:

- a tendency of the baby to eczema
- a tendency of the baby to seborrhoeic dermatitis
- rough-textured nappies
- detergents and other chemicals in nappies
- infection, especially monilia (thrush)
- plastic pants (aggravates wetness)
- excessive washing of the skin with soap

- too much powder over the nappy area (avoid talcum powders).[3]

Therapeutic Strategy

In managing nappy rash it is important to consider the following:[3]

- Keep the area dry. Change wet or soiled nappies frequently and as soon as you notice them.
- After changing, gently remove any urine or moisture with a light aqueous based cream or warm water.
- Wash gently with warm water, pat dry (do not rub) and then apply a calendula cream or ointment to help heal and protect the area.
- Expose the bare skin to fresh air wherever possible. Leave the nappy off several times a day, especially if the rash is severe.
- Thoroughly rinse out any bleach or disinfectant.

Aromatherapy Treatment

Add 5 drops of lavender, 2 drops of German chamomile and 5 mL of calendula-infused oils to 50 g of aqueous cream base, blend thoroughly and apply as recommended above.

Tinea

Tinea, or ringworm infections is caused mainly by *Trichophyton rubum* and is the commonest type of fungal infection. The symptoms include itchness and foot odour. Sweat and water make the epidermis white and soggy. There often is scaling, maceration and fissuring of the skin between the fourth and fifth toes and also third and fourth toes.[3]

Therapeutic Strategy

- keeping feet as clean and dry as possible
- carefully drying feet, especially between toes
- removing flaky skin from beneath the toes each day with dry tissue paper or gauze
- wearing light socks made of natural absorbent fibres, such as cotton and wool, to allow better circulation of air and to reduce sweating
- avoiding socks made with synthetic fibres
- wearing open sandals or shoes with porous soles and uppers
- going barefoot whenever possible.[3]

Aromatherapy Treatment

The antifungal properties of tea tree have been extensively documented and clinically proven. Tea tree oil is considered one of the most effective essential oils for the treatment of tinea. The oil can be applied neat, to the infected area.

Pruritus

Pruritus is another term for itching. It is one of the most important dermatological symptoms and is usually a symptom of a primary skin disease with a visible rash. The urge to itch arises from the same nerve pathway as pain, but pain and itching are two distinct sensations. The difference is the intensity of the stimuli.[3]

Aetiology

Primary skin disorders causing significant pruritus:

- atopic dermatitis
- urticaria
- scabies
- pediculosis
- asteatosis (dry skin)
- *Lichen planus*
- chicken pox
- contact dermatitis
- insect bites.[3]

Therapeutic Strategy

The basic principle of treatment is to determine the cause of the itch and treat it accordingly:

- apply cooling measures
- avoid rough clothes, wear light clothes
- avoid known irritants
- avoid overheating
- avoid vasodilation — for example, alcohol, hot baths/showers (keep showers short and not too hot)
- topical treatment
- emollient to lubricate the skin
- local soothing lotions.[3]

Aromatherapy Treatment

Essential oils that are soothing and anti-inflammatory will help to ease itching. It is very important to use the oils in very low dilutions (usually 1.0–0.5%). The most common essential oils are German chamomile and true lavender. Another essential oil that effectively reduces pruritus is peppermint oil. Once again, keep the dilution to 0.5%.

Jojoba oil is a very effective vegetable oil to use as a base. In some cases, it may be better to use an essential oil dispersant with the essential oils in a bath.

Scabies

Scabies is a highly infectious skin infestation caused by a tiny mite called *Saroptes scabiei*.

The female mite burrows just beneath the skin to lay her eggs. She then dies. The eggs hatch into tiny mites, which spread out over the skin and live for only 30 days. The excreta of the mites causes an allergic reaction. The mites are spread from person to person through close personal contact.

Therapeutic Strategy

Davis recommends dosing up on garlic capsules and making a preparation of lavender and peppermint.[12] Valnet quotes a formula that contains cinnamon, clove, lavender, lemon and peppermint in a cream or ointment at about 5% dilution. If you wish to try this, ensure that the percentage of cinnamon and clove is low to minimise irritation to the skin.[28]

It is extremely important to follow meticulous hygiene. Wash all clothing and bed linen in hot water and hang in the sun to dry. Take the mattress outside and air in the sun.

Jock Itch (Tinea cruris)

Jock itch is a term used to describe a common infection of the groin area in men that is commonly caused by a tinea infection.

Aetiology

There are other possible causes of a groin rash as listed below:

- skin disorders such as psoriasis, seborrhoeic dermatitis, eczema
- fungal conditions such as candida
- contact dermatitis.[3]

The dermatophytes responsible are *Trichophyton rubrum* (60%), *Epidermophyton floccosum* (30%) and *T. mentagrophytes*. The organisms thrive in damp, warm, dark sites. The feet should be inspected for evidence of *Tinea pedis*. It is transmitted by towels and other objects; particularly in locker rooms, saunas and communal showers.[3]

Clinical Features

- itchy rash
- more common with young males
- strong association with *T. pedis*
- usually acute onset
- more common in the warmer months
- more common in physically active people
- related to chafing in groin from tight pants
- well-defined border.[3]

Aromatherapy Treatment

Wash the area in a warm bath and dry thoroughly. Then apply an ointment containing tea tree oil.

References

1. Van de Graaff K, Fox S. *Concepts of human anatomy & physiology*. 3rd edn, Wm.C. Publishers, USA, 1992.
2. Cohen BJ, Wood DL. *Memmler's the human body in health and disease*. 9th edn, J.B. Lippincott Williams & Wilkins, USA, 2000.
3. Murtagh J. *General practice*. 2nd edn, The McGraw-Hill Companies Inc., Australia, 1998.
4. Gawkrodger D. *Dermatology*. 2nd edn, Churchill Livingstone, UK, 1997.
5. Hoffman D. *An elders' herbal*. Healing Art Press, USA, 1993.
6. Beckman N. *The family library guide to natural therapies*. Family Library, Australia, 1992.
7. Tubaro A et al. *Evaluation of anti-inflammatory activity of a chamomile extract topical application*. Planta Medica 1984; 50(4): 359.
8. Glowania HJ. *Effect of chamomile on wound healing — A clinical double-blind study*. Z Hautkz, 1987; 62(17): 1262.
9. Bassatt IB, Pannowitz DL, Barnetson RSC. *A comparative study of tea tree oil versus benzyl peroxide in the treatment of acne*. Medical Journal of Australia 1990; 153: 455–458.
10. Pizzorno J, Murray M. *A text book of natural medicine*. 2nd edn, Churchill Livingstone, UK, 1999.
11. Osiecki H. *The physician's handbook of clinical nutrition*. Bioconcepts Publishing, Australia, 1990.
12. Davis P. *Aromatherapy: An A–Z*. 2nd edn, The C.W. Daniel Company Limited, Great Britain, 1999.
13. Lavabre M. *Aromatherapy workbook*. Healing Art Press, USA, 1997.
14. Saunders S. *The use of aromatherapy in the treatment of acne*. The Aromatherapist 1997: 4(1): 4–17.
15. Balch J, Balch P. *Prescription for nutritional healing*. Avery Publishing Group, USA, 1997.
16. Willard T. *Text book of modern herbology*. Wild Rose College of Natural Healing, Canada, 1993.
17. Werner R. *A massage therapist's guide to pathology*. Lippincott Williams & Wilkins, USA, 1998.
18. *Australian first aid manual*. St John Ambulance, Australia, 1998.
19. Gattefosse RM. *Gattefosse's aromatherapy*. The C.W. Daniel Company Limited, Great Britain, 1993.
20. Mailhebiau P. *Portraits in oils*. The C.W. Daniel Company Limited, Great Britain, 1995.
21. Weiss R. *Herbal medicine*. Beaconsfield Publishers, translated from the 6th German edition of Lehrbuch der Phytotherapie by A.R. Meuss. English edition first published in 1988.
22. Tyler V. *Herbs of choice*. Haworth Press, USA, 1993.

23. Tisserand R. *In praise of melissa.* The International Journal of Aromatherapy 1989; 1(4) & 2(1): 10–11.

24. Bone K, Mills S. *Principles and practice of phytotherapy.* Churchill Livingstone, UK, 2000.

25. Guba R. *Wound healing Part I.* Aromatherapy Today, 1997; 3: 21–24.

26. Guba R. *Wound healing Part II.* Aromatherapy Today, 1997; 4: 5–8.

27. Price L, Price S. *Aromatherapy for health professionals.* 2nd edn, Churchill Livingstone, UK, 1999.

28. Valnet J. *The practice of aromatherapy.* The C.W. Daniel Company Limited, Great Britain, 1980.

The Nervous System

Objectives

After careful study of this chapter, you should be able to:

- outline a holistic strategy for the management of conditions associated with the nervous system
- identify, list and describe common pathophysiologies of the nervous system
- explain the aromatherapy treatment for specific conditions and disorders of the nervous system
- explain the role of other holistic strategies for specific conditions and disorders of the nervous system.

Introduction

The nervous system is the body's control centre and communication network. The nervous system serves three broad functions:

- it senses change inside the body and in the outside environment
- it interprets the changes
- it responds to the interpretation by initiating action in the form of muscular contractions or glandular secretions.[1]

The nervous system is divided into two principal divisions, the central nervous system and the peripheral nervous system, and several subdivisions. The *central nervous system* (CNS) is the control centre for the entire system, consisting of the brain and the spinal cord. The various nerve processes that connect the brain and spinal cord with receptors, muscles and glands are referred to as the *peripheral nervous system* (PNS).[1]

The peripheral nervous system may be divided into an afferent and an efferent system. The afferent system consists of nerve cells that convey information from receptors in the periphery of the body to the central nervous system The efferent system consists of nerve cells that convey information from the central nervous system to the muscles and glands.[1]

The efferent system is subdivided into the *somatic nervous system* and the *autonomic nervous system* (ANS). The somatic nervous system consists of efferent nerves that conduct nerve impulses from the central nervous system to skeletal muscle tissue. Since the somatic nervous system produces movement only in skeletal muscle tissue, it is under conscious control and therefore voluntary. The ANS contains efferent neurons that convey nerve impulses from the central nervous system to smooth muscle tissue, cardiac muscle tissue and glands. Since it produces responses only in involuntary muscles and glands, it is considered to be involuntary.[1]

The ANS is organised in two divisions, the sympathetic division and the parasympathetic division. In general, one division stimulates or increases an organ's activity, while the other inhibits or decreases activity.[1] The sympathetic nervous system is responsible for the fight or flight response. It produces the following effects:

- increase in the rate and force of heart contraction
- increase in blood pressure due partly to more effective heartbeat and partly to constriction of small arteries in the skin and the internal organs
- dilation of the blood vessels to skeletal muscles, bringing more blood to these tissues
- dilation of the bronchial tubes to allow more oxygen to enter
- stimulation of the medulla of the adrenal glands. This produces hormones, including epinephrine, that prepare the body to meet emergency situations
- increase in metabolism.[2]

The sympathetic nervous system also acts as a brake on those systems not directly involved in the response to stress, such as the urinary and digestive systems. The parasympathetic part of the ANS normally acts as a balance for the sympathetic system once a crisis has passed. The parasympathetic nervous system will cause constriction of the pupils, slowing down of the heart rate and constriction of the bronchial tubes. It also stimulates the formation and release of urine and activity of the digestive tract.[2]

General Considerations

A holistic approach to treating conditions associated with the nervous system and mental wellbeing must acknowledge the connection between the physical and the psychological aspects of our wellbeing. While the nervous system is part of the physical make-up of the body, all psychological processes also take place in the nervous system. Therefore, if there is disease on the psychological level, it will reflect in the physical; and when there is disease on the physical level, this will reflect in the psychological.

According to The Australian Institute of Health and Welfare, individuals differ in their sense of wellbeing and their behavioural functioning. However, in some people there are symptoms and behaviours that are distressing to them or others and which impair their social functioning. Mental problems account for much disability, incur high health costs and impose a heavy burden of human suffering including stigmatisation of people with mental disorders and their families.[3]

Breggin warns us of a biopsychiatry that is replacing psychotherapy in some psychiatric training programs:

> *As the medical and biological wing of the profession has taken over, compassionate psychologically oriented psychiatrists have been replaced by biochemists and lab researchers as department heads. Major journals devote nearly all their space to studies on the brains, blood, and urine of psychiatric patients — without so much as a passing mention of patients with thoughts and feelings relevant to their consideration and their recovery.*
>
> *People suffering from what used to be thought as 'neuroses' and 'personal problems' are being treated with drugs and shock. Children with problems that were*

once handled by remedial education or improved parenting are instead being subjected to medical diagnosis, drugs and hospitals. Old people who used to be cared for by their families are being drugged in nursing homes that find it more cost effective to provide a pill than a caring, stimulating environment.[4]

Aldridge agrees that the use of pharmaceutical drugs that work on the mind are the subject of controversy:

The role of psychotropic drugs in society continues to be controversial. There is evidence that 'talking treatments' — such as psychotherapy, cognitive therapy and counselling — are effective in treating mental illnesses.

The evidence comparing cognitive therapy with drugs for depression is equally impressive. In cognitive therapy — which is shorter in duration than conventional psychotherapy — the patient is taught to challenge the negative or aberrant thought patterns or beliefs that lie at the core of their condition.[5]

Beckman is concerned that the over-use of pharmaceutical sedatives and antidepressants does not often cure the problem, it only tends to dampen one's ability to think clearly. The result is that over a period of time the person concerned often loses the will to improve his or her general level of health and does not have the mental or physical energy to reduce the aggravating factors which probably caused the problem in the first place.[6]

While traditional allopathic medicine tends to reduce psychological problems to the mere biochemical level, many naturopathic techniques assume or imply the other extreme, namely that psychological factors are the cause of any disease and that treatment of the psyche is the only appropriate way of healing. Hoffman suggests that by bringing these two reductionist views together we come closer to a holistic approach. He says:

For our being to be wholly healthy, we have to take care of our physical health through right diet and right lifestyle, but we are also responsible for a healthy emotional, mental and spiritual life. The emotional atmosphere we live in should be fulfilling, nurturing and support emotional stability. Our thoughts should be creative and life enhancing, open to the free flow of intuition and imagination, not conceptually rigid. And equally, we have to stay open to the free flow of the higher energies of our soul, without which health is impossible.[7]

Hoffman says that we must also remember that we are part of the greater whole of humanity and that many of the mental disorders we encounter in today's Western society are normal responses to an abnormal environment. He says that many mental disorders are a reflection of the chaos and sickness in today's society. He suggests that:

Herbal medicine can be an ecological and spiritually integrated tool to aid the nervous system of humanity, so that humanity can help itself. It is an ideal counterpart on the physical level for therapeutic techniques on the psychological level, to help people embrace their wholeness.[7]

Holistic Therapeutic Strategy

A relaxed body and mind are better able to deal with life situations than when stressed. Learning to control and balance stress with relaxation is an essential part of holistic health.

While the care of oneself should involve a well-balanced nutritional diet, regular exercise and plenty of sleep and rest, it should also be a process of life enrichment by doing what brings one satisfaction and a sense of wellbeing.

A holistic approach to the treatment of problems associated with the nervous system may involve the use of:

- a well-balanced diet and nutritional supplements
- rest and sleep
- managing stress
- relaxation techniques
- aromatherapy and massage
- flower essences
- herbs
- and many other holistic therapies that address the body, mind and spirit.

It has been shown that attitude and behaviour can influence one's resistance to disease. For many years positive imagery and meditation have been used in the treatment of cancer. Meares poetically describes the benefits of meditation:

In meditation
There comes a calm,
a clarity,
which enlightens
the inner depths of our being,
brought to us
by the more harmonious function
of nerve and endocrine cell
which mastermind
the healing powers of the body.[8]

Aromatherapy Considerations

No other holistic health modality is able to offer us such a multidimensional approach to the management of conditions associated with the nervous system. This multidimensional approach involves:

- the pharmacological activity of the essential oils
- the therapeutic and nurturing benefits of the massage

- the caring professional relationship between the therapist and the client
- the powerful influence that olfaction has on the ANS memory and emotion

The benefits of essential oils and massage have been widely researched and documented. Farrow investigated the physical and psychological benefits of massage using 30 patients at St Mary's Hospital, London. The observed effects of the massage treatment included:

- reduction of pain levels
- reduction of anxiety
- reduction of muscle spasm and tension
- improved wellbeing and self-worth.[9]

In treating conditions associated with the nervous system the following properties of the essential oils are considered useful:

Analgesics

Analgesics provide relief from pain and can be used for the treatment of headaches and migraines. Essential oils that are analgesic include cajeput, eucalyptus, lavender, spike lavender, sweet marjoram, peppermint, rosemary and thyme.

Antidepressants

Essential oils such as basil, bergamot, clary sage, lavender, lemon, geranium, jasmine, neroli, rose otto and absolute, sandalwood and ylang ylang can be used to alleviate depression.

Antispasmodics

Essential oils such as Roman chamomile, clary sage, lavender, sweet marjoram and yarrow help prevent or alleviate spasms or convulsions and may be beneficial for treating headaches, migraines and muscular spasms caused by nervous tension.

Nervines

Nervines work to tone and strengthen the nerves. There are two types of nervines — stimulant nervines and sedative nervines.

Stimulant nervines strengthen the nervous system. They are useful in cases of shock, stress or nervous debility. Some excellent nerve tonics include angelica root, basil, clary sage, juniper berry, lemongrass, vetiver, rosemary and peppermint.

Sedative nervines can help alleviate stress and tension. Some excellent nervine relaxants include Roman chamomile, bergamot, lavender, sweet marjoram, neroli, sandalwood and valerian.

Soporifics

Essential oils such as lavender, sweet marjoram and valerian help to induce sleep.

Associated Conditions

Anxiety

Useful Oils

• basil • bergamot • Virginian cedarwood
• Roman chamomile • cypress • frankincense
• jasmine absolute • lavender • lemon • lime
• sweet marjoram • neroli • melissa • palmarosa
• patchouli • rose • rosewood • sandalwood
• vetiver • ylang ylang • sweet orange

Definition

Anxiety is an uncomfortable inner feeling of fear or imminent disaster. It has been defined as:

> *Generalised and persistent anxiety or anxious mood, which cannot be associated with, or is disproportionately large in response to a specific psychological stressor, stimulus or event.*[10]

Clinical Features

Anxiety is a normal human emotion and most of us experience some degree of anxiety in our lives as a normal reaction to stress or misfortune. However, some people are constantly anxious to the extent that it is abnormal and interferes with their lives. They suffer from an anxiety disorder, a problem that affects 5–10% of the population.[10]

Anxiety disorders are generally classified in the following categories:

- generalised anxiety disorder
- panic disorder, with or without agoraphobia
- phobia disorder, including social phobia
- obsessive compulsive disorder
- post-traumatic stress disorder.[10]

Generalised anxiety comprises excessive anxiety and worry about various life circumstances and is not related to a specific activity, time or event such as trauma, obsessions or phobias.[10] Clinical features include:

- persistent unrealistic and excessive anxiety
- worry about two or more life circumstances for 6 months or longer.[10]

The diagnostic criteria for generalised anxiety disorder are three or more of:

- irritability
- restless, 'keyed up' or 'on edge'
- easily fatigued
- difficulty concentrating or 'mind going blank'

- muscle tension
- sleep disturbance.[10]

Symptoms associated with anxiety include:

- psychological — apprehension, irritability, exaggerated startle response, sleep disturbance and nightmares, impatience, panic, sensitivity to noise and difficulty concentrating or 'mind going blank'
- physical — muscle tension/aching, trembling, shaky, twitching, restlessness and tiredness/fatigue
- ANS overactivity — dry mouth, palpitations, tachycardia, sweating, cold clammy hands, flushes, chills, difficulty swallowing or 'lump in throat', diarrhoea, abdominal distress, difficulty breathing, smothering feeling and dizziness or light-headedness.[10]

Therapeutic Strategy

In managing anxiety it is important to consider the following:

- Give careful explanation and reassurance.[10]
- Provide practical advice on ways of dealing with the problems.[10]
- Avoid aggravating substances such as caffeine, nicotine and other stimulants.[10]
- Recommend stress management techniques, relaxation programs and regular exercise and organise these for the patient.[10]
- Advise on coping skills: include personal and interpersonal strategies to manage difficult circumstances and people.[10]
- Recommend essential oils with relaxing properties in aromatherapy massages, baths and vaporisers.

Aromatherapy Treatment

Aromatherapy provides a valuable alternative to psychotropic drugs and muscle relaxants that are commonly used in treating anxiety allopathically.[11] Davis recommends using any of the essential oils with sedative properties. These oils include bergamot, chamomile, Atlas or Virginian cedarwood, clary sage, cypress, frankincense, geranium, hyssop, jasmine, juniper, lavender, marjoram, melissa, neroli, patchouli, rose, sandalwood and ylang ylang.[11]

Davis says that clients will often instinctively select the essential oil that most closely corresponds to their present state. There is no doubt that the caring approach of the aromatherapist is an integral part of the treatment. The aromatherapy massage should be the basis of the treatment because it will allow reassurance, love and concern expressed in the most direct, nonverbal way.[11]

Mailhebiau says that basil oil is remarkably relaxing, due to its methyl ether content and is recommended for people with schizoid tendencies as it soothes, calms and relaxes. He calls it *the anti-stress essence par excellence.*[12]

According to traditional Chinese medicine, anxiety is commonly linked to an energetic imbalance of the heart — the home of the mind (shen). When the heart is deficient in qi, blood or yin, the shen becomes disturbed and loses its settled state of residence. This results in emotional unease. The long-term emotional pressures that result in chronic anxiety also cause these energetic deficiencies that in turn lead to additional problems of a physiological nature. Anxiety, therefore, is classified as a cause or a symptom of the heart and fire element.[13]

Mojay recommends the following essential oils in the management of anxiety:[13]

- Lavender and melissa oil cool the heart, and are considered the most comforting oils for the mind. These two oils are best used for anxiety in those who feel oppressed and suffocated.
- Mojay recommends blending lavender oil with cypress and neroli for anxieties that are expressed through compulsive behaviour.
- Neroli is of benefit for those who cannot confront painful and disturbing emotions — feelings of shame, guilt or half-conscious hurt and rage. It also helps one find peace of mind.
- Rose and palmarosa are for the abandoned and those who cannot, during times of emotional distress, bear being left alone.
- Geranium oil calms the nervous anxiety of those not by nature 'emotional' but tend to be 'over-achievers' who have little time for their feelings.
- Vetiver helps to restore a sense of grounded stability in those who feel anxious and 'disembodied'.
- Jasmine oil combines a calming effect with an uplifting effect. It is especially beneficial for anxiety when it alternates with feelings of depression.
- Ylang ylang is beneficial for calming the restless mind.

Aromatherapy works in harmony with de-stressing techniques such as yoga, tai chi, meditation and simple relaxation techniques. As an aromatherapist you should become familiar with one or more of these techniques or you should know other therapists who can teach these techniques to your client.

Other Treatments

Nutrition

- Include in the diet apricots, asparagus, avocados, bananas, broccoli, brown rice, fish, garlic, green leafy vegetables, legumes, raw nuts and seeds, soya products, whole grains and yoghurt. These foods are a rich source of valuable minerals such as calcium, magnesium, phosphorus and potassium, which are all needed for a healthy nervous system.[15]
- Avoid foods containing refined sugar or other simple carbohydrates.[15]
- Limit your intake of animal protein. Concentrate on meals high in complex carbohydrate and vegetable protein.[15]

Herbs

- Catnip, chamomile, cramp bark, hops and passion flower promote relaxation and can be used to prevent panic attacks.[15]
- Scullcap and valerian root should be taken at bedtime to promote sleep and to prevent panic attacks at night.[15]

General Advice

- Get regular exercise. Any type of exercise will work — a brisk walk, bicycle riding, swimming, aerobics, or whatever fits your individual lifestyle. After a few weeks of exercise most people notice an improvement in anxiety symptoms.[14,15]
- Be sure to get adequate rest. If sleep is a problem, refer to the section on insomnia for advice.[14,15]
- Seek out sympathetic friends or family members for support.[14,15]
- Find some interesting activities, do something for other people.[14]
- Bach flowers are very useful for emotional problems.[14]
- Take up meditation, yoga, tai chi or stress management.[15]
- While coffee and alcohol give a temporary lift, their overall long-term effect is that they tend to increase anxieties.[14,15,16]
- To manage an acute anxiety attack, use breathing techniques. Inhale slowly to a count of four, hold your breath for a count of four, exhale slowly to a count of four and then do nothing for a count of four. Repeat this sequence until the attack subsides.[14]
- It is best to avoid drugs. Instead, look for factors in your lifestyle that cause you stress and anxiety and modify or remove them (if possible). Be on the lookout for solutions. Examples are changing jobs and keeping away from people or situations that upset you. Sometimes confronting people and talking things over will help.[10]
- Be less of a perfectionist, do not be a slave to the clock, do not bottle things up, feeling guilty, approve of yourself and others, express yourself and your anger. Resolve all personal conflicts. Make friends and be happy. Keep a positive outlook on life, and be moderate and less intense in your activities.[10]
- Seek a balance of activities such as recreation, meditation, reading, rest, exercise and family/social activities.[10]
- Learn to relax the mind and body: seek out special relaxation programs such as yoga, tai chi and meditation.[10]

Stress

Useful Oils

• basil • bergamot • Roman and German chamomile • Virginian and Atlas cedarwood • clary sage • frankincense • geranium • jasmine absolute • lavender • lemon • sweet marjoram • may chang • neroli • melissa • sweet orange • petitgrain • rose otto and absolute • rosemary • rosewood • sandalwood • tangerine • vetiver • ylang ylang

Definition

Stress is one of the major health problems in Western society today. It is responsible for many of our illnesses and any illness where stress is also present will be more difficult to treat.

Stress is defined as a negative differential between a series of demands and ability to cope with them. We each have a personal comfort level, which may vary from day to day. Everyone thrives and feels comfortable within this personal level, but placed outside of one's comfort zone, stress will quickly manifest.

It is important to realise that not all stress is bad, in fact a certain amount of stress is functional to maintaining optimal health. An environment totally devoid of stress would not be beneficial as some stress appears to be necessary for growth and change to take place and for the person to develop successful coping strategies.

The body's reaction to stress is controlled by the ANS, over which we have no direct voluntary control. The ANS has two branches:

- the sympathetic nervous system, which regulates the 'fight or flight' response

- the parasympathetic nervous system induces relaxation and helps the body compensate for periods of high arousal — for example, by lowering heart rate, blood pressure, and muscle tension.[1]

These relaxing responses are a biologically regenerative state, helping the body to recuperate. This reaction was called the relaxation response by Bensen of the Harvard Medical School, and all methods of managing acute and chronic stress aim to elicit this positive parasympathetic state.[18]

There is a wide range of causes of stress, most of which can be grouped under several major headings, namely physical stress, psychological stress and environmental stress.[17,19] When a threatening situation arises the human body is programmed to react with the 'fight or flight' response.

Clinical Features

Distress can cause psychobiological reactions which, initially, produce warning signs such as palpitations, insomnia, fatigue and mild depression. The first stage of distress may lead one to resort to quick fix remedies such as coffee, alcohol or tranquillisers, but the long-term effect of these remedies has no beneficial properties and may even damage health.

Hans Selye, a leading researcher into the effects of stress, has developed the notion of *General Adaption Syndrome*:[18]

- Stage 1 (alarm reaction) is the initial encounter with stress in which the body rises to meet the challenge of the stress.
- Stage 2 (resistance reaction) is when the body has adapted to stress and there is a considerable expenditure of the body's adaptive energy, notably the function of the adrenal cortex.
- Stage 3 (exhaustion) is finally one of exhaustion, in which many of the body functions become impaired.

Stress is a multidimensional syndrome because it involves mind, body and emotions. The symptoms of stress involve both behavioural and psychological problems, and the reason for the success of aromatherapy in dealing with stress is that it uses a multidimensional holistic approach.

Therapeutic Strategy

Effective stress management should involve the following activities:

- techniques to calm the mind and promote a positive mental attitude
- adopt healthy lifestyle factors
- regular exercise
- a healthy diet designed to nourish the body and support physiological processes
- herbs to support the body, especially the adrenal glands
- use of essential oils that are relaxing and nervines.[20]

Aromatherapy Treatment

It is not surprising that holistic aromatherapy excels in managing stress. Its success is due to the combined benefits of:

- the essential oils
- the massage
- the therapist/client interaction.[17]

The sensory aspect of aromatherapy is significant in the treatment of stress. This involves the sense of touch and smell. It is interesting to note that these are perhaps the most intimate and sensual of our senses, and they are usually not the ones being stimulated in our work or environment. The fact that aromatherapy is a sensory experience is inherent in its de-stressing action.[17]

Tisserand explains that to fully appreciate the benefits of aromatherapy we should consider a four dimensional model comprising cognitive, sensory, physiological and emotional aspects:

> *The cognitive aspect involves counselling and listening skills. When people receive massage they very often start to talk about their problems in a way that demands listening skills ... Some stressed individuals, however, would not feel comfortable visiting a counsellor or psychotherapist and would find an aromatherapy session more attractive and less confrontational. It is certainly one of the most pampering and cocooning of therapies, and this is of great importance in understanding the benefits of stress.*[17]

The essential oils may 'de-stress' through two routes; inhalation (primarily psychological effects) and dermal absorption (primarily physiological effects). The two possible mechanisms by which the essential oils work are:

- pharmacological effect
- triggering response via the olfactory–limbic–endocrine system.[17]

Many essential oils are available to help cope with stress:

- Essential oils to induce relaxation, reduce irritability, relieve headaches and overcome insomnia: bergamot, Roman chamomile, clary sage, frankincense, lavender, petitgrain, rosewood, sweet marjoram, sweet orange, sandalwood, tangerine and ylang ylang.[21]
- Essential oils to help relieve tiredness, and aches and pain: basil, black pepper, ginger,

lemon, lime, geranium, rosemary, peppermint, pine, and thyme.[21]

- Essential oils to help overcome depression, guilt, apathy, melancholy and feelings of helplessness: bergamot, mandarin, melissa, neroli, rose, jasmine.[21]

Other Treatments

Nutrition

Emotional, mental and psychological stress may affect nutritional needs. A balanced diet will help you cope with stress more effectively. This includes:

- eliminating or restricting the intake of caffeine
- eliminating or restricting the intake of alcohol
- eliminating refined carbohydrates from the diet
- eating a diverse range of whole foods
- eating regularly planned meals in a relaxed environment
- controlling food allergies
- avoiding foods that place stress on the body such as cola drinks, fried foods, junk foods, sugar and white flour products.[15,20]

Many disorders that arise from stress are a result of nutritional deficiencies, especially deficiencies of the B complex vitamins, which are very important for proper functioning of the nervous system, and of certain electrolytes that are depleted by the body's stress response. Stress also promotes the formation of free radicals that can become oxidised and damage body tissues, especially cell membranes.[20]

Herbs

Herbs can be effective in relieving the symptoms of stress. When used in conjunction with changes in nutrition and lifestyle, they form a very effective stress management programme.

- Skullcap has a relaxing and gentle sedative effect on the nervous system, as well as a restorative one, making it ideally suited to any condition associated with nervous tension and/or relaxation.[15]
- Passion flower is excellent for its sedative properties. It may be combined with valerian and skullcap to induce sleep. It is useful for relieving restlessness, irritability, wakefulness and symptoms of exhaustion.[15,25]
- Hops have a marked relaxant effect on the central nervous system. Hops can be used for the treatment of restlessness, headaches and insomnia. For insomnia, it may be blended with valerian and passion flower.[15]
- Oats are recommended in cases of nervous debility and exhaustion associated with depression.[15]
- Siberian ginseng is an adaptogen. It increases the body's capacity to cope with stress. It has a normalising action on the body. Unlike *Panax ginseng* it does not have the potential to cause over-stimulation.[15,20,22]
- Contrary to popular belief, valerian does not cause drowsiness or interfere with the reflexes or co-ordination. It keeps the nervous system from being overwhelmed. It also helps to ease stress-related headaches.[15]

General Advice

There are many different ways to relieve stress. The one that is best for the patient should be chosen. The following is a list of suggestions:

- Learn to relax — Relaxation is very difficult for people suffering from the effects of stress. It is a learned skill and it is not always something you can achieve on your own. Take up yoga, tai chi or meditation.[15,20]
- Get sufficient sleep each night — The less sleep you get, the more stress will affect you, the weaker your immune system becomes and the higher the risk of becoming ill.[15]
- Practise deep breathing — This can easily be done when facing a stressful situation. Holding your breath is also excellent for relieving stress. Inhale deeply with your mouth closed and hold your breath for a few seconds, then exhale slowly through your mouth. Do this four or five times, until you feel the tension disappear.[15,20]
- Monitor your internal conversations — Stop those futile inner conversations that keep telling you that you are not good enough or that you should have done better etc. The way we talk about ourselves has much to do with how we feel about ourselves and our environment.[15]
- Identify the sources of stress in your life — This can be an important first step in managing stress. Taking a stress inventory periodically helps you understand what is causing your problems.[15]
- Take a day off — That is what weekends are for. Take a drive, listen to music, a trip to the beach, read, do whatever you find rewarding and relaxing. Keep your thoughts in the present during this time so that you do not think about whatever is causing the stress.[15]
- Take up a hobby. Hobbies are great for relieving stress. Take time to do what you enjoy. Do

not feel guilty about spending time doing what you enjoy.[15]

- Do not repress or deny your emotions — This only compounds stress. Admit your feelings and accept them. Keeping strong feelings bottled up only causes them to resurface later as illness. Don't be afraid to cry.[15]
- Do not take life too seriously — Learn to laugh.[15]
- Have a positive image of yourself. Find work or a hobby which gives a feeling of satisfaction or accomplishment.[15]
- Physical activity can clear the mind and keep stress under control — Some people find running or walking beneficial; others prefer to play team sports. Any type of exercise will be ideal, as long as it is done regularly.[15,20]
- If you feel you cannot handle the stresses in your life consider seeking outside help. It may be worth consulting a qualified counsellor or other practitioner who may be able to help you handle your problems and teach you effective stress management techniques.[15]

Depression

Useful Oils

• basil • bergamot • Roman chamomile • clary sage
• cypress • frankincense • geranium
• jasmine absolute • lavender • lemon • mandarin
• sweet marjoram • may chang • melissa • neroli
• peppermint • pine • rose absolute or otto
• sandalwood • tangerine • ylang ylang

Definition

Depression is one of the most common human experiences. We may all experience it at some stage of our life or through those of our family and friends. We tend to think of depression as a natural response to the 'ups' and 'downs' of life. We are usually able to attribute depression to something specific, such as a death in the family, the loss of a job, a failure in love, feeling trapped or unproductive in one's life, or coping with a life-threatening or debilitating physical disease.

Many people will tend to deny that they have depression as there is often social stigma attached to signs of 'mental illness' or not coping with life. When the cause is not obvious, we often identify basic attitudes or personality traits that may help to explain the depression reaction. We might decide — *He has had a tough childhood and he's never got over it* or *She has had a string of bad luck.*

It is important to acknowledge depression as a very real illness that affects the entire mind and body. Depression can be a problem at any stage of life from childhood, adolescence, adulthood to old age. It has been found that women are more likely to experience depression than men.

Aetiology

In general, there are three major groups of depression, with similar symptoms in each group:

1. **Reactive:** Depression may occur in reaction to some outside (exogenous) adverse life situation, usually a loss of a person by death, divorce, financial reversal, loss of an established role etc. Anger and its repression are frequently associated with the situation, which in turn produces a feeling of guilt. The symptoms range from mild sadness, anxiety, irritability, worry, lack of concentration and discouragement.[23]
2. **Major affective disorders** are classified as:
   - **Major depressive episode:** A period of mood depression that occurs relatively independent of the client's life situation or events. Complaints vary widely but most frequently include loss of interest and enjoyment in living, withdrawal from activities and feelings of guilt. Symptoms also include inability to concentrate, feelings of worthlessness, somatic complaints, chronic fatigue and loss of sexual drive.[23]

     Physiological symptoms reported may include insomnia, anorexia with weight loss and constipation. Occasionally severe agitation and psychotic, paranoid thinking are present.[23]
   - **Manic episode:** A mood change characterised by elation with hyperactivity, over-involvement in life activities, low irritability threshold, flight of ideas, easily distracted and little need for sleep.[23]

     The over-enthusiastic quality of the mood and the expansive behaviour initially attracts others, but the irritability, mood swings, aggressive behaviour and grandiosity usually lead to marked interpersonal difficulties. Activities may occur that are later regretted — for example, excessive spending, resignation from a job, a hasty marriage, or exhibitionistic behaviour. Manic episodes usually occur earlier in life (teens or early adult life) than major depressive episodes.[23]
3. **Secondary to illness and drugs:** Any illness, severe or mild, can cause significant depression. Conditions such as rheumatoid arthritis, multiple sclerosis and chronic heart disease are likely to be associated with depression as are all other chronic illnesses.[23]

Clinical Features

Depression is considered an illness that seriously affects the following basic activities:

- energy for activity
- sex drive
- sleep
- appetite
- ability to cope with life.[10]

According to the *DSM-IV*, a manual of psychological problems that is used as a diagnostic guide, a patient with depression must have at least five of the following symptoms for 2 weeks (criterion 1 or 2 is essential):

1. depressed mood
2. loss of interest or pleasure
3. significant appetite or weight loss or gain
4. insomnia or hypersomnia
5. psychomotor agitation and retardation
6. fatigue or loss of energy
7. feelings of worthlessness or excessive guilt
8. impaired thinking or concentration, indecisiveness
9. suicidal thoughts.[10]

Murtagh suggests extending the criteria to include:

- feelings of not being able to cope with life
- continual tiredness
- loss of sense of humour
- tension and anger
- irritability, anger or fearfulness
- somatic symptoms such as headache, constipation, indigestion, weight loss, dry mouth and unusual pains or sensations in the chest or abdomen.[10]

Therapeutic Strategy

In managing depression it is important to consider the following:

- If symptoms are major and the patient is in poor health or is a suicidal risk, referral is appropriate.[10]
- Psychotherapy, including education, reassurance and support. All patients will require minor psychotherapy. Cognitive therapy teaches the patient new ways of positive thinking, which have to be relevant and achievable for the patient.[10]
- Use of botanical antidepressants.
- Use of essential oils with antidepressant properties.

Aromatherapy Treatment

Aromatherapy treatments have a wonderful energising, uplifting effect on the nervous system and help lift spirits. Essential oils can help balance, relax and restore the nervous system. Price lists a range of essential oils that may be used to treat depression:

- **General oils:** basil, bergamot, frankincense, Roman chamomile, geranium, lavender, sweet marjoram, neroli.
- **Agitation:** oils listed in general category, melissa.
- **Emotional instability:** any of the essential oils listed above.
- **Fatigue:** basil, cypress, peppermint.
- **Headaches:** Roman chamomile, lavender, lemon, sweet marjoram, peppermint.
- **Insomnia:** lavender, sweet marjoram, neroli.
- **Irritability:** frankincense, geranium, lavender, neroli, ylang ylang.
- **Sadness:** frankincense, mandarin, neroli, rose absolute or rose otto.[21]

The choice of essential oils for the treatment of depression is quite extensive. It is important to select the most appropriate oil or blend of oils for the client at any given time, as the client's needs may change from day to day.

Davis says that in helping people who are depressed it is important to pay attention to their preferences in regards to the oil or oils to be used, as this often will instinctively be the right choice at the particular time. The changing preferences give the therapist valuable clues to the changing moods and needs of the client.[11]

Other Treatments

Nutrition

- The body will react more quickly to the presence of sugar than it does to the presence of complex carbohydrates. The increase in energy supplied by sugar is quickly accompanied by fatigue and depression. Therefore increase complex carbohydrate intake and reduce sugar intake.[15]
- Vitamin B3 (niacin) deficiency is often associated with anxiety and depression. Vitamin B3 is metabolised into the amino acid tryptophan that has mild sedative qualities. Tryptophan is a precursor of serotonin, a neurotransmitter, which regulates the transmission of electrical impulses within the central nervous system. Irregular serotonin levels are associated with depression, mania and schizophrenia.[24]
- Mineral deficiencies of calcium and magnesium are likely to lead to nervousness and depression.[24]

- Avoid alcohol, caffeine and processed foods.[15]
- High fat intake can also contribute to depression through slowing the metabolism.[24]
- For women there is the additional complication of premenstrual syndrome. This may be the prime cause of depression and needs to be treated.

Herbs

- St John's wort *(Hypericum perforatum)* — Clinical studies show that hypericin, the active compound in St John's wort results in significant reduction in anxiety, depression and feelings of worthlessness. Duke suggests steeping one to two teaspoons of the dried herb in a cup of boiling water for 10 minutes and taking one or two cups a day for 4 to 6 weeks.[15,20,24]
- Liquorice root *(Glycyrrhiza glabra)* — While it doesn't have the same potency as St John's wort, according to Duke no other plant has more antidepressant compounds than liquorice. He says there are at least eight monoamine oxidase (MAO) inhibitors, which are compounds capable of potent antidepressant action.[15,20,24]
- *Ginkgo biloba* — Studies have shown that ginkgo may help to relieve depression, especially in the elderly who suffer reduced blood flow to the brain.[15]
- Siberian ginseng *(Eleutherococcus senticosus)* — Siberian ginseng has been shown to act as an MAO inhibitor. In people with depression, the herb helps to improve their sense of wellbeing.[15,24]

General Advice

- Depressed people need to talk about themselves, so a sympathetic ear is always useful, as is reassurance of worth, effectiveness and that bad times will pass. Cheerful companions can help bring depressed people out of their low state.[15]
- Exercise is a great boost, emotionally and spiritually.[15]
- Keep the mind active and get plenty of rest. Avoid stressful situations as much as possible.[15]
- Research has shown that the sun and bright light seem to trigger a response to a brain hormone known as melatonin (produced by the pineal gland), which is, in part, responsible for helping prevent depression.[15]
- Bach flowers such as mustard and gorse may be useful. Others may be needed according to the associated emotions.

Insomnia

Useful Oils

• bergamot • Roman chamomile • lavender • lemon • sweet marjoram • neroli • petitgrain • sweet orange • sandalwood • valerian

Clinical Features

Insomnia is usually considered to be sleep deprivation or a marked change in perceived sleep pattern. Insomnia can be divided into two categories:[16]

- Sleep-onset insomnia — difficulty in falling asleep.
- Maintenance insomnia — frequent or early wakening.

Aetiology

Factors contributing to insomnia include:

- sleep-onset insomnia — anxiety or tension, environmental change, emotional arousal, fear of insomnia, phobia of sleep, disruptive environment, pain or discomfort, caffeine, alcohol
- sleep-maintenance insomnia — depression, environmental change, sleep apnoea, hypoglycaemia, pain or discomfort, drugs, alcohol.[20]

Many patients respond to reassurance that their sleeplessness is a result of normal anxieties or a treatable physical disorder. Providing an opportunity to ventilate anxieties often will ease distress and help to re-establish normal sleep patterns.

While tension and anxiety are undoubtedly the main culprits there are a variety of secondary factors that should not be ignored. These may include sleeping in a poorly ventilated room, uncomfortable beds, droning noises, pick-me-up drinks such as coffee, tea and cola soft drinks. Many people with sleep disturbances have reported being 'cured' simply because they have stopped drinking these beverages.

Therapeutic Strategy

In managing insomnia it is important to consider the following:

- eliminate those factors that are known to disrupt sleep, such as coffee, tea, chocolate, alcohol, recreational drugs, many over-the-counter medications and some prescription drugs
- regular exercise that elevates heart rate 50–75% for at least 20 minutes a day
- relaxation techniques
- use of herbs and essential oils that are nervine relaxants.[20]

Aromatherapy Treatment

The calming, soothing, balancing and anxiety-reducing benefits of essential oils make aromatherapy very effective for treating insomnia. The most commonly used essential oil for relieving insomnia is lavender. Clinical trials have found lavender to be effective as a nocturnal sedative for elderly patients with sleeping disorders. According to observations made by the nursing staff at the Old Manor Hospital, Salisbury, England, lavender was found to be very effective:

> *After the aromatherapy started, residents exhibited less restlessness during the night, their sleep was deeper and so they would not be woken while staff made their rounds, there were fewer periods of simple insomnia and the mood of residents on waking was more pleasant.*[27]

Other useful essential oils include bergamot, Roman chamomile, sweet marjoram, mandarin, neroli, sandalwood, petitgrain, sweet orange, sandalwood and valerian. You can simply add a drop or two of any of these essential oils to your pillow or you may want to use these oils or a blend in a vaporiser, a warm bath before bedtime or in a massage oil.

It goes without saying that massage promotes relaxation and sleep. Most people with sleeping problems carry a tremendous amount of stress in the back and stomach areas, and massage will help to reduce tension in these areas.

Having a warm bath is very effective. Ensure that it is not too hot. Just more than lukewarm is ideal. This warms the blood a little, giving a soporific effect when it circulates to the brain. Trying adding a few drops (no more than 3 drops) of lavender or sweet marjoram to the bath.

Other Treatments

Nutrition

- Drink a cup of warm milk. Milk contains two natural nerve sedatives, the mineral calcium and the amino acid tryptophan.[15]
- Don't drink tea, coffee and cola drinks in the evening. They are full of caffeine that will not be inducive to a good night's sleep.[15,16]
- Vitamin B6, B3 and magnesium act as a co-factor in the conversion of tryptophan to serotonin which contributes to an improved sleep cycle.[16]
- Foods high in tryptophan such as bananas, figs, dates, yoghurt and wholegrain crackers promote sleep.[16]
- Avoid the consumption in the evening of caffeine, alcohol, sugar, cheese, chocolate, wine, ham, potatoes, spinach and tomatoes. These foods contain tyramine which increases the release of norepinephrine, a brain chemical stimulant.[15]

Herbs

Herbal teas such as valerian, skullcap, passion flower, chamomile, hops and catnip have all been used to reduce sleeplessness and induce relaxation.[7,15,20,24,25]

Hoffman recommends a valerian bath. He suggests pouring 2 litres of boiling water onto one or two handfuls of the dried root of valerian, leave it stand for half an hour, then strain the liquid and add it to the bath.[7]

General Advice

- Establish a regular sleep pattern. It seems very important to establish a regular going to bed and getting up time, so that the daily body rhythms accustom themselves to a routine.[15]
- Learn to relax. Meditation can open the doors to clarity and inspiration that is usually available to us during the dream state.[15]
- Avoid medication to induce sleep. Sleeping pills can be detrimental and should only be taken under strict medical supervision. They promote the wrong type of sleep, particularly a reduction in REM. Taken over a long period the drugs often have dangerous side-effects.[15]
- Listen to some soft music. Music can be a wonderful relaxation therapy.[15]
- Invest in a good comfortable bed. This is essential for a restful sleep.[15]
- Make sure the bed temperature is comfortable.[15]
- Dismiss negative emotions. Focus on thoughts that are uplifting and pleasant.[15,16]
- Physical exercise performed during the day does not increase the requirements for additional sleep. Instead, a physically tired body often relaxes quicker, thus encouraging deep sleep to occur easily.[15,16,20]
- Take a hot bath an hour or two before bedtime.[15]
- Avoid alcohol. A small amount can help to induce sleep initially, but it eventually disrupts deeper sleep cycles.[15,16,20]

Headaches and Migraines

Useful Oils
• cajeput • Roman chamomile • clary sage
• eucalyptus • lavender • spike lavender • lemon
• sweet marjoram • neroli • peppermint • rosemary
• thyme

Definition

Headaches are a common symptom that may be due to a wide variety of causes such as stress, tension, anxiety, allergies, constipation, coffee consumption, eyestrain, hunger, sinus pressure, muscle tension, hormonal imbalance, temporomandibular joint (TMJ) syndrome, trauma to the head, nutritional deficiencies, the use of alcohol, drugs or tobacco, fever, and exposure to irritants such as pollution.

Clinical Features

Headaches can be divided into three basic categories:

Vascular headaches: These include classic and common migraines, cluster headaches and possibly sinus headaches. They account for approximately 6 to 8% of all headaches.[14]

Muscular contraction headaches: These are by far the most common type of headache people experience (approximately 90 to 92%). Usually brought on by muscular tension and musculoskeletal misalignment.[14]

Traction-inflammatory headaches: These account for approximately 2% of headaches, and generally are indicative of severe underlying pathology such as tumours, aneurysm or infection in the central nervous system.[14]

85% of the population will have experienced a headache within 1 year and 38% of adults will have had a headache within 2 weeks.[10]

Migraines affect at least 10% of the adult population and 25% of these patients require medical attention for their attacks at some stage.[10]

The pain of a headache comes from outside the brain because the brain tissue itself does not have sensory nerves. Pain arises from the meninges and from the scalp and its blood vessels and muscles when these structures are stretched or tensed.[23]

Many headaches previously considered to be tension are secondary to disorders of the neck, eyes, teeth, TMJ or other structures.[10]

Aetiology

The major causes of tension headaches have been identified as:

- Muscular, tendinous or ligamentous injury to the head or neck structure. Simple muscular tension in the suboccipital triangle or the jaw flexors can cause headaches. These muscles are especially vulnerable to the effects of emotional stress. When people worry or are angry they tend to clench their jaws and tighten their necks.[14]
- Subluxation or fixation of cervical vertebrae can irritate ligaments or cause muscular spasms, both leading to headaches.[14]
- Structural problems in the alignment of the cranial bones or in the TMJ can cause headaches.[14]
- Trigger points in the muscles of the neck and head can refer pain to the head.[14]
- Any kind of ongoing mental or physical stress can change postural and movement patterns.[14]

A number of triggers have been identified in initiating migraines:

- injury to the head associated with football or boxing
- weather — sudden changes in weather, particularly thunderstorms or hot dry winds, may trigger headaches
- stress — emotions, glare and noise
- missing meals and hypoglycaemia
- fluctuations in hormonal levels — drops in oestrogen levels, particularly prior to menses, appears to be the major trigger in women
- food allergies and intolerances.[16]

A migraine can be preceded by vague mood changes, food or sugar craving, uncontrolled and repeated yawning and changes in sexual drive.[16]

Therapeutic Strategy

In the management of a migraine it is important to consider the following:

- keep a food diary of foodstuffs or drinks that may be trigger factors
- consider a low-amine diet
- practise a healthy lifestyle, relaxation therapy, meditation techniques and biofeedback training
- acupuncture or hypnotherapy may be effective.[10]

In the management of a tension headache it is important to learn stress management techniques, relaxation therapy, yoga and meditation.[10]

It is also recommended to use compresses with analgesic essential oils.

Aromatherapy Treatment

The most effective essential oils to treat headaches are lavender, peppermint and rosemary.[11] When using essential oils to treat a headache it is important to identify the cause of the headache before selecting the essential oils and method of application. For example:

- A headache that has been triggered by a long period of mental effort would best be treated using rosemary oil.
- A headache associated with anxiety and stress would best be treated using lavender.
- A headache associated with allergies and sinus congestion would best be treated with Roman chamomile and eucalyptus.

The method of application is equally important. Often massage may aggravate a headache, hence a compress or inhalation would be more suitable. When treating migraines, Davis warns that many people are often unable to tolerate the smell of essential oils or anyone touching their heads.[11]

Migraine headaches may be treated by cold compresses of peppermint and lavender essential oils. Many migraines are due to restricted blood supply to the brain, and hot or warm compresses with sweet marjoram or lavender on the back of the neck will increase the blood flow to the head. Sweet marjoram is a vasodilator, and warmth itself also helps.

Other Treatments

Nutrition

- Eat a well-balanced diet. Avoid chewing gum, ice cream, iced beverages, salt, and excessive sunlight.[15]
- Foods such as chocolate, cheese, beer and red wine precipitate migraine attacks in many people because they contain histamine and/or other vasoactive compounds that can trigger a migraine.[20,24]
- Eliminate foods containing tyramine and the amino acid phenylalanine. Then, reintroduce one food at a time and see which ones produce headaches. Phenylalanine is found in aspartame, monosodium glutamate (MSG), and nitrates (preservatives found in salami and small goods). Foods containing tyramine include alcoholic beverages, bananas, cheese, chicken, chocolate, citrus fruits, cold cuts, herring, onions, peanut butter, pork, smoked fish, sour cream, vinegar, wine and freshly baked yeast products. Tyramine causes the blood pressure to rise, resulting in a dull headache.[15,20,24]
- Avoid nitrates (preservative found in hot dogs and salamis), aspirin and MSG, a common seasoning.[15]

Herbs

- The following herbs are recommended for the relief of headache pain: burdock root, fenugreek, feverfew, goldenseal, lavender, marshmallow, peppermint, rosemary, skullcap, valerian and thyme.[15]
- Balch recommends making an ointment from ginger, peppermint and wintergreen essential oils for the relief of headaches.[15]
- Ginkgo biloba improves the circulation to the brain and may be helpful for certain types of headache.[15,16]
- Feverfew is very effective for the treatment of migraines. 70% of migraine sufferers who had eaten feverfew daily for prolonged periods claimed that the herb decreased the frequency of their migraine attacks.[15,20]

Acupressure

Acupressure will provide relief for headaches. The following acupressure points are recommended for the treatment of headaches.

- Frontal headaches can be relieved by pressing LI 4 which is located in the webbing between the thumb and the index finger.[28]
- GB 20, Bl 2, Tai Yang and Lv 3.[28]
- Yin tang, located between the eyebrows, in the indentation where the bridge of the nose meets the forehead relieves hay fever, headaches and eye strain.[28]

General Advice

- Apply cold compresses to the spot from which the pain is radiating. This helps relieve headaches by constricting blood vessels and easing muscle spasms. Leave a damp wash cloth in the freezer for 10 minutes or use a cold gel pack.[15]
- Use a hot water bottle or a hot towel to relax the neck and shoulder muscles, which can cause muscle contraction headaches when they are too tight.[15]

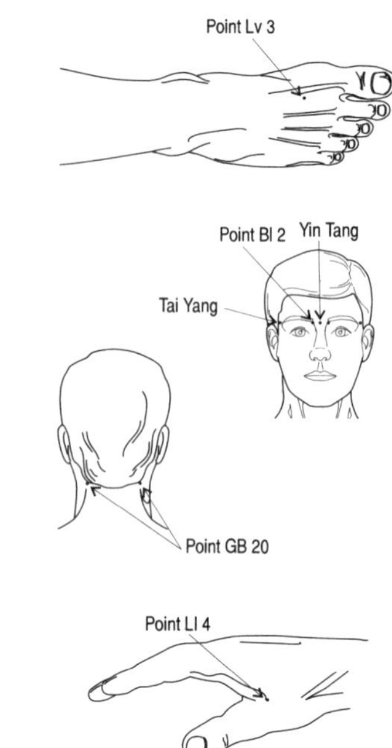

Acupressure points used to relieve headaches.

- For headaches caused by sinus congestion, facial massage techniques can help to drain the sinuses and ease tension. Apply heat to the sinuses, either with compresses or with steam inhalations.[15]
- Eating smaller meals and eating between meals may help to stabilise blood sugar levels which may prevent headaches.[15]
- It is important to obtain enough sleep.[15]
- Practise deep breathing exercises. A lack of oxygen can cause headaches.[15]
- Poor vertebral alignment may cause reduced blood flow to the brain. This is often caused by flat feet or wearing high heels. Chiropractic adjustment can help.[15]
- Acupuncture appears to have some success in reducing the frequency of migraine attacks.[20]
- Regular exercise can help prevent tension headaches and may reduce the severity and frequency of migraines. If the headache has organic causes it can be made worse by exercise.[15]

Epilepsy

Useful Oils
• Roman chamomile • lavender • sweet marjoram
• neroli • melissa • ylang ylang

Definition

Epilepsy is defined as a 'tendency to recurrence of seizures.' It is a symptom and not a disease. A person should not be labelled 'epileptic' until at least two attacks have occurred.[10]

Clinical Features

There are several types of seizures classified as follows:

Absence (petit mal): Most common in children and is characterised by a blank stare. During these seizures children are unaware of their surroundings.[15]

Atonic (drop attack): A childhood seizure in which the child loses consciousness for about 10 seconds after the legs have collapsed.[15]

Complex partial (temporal lobe): Blank stares, random activity, and chewing motion are characteristic of this type of seizure. The person may be dazed and unaware of the surroundings, and may act oddly. There is no memory of this seizure.[15]

Generalised tonic-clonic (grand mal): Characterised by sudden cries, a fall, rigidity and muscle jerks, shallow breathing and bluish skin. Loss of bladder control is possible. The seizure usually lasts 2 to 5 minutes and is followed by confusion, fatigue or memory loss.[15]

Myoclonic: Brief, massive muscle jerks.[15]

Simple partial (Jacksonian): Jerking begins in the fingers and toes and progresses through the body while the person is conscious.[15]

Simple partial (sensory): The person may see, hear, or sense things that do not exist. May occur as a preliminary symptom of a generalised seizure.[15]

Aetiology

In 75% of cases, the seizures begin in childhood and are characterised by staring spells and a few seconds of mental absence. In the remaining 25% of cases, seizures start later in life. The cause of most cases of epilepsy is unknown.[15]

Seizures may occur for no apparent reason, or they may be triggered by a wide range of factors such as exposure to allergens, flashing lights, drugs or alcohol, hypoglycaemia, infection, lack of sleep, metabolic or nutritional imbalances, trauma or head injury.[15]

An accurate medical diagnosis is based on the observation of a witness to the seizures, a general and neurological examination, an electroencephalogram (EEG) and a computerised tomography scan (CT) or preferably magnetic resonance imaging (MRI).[10]

Murtagh stresses that successful management of epilepsy requires an accurate diagnosis of the type of seizure, identification of the cause and appropriate investigation, the use of first-line drugs as the therapy for some weeks and the adjustment of the dose, according to clinical experience and plasma levels, to give maximum benefit.[10]

Therapeutic Considerations

Murtagh emphasises the following:

- most patients can lead a normal life
- a seizure in itself will not usually cause death or brain damage unless in a risk situation such as swimming
- patients cannot swallow their tongue during a seizure
- take care with open fires
- encourage patients to cease intake of alcohol
- adequate sleep is important.[10]

Avoid trigger factors such as fatigue, lack of sleep, physical exhaustion, stress, excess alcohol and prolonged flashing lights if photosensitive.

First Aid for Seizures

- move sharp or dangerous objects away from the person

- place the person on a bed or the floor
- loosen tight clothes
- turn the person on the side — if possible
- do not put anything in the person's mouth. Swallowing objects is more dangerous than biting the tongue
- stay calm and remember that the person does not feel anything during the seizure.[10]

Aromatherapy Treatment

There are a number of essential oils that should be avoided. These oils include: *Salvia officinalis, Foeniculum vulgare, Hyssopus officinalis* and *Rosmarinus officinalis*.[11,29]

Essential oils such as lavender or Roman chamomile are antispasmodic and may be beneficial for patients with epilepsy. However, I agree with Davis, who says that she would counsel against attempting to treat epilepsy by aromatherapy alone.[11]

Tim Betts, Senior Lecturer at the University of Birmingham and Consultant Neuropsychiatrist to South Birmingham Mental Health Trust, says that despite the conventional medical view, epilepsy behaves more like a psychosomatic illness.[30]

Once a seizure activity has started in a part of the brain it shows a conspicuous tendency to spread. He says there is good evidence that the ease with which the seizure activity spreads to the rest of the brain is dependent on the level of arousal in the part of the brain that surrounds the discharging focus. By controlling the level of arousal by altering life events, stress and by efforts of will and concentration, arousal responses can be modified. Thus it is possible that aromatherapy can be used to help modify psychological factors, which can minimise the event of epileptic seizures. As Betts says:

> *However to treat epilepsy solely as a medical condition just with drugs or surgery ignores the important fact that in many people epilepsy is made worse by stress and definite emotional factors ... Over medicalising epilepsy ignores the emotional needs of the person who has to live with it.*[30]

Betts says that it is possible for at least 30% of people with epilepsy to successfully control epilepsy using complementary methods. This involves the use of psychological counter measures, which a person applies either when the seizure activity appears to be about to start or in specific situations, which the person has learned to recognise as likely to lead to seizure activity.[30]

His work has shown that patients who:

- have a reliable prodrome, aura or precipitant
- have a clear association with the stress factor/life event, and
- are clearly able to identify stress and anxiety

are able to use aromatherapy together with auto-hypnosis to effectively control seizures.[30]

The essential oils chosen were ylang ylang (by far the most popular oil), lavender, chamomile, sweet marjoram, jasmine and bergamot.

Initially, the essential oils were introduced by a series of massages; however, they found that with time the person is able to instantly associate the particular aroma of the oil with the desired change in arousal. The person then practices changing arousal quickly by just using the aroma of the essential oil.[30]

Other Treatments

Nutrition

- Include beet greens, eggs, green leafy vegetables, raw cheese, raw milk, raw nuts, seeds and soya beans in the diet.[15]
- Drink fresh juices made from beets, carrots, green beans, green leafy vegetables, peas, red grapes, and seaweed.[15]
- Avoid alcoholic beverages, animal protein, fried foods, artificial sweeteners such as aspartame, caffeine and nicotine.[15]

General Advice

- Get regular moderate exercise to improve circulation to the brain.[15]
- Stay away from pesticides.[15]
- As much as possible, avoid stress and tension. Learn stress management techniques.[15]
- Consider having a hair analysis to rule out metal toxicity as the cause of seizures.[15]
- Other types of drugs can interfere with anti-seizure medications. Alcohol, birth control pills, the antibiotic erythromycin and some types of asthma, ulcer and heart medications are known to interact with certain epilepsy drugs.[15]

Shingles

Useful Oils

• bergamot • lavender • melissa • rose • tea tree

Definition

Herpes zoster or shingles is an acute infection of the sensory nerve roots. The condition is caused by a virus that is closely related to the chicken pox virus. It most commonly affects middle-aged or elderly people. The virus affects the sensory nerves before they enter the spinal cord and causes clusters of blisters on the area of skin served by the affected nerves. The pain is usually felt before the blisters appear and will sometimes persist for weeks or months after the blisters have disappeared.

Aetiology

Shingles is a disease caused by the varicella-zoster virus, the same virus that causes chicken pox.[15] The chance of an attack of shingles is increased by factors such as stress, cancer, and people with immune system deficiencies.[15]

Clinical Features

Shingles is often preceded by 3 or 4 days of chills, fever and aches. There may also be pain in the affected area. Then crops of tiny blisters appear. The affected area becomes excruciatingly painful and sensitive to touch. Other symptoms can include numbness, depression, tingling sensations, shooting pains, fever and headaches. The blisters eventually form a crusty scab and drop off.[15]

The skin of the affected area may become insensitive, although pain may persist for several months.

The trunk and the face are the regions most commonly affected. When the trigeminal nerve is affected, eruptions may appear on the cornea of the eye. Unless treated promptly, blindness may ensue.

Therapeutic Strategy

In managing shingles it is important to consider the following:

- Treat the rash with anti-inflammatory, antiviral and analgesic essential oils.
- Tonify the immune system.
- Dispel myths: Explain that it is not a dangerous disease, and that the patient will not go insane or die if the rash spreads from both sides and meets in the middle.[10]

Aromatherapy Treatment

The analgesic and antiviral properties of bergamot, lavender and tea tree are very beneficial in easing the pain, soothing the irritation, combating the virus and drying the blister. Davis recommends applying a 50/50 blend of bergamot and tea tree neat onto the blisters.[11]

Bergamot not only is one of the most active essential oils in inhibiting the herpes virus, it also has the benefit of being an antidepressant.

Schnaubelt recommends that once the blisters have disappear, but the pain still persists, a frequent application of aromatic hydrosol of Roman chamomile will bring relief.[31]

If large areas are affected use the essential oils in a bath. When the pain persists long after the blisters have disappeared use lavender and German chamomile in a hypericum-infused oil base.

Other Treatments

- The amino acid L-lysine is important for healing and for fighting the virus that causes shingles.[15]
- Keep stress to a minimum.[15]
- Passion flower is a mild tranquilliser and is recommended if there is neuralgic pain.[24]
- Valerian root calms the nervous system. It should be taken at bedtime, to promote sleep and rest.[15]

References

1. Tortora G, Anagnostakos N. *Principles of anatomy and physiology*. 4th edn, Harper & Row Publishers, New York, 1984.
2. Cohen BJ, Wood DL. *Memmler's: The human body in health and disease*. 9th edn, Lippincott, Williams & Wilkins, USA, 2000.
3. Australian Institute of Health & Welfare, *Australia's Health: 1998*. Commonwealth of Australia, 1998.
4. Breggin P. *Toxic psychiatry*. St Martins Press. New York, 1991.
5. Aldridge S. *Magic molecules: How drugs work*. Cambridge University Press, United Kingdom, 1998.
6. Beckman N. *The family library guide to natural therapies*. Family Library, Australia, 1992.
7. Hoffman D. *The new holistic herbal*. USA, Element Books Limited, 1983.
8. Meares A. *A way of doctoring*. Hill of Content, Australia, 1985.
9. Farrow J. *Massage therapy and nursing care*. Nursing Standard, 1990; 7(17): 26–28.
10. Murtagh J. *General practice*. 2nd edn, The McGraw-Hill Companies Inc, Australia, 1998.
11. Davis P. *Aromatherapy: An A–Z*. 2nd edn, The C.W. Daniel Company Limited, Great Britain, 1999.
12. Mailhebiau P. *Portraits in oils*. The C.W. Daniel Company Limited, Great Britain, 1995.
13. Mojay G. *Aromatherapy for healing the spirit*. Hodder & Stoughton, United Kingdom, 1996.
14. Werner R. *A massage therapist's guide to pathology*. Lippincott Williams & Wilkins, USA, 1998.
15. Balch J, Balch P. *Prescription for nutritional healing*. Avery Publishing Group, USA, 1997.
16. Osiecki H. *The physician's handbook of clinical nutrition*. Bioconcepts Publishing, Australia, 1990.
17. Tisserand R. *Success with stress*. International Journal of Aromatherapy 1992; 4(2): 14–16.
18. Bensen H. *The relaxation response*. William Morrow and Company, USA, 1975.

19. Worwood VA. *The fragrant pharmacy*. Macmillan London Limited, England, 1990.
20. Pizzorno J, Murray M. *A text book of natural medicine*. 2nd edn, Churchill Livingstone, UK, 1999.
21. Price L, Price S. *Aromatherapy for health professionals.* 2nd edn, Churchill Livingstone, UK, 1999.
22. Bone K, Mills S. *Principles and practice of phytotherapy.* Churchill Livingstone, UK, 2000.
23. Krupp M. Chatton M. *Current medical diagnosis and treatment 1980.* Lange Medical Publications, USA, 1980.
24. Davies S, Stewart A. *Nutritional medicine*. Pan Books, Great Britain, 1987.
25. Duke J. *The green pharmacy*. Rodale Press, USA, 1997.
26. Tyler V. *Herbs of choice.* Haworth Press, USA, 1993.
27. Hardy M. *Sweet scented dreams*. The International Journal of Aromatherapy 1991; 3(1): 12–13.
28. Reed Gach M. *Acupressure's potent points*. Bantam Books, USA, 1990.
29. Lawless J. *The encyclopaedia of essential oils*. Element Books Limited, Great Britain, 1992.
30. Betts T. *Sniffing the breeze*. Aromatherapy Quarterly 1994; 40: 19–22.
31. Schnaubelt K. *Medical aromatherapy*. Frog Ltd, USA, 1999.

The Lymphatic System

Objectives

After careful study of this chapter, you should be able to:

- explain the structure and function of the lymphatic system
- explain the effects of poor lymphatic performance
- explain how aromatherapy can assist the lymphatic system
- identify, list and describe common pathophysiologies of the lymphatic system
- explain the aromatherapy treatment for specific conditions and disorders of the lymphatic system
- explain the role of other holistic strategies for specific conditions and disorders of the lymphatic system.

Introduction

The role of the lymphatic system has always been of paramount importance in holistic therapies. The tissues of the body and organs excrete waste products as a result of their daily work. The waste products must be quickly removed or the tissues will suffer damage. The cleansing process of the body is performed by a mechanism called lymphatic circulation.

This chapter will investigate the structure and the function of the lymphatic system and how aromatherapy can increase its efficiency.

Structure of the Lymphatic System

The lymphatic system comprises a network of superficial and deep vessels which are found in all parts of the body except the brain, spinal column and areas such as bone marrow and cartilage that receive nutrition through diffusion rather than from blood vessels.

The two main structures of the lymphatic system are the lymph capillaries, vessels and large ducts which make up the network for the transport of lymph, and the lymph nodes, which are the filtering devices. Unlike the circulatory system, the lymphatic system has no pump and relies on muscular compression and general body activity for moving the lymphatic fluid around the body.[1]

The lymph nodes are the filtering sites for the lymphatic fluid, which resembles blood plasma but contains less protein and more lymphocytes. The lymph nodes are composed of lymphoid tissue, and are found near veins. There are about 600 to 700 lymph nodes found singly or in groups throughout the body. Those most easily felt on the body surface are the cervica (in the groin), the popliteal fossa (behind the knee), the occipital area (base of the skull), and the cupital area (at the elbow).[1, 2]

The spleen, thymus and tonsils are considered lymphatic organs, and the breast is largely made up of lymphatic glands and vessels.[1, 2]

Functions of the Lymphatic System

The lymphatic system serves three major functions in the body:

- it transports interstitial fluid which was initially formed as a blood filtrate back into the bloodstream
- it serves as the route by which absorbed fat from the small intestine is transported to the blood
- its cells — called lymphocytes (produced in the bone marrow, lymph organs, and other lymphatic tissue) — help to provide immunological defences against disease-causing agents.[1]

One of the main functions of the lymphatic system is to control the volume of fluid circulating in the body. Interstitial fluid consists of blood plasma, which filters through the thin walls of the capillaries into the surrounding connective tissues. Most of the proteins in the plasma remain in the blood, and this helps to draw some of the fluid back into the capillaries by osmosis.[3]

The interstitial fluid is vital to the cells. It brings moisture and nutrients, picks up waste products of cell metabolism, excess proteins, bacteria, viruses and inorganic materials such as chemicals to be transported to the organs of elimination. At rest the lymph system will drain away about 1.2–2.0 mL of 'dead fluid' per minute. Not all the fluid is drawn back into the capillaries, and this becomes lymph, which is absorbed into the lymphatic vessels and transported to the lymph nodes for filtering. During physical activity, the lymph system can drain away about 20 mL of 'dead fluid' per minute.[4]

Poor lymphatic drainage results in excessive fluid in the tissue, which causes oedema and a strain on all the organs responsible for excretion of fluids. Pronounced oedema may in fact be a sign of heart disease or kidney disease and should not be neglected. If this is suspected, a medical practitioner should be consulted.

Because the lymph system does not have a pump like the heart it can become sluggish and inefficient, particularly if we get little exercise and have a poor diet, which strains the cells with waste products that are difficult to eliminate.

Lymph nodes are responsible for manufacturing lymphocytes. Lymphocytes in turn manufacture antibodies, which are complex proteins with the capacity to neutralise invading organisms. The enlargement of lymph nodes indicates the production of large number of lymphocytes when an infection is present, or when the body is on the defensive. Granulocytes, which are white blood cells made in the bone marrow, also help in this process, and ingest foreign bacteria in a process known as phagocytosis. They migrate out of the capillaries and accumulate around areas of infection to engulf the invading microbes.

Lymphocytes and antibodies are also produced in the spleen and thymus gland. The spleen also filters lymph like a large lymph node, and contains considerable lymphoid tissue.

Lymph nodes also filter the lymphatic system. They comprise a network of fibres in which are

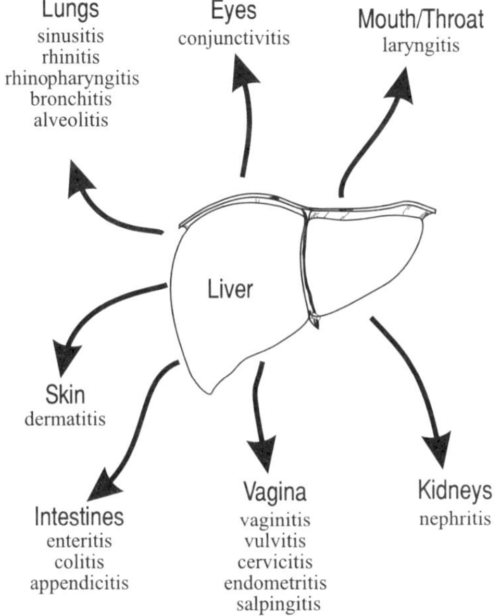

When the liver is overloaded with toxins the above emergency pathways are utilised.

found white blood cells called macrophages that ingest foreign bodies as the lymph passes through the nodes.

Effects of Poor Lymphatic Performance

When the lymphatic system does not work well, the resulting condition is known as congestion. Congestion is a form of lymphatic stagnation. The lymph is filled with waste products that pass through the lymph nodes. The lymph nodes fulfil the function of filter beds. These nodes form secretions and possess cells which have the ability to neutralise, dissolve, destroy or take up debris or waste products which may be in the body.

The liver is one of the largest organs responsible for detoxification; it neutralises and eliminates a large number of toxins. However, when the lymph nodes and the liver are unable to cope with the toxins, the toxins are diverted towards and can ooze through mucous membranes and other emergency elimination sites. This 'oozing' is a common condition known as catarrh or inflammation of the mucous membranes and is the cause of every form of 'itis'.

This serves as a basis for understanding how essential oils and naturopathic principles can be applied in eliminating toxins from the body, treating many conditions associated with toxic overload and restoring the body to good health.

Even though the lymph system acts as a modern sewage treatment plant, it is vital for the maintenance of life because when this system fails to function properly, excessive fluid and toxins build up in the body causing pain, loss of energy, infection and various diseases.

How Aromatherapy Can Assist Lymphatic Problems

Essential oils with the following properties can help to overcome some of the problems associated with the lymphatic system:

Alteratives, Blood Purifiers or Detoxifiers

Most essential oils will to some degree stimulate phagocytosis, that is, the ability of the white blood cells to 'gobble up' and clean up microbes and toxins.

According to Mills, tissues may be cleansed by improving the function of the major eliminatory channels in the body. These remedies are classified as blood purifiers, depuratives or alteratives. They may of course have conventional anti-inflammatory action or may otherwise change metabolic functions. All of these help in the elimination of excess waste products and make the job of the lymphatic system easier.[5]

Oils such as angelica root, carrot seed, cypress, grapefruit, fennel seed, geranium, juniper berry, lemon, mandarin and rosemary may be used.

Antiseptics

Valnet speaks at great length of the antiseptic powers of essential oils. He lists essential oils of eucalyptus, clove, niaouli, thyme, sandalwood, lemon, cinnamon, lavender, German chamomile and peppermint as being particularly beneficial.[6]

Circulatory Stimulants

Stimulating the circulation will also stimulate the flow of lymph. Essential oils such as black pepper, cinnamon bark or leaf, clove bud, cardamom, ginger and rosemary may be used in a lymphatic massage blend to stimulate the circulation.

Diuretics

Any essential oil that increases the flow of urine has diuretic properties. Diuretics stimulate the kidneys and accelerate the detoxification process. Typical essential oils include grapefruit, fennel seed, juniper berry, lemon, mandarin, sweet orange and tangerine.

Increasing Leucocytosis

Gattefosse first commented on the cytophylactic property of essential oils. He comments on observations made by Dr P. Sassard, who used lavender oil:

> *Wounds to the scalp: healed in 10 days; Infected herpes vesicle: healed in 5 days; Firearm wound: healed in 15 days; Sacral bedsore due to a high fracture in a 68 year old woman: healed in 11 days.*[7]

In all cases, the following was noted: rapid disappearance of pus; decrease in the number of bacteria; powerful stimulation of healing; recovery in a very short time. Apart from lavender; essential oils such as bergamot, lemon, rosemary, tea tree and thyme will increase the body's ability to manufacture white blood cells.

Lymphatic Stimulants

Many essential oils such as grapefruit, cold-pressed lime, sweet orange, tangerine, peppermint and rosemary are reputed to stimulate lymph and tissue fluid circulation.

According to Gumbel, peppermint is an important oil for stimulating the lymphatic system:

> *... has a special connection to everything aqueous, to the blood, to tissue fluid, lymph, spinal and cerebral fluid. The refreshing effect on all tissues lies in liberating influence on the lymphatic stream ... The oil has a cleansing, purifying and antiseptic effect on mucous membranes. It accelerates and increases their resorption ability.*[8]

Other Considerations

Lymphatic problems can be helped by using specific lymphatic drainage massage techniques. The aromatherapy massage techniques developed by Maury and Arcier incorporate lymphatic drainage.

The Micheline Arcier aromatherapy massage technique described in this book uses the neuro-lymphatic reflexes. These reflexes are also referred to as 'Chapman's reflexes'.[9] The position of the reflex points does not necessarily correspond to the positions of the lymph glands. The reflex points act like circuit breakers in that they 'turn off' when the system is overloaded. By gently massaging these points the lymphatic function will be stimulated.

The best-known system of lymphatic massage was developed by Dr Emil Vodder. It is important that the contra-indications of lymphatic massage be observed rigidly. Lymphatic massage should not be performed on anyone who has active cancer, heart problems, thrombosis, phlebitis, high blood pressure, varicose veins, pregnancy, any acute inflammation or infection, or any other severe medical problem. Do not use these techniques on anyone who has recently undergone chemotherapy, since the toxins stored in the blood and liver will be released into the bloodstream and make the person feel very ill.

Diet is of utmost importance, because a highly refined diet makes the job of waste removal much more difficult. An exercise program is also important. Baths with the detoxifying essential oils and magnesium sulphate can be useful and brisk friction rub over the body using a loofah or body brush should also be incorporated.

Mills suggests in his 'toxic thesis of disease' that:

> *The process of removing waste materials from the body is essential to health; several eliminatory functions share the task: failure in suppression of one will lead to extra burdens and possible signs of distress in others, and will have potentially widespread implications for general health.*[5]

Associated Conditions

Cellulite

Useful Oils

- carrot seed • cypress • sweet fennel • ginger
- juniper berry • grapefruit • geranium • lemon
- cold-pressed lime • mandarin • sweet orange
- rosemary • tangerine • sage

Definition

Cellulite is an accumulation of water and toxic wastes in the connective tissue surrounding the fat cells, which in turn form nodules. It starts with a build-up of toxins that causes the body to react via water retention in an effort to dilute the toxins and prevent self-poisoning. The tissue around the fat cells tends to harden, imprisoning the water and causing the unsightly bulges.

Medical practitioners use the term *cellulitis* to describe a diffuse, inflammatory or infectious process involving the subcutaneous structures.[10]

Clinical Features

Cellulite is classified in four major stages:[10]

Stage 1: the skin around the thighs and buttocks has a smooth surface when the subject is standing or lying. When the skin is pinched, it folds and furrows but does not pit or bulge. This stage is considered normal.

Stage 2: the skin surface is smooth while the subject is standing or lying, but the pinch test is clearly positive for the mattress phenomenon (pitting, bulging and deformity of the affected skin surfaces).

Stage 3: the skin surface is smooth while a subject is lying, but when standing there is pitting, bulging and deformity of the affected skin surfaces. This stage is common in women who are obese or over 35–40 years of age.

Stage 4: the mattress phenomenon is apparent when a subject is lying or standing. It is very common after menopause and in obesity.

Aetiology

Cellulite is seen almost exclusively in women. The reason for this is the basic structure of the subcutaneous tissue that is distributed in cellulite.

In women, the uppermost subcutaneous layer consists of what are referred to as 'large standing fat-cell chambers', which are separated by radial and arching dividing walls of connective tissue anchored to the overlying connective tissue of the skin (epidermis).

In contrast, in men the uppermost part of the subcutaneous tissue is thinner and has a network of crisscrossing connective tissue walls. The epidermis is also thicker in men.[10]

A simple test to demonstrate this difference is the 'pinch test'. Pinching the skin will result in the 'mattress phenomenon', pitting, bulging and deformation of the skin.

As women age, the epidermis becomes progressively thinner and looser. This allows the cells to migrate to this layer. In addition, the connective tissue walls between the fat cell chambers also become thinner, allowing the fat cell chambers to enlarge excessively. The breakdown or the thinning of connective tissue structures is a major contributor to the development of cellulite. Histological examination reveals distension of the lymphatic vessels of the upper epidermis and a decrease in the number of subepidermal fibres.[10]

Other contributing factors to cellulite include:

- hormonal imbalance
- poor blood circulation
- accumulation of wastes
- unbalanced diet
- abuse of stimulants (coffee, tea, cigarettes, alcohol)
- lack of correct exercise
- stress and emotional upheaval
- poor breathing
- constipation
- incorrect posture.

Research has identified that when there is greatest hormone fluctuation, cellulite may occur in women.[11] Typically this is:

- at the onset of puberty — 12%
- when first going on the contraceptive pill — 19%
- during pregnancy — 17%
- during menopause — 27%.

Oestrogen is responsible for female sexual development. Another important role of oestrogen is that it helps to eliminate waste materials from the vital organs and deposits them into areas where they will be relatively harmless. Therefore, it may be assumed that cellulite forms when there is a general circulatory problem in the body because the lymphatic system is unable to dispose of the body's wastes in the normal way.[11]

With the introduction of the contraceptive pill and hormone replacement therapy for postmenopausal women, the amount of oestrogen present in women's bodies has increased enormously. The more oestrogen present, it seems the more likely it is that cellulite will develop.[11]

Therapeutic Strategy

It must be kept in mind that cellulite is not a 'disease' per se. The holistic approach to the treatment of cellulite is to reduce the level of toxins by incorporating the following techniques into the treatment regime:

- exercise
- massage
- diet
- aromatherapy.[10,11,12]

Exercise

Exercise can be very effective once most of the cellulite has been eliminated. Although cellulite is partly caused by a sedentary lifestyle, vigorous exercise will not make the slightest difference to cellulite deposits that are already there. In fact, many forms of exercise, particularly impact sports such as jogging or aerobics, may place extra pressure on the joints and encourage the cellulite to harden and become even more compacted.

Massage

Massage, particularly lymphatic drainage massage, is very beneficial. The physical effects of massage improve circulation of the blood and lymph. The direction of the massage should always be from the periphery to the heart.[10]

Diet

A diet high in complex carbohydrates and low in refined carbohydrates and fats is very important. It is important to cut out junk food, anything greasy, fatty, refined, sugary or salty. A diet should follow these general rules:

- To make digestion easier, eat a limited number of foods at each meal.

- Reduce salt intake as salt tends to promote the retention of fluids in the tissues.
- Avoid taking fluids with meals or for half an hour afterwards, as liquids cause food to pass into the bloodstream before it has been efficiently digested. Drink liquids 20 minutes before or between meals.
- Drink purified water or mineral water with low salt content, and fresh vegetable and fruit juices.
- Celery juice and lemon juice are also worthwhile taking daily.
- The following foods are recommended as they are easily digested and provide varied nutrition needed for maintenance, regrowth, repair and detoxification:
  - Proteins of animal origins — should be lean and prepared by roasting or grilling.
  - Proteins of vegetable origins — wholegrains, cereals, legumes, lentils, soyabeans.
  - Dairy products — skim milk, natural cottage and feta cheese, natural yoghurt.

Aromatherapy Treatment

Essential oils which are detoxifying, stimulating to the lymphatic system, hormone balancing and which have diuretic properties should be used. The essential oils must be used in a massage and bath. While daily self-massage will be necessary, regular professional aromatherapy massage which uses lymphatic drainage techniques is also recommended.[11]

Essential oils such as cypress, fennel seed, geranium, grapefruit, juniper berry, lemon, cold-pressed lime and rosemary can be used in a massage or a bath.

Lymphoedema

Useful Oils
• carrot seed • sweet fennel • juniper berry
• grapefruit • geranium

Definition

Oedema is an excessive accumulation of fluid in tissue spaces. It may be generalised or localised.

Aetiology

According to Mills, the origins of oedema give significant insight into the normal mechanisms for draining tissues. They fall into five main categories:[5]

- **Obstruction to venous flow**. Notably seen in heart failure and accumulated back pressure in the venous system. Oedema in this case is seen in the most gravity-dependent regions first — that is, in the ankles.
- **Low levels of plasma protein**. This means that the colloid osmotic pressure in the capillaries, which effectively acts as a brake on fluid movement into the tissues, is reduced. This loss is extreme and is only seen locally with severe burns, and systemically with terminal kidney diseases or near starvation.
- **Lymphatic obstruction**. This is seen most dramatically in the tropical infection filariasis, in which nematode worm larvae are introduced into the lymphatic system following bites from infected mosquitoes. If untreated, the subsequent inflammations can lead to scarring and eventual occlusion of the lymphatics in the region. The consequences have been given the name elephantiasis.
- **Increased capillary fragility leading to passage of protein from blood cell to tissue**. The dramatic change in the balance of osmotic pressure can lead to tissue oedema. Burns, allergic reactions and radiation damage can all lead to fluid swelling in the tissues affected through this cause.
- **Kidney failure**. Fluid retention at the kidneys will inevitably lead, if serious, to extensive oedema.

Mills is implying that oedema is not a common condition and that in health there is a considerable safety margin built into tissue hydraulics to ensure that all excess fluid is easily mopped up.[5]

According to Kahn, lymphoedema may be due to a primary (congenital) cause or a secondary cause (caused by a known condition), including removal of lymph nodes, radiation or trauma. Lymphoedema can occur at any time in the years following mastectomy, lumpectomy followed by radiation, or after lymph nodes have been removed due to melanoma, radical hysterectomy or prostate cancer. The build-up of proteins in the interstitial tissue, due to inadequate functioning of the lymph vessel system, leads to chronic inflammation and a compromised local immunity that leads to bouts of cellulitis (infection).[13]

The impact of lymphoedema on the patient can be enormous due to decreased mobility, heaviness, discomfort and the threat of infection. It is a chronic condition which, left untreated, worsens with time. Patients often have to be hospitalised with multiple infections.

Therapeutic Strategy

Kahn recommends a *Complex Decongestive Therapy* which is a four-step process carried out over a 2–4 week period followed by a second maintenance phase.[13] She says it is a highly effective approach to decongest and maintain the affected limb or area. The treatment comprises:

- manual lymphatic drainage techniques
- compression therapy
- remedial exercises
- meticulous skin care.[13]

The aromatherapy treatment strategy is the reduction of the swelling by stimulating the lymph flow by using lymphatic drainage massage techniques and using cool compresses of essential oils such as juniper berry, fennel seed and cypress. The legs should be elevated and the use of firm elastic support to be worn during the day is also recommended.

The goal of the treatment is to reduce the swelling, facilitate lymph fluid and venous circulation to the affected area and reduce the risk of infection. Kahn also suggests incorporating self-massage, yoga, deep breathing, nutritional and lifestyle advice.[13]

It is important to ensure that if your patient has aromatherapy baths, which will be most beneficial, they should not be too hot. The heat can cause filtration of fluids into the tissue and further exacerbate the lymphoedema condition.

Kahn says that tension and stiffness can occur in the muscles of the shoulder and neck, as a result of arm oedema, and lower lack pain can result from leg oedemas, as the patients often have to compromise their posture to accommodate pain or discomfort.[13] The accompanying muscle tension further restricts the flow of lymph and contributes to the condition. Kahn recommends using an essential oil blend with sweet marjoram, juniper and Roman chamomile.[13]

Patients are also at risk of infections due to a compromised immune system. Patients with lymphoedema of the leg are at risk of dry, flaky skin and fungal infections, and patients with lymphoedema of the arm are at risk of dry, cracked skin and skin infections. These local infections can become systemic and endanger patients' lives. Kahn says it is important to use pH-balanced moisturising lotions with essential oils such as lavender, for its healing and antiseptic properties, and tea tree, for its antiseptic properties.[13]

It is very important for someone with lymphoedema to take special care to prevent cellulitis which is systemic and can be severe.[14] The symptoms are similar to those of influenza. The limb becomes fiery red and painful, and hospitalisation is often necessary. The treatment involves intravenous antibiotics. Patients are cautioned to avoid any cuts or scratches in the skin where bacteria or viruses can enter. The emphasis must be on moisturising the skin, protecting it with clothing and avoiding direct heat of any type.[14]

Lymphatic Drainage Massage

Manual lymphatic drainage is a gentle rhythmical massage to assist the lymph flow, boost immunity, decrease pain and balance the central nervous system. For this Kahn recommends essential oils such as lemon, *Laurus nobilis,* grapefruit, rosemary and peppermint which can all assist with lymph fluid circulation and elimination of wastes from the interstitial tissue.[13]

References

1. Van de Graaff K, Fox S. *Concepts of human anatomy & physiology.* 3rd edn, Wm.C. Publishers, USA, 1992.
2. Tortora G, Anagnostakos N. *Principles of anatomy and physiology.* 4th edn, Harper & Row Publishers, New York, 1984.
3. Cohen BJ, Wood DL. *Memmler's the human body in health and disease.* 9th edn, J.B. Lippincott Company, USA, 2000.
4. West C. *The golden seven plus one.* Samuel Publishing Co, USA, 1981.
5. Mills S. *The essential book of herbal medicine.* Penguin Books, England, 1991.
6. Valnet J. *The practice of aromatherapy.* The C.W. Daniel Company Limited, Great Britain, 1980.
7. Gattefosse R. *Gattefosse's aromatherapy.* The C.W. Daniel Company Limited, Great Britain, 1993.
8. Gumbel D. *Principles of holistic skin therapy with herbal essences.* Karl F. Haug Publishers, Germany, 1986.
9. Chaitow L. *Soft-tissue manipulation.* Thorson's Publishers Limited, England, 1988.
10. Pizzorno J. *A text book of natural medicine.* 2nd edn, Churchill Livingstone, UK, 1999.
11. Hodgkinson L. *How to banish cellulite forever.* Grafton Books, UK, 1989.
12. Davis P. *Aromatherapy: An A–Z.* The CW. Daniel Company Limited, Great Britain, 1988.
13. Kahn L, *Complementary care for the lymphedema patient.* Aromatherapy Today 2001; 17: 22–23.
14. Lunken A. *Lymphoedema and aromatherapy.* Aromatherapy Today 1998; 5: 26.

The Digestive System

Objectives

After careful study of this chapter, you should be able to:

- identify, list and describe common pathophysiologies of the digestive system
- explain the aromatherapy treatment for specific conditions and disorders of the digestive system
- explain the role of other holistic strategies for specific conditions and disorders of the digestive system.

Introduction

Food is vital to life. Every living cell in the body must have food to obtain energy and the building components it needs to live. However, the food that the cells use is quite different from the food that an individual ingests. Most foods we eat are simply too large to be absorbed through the plasma membranes of the cells. The process of changing insoluble and non-diffusible substances into soluble and diffusive forms which may be absorbed into the circulatory system is called digestion.[1]

The organs which collectively perform this function and break down food molecules for use by body cells comprise the digestive system.

The digestive system is generally divided into two groups of organs:

The *digestive tract*, a continuous passageway beginning at the mouth, where food is ingested, and terminating at the anus, where the waste products of digestion are expelled from the body.

The *accessory organs*, which are necessary for the digestive process but are not a direct part of the digestive tract. They release substances into the digestive tract through ducts. These organs are the salivary glands, liver, gall bladder and the pancreas.[2]

The digestive system prepares food for consumption by the cells through five basic activities:[2]

1. **Ingestion.** Taking food into the body (eating).
2. **Peristalsis.** The movement of food along the digestive tract.
3. **Digestion.** The breakdown of food by chemical and mechanical processes.
4. **Absorption.** The passage of digested food from the digestive tract into the cardiovascular and lymphatic systems for distribution to cells.
5. **Defecation.** The elimination of indigestible substances from the body.

While it is convenient to divide the functions of the digestive system into motility, secretion, digestion and absorption, it needs to be emphasised that these divisions are artificial and that these processes occur together.

Our health and vitality depend on our digestive system's ability to provide nutrients for our body. It is not just a matter of what substances we are putting in our mouth, but essentially one of what is properly processed so that it can be assimilated and used by the body. If there is a functional problem in the digestion, then no matter what is eaten it will not be properly absorbed, and a deficiency will occur.[3]

An example of a functional problem, as opposed to an organic problem, is eating rapidly and at irregular intervals. This leads to indigestion; the food enters a unprepared gut too fast causing malabsorption and thus a discomfort. The fault can lie in the eating habits, the content or amount of digestive juices or in a dysfunction of the intestinal walls, so that the food is not properly absorbed through the lining of the gut.[3]

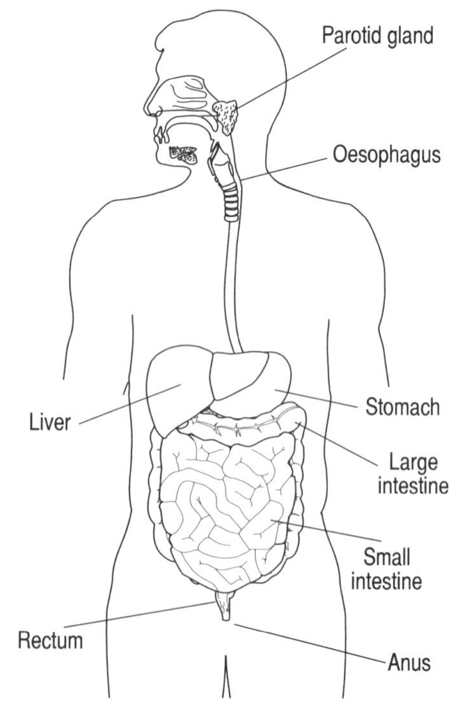

The digestive system.

Besides the function of assimilation, an equally important activity of the digestive system is elimination. Not all food that is eaten is absorbed. Some is not digestible and needs to be disposed of. The body also produces a lot of metabolic waste products that it has to eliminate, partly through the digestive system. The condition of the bowel and the state of its contents will affect the rest of the body.[3]

In addition to the physiological influences affecting the functioning and the health of the digestive system, there is a profound influence by the emotions and state of the mind. There is an immediate response to anger, anxiety, fear and all forms of stress and worry. To treat digestive problems in a holistic way, an appreciation of these psychological influences must also be considered. Most digestive problems that commonly occur are easily avoidable by changes of lifestyle and habits.[3]

General Considerations

The holistic treatment revolves around soothing and healing, supporting nervous balance, restoring digestive and absorptive mechanisms, correcting liver and gall bladder functions and cleansing and correcting eliminative functions. Some general guidelines include:

- Avoid over-eating, particularly rich, fatty and fried foods.
- Do not eat too fast, as this taxes the system.
- A number of commonly ingested substances and drugs may cause or aggravate digestive problems — for example, coffee, smoking, alcohol, excess orange juice and certain pharmaceutical drugs.
- Avoid drinking with meals. It does not seem sensible to dilute the gastric juices more than necessary, especially if there is a digestive problem.
- Regular exercise is essential to the health of the digestive system.
- Meals should be eaten in a relaxed environment and all food should be chewed thoroughly.
- The diet should be as natural and as high in roughage as possible.
- Artificial chemical additives should be avoided.
- Changes in bowel patterns and rectal bleeding must always be checked.
- Beware of fad diets and restrictive dietary recommendations.

Hoffman says that herbs are very effective in the treatment of digestive disorders. Most herbs are taken by the mouth and therefore easily absorbed through the digestive system where the therapeutic benefits will be effective immediately.[4] Weiss says that herbal teas have been used for centuries and are most useful for the management of digestive problems.[5]

Tyler says that herbs containing volatile oils are considered the most effective for treating gastrointestinal problems.[6] He says that it is surprising that herbal teas are commonly recommended, as volatile oils are relatively insoluble in water. He says that fluid extracts or tinctures of the herbs are much more effective. He also recommends alcoholic solutions of essential oils.[6]

Aromatherapy Considerations

The first act of digestion is olfaction. The aroma of food stimulates the secretion of saliva and digestive juices, in preparation for the act of eating.[7]

Tisserand recommends that essential oils for digestive disorders may be given orally, by enemas, by massage — especially over the dorsal and lumbar areas and by local compresses over the stomach area and the abdomen.[7]

Schnaubelt says that many complaints of the digestive tract are an expression of the autonomic nervous system.[8]

The antispasmodic, carminative and digestive stimulating properties of essential oils are well known, and many essential oils are currently used in pharmacopoeias.[6,7]

Research has proven that peppermint can be effectively used to treat irritable bowel syndrome.[9,10] These tests concluded that peppermint oil was a carminative with potent antispasmodic properties, and is particularly valuable for the symptomatic treatment of irritable bowel syndrome.

Lavender, peppermint, spearmint, fennel, coriander, thyme and German chamomile are pronounced cholagogues.[11]

Mills suggests that many of the herbal remedies used for treating the digestive system fall into two categories, the 'cooling and drying' bitters and the 'warming and drying' aromatic digestives, chosen according to the wider needs of the body. The emphasis on 'drying' is not surprising as the main organ responsible for digestion in Chinese medicine is the spleen and it is particularly vulnerable to *damp*.[12]

Essential oils which have a 'warming and drying' effect such as black pepper, fennel, coriander, sweet marjoram, myrrh and peppermint have traditionally been used to tonify the digestive system.[13,14]

The therapeutic properties of essential oils which have a particular affinity for the digestive system include:

Antimicrobials

Infections can be the cause of many digestive problems. Schnaubelt recommends strong antimicrobial essential oils such as cinnamon bark and clove bud for clearing the intestinal tract of pathogenic bacteria. He says that unlike antibiotics, these oils will not destroy the flora of the intestinal tract. He recommends one drop of the oil into a tablespoon of edible vegetable oil and to ingest this mixture in a gelatine capsule. He says that internal application is usually safe and effective.[8]

Antispasmodics

Antispasmodics or spasmolytics affect the smooth muscle, the intestine is relaxed, facilitating the passage of intestinal gas.[6]

Essential oils which are antispasmodic include angelica root, aniseed, bay laurel, black pepper, Roman chamomile, cinnamon bark and leaf, clove bud, dill, sweet fennel, ginger, nutmeg, sweet orange, peppermint, rosemary and rose.

Astringents

The action of astringents lies mainly in their ability to contract cell walls, thus condensing the tissue and making it firmer and arresting any unwanted discharge.[3]

Essential oils with astringent properties most suitable for the digestive system include cypress, juniper berry, lemon, myrrh, rosemary and sage.

Carminatives

Tyler cites Schilcher, who says that the carminative effects on the stomach, gall bladder and intestinal tract result from at least five different activities:[6]

1. Local stimulation of the stomach lining, leading to an increase in tonus and an intensification of rhythmic contractions facilitating the eructation of air from that organ; this is promoted by relaxation of the lower oesophageal sphincter.
2. Reflexive increase in stomach secretions resulting in improved digestion.
3. Antispasmodics affect the smooth muscles; the intestines are relaxed, facilitating the passage of intestinal gas.
4. Antiseptic action, limiting the development of undesirable micro-organisms.
5. Cholagogues, which promote bile flow, facilitating digestion and absorption of nutrients.

Essential oils that are carminatives include aniseed, basil, black pepper, carrot seed, cinnamon bark and leaf, clove bud, cardamom, Roman and German chamomile, coriander, dill, sweet fennel, ginger, nutmeg, sweet orange, peppermint and rose.

Cholagogues

Cholagogues increase the flow of bile and stimulate the gall bladder. Essential oils such as Roman and German chamomile, everlasting, lavender, peppermint, rosemary, rose and spearmint are recommended.

Hepatics

Hepatics strengthen, tone and stimulate the secretions of the liver. This causes an increase in the flow of bile. Hepatics include essential oils such as carrot seed, Roman and German chamomile, everlasting, lemon, rosemary, spearmint, turmeric and peppermint.

Laxatives

While some essential oils can be effective in the management of constipation, this does not imply that they have a laxative effect. Generally there are two types of botanical laxatives, the bulk-producing laxatives such as psyllium seeds and stimulating laxatives which contain anthraquinones such as cascara sagrada, senna and aloe.[6]

Associated Conditions

Periodontal Disease

Useful Oils

• sweet fennel • manuka • myrrh • peppermint
• tea tree

Definition

Periodontal disease is an inclusive term used to describe an inflammatory condition of the gingiva (gingivitis) and/or periodontium (periodontitis).[15]

Clinical Features

The gums become red, soft and shiny, and they bleed easily. Gingivitis is essentially painless; however, in some cases, there can be pain. If left untreated, gingivitis can lead to a condition called *periodontitis*. This is an advanced stage of periodontal disease in which the bone supporting the teeth begins to erode as a result of the infection. Periodontitis causes halitosis, with bleeding and often painful gums.[16]

Aetiology

Gingivitis is caused by plaque, sticky deposits of bacteria, mucus and food particles that adhere to the teeth. The accumulation of plaque causes the gums to become infected and swollen.[16]

Other factors contributing to gingivitis include breathing through the mouth, poorly fitted fillings and a diet consisting of too many soft foods that rob the teeth and gums of much-needed 'exercise'.[16]

Therapeutic Strategy

Treatment should be directed at the underlying cause.

- Thorough brushing of the teeth after every meal and the use of antiseptic rinses to reduce the number of micro-organisms will help to decrease odour formation.[16]
- A diet high in dietary fibre may have a protective effect by increasing salivary secretions.[15]
- Avoidance of sucrose and all refined carbohydrates is very important.[15]

Aromatherapy Treatment

Tea tree and thyme are the most useful essential oils for treating gum infections. Fennel and mandarin essential oils can be used to strengthen the gums, and myrrh is excellent for its healing and tonic properties.[17] Davis recommends the following mouthwash:[17]

250 mL of brandy
30 drops of thyme
30 drops of peppermint
10 drops of myrrh
10 drops of sweet fennel

To use, add 2 or 3 teaspoons to half a glass of warm water and rinse.

Other Treatments

Herbs

- Echinacea, myrrh and rose hips help to keep down inflammation and enhance immune function. These herbs should be taken as a tea or used as a poultice.[16]
- Apply aloe vera gel directly to inflamed gums to ease discomfort and soothe the tissues.[16]

Nutrition

- Eat a varied diet of fresh fruit, green leafy vegetables, meat and whole grains to provide the teeth and gums with the needed exercise.[16,18]
- Avoid sugar and all refined carbohydrates. Sugar causes plaque build up.[16]
- Vitamin A controls the development and general health of the gums, lack of vitamin A results in gum infection.[15,16]
- Adequate intake of vitamin C is particularly important for the prevention of gingivitis.[15,16]

Constipation

Useful Oils

• black pepper • carrot seed • cinnamon bark
• sweet fennel • sweet marjoram • sweet orange
• peppermint • pine • rosemary

Definition

Constipation is the difficult passage of small hard stools. It has also been defined as infrequent bowel actions or as a feeling of unsatisfied emptying of the bowels.[20]

Clinical Features

The frequency of defecation and the consistency of stools vary greatly in normal individuals. A client should be considered to be constipated only if defecation is unexplainably delayed for a matter of days or if the stools are unusually hard, dry and difficult to express. If constipation is a regular problem, the possibility of cancer or another obstruction in the lower bowel should not be dismissed unless a thorough medical examination has been conducted.[20]

Individuals with constipation develop a variety of symptoms, such as bowel pain, rectal discomfort, abdominal fullness, nausea, anorexia and general feeling of malaise.[19] Bleeding suggests carcinoma, haemorrhoids, diverticular disease or inflammatory bowel diseases.[20] Constipation is also a common problem in pregnancy.

Aetiology

The cause of constipation could be something simple such as stress, insufficient dietary fibre, excess protein, refined foods or poor bile flow. It could also be related to liver or thyroid underactivity. Other causes include inadequate fluids, pregnancy, antacids, metabolic disorders, tumours, strokes, old age and constant use of enemas and laxatives.[19]

Therapeutic Strategy

In the management of constipation it is important to consider the following:

- The most important treatment strategy for the management of constipation is dietary.[20]
- Check for the possible cause of constipation. If it is due to drug or laxative abuse, restrict the intake if possible.[19]
- Get adequate exercise. Physical exercise speeds movement of waste through the intestines. A 20-minute walk can often relieve constipation. Regular exercise is important for preventing constipation in the first place.[16,20]
- Heavy laxative users should take acidophilus to replace the ‘friendly’ bacteria. The continued use of laxatives cleans out the intestinal bacteria which eventually makes constipation worse.[16]
- Go to the toilet the same time every day, even if the urge does not exist, and relax. Stress tightens the muscles and can be the cause of constipation. Never repress the urge to defecate.[16,20]
- If constipation is persistent it may be recommended to take a enema.[16]

It is important to ask the patient to define exactly what they mean by constipation. The following questions should be useful:[20]

- How often do you go to the toilet?
- What are your bowel motions like?
- Is there pain on opening your bowels?
- Have you noticed any blood?
- What medications are you taking?

Aromatherapy Treatment

The most effective application of aromatherapy for constipation is massage of the abdomen, always in a clockwise direction. This is something that the patient can be easily taught to carry out daily at home. The most effective oils to use for massage are sweet marjoram and rosemary, together or on their own. Black pepper should also be used as it stimulates peristalsis. Fennel can also be considered.

If stress and anxiety are part of the clinical picture, include essential oils that will help to alleviate these emotional states.

Mailhebiau suggests blending peppermint oil with cinnamon bark, pine and rosemary essential oils for constipation, especially when it is due to certain psychological and emotional blockages. He says that cinnamon bark essential oil is an excellent gastrointestinal stimulant, which resorbs flatulence and enhances regular bowel movement.[21]

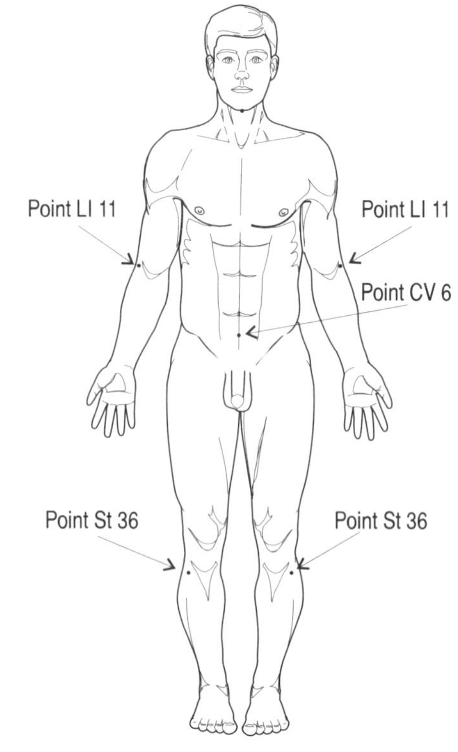

Acupressure points to relieve constipation.

Other Treatments

Nutrition

- Increase fluid intake to 2 litres per day.[19]
- Avoid all tea and coffee.[19]
- Increase the intake of fibre-rich foods, such as whole grains and raw fruit and vegetables.[19]
- Eat foods that have a natural laxative effect such as figs, prunes, apricots and paw paw seeds.[19]
- Linseed or olive oil taken regularly can also help.[19]
- Avoid foods that stimulate secretions of mucous membranes. Eat fresh fruits, raw leafy vegetables and brown rice daily. Avoid dairy products, white flour and sugar.[16]
- Consume plenty of foods that are high in pectin, such as apples, carrots, beets, bananas, cabbage and citrus fruits.[16]
- Some people find that a glass of hot water with the juice of half a lemon is helpful when taken first thing in the morning.[16]
- Follow a low-fat diet. Do not eat fried food.[16]
- Eat smaller meals — no large, heavy meals.[16]
- Consume barley juice or wheat grass for chlorophyll.[16]

Herbs

- Herbs are often very effective in treating constipation. Some herbs such as psyllium seed are classified as bulk-producing herbs which, when consumed with sufficient liquid, expand in volume, thereby stimulating peristalsis and emptying the bowel. They are probably the safest laxatives to take as they function the same as high-residue foods.[6, 23]
- A large number of herbs such as aloe vera, cascara and senna are stimulants, due to their content of anthraquinones. These do increase the motility of the colon and induce changes in its surface cells, promoting the accumulation of water and electrolytes. Drawbacks to the use of such medications are their tendency to promote over-emptying and reduction of spontaneous bowel function, thus leading to the development of the so-called laxative habit.[6, 23]
- Flaxseed or linseeds are well known as a treatment for constipation. Take one to three tablespoons of the whole crushed flaxseeds two to three times a day for chronic constipation.[16, 23]
- Aloe vera has a healing and cleansing effect on the digestive system and aids the formation of soft stools. Drink a cup of aloe vera juice in the morning and at night.[16, 23]
- Use milk thistle herbal extract to aid the liver function and stimulate bile to soften the stools.[16]
- Fenugreek contains fluid-absorbing mucilage. When taking fenugreek seeds, ensure drinking plenty of water. Do not take more than two teaspoons at a time.[22]

General Advice

- If you have been a heavy laxative user, it will have cleaned out the intestinal bacteria, causing chronic constipation. Take acidophilus yoghurt to replace the friendly gut bacteria.[16]
- According to Harrison, relief of physical constipation will rapidly follow relief of mental constipation. Flexible minds make flexible bodies, capable of adjusting to environmental change.[24]
- Hay suggests that people with constipation refuse to release old ideas and are stuck in the past.[25]
- Acupressure points CV 6, St 36, Li 11 and Li 4 are used to relieve abdominal pain, constipation and stomach disorders.[26]

Diarrhoea

Useful Oils

• black pepper • cajeput • carrot seed • German and Roman chamomile • cinnamon bark • cypress • eucalyptus • sweet fennel • ginger • mandarin • neroli • peppermint

Definition

Diarrhoea is a symptom characterised by abnormally frequent watery bowel movements. Normal bowel function varies from individual to individual, and the definition of diarrhoea must take this variation into account.

Clinical Features

Essential clinical features include:

- an increase in frequency of bowel action
- an increase in softness, fluidity or volume of stools.[20]

The danger of diarrhoea is dehydration and loss of salts, especially in infants. Diarrhoea may result from excess activity of the colon, faulty absorption, or infection and food poisoning. Central colicky abdominal pain indicates involvement of the small intestine, while lower abdominal pain indicates the large intestine.[20]

The characteristics of the stool provide a useful guide to the site of the bowel disorder:[27]

- Small volume indicates inflammation or carcinoma of the colon, while large volume indicates possible laxative abuse and malabsorption.
- Diseases of the upper gastrointestinal tract tend to produce diarrhoea stools that are copious, watery or fatty, pale yellow or green.
- Colonic diseases tend to produce stools that are small, of varied consistency, brown and may contain blood or mucus.

Aetiology

The relationship of the diarrhoea to the recent history of the client is important. For example, correlation with a particular food such as milk may indicate either lactose deficiency or sensitivity to milk protein. The relationship to emotional upheaval suggests irritable colon syndrome. Nocturnal diarrhoea suggests an organic cause. Relationship of diarrhoea to travel experience suggests a bacterial infection, an enterotoxigenic bacterial infection, amoebiasis or giardiasis.

The presence of pus in the stool suggests inflammatory bowel disease or infection, but not viral diarrhoea or irritable colon syndrome.

Most cases of diarrhoea are self-limiting and pose no special problem. They are often due to dietary indiscretions or mild gastrointestinal infections. Other causes of diarrhoea include:[27]

- psychogenic disorders: 'nervous diarrhoea'
- intestinal infections: viral enteritis, salmonellosis, cholera, giardiasis, amoebiasis or staphylococcal infections
- other intestinal factors — heavy metal poisoning, antibiotic therapy, faecal impaction, inflammatory bowel diseases, carcinoma
- malabsorption: coeliac sprue, short bowel syndrome
- pancreatic diseases: pancreatic insufficiency, pancreatic endocrine tumours
- reflex from other viscera: pelvic disease (extrinsic to gastrointestinal tract)
- neurological disease: diabetic neuropathy
- metabolic disease: hyperthyroidism
- immunodeficiency
- malnutrition: marasmus
- food allergies
- dietary factors: excessive fresh fruit intake.

Therapeutic Strategy

In the management of diarrhoea it is important to consider the following:

- the basic principle is to achieve and maintain adequate hydration until the illness resolves
- determine the cause
- check for food sensitivities
- improve digestion
- reduce anxiety and stress. Both can cause looseness of the bowel.[20]

Aromatherapy Treatment

Essential oils are useful in helping diarrhoea because of their calming and soothing effect on the intestinal lining, some because they have an antispasmodic action on the intestinal muscles, some because of their astringent properties and others because of their ability to calm the nervous system.

German and Roman chamomile, cypress, sweet fennel, ginger, lavender, neroli and peppermint are among the most effective antispasmodics and can be used to treat diarrhoea.

German Chamomile is an anti-allergenic oil, and would be my first choice if a food allergy was involved. Warming and carminative essential oils, such as ginger, sweet fennel or black pepper are used to relieve the pain in diarrhoea. Massaged gently over the abdomen, these can be helpful in easing the griping pains caused by spasmodic contractions of the intestinal walls.

Often when an infection is present, it is best to use essential oils with antimicrobial properties such as eucalyptus, cajeput or thyme.

When diarrhoea is provoked by stress and anxiety it is particularly useful to use essential oils that may help to minimise the client's reaction to stress by using essential oils such as chamomile, neroli or lavender in an inhalation, a massage oil blend or in a bath before the stressful event.

Gravett used essential oils to treat patients suffering from diarrhoea who were undergoing chemotherapy.[28] The essential oils used in his aromatherapy protocol were German chamomile, patchouli and turmeric. Initially the essential oils were applied by abdominal massage twice a day, but patients with abdominal problems such as nausea and diarrhoea do not often enjoy having their stomachs massaged. They resorted to administering the essential oils internally, using a small amount of an alcoholic vehicle, usually sherry.[28]

Mailhebiau says that cinnamon bark oil is an excellent gastrointestinal stimulant, which resorbs flatulence and enhances regular bowel movement. It increases peristalsis in cases of diarrhoea and should be blended with carrot seed.[21]

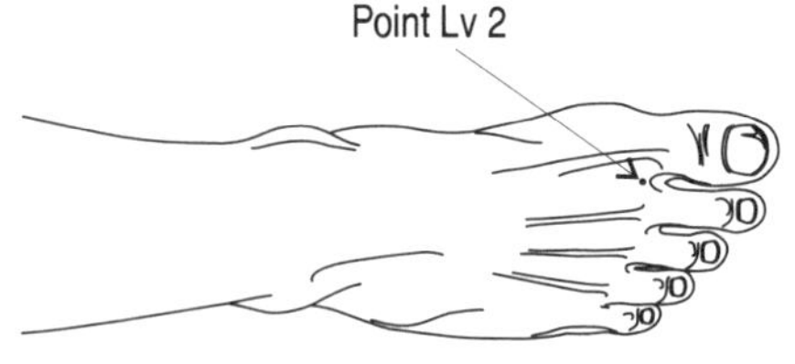

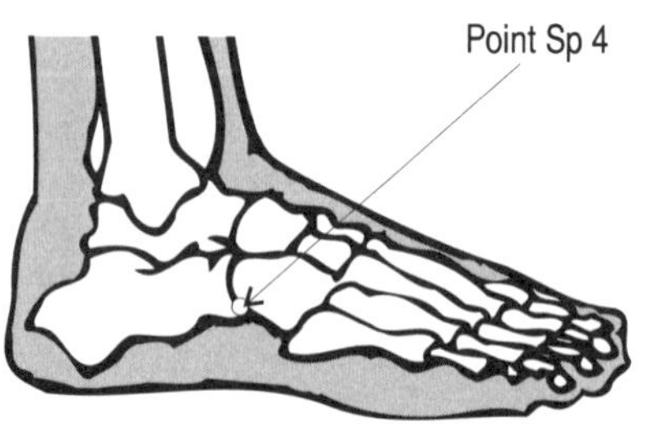

Acupressure points to relieve diarrhoea.

Other Treatments

Nutrition

- A high-fibre diet is important. Eat oat bran, rice bran, raw foods, yoghurt daily.[16]
- Do not eat dairy products (unless they are soured products). Dairy products are often allergenic. Diarrhoea also causes a temporary loss of the enzyme needed to digest lactose (milk sugar).[16]
- Eat a bland low-fibre diet while stools are loose. Avoid irritants such as coffee, alcohol and hot spices.[16]
- Eat oat bran, rice bran, raw foods, yoghurt and soured milk products daily.[16]
- Drink three cups of rice water daily. To make rice water, boil a cup of brown rice in three cups of water for 45 minutes. Strain out the rice and drink the water. Eat the rice as well, it helps to form stools and is a good source of vitamin B group.[16]
- Recolonise the gut by supplementing with *Lactobacillus acidophillus* and *L. bifidus*.[19]

Herbs

All of the herbs that are beneficial contain one or more of three natural ingredients, tannin, pectin and mucilage.

Tannins are constituents that give herbs their astringency — that is, the ability to bind or contract tissues. Tannin's astringent action reduces intestinal inflammation. The tannins bind to the protein layer of the inflamed mucous membranes and cause them to thicken, hence slowing resorption of toxic materials and restricting secretions.[22]

Pectin is a soluble fibre that adds bulk to stools and soothes the gut. Mucilage soothes the digestive tract and adds bulk to stools by absorbing water and swelling considerably.[22]

- Dandelion tea (two cups) and watermelon juice should be taken regularly.[19]
- Ginger tea relieves cramps and abdominal pain.[16]
- Slippery elm bark taken as a tea is soothing to the digestive tract.[16]

General Advice

- Diarrhoea is especially serious in babies and old people, as it causes dehydration. Make them drink plenty of water.[16,20]
- The abdominal acupressure points St 16 and CV 6 tone the abdominal area, while St 36, Sp 4 and Lv 2 on the legs and feet harmonise the digestive system. These points should be pressed three to four times a day to alleviate diarrhoea.[26]

Dyspepsia

Useful Oils

• aniseed • black pepper • cardamom
• German and Roman chamomile
• cinnamon bark and leaf • sweet fennel • ginger
• mandarin • sweet marjoram • neroli • nutmeg
• sweet orange • peppermint • rosemary • spearmint

Definition

Dyspepsia is pain or discomfort centred at the upper abdomen that is chronic or recurrent in nature.

Clinical Features

Indigestion may be a symptom of a disorder in the stomach or the intestines, or it may be a disorder in itself. It may include the following:

- nausea
- heartburn/regurgitation
- upper abdominal discomfort
- lower chest discomfort
- acidity
- epigastric fullness or unease
- abdominal distension.[20]

Aetiology

If food is not properly digested, it may ferment in the intestines, producing hydrogen and carbon dioxide. Foods high in complex carbohydrates, such as grains and legumes, are the primary foods responsible for gas because they are difficult to digest. Indigestion can be caused by excessive consumption of spicy or fatty and fried foods, alcohol, coffee, citrus fruit, chocolate and tomato-based foods.[16]

Psychological factors such as stress, anxiety, worry or disappointment can disturb the nervous mechanism that controls the contractions of stomach and intestinal muscles. A lack of digestive enzymes can also cause intestinal problems. Heartburn often accompanies indigestion.[16]

Other situations that can cause indigestion include cancer of the stomach, coronary heart disease (angina) and acute pancreatitis. These should be referred to a medical practitioner.

Therapeutic Strategy

Mojay says that unless the dietary factors that cause dyspepsia are removed very little progress will be made in the management of dyspepsia.[29]

There are many ways of treating indigestion. More importantly, there are many ways of preventing indigestion.

- **Eating slowly**
  Many cases of indigestion are caused by eating quickly, which sets up several imbalances leading directly to indigestion. Eating quickly results in a tendency to swallow quantities of air, which in turn cause gas and abdominal bloating.

  The other problem is that eating quickly overloads the stomach, causing much of the food to pass through to the intestine without receiving adequate enzyme breakdown. This results in further trouble when the food reaches the lower bowel.
- **Chewing food well**
  The process of digestion begins in the mouth. By carefully masticating food, the enzymes in the saliva are able to do their job thoroughly so that by the time the food reaches the stomach it is in an easily assimilated form.
- **Not drinking liquids with meals**
  Enzymes secreted in the saliva have a specific digestive function to perform. This process can be impaired by a surplus of liquids. The liquids will dilute the digestive enzymes, impairing the efficiency of the saliva.
- **Avoiding unhealthy or gas-producing food**
  Indigestion also results from eating unhealthy foods such as fried foods, carbonated beverages, fats, sugars, processed foods or spicy or highly seasoned foods.

  Certain gas-producing foods such as onions, beans and peas, which are normally considered healthy, may also cause indigestion. Avoid fatty meat as it is a primary cause of bloating.
- **Eating good foods**
  All soured milk products such as yoghurt are helpful for stomach and intestinal bacteria. Food combining is important. Protein and starch are a poor combination, as are vegetables and fruits.

Milk should not be consumed with meals. Sugars must not be consumed with proteins or starches.

- **Avoiding iced drinks with meals**
  Whether one takes liquid with a meal or not, it is not wise to drink iced liquids with meals.
- **Not over-eating**
  Over-eating accounts for many cases of indigestion. The best practice is to leave the table feeling slightly hungry.
- **Not eating when emotionally upset**
  Eating when nervous, angry, overtired or depressed can cause indigestion. It may not be easy to make these emotional states disappear just in time for dinner, thus when eating food in a stressed state the best procedure is to eat the food as slowly as possible and to eat little.
- **Not smoking**
  Smokers should not smoke immediately before a meal. Smoking slows down the peristaltic action of the stomach and intestines, and hence makes food stagnate throughout the alimentary system. The final result can be constipation, diarrhoea or both.

Aromatherapy Treatment

The antimicrobial, antispasmodic, carminative and cholagogue effects of essential oils will help to alleviate indigestion.

Peppermint is a digestive stimulant and carminative that will help to relieve the discomforts of epigastric distension from over-eating and improper dietary habits. The antispasmodic and cholagogue properties of German and Roman chamomile, neroli, sweet or bitter orange and mandarin make these essential oils useful in a variety of cases.

Warming and carminative essential oils such as aniseed, black pepper, cardamom, cinnamon bark and ginger oils are useful in the treatment of indigestion.

Other Treatments

Nutrition

- If you are prone to indigestion, consume a well-balanced meal with plenty of fibre-rich foods such as fresh fruits, vegetables, and whole grains.[16]
- Include a diet of fresh papaya (which contains papain) and fresh pineapple (which contains bromelain). These are both good sources of beneficial digestive enzymes.[16]
- Add acidophilus to the diet. Acidophilus can be useful for indigestion, because a shortage of the 'friendly' bacteria is often the cause.[16]
- Avoid refined cereal products, caffeine, carbonated beverages, citrus juices, fried and fatty foods, pasta, peppers, potato chips and other snack foods, red meat, refined carbohydrates, tomatoes and salty or spicy foods.[16]
- Do not eat dairy products, junk foods or processed foods. These cause excess mucus formation, which results in inadequate digestion of protein.[16]
- Drink the juice of a lemon first thing in the morning. It is a good healer and blood purifier.[16]

Herbs

- Aloe vera is good for heartburn and other gastrointestinal symptoms. Take a cup of aloe vera juice on an empty stomach in the morning and again at bedtime.[16]
- Catnip, chamomile, fennel, fenugreek, goldenseal and peppermint are all excellent herbs for indigestion.[16]
- Slippery elm is good for inflammation of the colon.[16,22]
- Garlic has antiseptic qualities, it stimulates gastric juices, relieves flatulence, helps detoxify the intestines and serves as a general aid to the digestive system.[16]

General Advice

- Do not lie down immediately after eating.[19]
- Stop smoking.[19]
- Insufficient levels of hydrochloric acid can lead to indigestion. This can be relieved by sipping one tablespoon of apple cider vinegar, mixed with water, while eating a meal.[16]
- Acupressure is very effective for treating indigestion that results from emotional or psychological problems. The acupressure points commonly used for relieving abdominal pain and preventing indigestion are CV 12, St 36, Pe 6 and Sp 4. Precaution: Use CV 12 only before eating.[26]

Eating Disorders

Useful Oils

• bergamot • Roman chamomile • clary sage • neroli • rose otto • ylang ylang

Anorexia Nervosa

Anorexia nervosa is a disorder characterised by loss of appetite. The subconsciously self-imposed starvation seems to be a response to emotional conflicts about self-identification and acceptance of a normal adult sex role. This disorder is found predominantly in young females. The physical consequences of this disorder are severe. Amenorrhoea and a lowered basal metabolic rate reflect the depressant effects of starvation.[16]

Even though they become emaciated, sufferers are obsessed with the idea that they are fat. This can result from excessive teasing by their peers or parents. Anorexics often display great fear at the prospect of growing up and with female anorexics there is frequently a very difficult mother/daughter relationship. All forms of treatment are normally rejected.[30]

Signs of anorexia include erosion of the enamel on back teeth from excessive vomiting, broken blood vessels in the face, underweight, extreme weakness, dizziness, cessation of menstruation and low pulse rate and blood pressure.[16]

Symptoms include self-starvation, vomiting deliberately and/or taking huge doses of laxatives. 30% of all anorexics struggle with the disorder all their lives, while 40% outgrow it and 30% have at least one life-threatening bout with it.[16]

Bulimia

Unlike the starvation tactics employed by the anorexic, the bulimic patient characteristically has abnormal increases in hunger, binges several times a day then induces vomiting. People with bulimia can hide their disorder for long periods, even years, because their weight is usually in the normal range.[16]

The cause of bulimia is often of a psychological origin and stress-related. Binging may be a means by which individuals with bulimia manage their emotions; they allow them to focus attention away from unpleasant or uncomfortable emotional problems. People with bulimia may also be obsessed with exercise as a means of controlling weight.

Many individuals who suffer from this disorder have come from families in which they were subjected to physical or sexual abuse. In some families, substance abuse is also a factor. Others are perfectionists and over-achievers with high standards but low self-esteem.[16]

Physical signs of bulimia may be swollen glands in the face and neck, erosion of the enamel of the back teeth, broken blood vessels in the face, swollen salivary glands, constant sore throat, inflammation of the oesophagus and hiatus hernia. All of these are consequences of induced vomiting.[16]

People with bulimia often feel extremely guilty about their behaviour, which is why they can often hide the disorder for years.[16]

Treatment Strategy

In the management of eating disorders it is important to consider the following:

- there are often problematic family interrelationships that require exploration
- establish a good and caring relationship with the patient
- resolve underlying psychological difficulties
- restore weight to a level between ideal and the patient's concept of optimal weight
- for anorexia nervosa provide a balanced diet of at least 3,000 calories per day.[20]

Aromatherapy Treatment

Anorexia Nervosa

Treatment of anorexia nervosa is difficult and is best carried out by individuals trained and experienced in the care of patients with the condition. Many cases of anorexia may require hospitalisation for the initial restoration of adequate nutritional status.

Aromatherapy is very beneficial for the management of anorexia nervosa. If aromatherapy is combined with skilled counselling or psychotherapy, the aromatherapy treatment can be very beneficial. Davis says that the massage will help to bring sufferers into contact with their body. This is important, since many sufferers are alienated from their physical bodies.[17]

The choice of essential oils varies according to the individual's need. Certainly, it would be useful to select essential oils such as bergamot, Roman chamomile, clary sage, neroli and ylang ylang, which are calming, emotionally soothing and antidepressant.

When patients with anorexia nervosa display conflict with their sexuality, rose oil is an excellent choice as it relates to a woman's sexuality at a physical and emotional level. Baths using the essential oils between massage sessions are also recommended, and here again the idea of pampering and nurturing is important.[17]

Bulimia

As with anorexia nervosa the aromatherapy treatment of bulimia will be most effective if we address the underlying psychological factors that are the cause of the bulimia.

Other Treatments

Counselling

- Recommend your client to a practitioner who specialises in the treatment of eating disorders and who can address the complex of physical and psychological elements involved.[16]

- Address levels of low self-esteem. Individuals with a lower self-esteem will tend to engage in self-destructive behaviours such as entering into abusive relationships, compulsive sexual behaviour and eating disorders.[16]

Herbs

- Appetite-stimulant herbs such as ginger, ginseng, gotu kola and peppermint are recommended.[16]
- Tonify and rebuild the liver and cleanse the bloodstream with herbs such as dandelion, milk thistle, red clover and wild yam.[16]

Nutrition

- While a normal eating pattern is being established, eat a well-balanced diet that is high in fibre. Eat plenty of fresh fruit and vegetables. These foods are cleansing to the system. When the body is cleansed the appetite tends to return to normal.[16]
- Do not consume any sugar in any form. Avoid junk foods and white flour products.[16]

Flatulence

Useful Oils

• angelica seed • aniseed • black pepper • caraway • cardamom • cinnamon bark • dill seed • sweet fennel • lavender • sweet marjoram • peppermint • spearmint

Clinical Features

Flatulence is the medical term for excessive production of wind, which is then passed anally or orally. The amount of intestinal gas varies from individual to individual. It can cause abdominal distension, pain and disturbed bowel function.

Aetiology

Intestinal gas comes from air swallowed unavoidably during eating and drinking, from gases in foods, disaccharidose deficiency, and as a result of fermentation by bacteria in the gastrointestinal tract, which produces gas. Increased fermentation can occur as a result of bacterial overgrowth of the gastrointestinal tract, constipation, irritable bowel syndrome, inflammatory bowel syndrome, food intolerance, chronic gastrointestinal candidiasis and chronic gut infections and parasites.[27]

Certain foods, especially beans, can cause flatulence. All of these conditions are made worse by inadequate digestive juice secretion by the stomach, pancreas and gall bladder. Therefore flatulence can be either normal or a manifestation of almost any gastrointestinal disease.

Therapeutic Strategy

In the management of flatulence it is important to consider the following:

- eliminate specific cause if known
- anxiety states are often associated with deep breathing and sighing and consequent swallowing of considerable amounts of air. When possible, treat underlying anxiety
- good hygiene and eating habits. Instruct the client to avoid dietary indiscretions, eating too rapidly and too much, eating while under emotional strain, drinking large quantities of liquids with meals, taking laxatives and chewing gum.

Aromatherapy Treatment

Aromatherapy in conjunction with the advice given above will help to reduce flatulence. Any essential oil that is a carminative will help to alleviate flatulence. The essential oils may be used in a 3% dilution in a suitable carrier oil and massaged into the abdomen in a clockwise direction.

The following essential oils may be used: angelica root, aniseed, black pepper, cardamom, caraway, cinnamon, sweet fennel, ginger, sweet marjoram, nutmeg, peppermint, spearmint.

Other Treatments

- Eliminate specific causes if known. For example, people who experience flatulence after eating beans may experience relief if the beans are soaked in water for 24 hours before removal of the husks and thorough cooking.[16]
- Milk and milk products and certain other foods (for example, beans, aromatic vegetables, carbonated beverages) may lead to excessive flatulence in susceptible individuals.[16]
- Any herb that is known as a carminative will help to reduce flatulence. The most notable herbs are fennel seed, dill seed, caraway, cardamom, chamomile, coriander, marjoram and peppermint.[16]

Irritable Bowel Syndrome

Useful Oils

• bergamot • German or Roman chamomile • geranium • lavender • peppermint

Definition

In irritable bowel syndrome, the normally rhythmic muscular contractions of the digestive tract become irregular and uncoordinated.[16] Irritable bowel syndrome is considered the most common gastrointestinal disorder seen in general practice.[15,16]

Clinical Features

Irritable bowel syndrome is characterised by a combination of:

- abdominal pain
- altered bowel function, constipation or diarrhoea
- hypersecretion of colonic mucus
- dyspeptic symptoms (flatulence, nausea, anorexia)
- varying degrees of anxiety or depression.[16]

It is important to differentiate between irritable bowel syndrome with other disorders that can have similar symptoms such as Crohn's disease, diverticulitis, lactose intolerance and ulcerative colitis. A medical practitioner may recommend a barium enema, colonoscopy, rectal biopsy, sigmoidoscopy and stool examination to make an accurate diagnosis.[15]

Aetiology

Three main factors appear significant in the pathogenesis of irritable bowel syndrome:

Colonic motor activity: Colonic motor activity is abnormally high in patients with colonic pain, for example, after meals or emotional stress.

Psychological stress: Many patients with irritable bowel disease exhibit colonic symptoms at times of stress. It is very often associated with a nervous disorder and anxiety.

Diet: Irritable bowel syndrome has been linked to allergies to certain foods. A food sensitivity test is advised. The foods which commonly provoke symptoms are wheat, corn, dairy products, coffee and tea and citrus fruits.

Therapeutic Strategy

Once other conditions have been ruled out, there are three major treatments to consider when developing a therapeutic strategy:

- increase dietary fibre
- eliminate allergic/intolerant foods
- control psychological components.[15,19]

Aromatherapy Treatment

Essential oils with analgesic and antispasmodic properties will be beneficial in an abdominal massage blend. There is often much stress associated with irritable bowel conditions so essential oils which also help to alleviate stress and anxiety will be most suitable.

Peppermint oil aids digestion. It must be taken in an enteric-coated capsule to prevent the oil being released before it reaches the colon. Most studies have recommend 0.2 mL twice daily between meals.[15,16]

Other Treatments

Herbs

- Balm, chamomile, fenugreek, ginger, goldenseal, marshmallow and slippery elm herbal extracts or tea are beneficial for irritable bowel syndrome.[16]
- Aloe vera aids in healing the colon, thereby easing pain. Drink a cup of aloe vera juice in the morning and again in the evening.[16]
- Skullcap and valerian root are beneficial for the nerves that regulate intestinal muscle function. Best taken at bedtime or when an upset occurs.[16]
- Tea (*Camellia sinensis)* contains tannins which are astringent and beneficial for relieving gastrointestinal distress.[22]

Nutrition

- Eat a high-fibre diet including plenty of fruits and vegetables, as well as whole grains and legumes.[16,19] Patients with constipation are more likely to respond to dietary fibre than those with diarrhoea.[15]
- Avoid animal fats, butter, all carbonated beverages, coffee and any other substance containing caffeine, candy, chocolate, all dairy products, fried foods, ice cream, all junk foods, the additives mannitol and sorbitol, all processed foods, seeds, spicy foods, sugar, sugar-free chewing gum, and wheat bran and wheat products. These foods encourage the secretion of the mucus by the membranes and prevent the uptake of nutrients.[16]
- Avoid alcohol and smoking; these irritate the linings of the stomach and colon.[16]
- When an intestinal upset occurs, switch to a bland diet.[16]
- Eliminate allergenic foods from the diet.[16]
- Chew food well, do not overeat or eat in a hurry.[16]

General Advice

- Irritable bowel syndrome should not be confused with more serious bowel conditions such as Crohn's disease and ulcerative colitis. These are also inflammatory bowel diseases, but unlike irritable bowel syndrome they result in demonstrable lesions in the digestive tract.[16]

- Breathing exercises can control irritable bowel syndrome. Stress management also relieves symptoms.[15, 16]

Nausea and Vomiting

Useful Oils
- black pepper • cardamom
- Roman and German chamomile • fennel
- ginger • peppermint

Definition

Nausea is defined as the unpleasant sensation that can indicate the onset of vomiting or can be present without vomiting. Vomiting or emesis is the forceful expulsion of gastric contents through the mouth.[20]

Aetiology

Nausea and vomiting may be due to a wide variety of causes. The vomiting centre of the medulla may be stimulated by afferent impulses from gastrointestinal structures or other viscera.

Simple acute vomiting that may occur following dietary or alcoholic indiscretion or in the morning sickness of early pregnancy may require little or no treatment. Severe or prolonged nausea and vomiting requires careful management.[20]

Nausea and vomiting are common symptoms that may arise from local disease of the gastrointestinal tract, but can also be associated with systemic illnesses such as diabetes, liver disease or kidney failure. It is also associated with disturbances of labyrinthine function, such as motion sickness and acute labyrinthitis.[30]

Treatment Strategy

The treatment strategy is to ensure that any fluid and electrolyte imbalance is corrected and that the underlying cause is identified and treated.[20]

Aromatherapy Treatment

Davis recommends very gentle massage over the stomach area, or the application of a warm compress to that area. The most appropriate essential oils are sweet fennel, ginger and peppermint.[17]

Mailhebiau recommends using dill seed oil for children. He says that it is a excellent stimulant and digestive antispasmodic for children with a delicate stomach — those who have been given food which is too rich and whose troubles manifest through vomiting, colic, nausea and feelings of bloating. He recommends blending it with lemon, rosemary and basil.[21]

While nausea may be relieved by the diluted essential oils over the abdomen, patients may find the massage uncomfortable. In this case a compress may be preferred or, as Gravett found out, inhalation of essential oils is effective in relieving nausea and increasing appetite in patients undergoing high dose chemotherapy. The essential oils used were turmeric, ambrette seed, carrot seed and nutmeg.[28]

Other Treatments

- Tyler cites clinical studies that have confirmed the anti-emetic properties of ginger. However, while most of the studies involve using the whole rhizome, he says that the active constituents may be attributed to the volatile oils and oleoresin. The principal components of ginger essential oil are the sesquiterpene hydrocarbons zingiberene and bisabolene while the non-volatile pungent components not found in the distilled essential oil but found in the CO_2 extract ginger oil include the shogaols and gingerols.[6]
- Duke recommends taking cinnamon or peppermint tea to alleviate nausea.[22]
- The acupressure point Pe 6 is used to relieve nausea.[26]

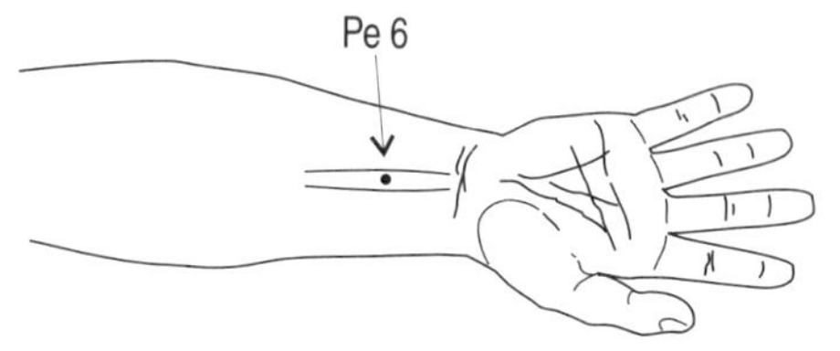

Acupressure point used for treating nausea.

References

1. Tortora G, Anagnostakos N. *Principles of anatomy and physiology*. 4th edn, Harper & Row Publishers, New York, 1984.
2. Cohen BJ, Wood DL. *Memmler's: The human body in health and disease*. 9th edn, J.B. Lippincott Company, USA, 2000.
3. Hoffman D. *An elders' herbal*. Healing Art Press, USA, 1993.
4. Hoffman D. *The new holistic herbal*. 3rd edn, Element, Great Britain, 1990.
5. Weiss R. *Herbal medicine*. Beaconsfield Publishers, translated from the 6th German Edition of Lehrbuch der Phytotherapie by A.R. Meuss. English Edition first published in 1988.
6. Tyler V. *Herbs of choice*. Haworth Press, USA, 1993.

7. Tisserand R. *The art of aromatherapy*. The C.W. Daniel Company Limited, Great Britain, 1977.
8. Schnaubelt K. *Medical aromatherapy*. Frog Ltd, USA, 1999.
9. Somerville KW et al. *Delayed release peppermint oil capsules for spastic colon syndrome: A pharmacokinetic study*. British Journal of Clinical Pharmacology 18(4): 638–40.
10. Rees WD et al. *Treating irritable bowel syndrome with peppermint oil*. British Medical Journal 2(6194): 835–6.
11. Rangelov A. *An experimental characterisation of cholagogic and cholesteric activity of a group of essential oils*. Folia Med 31(1): 46–53.
12. Mills S. *The essential book of herbal medicine*. Penguin Books, England, 1991.
13. Holmes P. *The energetics of western herbs Vol.1*. Artemis Press, USA, 1986.
14. Mojay G. *Aromatherapy for healing the spirit*. Hodder & Stoughton, United Kingdom, 1996.
15. Pizzorno J, Murray M. *A text book of natural medicine*. 2nd edn, Churchill Livingstone, UK, 1999.
16. Balch J, Balch P. *Prescription for nutritional healing*. Avery Publishing Group, USA, 1997.
17. Davis P. *Aromatherapy: An A–Z*. The C.W. Daniel Company Limited, Great Britain, 1988.
18. Beckman, N., *The family library guide to natural therapies*. Family Library, Australia, 1992.
19. Osiecki H. *The physician's handbook of clinical nutrition*. Bioconcepts Publishing, Australia, 1990.
20. Murtagh J. *General practice*. 2nd edn, The McGraw-Hill Companies Inc., Australia, 1998.
21. Mailhebiau P. *Portraits in oils*. The C.W.Daniel Company Limited, Great Britain, 1995.
22. Duke J. *The green pharmacy*. Rodale Press, USA, 1997.
23. Schul V, Hansel R, Tyler V. *Rational phytotherapy: A physician's guide to herbal medicine*. Springer, Germany, 1998.
24. Harrison J. *Love your disease: It's keeping you healthy*. Angus & Robertson Publishers, Australia, 1984.
25. Hay L. *You can heal your life*. Specialist Publications, Australia, 1987.
26. Reed Gach M. *Acupressure's potent points*. Bantam Books, USA, 1990.
27. Krupp M. Chatton M. *Current medical diagnosis and treatment 1980*. Lange Medical Publications, USA, 1980.
28. Gravett P. *An investigation of the use of essential oil*. Aroma'95 Conference Proceedings, Aromatherapy Publications, 1995.
29. Mojay G. *Dyspepsia & gastritis*. Aromatherapy Quarterly 1998; 58: 23–26.
30. Macpherson G, ed, *Black's medical dictionary*. 40th ed, A & C Black Publishers Limited, London, 2002.

The Immune System

Objectives

After careful study of this chapter, you should be able to:

- discuss the role of microbes
- explain the organisation of the immune system
- identify, list and describe common pathophysiologies of the immune system
- explain the aromatherapy treatment for specific conditions and disorders of the immune system
- explain the role of other holistic strategies for specific conditions and disorders of the immune system.

Introduction

Twenty-four hours a day our body is at war. Millions of microorganisms are continually attempting to invade and occupy our organs and tissues. If it were not for the highly sophisticated immune system, we would succumb.

The job of protecting us from these harmful agents belongs in part to certain blood cells and the lymphatic system, which together make up our immune system.

The immune system is part of our general body defences against disease. Some of these defences are non-specific; that is, they are effective against any harmful agent that enters the body. Other defences are referred to as specific — that is, they act only against a certain agent and no other type.

The Body at War

According to Aldridge, the war against infection will never be over. The latest figures issued by the World Health Organisation (WHO) show that in 1995, 17 million people, mostly children, died of infectious diseases. Pneumonia topped the list with four million deaths, followed by TB and malaria with 3.1 million deaths each year. Cholera, typhoid and dysentery between them claimed another three million lives, while hepatitis B, HIV/AIDS and measles were each responsible for a further million deaths. Finally, a million deaths were from tetanus, whooping cough or intestinal worms.[1]

The pattern of infectious disease throughout the world changes constantly. The WHO estimates that there have been at least 30 new diseases over the last 20 years. These include the Ebola virus which appeared in 1976, AIDS which was first reported in the early 80s, hepatitis C in 1989 and legionnaire's disease in 1977.[1]

Why are we encountering many problems that the immune system cannot cope with? Should we view microbes that are responsible for so much human suffering as malevolent life forms that should be totally eradicated from existence?

The Role of Microbes

Before we go any further, it is necessary to define what we actually refer to as microbes. Microbes may actually be:

- viruses
- bacteria
- fungi
- parasites.

Mills suggests microbes, like all living things, play an important role in the ecology of our planet:

> *There is an ecological view of bacteria, viruses and other disease causing organisms that is rarely explored. In any balanced ecosystem all living things have to find a niche that fits with the whole.*
>
> *... Every creature is part of a food cycle; every excretion, every demise, creates a source of nutrients for some other organism; every act of predation creates an opportunity for more prey to fill the gap. Thus all bacteria, fungi, viruses, every form of mosquito, fly and other pest, must have their positive roles in the balance of life. An attitude that says that any of these life forms is always evil, always to be attacked, is unimaginative and counter-productive as any jingoistic nationalism.*[2]

For example, as trees in a forest die and fall they leave large carcasses of relatively tough wood that would potentially litter the forest floor; the minerals and other nutrients they contain would be locked up and unobtainable for other plants; eventually choking life off. It is therefore the fungi and wood-boring insects that exist to recycle the wooden logs back into the ecosystem. They may marginally affect, but they do not damage, healthy living trees. Such organisms are termed 'saprophytic'. The naturopathic view is that most so-called pathogens are in fact saprophytes. Germs do not arrive 'out of the blue' to strike down an unwary victim. Rather, they will colonise only where there is unhealthy tissue.[2]

Indeed, the majority of the microbes which share our world are harmless — in fact, some are positively beneficial to us. There are microbes in the air, the soil, the food and water we consume and on our bodies. In fact, there are as many bacteria on the surface of your skin as there are people on the planet. The staphylococci which live on your skin produce acid secretions which help to repel potentially harmful bacteria. In return, the staphylococci benefit from feeding off dead skin cells.[1]

To understand how the immune system deals with these pathogens, it is necessary to discuss each of them individually.

Viruses

Viruses are very adaptable and successful life forms (or near-life forms, they can not survive on their own). For a virus to grow and multiply it must enter an environment of specific cells that will become unwilling hosts. Viruses are therefore parasites, living off other organisms.

A virus is composed of genetic material in the form of DNA. Once it has invaded a cell, it can then reprogram the cell's DNA inside the nucleus to manufacture copies of the virus. The infected cell then fills up with new viral particles and the cell membrane bursts, releasing the viruses, which

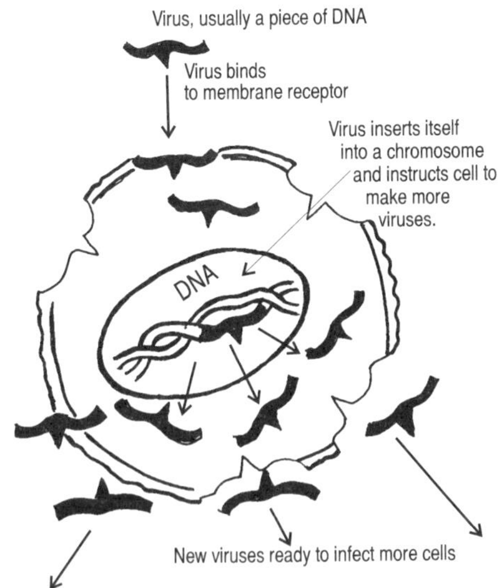

A virus invading a host cell.

happily go on invading other cells, causing extensive damage. When a virus is reproduced by a cell it has just invaded it is often wrapped in an envelope made of a combination of protein and fatty material. This often allows the virus to live undamaged for extended periods of time outside the body.[3]

The most common way that a virus can enter the human body is through direct contact with the infected secretions of another infected organism. We can easily inhale viral particles, as a good sneeze will often expel millions of viral particles.[3]

While vaccines have been relatively successful in taming viral organisms such as smallpox, measles and polio, many viruses that have gone undetected for centuries keep being discovered. Viruses such as the Ebola virus have made the jump from monkeys to humans, simply because people are slowly destroying the natural habitat of the animals and the viruses. Dr Robert Shope, a Yale epidemiologist, says:

> *We know of at least 50 different viruses that have the capacity of making people sick that inhabit the Brazilian rainforest. There are probably hundreds more that we have not found.*[4]

Bacteria

Bacteria are very different from the viruses discussed previously, mainly because bacteria are complete life forms. Unlike viruses, they are not parasites and do not need a host to reproduce. The bacteria that cause tetanus by secreting a toxin that can paralyse nerves live just as happily in the soil as they do inside the human body. Bacteria consist of one or more cells, and are much bigger than viruses. Bacteria just eat and divide constantly, and they thrive when the conditions are right. Bacteria can harm us in at least three ways:[3]

- As they multiply in the body, they may excrete poisonous chemicals and disturb one or more bodily functions. Some may block the ability of the cells in our intestinal tract to absorb water, which may lead to diarrhoea, or others may lead to paralysis.
- Bacteria may invade body tissue such as the lungs and multiply so quickly that staggering numbers of them can accumulate, interfering with the function of the lungs, causing pneumonia.
- When our immune system comes to the rescue and mounts a vicious attack on the invading bacteria, our own tissue is often caught up in the battle and may be damaged. Such tissue destruction results in an abscess, and the chemically digested remains of the bacteria and those parts of our cells that were accidentally destroyed are known as pus.

Antibiotics have been used to treat bacterial infections. However, many bacteria have developed resistance to antibiotics. In 1941, less than 1% of *Staphylococcus aureus* strains were resistant to the newly introduced penicillin. By 1946, 14% of *S. aureus* strains were resistant and by 1948, 38%. Today less than 1% of all strains of this species, which is responsible for pimples, boils, food poisoning and respiratory infections, are sensitive to penicillin.[1]

Aldridge says that there are several issues which have led to antibiotic resistance:

> *Suppose you take a course of ampicillin for a throat infection. You start off with a normal population of, say, Staphylococcus aureus in your throat. Inevitably some of the microbes will be more resistant to the ampicillin than others. The more sensitive ones will be killed within the first couple of days of the ampicillin treatment, and the population then in your throat will be relatively more resistant to the drug. Suppose you then feel better and forget to take the rest of the course — which would have been needed to kill off the resistant bugs in the population. You have now shifted the balance in favour of resistant bacteria. Next time you have a throat infection it will be harder to cure, because you did not complete the course the first time.*[1]

According to a report in *The Lancet*, up to 40% of patients visiting their GP with a 'cold' get antibiotics. A cold is a viral infection, therefore it is not affected by antibiotics. In a minority of colds — say one in five — there is a co-existing bacterial infection in the upper respiratory tract and this may respond to the antibiotic. In time the immune system would probably throw off both infections. Prescription of an antibiotic for a cold, according to Aldridge, is usually unnecessary and, in the long-term, actually harmful — because it encourages the emergence of resistant bacteria.[1]

Doctors have tended to use broad-spectrum antibiotics, which attack a wide range of bacteria, while they wait for laboratory results to confirm which organism is responsible for the infection. It might be wiser to wait, and then prescribe something more specific, which will exert selective pressure on fewer species than a broad-spectrum drug.[1]

The widespread use of antibiotics as a prophylactic in agriculture also creates a selective pressure on resistant microbes just as their clinical use in humans does. Resistant bacteria start to turn up in poultry, beef and lamb, which are then consumed by the fast food market.[1]

Fungi

Everyone has come in contact with fungi. Moulds are fungi and they can grow on a piece of bread or crawl up a shower curtain. There are thousands of fungi, the great majority of which are harmless to humans. Fungi possess a simple membrane-bound nucleus, which contains their genetic information and the walls of the fungi are made up of polysaccharides.[3]

As is true of bacteria, not all fungi cause disease, in fact some can be beneficial, such as the fungi that are used to make cheeses, yoghurt and fermented drinks. More than 200 species of fungi are known to cause disease in humans. In people with depressed immune systems fungal infections of the skin, intestinal tract, lungs and brain are frequent.[3]

One particular fungus, known as candida, has come under the spotlight. This fungus happily inhabits your intestinal tract. Defence mechanisms have been developed to ensure that bacteria found in the intestines will not harm us but work in our favour. The bacteria make vitamins for us and break down proteins to help us digest and reassimilate the essential nutrients that we eat.[3]

However, bacteria can get out of hand very easily and may grow so rapidly in our intestinal tract that they swamp our defence mechanisms. To prevent this from happening the candida organism, which is naturally found in human intestines, competes with bacteria for essential nutrients. An ecological balance is maintained that prevents excessive growth of either bacteria or fungi.[3]

It is common for anyone who has been treated by antibiotics that the bacteria in the gastrointestinal tract may have been killed. As a result the

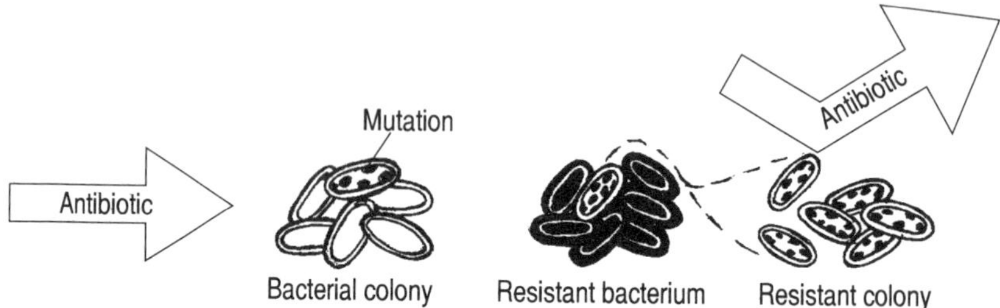

When a colony of bacteria is treated with an antibiotic, most of the microbes are killed. However, there may be a microbe with a mutation that makes it resistant to the drug. When the colony grows back, all of the new bacteria will have the same drug-resistant properties of the original mutant.

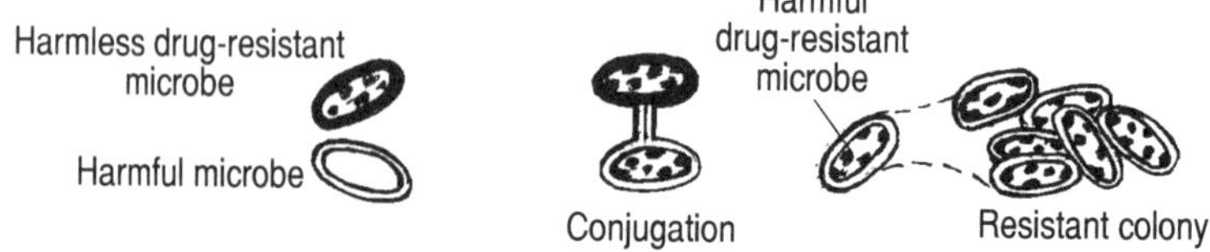

Antibiotics will attack harmless microbes as well as harmful ones. Drug resistance that develops in harmless bacteria may be transferred to harmful microbes. One microbe attaches itself to another, and a process known as conjugatio occurs. A copy of the genes that make the microbe resistant can then be passed from one to the other.

Development of drug-resistant bacteria.[5]

candida organism can spread up and down the intestinal tract.[3]

Parasites

A parasite is anything that depends on others in one way or another for its ability to survive without contributing to the wellbeing or the survival of the organism on which it depends. In biological terms, a virus could be a parasite. However, the term parasite often refers to those usually large and complicated organisms that produce long-standing infections in humans and animals, particularly in the developing countries.

According to Dwyer, one of the world's most experienced immunologists, diseases such as malaria, trypanosomiasis, leishmaniasis and filariasis are responsible for most human sickness and death.[3]

Parasites can be divided into two major groups, the protozoans and the helminths. The protozoan family is made up of many different types of organism. One of these is responsible for malaria, which is one of the world's most serious infectious diseases, although the hepatitis B and AIDS viruses are closing in on the title.[3]

Helminth is the technical term for worms. There are three major types of worms that are found in humans — round worms, tapeworms and flukes.[3]

The parasite that causes malaria matures in the salivary glands of a particular family of mosquito that is the host. When the mosquito bites, it secretes and injects saliva, which contains a substance that prevents the blood from clotting before it begins to feast on the blood. The parasite that is in the mosquito's saliva now finds itself in the victim's bloodstream. Many deaths from malaria occur because the parasitic organism produces severe anaemia, destroying too many red blood cells. Most victims develop an uneasy truce with the parasite. It does not kill them, nor are they able to kill it and a chronic state of ill-health is established.[3]

The Organisation of Defence

The body's protection against intrusion from outside may be compared to a high-security system for a very important industrial complex. This system is designed to keep intruders out and to immediately detect any that do make it into the complex. The security problem is made more difficult by the fact that, during the day, the complex employs thousands of people. These employees need to be easily identifiable and, of course, provoke no response from the security forces.[3]

The human body continually attempts to maintain balance by counteracting harmful stimuli in the environment. These harmful stimuli are often disease-producing organisms, referred to as pathogens. Defence against pathogens is grouped into two broad areas:

- non-specific resistance
- specific resistance — immunity.[6]

Non-specific Resistance

Chemical and Mechanical Barriers

The first line of defence is the skin, which serves as a mechanical barrier as long as it remains intact. Unfortunately, if the skin has been damaged, intruders are easily able to enter the body. The mucous membranes and mucus also inhibit the entrance of many other intruders and trap microbes in the respiratory system and digestive tract.[7]

Chemical barriers such as the high acidity of gastric juice, which is a collection of hydrochloric acid, enzymes and mucus produced by the glands of the stomach, are sufficient to preserve the usual sterility of the stomach and destroy almost all bacterial toxins.[7]

The acid pH of the skin, the unsaturated fatty acids and lysosomes (antimicrobial substance in perspiration, tears, saliva, nasal secretions and tissue fluids) also discourage the growth of many microbes that come into contact with the skin.[7]

Phagocytosis

Phagocytosis is part of the second line of defence against invaders. In the process of phagocytosis, white blood cells take in and destroy microbes and foreign material. Neutrophils and macrophages are the main phagocytic white blood cells. Neutrophils are a type of granular leukocyte. Macrophages are derived from monocytes. Both types of cells travel in the blood to sites of infection. Some of the macrophages remain fixed in the tissues, to fight infection and remove debris.[6]

Natural Killer Cells

The natural killer (NK) cell is a type of lymphocyte different from those active in immunity. NK cells can recognise body cells with abnormal membranes, such as tumour cells and cells infected with a virus, and, as the name suggests, can destroy them on contact. NK cells are found in lymph nodes, spleen, bone marrow and blood. They destroy abnormal cells by secreting a protein that breaks down the cell membrane.[6]

Interferon

Cells infected with viruses produce a substance called interferon, a substance that prevents the infection of other cells.[6]

Immunity

Immunity is described as the final line of defence against disease. Immunity is a selective process, meaning that immunity to one disease does not necessarily mean immunity to another. There are two main categories of immunity:

- inborn immunity is inherited along with other characteristics in an individual's genes
- acquired immunity developed after birth, by natural or artificial means.[6]

Inborn Immunity

There are three forms of inborn immunity, they are:

Species immunity — Some diseases found in animals may be transmitted to humans. However, many infections that affect humans do not appear to affect animals in contact with humans who have these illnesses.[6]

Population immunity — Some groups appear to have greater inborn immunity to certain diseases than others. Although measles is generally considered a mild disease in Europeans, it can be a serious and often fatal disease among people of the Pacific islands when Europeans brought it there. These populations had never been exposed to the measles virus and had not developed genetic resistance to the disease over time.[6]

Individual immunity — Some members of a same group may have a more highly developed immunity to specific diseases.[6]

Acquired Immunity

Acquired immunity develops during a person's lifetime as that person encounters various harmful agents.

Antigens

An antigen is any foreign substance that enters the body and induces an immune response. Antigens stimulate the activity of T and B cells.

T Cells

Both T and B cells come from stem cells in bone marrow. However, they differ in their development and their actions. Some of the immature stem cells migrate to the thymus gland and become T cells, which make up about 80% of the lymphocytes in the circulating blood. While in the thymus, these T lymphocytes multiply and become capable of combining with specific foreign antigens, at which time they are described as being sensitised.[3]

These thymus-derived cells produce an immunity which is referred to as cell-mediated immunity. There are several types of T cells, each with different functions. These include:

- killer T cells are designed to destroy foreign cells directly
- helper T cells release substances known as interleukins that stimulate other lymphocytes and macrophages
- suppressor T cells may inhibit or destroy active lymphocytes
- memory T cells remember an antigen and start a rapid response if that antigen is encountered again.[3]

The T cells are generally responsible for the defence against cancer, certain viruses and other pathogens that grow within cells.[3]

B Cells and Antibodies

An antibody, known as an immunoglobulin, is a substance produced in response to an antigen. Antibodies are manufactured by B cells.

B cells have surface receptors that bind with a specific type of antigen. Exposure to the antigen stimulates the cells to multiply rapidly and produce large numbers of plasma cells. Plasma cells produce antibodies against the original antigen and release these antibodies into the blood, providing humoral immunity. Humoral immunity protects against

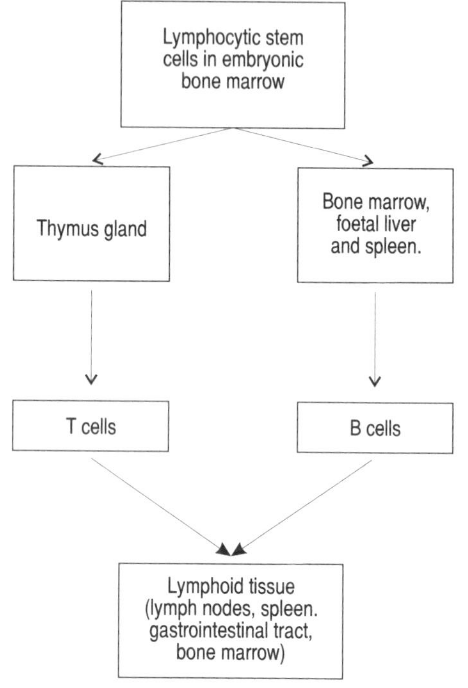

Origin and differentiation of T cells and B cells.

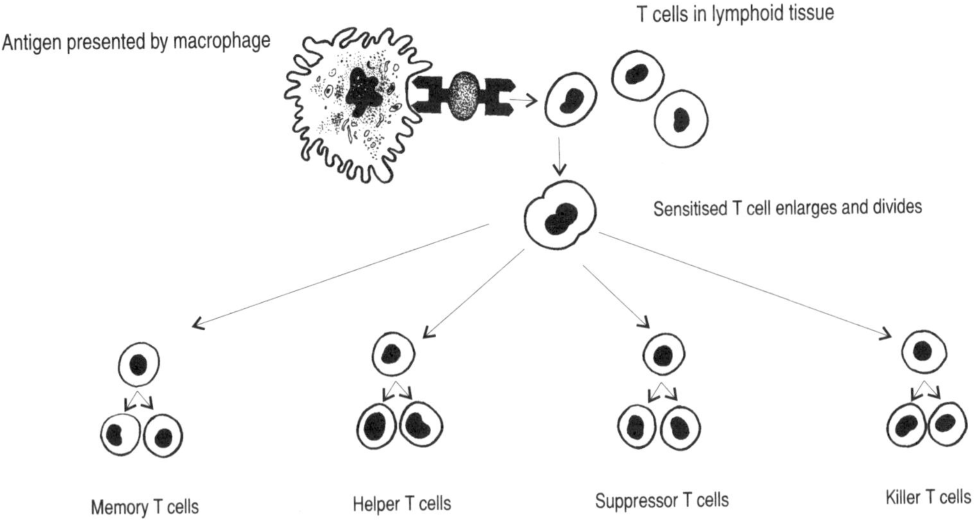

The role of T cells in cellular immunity.

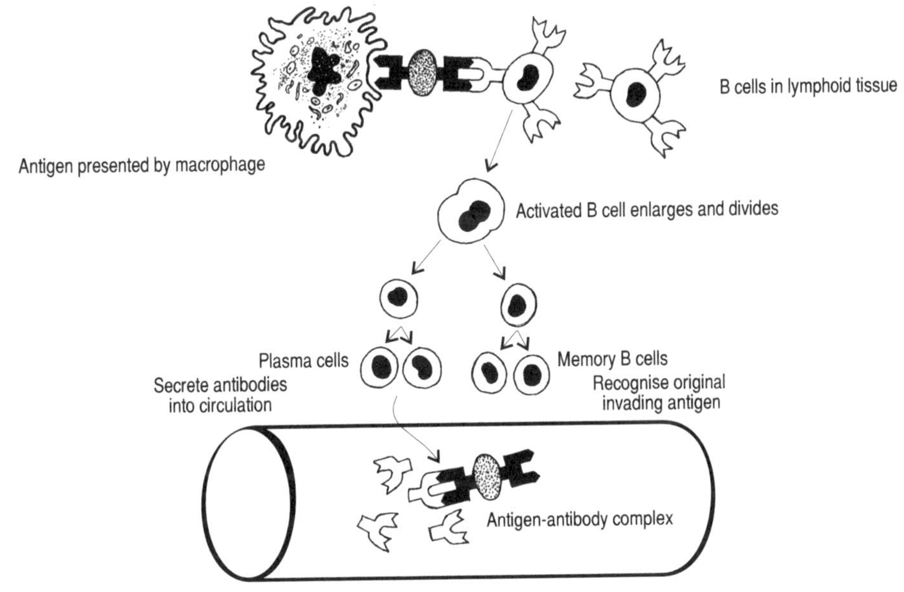

The role of B cells in humoral immunity.

circulating antigens and bacteria that grow outside the cells. Some antibodies produced by B cells remain in the blood to give long-term immunity.[3]

Some B cells become memory cells. On repeated contact with an antigen, these cells produce antibodies. Because of this, one is usually immune to childhood diseases.[3]

A Holistic Basis for the Cause of Infections

To understand how colds and flu can be prevented, we need to know what causes a cold or flu in the first place. There are two general theories: the germ theory and the traditional naturopathic theory. The germ theory is embraced by many doctors who maintain that any one of the thousand or more viruses is responsible for infection. On the other hand, the fundamental naturopathic theory of infectious disease stresses a totally different approach.

Poor nutrition, lack of exercise, stress, negative attitudes and other lifestyle problems all combine to place a heavy strain on the body's functional abilities. The result is that waste products are created more rapidly than they can be eliminated by the liver, kidneys, lungs and skin, so they build up in the body. These wastes are toxic and the condition is referred to in naturopathy as toxaemia.

The accumulation of toxins further interferes with most of the bodily functions, leading to a depletion of nerve energy, and the tissues become exhausted. This becomes a vicious circle which seriously interferes with most of the bodily functions and provides the basis of most acute and degenerative diseases.

If the toxins were to build up indefinitely, they would eventually become life-threatening. However, the body has great resources for self-preservation and self-healing and, when the limits of tolerance are reached, emergency elimination is required. Toxic wastes are then eliminated through the mucous membranes. The membranes may become highly irritated, swollen and painful and the mucus is often copious to literally wash the toxins out of the body.

Influenza is a severe cold in which a fever is present to speed up the eliminative processes. When the same process occurs in other parts of the body, it is given different names, such as bronchitis in the air passages or sinusitis in the nasal passages. These are not really different diseases, but different manifestations of one basic disease, toxaemia.

If the emergency elimination is completed, the body is able to once again function at a normal level with renewed vitality, provided the cold has run its course. If, however, the process has been suppressed in some way, then the body's self-cleaning mechanisms will have been lost.

While the germ theory views bacteria, viruses, fungi and protozoa as the primary cause of infectious disease, the natural health theory sees the role of these organisms as being the secondary agent of disease, being able to gain a foothold only in living tissue which is already congested with toxic wastes. In other words, germs cannot and do not attack healthy tissue. Germs may therefore be likened to nature's scavengers, 'feeding' on waste products and helping directly to lower the level of toxaemia.

This explanation is a simplification of the theory. However, it does make more sense than the orthodox germ theory which has many inconsistencies. If, for example, germs can attack healthy tissue, we should be sick all the time because there are always pathogenic germs in all of us.

The common cold can therefore be thought of as an alarm mechanism. It will evoke inflammatory and febrile response that in most cases is completely resolved.

Aromatherapy Considerations

Essential oils can be used in treating infections by:

- their antimicrobial action working directly against micro-organisms
- their immune-stimulant action boosting the body's own defences
- their depurative properties eliminating accumulated waste material and toxins that become a prime environment for microbes to breed.

According to Dr Pénoël, who uses essential oils in the medical treatment of infectious diseases, the following conclusions can be drawn:

- There is a close relationship between the bacteria that live inside the organism and the general state of health, not only physically, but also psychologically.
- Essential oils respect the protective commensal flora of the organism.[8]

Antimicrobial Properties

The antimicrobial activity of many essential oils has been known for a long time and many microbiological studies have been performed on essential oils. However, little is known about the mechanism of action of essential oils. It has been shown that essential oils cause damage to a biological membrane due to their lipophilic properties (their solubility in the phospholipid bilayer of cell membranes).

The terpenoid constituents have been found to interfere with enzymatic reactions of energy metabolism. Much of the primary energy metabolism takes place in the cell membranes of bacteria. Low concentrations of different terpenoid compounds were able to significantly inhibit oxygen intake and formation of adenosine triphosphate (ATP) in the cell wall.[9]

According to Knobloch, the oxygen intake was completely inhibited by functional groups such as phenols (thymol and carvacrol) and alcohols also revealed the strong inhibitory effects, followed by aldehydes and ketones.

The values of inhibition of oxygen uptake and ATP formation given in the table below were determined by Knobloch using the bacterium *Rhodopseudomonas sphaeroides* as a test organism. This non-pathogenic, gram-negative bacterium was accepted as a test organism for its wide distribution and its ability to grow anaerobically or aerobically on numerous organic compounds.[9]

Compound	% Inhibition of ATP Formation	% Inhibition of O_2 Uptake
Thymol	100	100
Menthol	85	86
Borneol	89	88
Borneol acetate	65	64
Camphor	66	65
Eugenol	90	93
Cymene	24	21

The antimicrobial properties of tea tree oil have been extensively researched.[10] Studies on tea tree oil have highlighted the oil's excellent antibacterial properties. A case was reported of a woman suffering from anaerobic vaginosis who refused antibiotics and treated herself with tea tree pessaries. Re-examination by her doctor a month later showed normal vaginal secretions and bacterial flora. It was discussed that tea tree oil may be a preferable treatment for the condition rather than nitroimidazoles.[11]

Antiviral Properties

While antibiotics have played an important role in modern medicine against the battle of bacterial infections, the development of antiviral drugs has not lived up to the same expectations. This is largely due to the fact that a virus does not show all the qualities of a living organism until it invades a host cell. This means that:

- viruses are difficult to inactivate chemically and usually require highly toxic agents to do so
- once a cell is infected it is difficult to selectively inhibit the virus without harming the cell.

While much research has been conducted on the antibacterial properties of the essential oils, very little work has been conducted in the use of the antiviral properties of essential oils. However anecdotal evidence indicates that essential oils may successfully contribute to the treatment of viral infections.

This has been confirmed by the clinical successes of Drs Pierre Franchomme and Daniel Pénoël. Franchomme proposes that viruses with a hull are sensitive to essential oils with a predominance of monoterpene alcohols and phenols. Unhulled or naked viruses are sensitive to essential oils with a large proportion of terpenoid ketones.[12]

Dr Pénoël suggests that essential oils with a portion of terpene alcohols and cineole such as bay, cajeput, eucalyptus and niaouli are suited to treating influenza-causing myxovirus influenza.[8]

The suggested treatment is a combination of essential oils applied externally. Pénoël suggests that if the treatment is begun right at the onset, the disease can be stopped on the first day. It is also suggested that these measures can be taken as a preventative measure during flu epidemics.[8]

The rapid action of the essential oil is a result of the action of the essential oil on the pathogen and the powerful stimulating effect on the immune system of the host. Pénoël suggests that essential oils alter the pH and the electrical resistance of the terrain in a way which is unfavourable to the viral organism. He also cites studies which have shown that patients who received essential oils of tea tree, oregano, niaouli and thyme chemotype thuyanol-4 had higher levels of immunoglobulin A after the test period compared to before.[8]

Pénoël suggests the importance of using sufficient amounts of essential oil and is unconcerned with overdoses as the bulk of the essential oil is applied externally:

> *When the organism is under siege there is no fear of overdoses, for instance the total amount of essential oil applied in the course of the day may reach 12 ml without any problems.*[8]

Immunostimulants

It is often suggested that many essential oils are immunostimulants simply because they have bactericidal, antiseptic or antiviral properties. While the research and clinical evidence for the antimicrobial properties of the essential oils are well documented, the term *immunostimulant* has often been misused.

According to Tyler, immunostimulants affect either the cellular or humoral immune system or both. Of all the non-specific immunostimulants of plant origin, the most comprehensively researched is echinacea. Echinacea has no direct bactericidal or bacteriostatic properties; however, it is known to increase phagocytosis and promote the activity of the lymphocytes.[38]

There are a wide variety of essential oils that are reputed to strengthen the immune system. The reasons given are because so many essential oils possess a wide range of properties (for example, antifungal, antibacterial, antiseptic, antiviral) that are beneficial to the immune system. Essential oils which have been described as immunostimulants or are of benefit to the immune system include:[8,13]

- *Boswellia carteri* is an uplifting essential oil which strengthens the immune system.
- *Citrus bergamia* will recharge the central nervous system with energy, indirectly helping to strengthen the immune system.
- *Melaleuca viridiflora* is uplifting and an immunostimulant.
- *Rosmarinus officinalis ct. bornyl acetate, verbenone* encourages the work of clearing excretory ducts and organs, draining the hepatobiliary area and strengthening natural immunity.
- Cineole-rich essential oils such as the eucalyptus species stimulate the immune system because they have an enhancing effect on gamma- and beta-globulins. They reduce the inflammatory reaction and therefore their effect is said to be immunomodulant.

Davis says that essential oils are effective in dealing with infectious illnesses because they:

- increase the body's ability to combat infection from micro-organisms
- inhibit micro-organisms
- prevent the spread of infection.[14]

Schnaubelt says that genuine research into the immunostimulant properties of essential oils on the immune system is still quite limited:

> *Precise statements about the specific interaction between essential oils and the various functions of the immune system are not possible at this time. It is probable that, with the increasing popularity of aromatherapy, in the near future a field known as "aroma-immunology" may arise because certain conclusions about the relationship between oils and their effects on the immune system can already be drawn. Immunoglobin levels in the bloodstream, for example, can be positively influenced by treatment with essential oils.*[15]

Various terpene alcohols have the ability to correct pathologically elevated or depressed gamma-globulin counts to their proper level. A depressed gamma-globulin level, as encountered with chronic bronchitis, can be corrected by using essential oils such as savory, thyme (linalool chemotype), spike lavender and eucalyptus globulus.[15]

Tisserand says that there are two ways in which essential oils may have an effect on the immune system. One is a pharmacological effect and the other is a psychological effect. He cites Burger, who found that a fraction of garlic oil rich in allicin stimulated NK cells in vitro. However, it is not surprising that while garlic's immunostimulant properties are well known it is of very little value as an essential oil used in holistic aromatherapy.[16]

According to research cited by Tisserand, coumarin, a trace component in several essential oils, has been found to stimulate lymphocyte transformation values in cancer patients. Research has also found that benzaldehyde, a major constituent in bitter almond oil, has antitumoral effects and stimulates NK cells (cells of the immune system which have a dual function — to kill viruses and to kill diseased cells such as cancer cells.)[16]

Psychoneuroimmunology

There is now considerable scientific evidence that immunity and resistance to disease are linked to attitudes and behaviour. Felton, a Professor of Neurobiology and Anatomy, discusses the physical link between the nervous system and the immune system:

> *Why would a lymphocyte have a receptor for a neurotransmitter? So we started studying immunologic changes that occur when you use drugs to affect the neurotransmitters. Much to our surprise, we found that if you took the nerves away from the spleen or the lymph nodes, you virtually stopped immune responses in their track … the practical implication was that many stressors we face in life, which affect the autonomic nervous system, might have an impact on the immune system.*[17]

The immune system can be conditioned by olfactory stimuli, and therefore suggests that there is a connection between the olfactory receptors, the central nervous system (CNS) and the immune system. Tisserand cites a study which found that the conditioned immune response resulted in stimulation of NK cell activity. It has been suggested that the mechanism of the conditioned immune response involves interferon–beta stimulating NK cells (IFN), and that IFN interacts in some way with the CNS.[16]

Adrenalin and cortisol are two of the many neurotransmitters whose release can be triggered by negative emotions associated with sudden or long-term stress. According to research cited by Price, these two hormones influence the immune system directly to switch it off. It is therefore possible that emotional states can translate into altered responses in the immune system.[13]

There is no doubt that holistic aromatherapy is therefore capable of having a major influence on the immune system:

- there is a significant feel-good factor in aromatherapy
- the feel-good factor is an important part of psychoneuroimmunology — feeling good can strengthen immunity
- it is therefore likely that the feel-good factor in aromatherapy strengthens immunity and thereby improves health.[16]

Fever

Useful Oils

• cinnamon bark • German chamomile • eucalyptus • ginger • peppermint • spearmint

Clinical Features

Fever is often associated with viral and bacterial infections such as the flu, measles, rubella, rheumatic fever, pneumonia, malaria, scarlet fever, polio, tuberculosis and meningitis.[18]

It is essential that the diagnosis of someone with a fever is accurate as possible, especially in the very young and elderly, pregnant women, among overseas travellers and those with immune disorders.[18]

Fever can promote much fear in a patient and can be equally troubling to the practitioner. Fevers have in the past been the common cause of death, and in some, such as the plague, smallpox, typhoid and cholera, have been notoriously destructive.

The traditional naturopathic approach is that fever plays a major role in the body's defence against infection. Its effect up to a point is beneficial. The higher temperature is believed to inhibit the growth of some bacteria and viruses. The heat also stimulates the activity of some white blood cells.

According to Mills, the following points will assist in interpreting a fever:[2]

- Feeling cold, having a pale cyanosed skin and shivering means that the body temperature is lower than the thermostat setting in the hypothalamus, and is most likely to be still rising.
- Feeling hot, having a flushed skin and sweating means that the body temperature is higher than the thermostat setting, and is most likely coming down.
- Having no dominant feeling of being hot or cold suggests relative equilibrium between thermostat and body temperature.

If the fever is in the safe and optimal range (38 to 39.4°C), or if a high fever (above 39.4°C) is accompanied by sweating, which is a sign that the temperature is dissipating, and there are no contraindications, the fever is best left to run its course naturally. When treatment is indicated, the approaches described in the therapeutic strategy are recommended.[2]

The nature of the fever is dependent upon the virulence of the pathogen and the vigour of the individual's own immune system response. If the defences are weak, then no matter what the virulence of the offensive pathogen, the result will be a slight fever. If on the other hand active defence response is good, then the fever will accurately reflect the virulence of the pathogen itself. The pathogen merely triggers the immune system.

Fevers can be dangerous. They can change rapidly and initial diagnosis can be wrong. It would be irresponsible to take responsibility for managing a fever without the necessary medical qualifications and experience unless supported by a medical team.[20]

Therapeutic Strategy

It is known that a high temperature actually assists in the struggle against micro-organisms, while the act of sweating itself not only keeps the temperature under control, but also speeds up the removal and elimination of toxic debris resulting from the conflict. The treatment strategy for resolving external conditions is to support the body's own active defences.

Since the initial stage involves a fever, it follows that diaphoretics or sudorifics are required. Sweat-inducing remedies are divided into warming and cooling types.

When fever management is called for, the following approaches are recommended:

- Bed Rest: The classic treatment of acute illness is sometimes the most difficult to achieve.[19]
- Diet and Nutrition: The digestive system rests when the temperature exceeds 37°C. Gastric secretion decreases as the fever intensifies. Fasting, which febrile people tend to do spontaneously, is the treatment of choice in moderate to high fevers. Clinical evidence shows the fasting prevents the temperature from rising too high. If fasting is contraindicated or dehydration is imminent, a light diet is advised, preferably dilute juices and vegetable broths.[20]

- Increase water intake to prevent dehydration.[19,20]
- Avoid exposure to cold.[20]
- Use diaphoretics such as ginger and yarrow to promote heat elimination through perspiration.[20]
- Support the immune system by using herbs such as echinacea and garlic.[20]
- If a patient starts to sweat, decrease thermal support to control the fever. Sweating indicates that the patient is becoming overheated. Control of the fever is necessary. Use the usual techniques for bringing the temperature down, such as a cool wet flannel or tepid bath.

Aromatherapy Treatment

According to Holmes, remedies that induce sweating to release external conditions are used to treat fever. External conditions are acute conditions with rapid onset, which are triggered by bacterial or viral infection and are said to belong to the initial or alarm stage of general adaptation. These symptoms are typically found at the onset of colds, influenza, laryngitis and other acute upper respiratory infections.[21]

Holmes states that rubefacients such as peppermint, ginger and cinnamon are known as warm circulatory diaphoretics because they generate warmth. He states that essential oils such as eucalyptus, spearmint and German chamomile are known as warm peripheral vasodilatory diaphoretics, and are used to control and resolve the warmth response.[21]

The body temperature will need to be monitored, and many other symptoms of fever will also need to be observed. Nausea, vomiting, diarrhoea, headaches, coughing, pain and spasms may be managed by using the appropriate essential oils.

Other Treatments

Herbal teas such as yarrow, elderflower and catnip are sudorifics that encourage perspiration and will help manage a fever.[19,20,22]

Inflammation

Useful Oils

• German chamomile • clove bud • cinnamon bark • everlasting • ginger • lavender • nutmeg • thyme • yarrow

Clinical Features

Many disease states have inflammation as a component of distress. To successfully deal with inflammation it is necessary to understand the actual process that leads to it. The initial stages of inflammation are:

- dilation of blood vessels in the area with consequently greatly increased blood flow
- increased permeability of the capillaries in the area allowing fluid to leak into the tissues
- migration of leucocytes (and later macrophages) through the leaky capillary wall into the tissues.[2]

The total effect leads to the breakdown of damaged tissue and foreign material with sufficient pain and immobility, so that the area is protected from further damage. If this is successful healing occurs.

If on the other hand, healing cannot keep pace with the rate of damage, the inflammation becomes chronic and the inflammatory and repair processes occur simultaneously. The inflammation becomes increasingly counter-productive. This can often result from:

- persistence of some foreign material at the inflamed site, such as chemicals, metabolites (for example, uric acid), insoluble particles such as silica and asbestos
- infection by certain pathogens, such as tuberculosis or syphilis, where phagocytic activity is compromised and hypersensitivity develops to persistent allergens
- autoimmune diseases, also marked by hypersensitivity to persistent antigens.[2]

In all cases of chronic inflammation there is a shift in the population of phagocytes. The neutrophil leucocytes that are responsible for resolving acute inflammation are replaced by macrophages, and also by eosinophil leucocytes. Most cases of inflammation are conditions whose names end in 'itis'. Chronic conditions such as arthritis, bronchitis, sinusitis, rhinitis, colitis, gastritis, hepatitis and dermatitis, to name a few, are the most common problems in clinical medicine.[2]

Modern medicine is primarily concerned with treating the 'itis' as if inflammation is the core of the problem. In traditional natural therapies, inflammation is an indication that the body has recognised a problem and is engaging it. It is a call for support of the active participants in inflammation, those mediators responsible for increasing blood flow, and the phagocytes responsible for resolving the damage. It may be seen as the body resolving what could possibly be a long-standing malady.

Unfortunately chronic inflammations are usually resistant to conventional drug treatment. Anti-inflammatory drugs such as steroids and aspirin-derived drugs often alleviate the symptoms while they are being administered but have possible negative long-term effects. The prospects for a sufferer of chronic arthritis, ulcerative colitis or sinusitis are not improved by conventional medicine, although the symptoms may be eased, and patch-up surgery is often used to repair damaged tissue.

Therapeutic Strategy

Mills describes the traditional 'natural cure' view of unresolved inflammation as a sign of persisting toxicity or damage to the tissues affected. He doubts the very notion of the term 'anti-inflammatory', and says that the best way to help the situation is to support the inflammatory response. This may mean mobilising the body's eliminative activity and increasing the circulation, phagocyte activity and tissue repair.[2]

Aromatherapy Treatment

Traditional remedies used in inflammatory diseases have been found to possess circulatory stimulating, diuretic, laxative, choleretic, digestive stimulating or any other eliminative effects.[2]

The topical application of German chamomile has been well documented for its anti-inflammatory properties. The presence the hydrophilic (principally the flavonoids) groups greatly contributes to the anti-inflammatory action.[23] The flavonoids in particular are involved in the suppression of histamine release. (-)-α-bisabolol promotes granulation and tissue regeneration. Originally much attention was paid to the presence of chamazulene as the primary anti-inflammatory constituent, but in recent years flavonoids and (-)-α-bisabolol have been acknowledged as the primary constituents.[24]

Other essential oils such as nutmeg, thyme, clove and cinnamon oil have been reported as having pronounced anti-inflammatory effects.[25] It seems that through skin irritation the skin reflexes release binding endogenous substances, whereby the local inflammation process is influenced.

Other Treatments

A holistic approach should also consider the following:

- avoiding all processed and refined foods
- not smoking and avoiding all tea, coffee and alcohol
- taking supplements of vitamin C and E
- taking supplements of evening primrose oil and fish oil
- taking supplements of fresh or dried ginger.[26]

Allergies

Useful Oils
• German and Roman chamomile • everlasting • lavender • yarrow

Clinical Features

An allergy is an inappropriate response by the body's immune system to a substance that is not normally harmful. The immune system is a highly complex defence mechanism that helps us combat infection. It does this by identifying 'foreign invaders' and mobilising the body's white blood cells to fight them. In some people, the immune system incorrectly identifies a non-toxic substance as an invader, and the white blood cells overreact and do more damage to the body than the invader. This allergic response becomes the disease in itself. Common responses are nasal congestion, coughing, wheezing, itching, hives and other skin rashes, headaches and fatigue.

Allergic disorders affect approximately 20% of the population. The most common allergies are those associated with IgE mediated hypersensitivity such as hay fever, atopic dermatitis and allergic asthma.[27]

Aetiology

A substance that provokes an allergic reaction is called an allergen. Allergens can be divided into three common groups:

- food
- chemicals
- inhaled allergens.

Sources of common allergens causing immediate hypersensitivity are listed below:[29]

Inhalants	Pollens, domestic animals, house dust mites, mould spores, cockroaches
Foods	Peanuts, shellfish, milk, eggs, wheat
Other	Drugs, latex, insect venoms, occupational

Do not confuse food allergies with food intolerances.[19,27] A person with a food intolerance is unable to digest and process that food correctly, usually due to a lack of a certain enzyme or enzymes.[19] A food allergy, on the other hand, occurs when a person's immune system produces an antibody response to ingested food.[19]

Balch says that allergies run in the family, and it is believed that babies who are not breastfed are more likely to develop allergies. Emotional factors such as stress and anger may also be contributing factors.[19]

Therapeutic Strategy

The following recommendations should be considered in the management of allergies:

- Maintain a healthy well-balanced diet, avoid 'junk food' and live sensibly with balanced exercise, rest and recreation.[28]
- The suspected allergens should be totally withdrawn at least initially.
- If food allergies exist, a food diary should be maintained.
- Seek advice on keeping your bedroom or house dust-free, especially if you have perennial rhinitis.[19]
- Pets, especially cats and dogs, should be kept outside.
- Avoid food products that contain artificial colourings. Many people have allergies to food colourings.[19]
- Promote relaxation and removal of stressors which are known to trigger allergic reactions.[28]
- Promote elimination using depuratives.[2]
- Promote immunostimulation.[2]
- Support the liver with hepatics.[2]

Aromatherapy Treatment

Often people who develop asthma, eczema or other allergic reactions to various allergens when under stress can come into contact with the same allergen without any reaction when they are feeling relaxed and happy. Therefore, aromatherapy is an excellent holistic approach to the management of stress and any essential oil which can be used to treat stress can also help to reduce an allergic reaction.

The aromatherapist's approach to allergies should employ essential oils that are calming and soothing. Davis says that essential oils such as chamomile, lavender and melissa are the ones most often used successfully to help allergies.[14]

For specific aromatherapy treatment refer to the appropriate sections such as hay fever, sinusitis and psoriasis.

Other Treatments

- Exercise plays an important role in the management of allergies. Regular exercise will stimulate metabolism and improve a sense of wellbeing.[28]

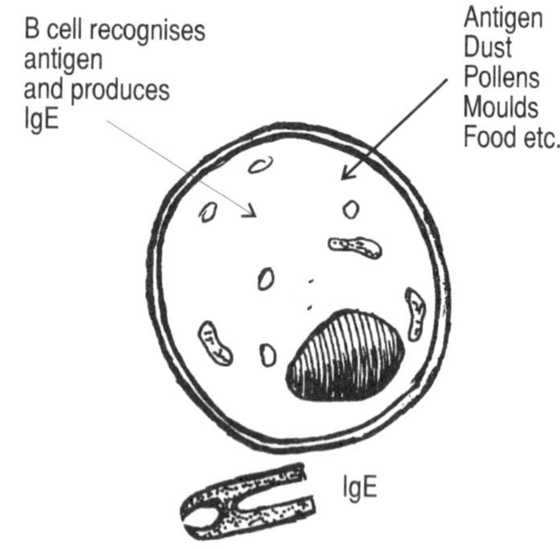

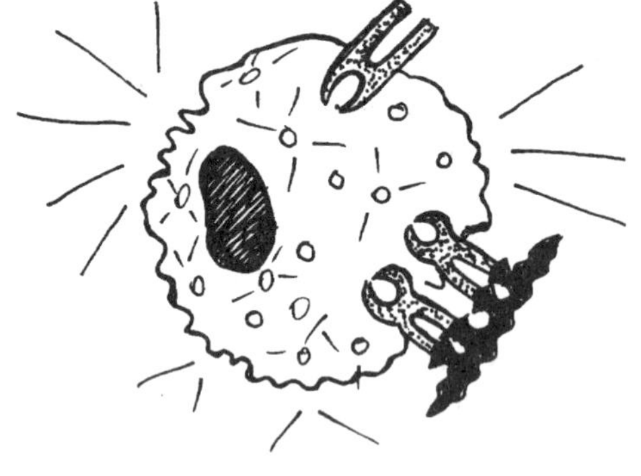

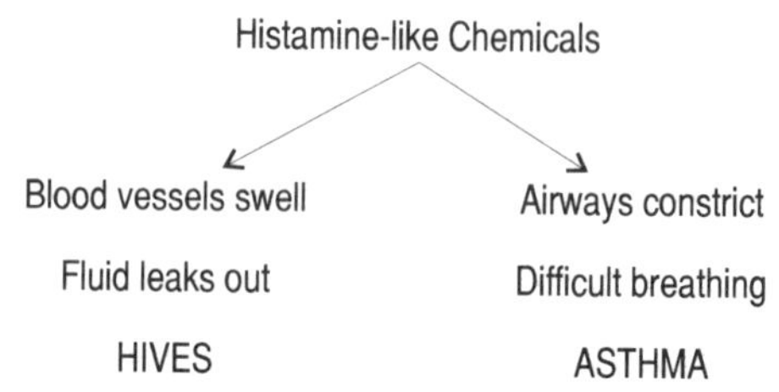

Immediate hypersensitivity.

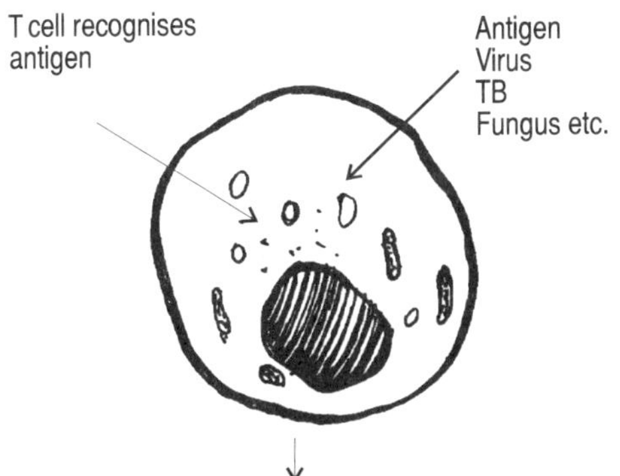

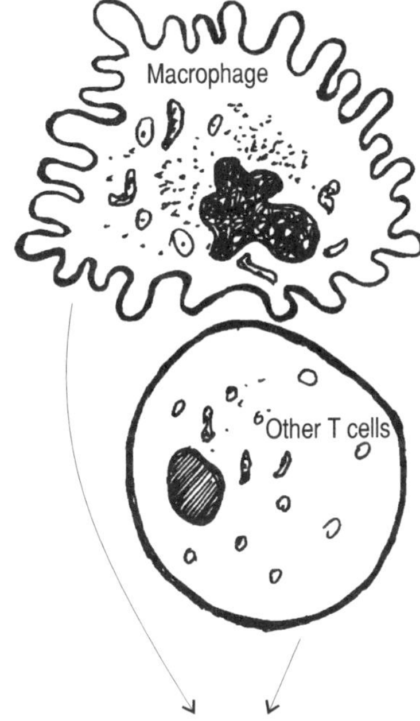

6-12 hours: Antigen
↓
12-24 hours: Attack starts
↓
24-48 hours: Maximum intensity

Delayed hypersensitivity.

- Reduce exposure to toxins. It may be worth while screening for excess toxic metals by having a hair mineral analysis.[28]
- Adequate sleep, rest and relaxation are all important factors to reduce the impact of allergies.[28]
- Evening primrose and linseed oil contains gamma-linolenic acid, which can reduce food intolerance symptoms.[28]

Candidiasis

Useful Oils

• bergamot • German chamomile • lavender
• lemongrass • melissa • myrtle • myrrh • rosemary
• tea tree

Description

Candida albicans infection is a yeast-like fungus that inhabits the intestine, genital tract, mouth and throat. Normally this fungus lives in healthy balance with the bacteria and other fungal yeasts in the body; however, certain conditions can cause this fungus to multiply, weakening the immune system and causing the infection candidiasis.[19,29]

Clinical Features

Because candidiasis travels through the blood to many parts of the body, various symptoms may develop. When it infects the oral cavity, it is called thrush. White sores may form on the tongue, gums, and inside the cheeks. When it infects the vagina, it results in vaginitis, also commonly known as thrush. The most common symptoms include a large amount of white discharge and intense itching.[19]

If candidiasis persists, other symptoms may develop such as depression, poor memory, pre-menstrual syndrome, recurrent cystitis and fungal infections such as athlete's foot. It can also cause food intolerances, which result in abdominal distension, bloating, diarrhoea or constipation.[19,28]

Aetiology

Candidiasis is defined as a classic example of a 'multifactorial' condition. The predisposing factors to *C. albicans* overgrowth include:

- decreased digestive secretions
- dietary factors
- impaired nutrition
- nutrient deficiency
- drugs — particularly antibiotics
- impaired liver function

- underlying disease states
- altered bowel flora
- prolonged antibiotic use.[29]

The most effective treatment needs to address the factors which predispose to *C. albicans* overgrowth and is far more involved than simply using antifungal agents.[29]

Therapeutic Strategy

There are several important steps in the successful treatment *C. albicans*:

- Eliminate the use of antibiotics, steroids, immune-suppressing drugs and birth control pills (unless a medical necessity).[19,29]
- Follow a strict diet which will help control candida.[26,29]
- Improve digestion.[26,29]
- Improve immune function.[26,29]
- Promote detoxification, it is necessary to improve liver function.[26,29]
- Recommend probiotics.[26,29]
- Use herbs and aromatherapy, which will help to control *C. albicans* and promote a healthy bacterial flora.

Aromatherapy Treatment

Schnaubelt cites the work done by Belaiche, who has done extensive research on the clinical efficacy of tea tree oil in the treatment of candidiasis. Belaiche attributed these noteworthy results to two factors:

- The strong antimicrobial effects of tea tree oil itself, which are evident in the aromatogram
- Tea tree oil's extreme tolerability, which allows its use for longer periods of time without the slightest irritation to mucous membranes.[15]

Other essential oils which have been found to be effective include German chamomile, melissa, *Eucalyptus citriodora,* rosemary, lemongrass and myrtle.[30,31,32,33,34]

Worwood suggests blending the following:[35]

German chamomile	5 drops
Lavender	5 drops
Tea tree	5 drops.

These essential oils are added to 100 g of acidophilus yoghurt and mixed well. Then use an applicator for inserting pessaries or a tampon applicator to get the mixture into the vagina. This method is very effective if there is a lot of soreness and itching.[35]

Another way of using yoghurt is to dilute it in warm spring water until it is a thin fluid. Then add the essential oils. This mixture is added to a douche and the vagina is washed once a day.

For oral thrush, gargle and mouthwash using 2 drops of tea tree in warm water after meals.

Immune-stimulating essential oils such as lavender, lemon and rosemary may also be used in a massage. If the patient suffers from depression, as is often the case, uplifting oils such as grapefruit, clary sage or bergamot can be used in massage, baths or oil burners.

Other Treatments

Nutrition

- Avoid all yeast-containing foods such as vegemite, melons, yeast breads, fermented beverages, mouldy cheeses, fermented vinegars, salad dressings, nuts, biscuits, old cereals, apple cores, canned citrus fruit juices, cake mixes, hamburgers, ice cream, all dried fruits, oranges, pickles, tomato sauce, fungi, yeast powder, buttermilk, sour milks, processed and smoked meats, malt products, barbecue sauce, olives, mayonnaise and chillies.[19,26]
- Avoid all refined carbohydrates such as refined sugar, soft drinks, pastries, fruit juices, honey and canned fruit.[19,26,28,29]
- Avoid all known or suspected allergic foods.[28,29]
- Avoid milk and milk products with a high content of lactose. High lactose products promote the overgrowth of *C. albicans*.[29]
- Take one clove of garlic and one teaspoon of olive oil daily. Garlic is especially active against *C. albicans*.[26]
- The intestinal flora plays a major role in our health. Therefore *L. acidophilus* and *B. bifidum* are considered important in promoting proper intestinal environment, post-antibiotic therapy, vaginal yeast infections and urinary tract infections.[29]

Herbs

- Gentian aids gastric secretions and is a good digestive stimulant.[22]
- Other herbs that are recommended include barberry and goldenseal. These herbs contain berberine and have been used in herbal medicine as anti-diarrhoeal and anti-infective agents. Berberine is an effective antimicrobial agent against a wide range of organisms, including *C. albicans*. Its action on candidiasis prevents the overgrowth of yeast that commonly follows antibiotic use.[29]

Chronic Fatigue Syndrome

Useful Oils

• basil • geranium •lavender • lemon • sweet orange • rosemary

Definition

This complex syndrome, which causes profound and persistent tiredness, is also known as myalgic encephalomyelitis, chronic neuromuscular viral syndrome, post-viral syndrome, chronic Epstein-Barr viral syndrome, viral fatigue state, epidemic neuromyasthenia, neurasthenia and Royal Free disease.

Clinical Features

Chronic fatigue syndrome (CFS) is not to be confused with tiredness and depression that follow a viral infection such as infectious mononucleosis, hepatitis or influenza. These post-viral tiredness states are certainly common but resolve within 6 months or so. Typical features of CFS are:

- extreme exhaustion (with minimal physical effort)
- headache or a vague 'fuzzy' feeling in the head
- aching in the muscles and legs
- poor concentration and memory
- hypersomnia or other sleep disturbances
- waking feeling tired
- depressive-type illness
- sore throat
- subjective feeling of fever (with a normal temperature)
- tender swollen lymph glands
- usually occurs between 20 and 40 years of age.[27]

In approximately 2 out of 3 patients the illness follows a clearly defined viral illness. However, no single virus has been consistently associated with the syndrome.[27]

Diagnostic criteria for CFS includes:[27,29]

Major criteria (must meet both)

1. New onset of persistent or relapsing debilitating fatigue (of muscular type) that impairs daily activity to below 50% of the premorbid level for at least 6 months.
2. Complete exclusion of other physical or psychiatric disorders that may produce similar symptoms.

Minor criteria (must have 6 + 2 physical criteria or 8 of 11 symptoms). Symptom criteria:

1. mild fever (37.5–38.6°C)
2. recurrent sore throat
3. painful lymph nodes
4. muscle pain
5. muscle weakness
6. prolonged fatigue after exercise
7. generalised headache
8. neuropsychiatric complaints (poor concentration, confusion, excessive irritability, depression)
9. migratory joint pain
10. sleep disturbances
11. rapid onset of symptom complex.

Aetiology

The causes of chronic fatigue syndrome are not well understood. Many believe that it is not a condition as such, but a set of symptoms which can be produced by more than one causative factor.

Research has identified the Epstein-Barr virus (EBV) to be connected with chronic fatigue syndrome, but this connection has not been conclusively proven.[19,29] EBV is a member of the herpes group of viruses, which includes *Herpes simplex* types 1 and 2, varicella zoster virus, cytomegalovirus and pseudorabies virus.[29]

A number of immune system abnormalities have been reported in CFS patients. The most consistent abnormality is a decreased number or activity of natural killer (NK) cells.[29]

Other possible causes include anaemia, chronic mercury poisoning from amalgam dental fillings, hypoglycaemia, hypothyroidism, *C. albicans* and sleep problems.[19]

Therapeutic Strategy

Chronic fatigue syndrome is a multifactorial condition, which requires a therapeutic strategy that involves multiple therapies. The most effective treatment is a comprehensive program designed to address the following issues where applicable:

- Depression is one of the major features of CFS.[29]
- Stress is another factor to consider in individuals with CFS. Stress is the underlying factor in the patient with depression and low immune function.[29]
- Impaired liver function: Exposure to food additives, solvents (cleaning materials, formaldehyde, toluene, benzene), pesticides, herbicides, heavy metals (lead, mercury, cadmium, arsenic, nickel and aluminium) and other toxins can impair the liver.[29]

- Impaired immune function: When the immune system is impaired, infections can linger and fatigue persist.[29]
- Food allergies: Chronic fatigue has been long recognised as a key feature of food allergies.[29]
- Chronic candidiasis infection: One of the most common findings in individuals with impaired immune function is gastrointestinal overgrowth of *Candida albicans*.[29]
- Excessive gastrointestinal permeability is a common finding of CFS. A treatment program utilising food allergy control, nutrients to stimulate intestinal regeneration and support hepatic function has been found to be effective in the treatment of CFS.[29]
- Hypothyroidism is a common cause of chronic fatigue.[29]

Aromatherapy Treatment

Aromatherapy is considered one of the most consistently successful therapies for treating CFS.[36] Lemon and sweet orange oil are recommended for their uplifting and refreshing effects on the mind. Rosemary and basil are recommended for lethargy. Geranium for its harmonising influence on the body and mind. Lavender is ideal as it has a soothing and relaxing influence suitable for physical and mental fatigue. The essential oils used for the treatment of CFS address the problem at all levels.

Other Treatments

Nutrition

- Eat a well-balanced diet of 50% raw foods and fresh juices. The diet should consist mostly of fruits, vegetables, and whole grains, plus raw nuts, seeds and deep water fish. These foods supply nutrients that renew energy and build immunity.[21]
- As many people with chronic fatigue syndrome are infected with candidiasis, add some form of acidophilus to the diet.[19]
- Vitamin C is important for the functioning of the immune system, and when it is offered intravenously it bypasses the digestive system, which may be faulty in CFS sufferers. Some CFS patients have shown only 20% of normal levels of vitamin C.[19,29]
- Consume plenty of water (at least 8 glasses a day). This will help to flush out toxins and aid in the reduction of muscle pain.[19]

Herbs

- Duke recommends a combination of echinacea, goldenseal, liquorice, lemon balm and ginger. He suggests making a blend of equal amounts of these herbs and making a cup of tea using a teaspoon or two and having at least three cups a day.[37]
- Panax ginseng and Siberian ginseng are both beneficial as a tonic to combat feelings of lassitude and debility, lack of energy and ability to concentrate, and during convalescence. Ginseng stimulates the immune system, and is known as an adaptogen which increases general resistance to all types of stress.[29,37]
- Herbs such as garlic and echinacea should be used to boost the immune system.[37]
- Ginkgo biloba may be used to stimulate circulation, thus improving memory and concentration.[37]
- Teas brewed from burdock root, dandelion, and red clover promote healing by cleansing the blood and enhancing immune function.[19]
- Liquorice root supports the endocrine system.[19]
- Milk thistle protects the liver.[19]
- St John's wort has antiviral properties.[19]
- Skullcap and valerian root will improve sleep.[19]

AIDS

Useful Oils

• bergamot • Roman chamomile • lavender • lemon • neroli • sandalwood • tea tree • thyme • vetiver

Definition

HIV (Human immunodeficiency virus) undermines the immune system, leading to AIDS (Acquired Immune Deficiency Syndrome). This makes the body vulnerable to a range of infections and other diseases that are characteristic of the condition.

Clinical Features

Over 21 million people are infected with HIV, making it the greatest pandemic of the second half of the 20th century.[3] More than 90% of AIDS cases are in developing countries. HIV is transmitted during exposure of the victim's bloodstream to infected body fluids (such as blood or semen) via sexual intercourse, blood transfusion, needle stick injury, or from the mother to the foetus.[3]

Aetiology

It is spread primarily through sexual or blood-to-blood contact. It can be spread by blood transfusion or use of blood products such as clotting factors, if the blood used for these purposes is infected.[19]

Many people who are infected with HIV are not aware that they have it. While some people may experience flu-like symptoms within 2 to 4 weeks of exposure to the virus, it may take up to 5 years before any symptoms of HIV infection appear. The first symptoms are usually non-specific and variable. They often include diarrhoea, fever, fatigue, inflamed gums, loss of appetite and weight, mouth sores, swollen lymph nodes and an enlarged liver and/or spleen. If such symptoms become chronic a person is said to have AIDS-related complex (ARC).[19]

HIV is a retrovirus, its genetic material is ribonucleic acid (RNA) rather than deoxyribonucleic acid (DNA). It infects a range of white blood cells, the most important being the CD4 or T helper cells. These are so called because they bear molecules of protein called CD4 on their surface. The CD4 cells trigger antibody production as part of the immune response to infection.[1]

The risk of developing AIDS is proportional to the degree of immune suppression and the amount and duration of exposure to HIV. If the immune system is healthy it may be possible to avoid developing AIDS, even if one is a member of a high-risk group. Studies have clearly shown that immune-compromised persons are at the greatest risk of contracting AIDS.

Balch cites studies at the Pasteur Institute that indicate the virus may be more hardy and virulent than we ever suspected it to be. We have always been told that the AIDS virus cannot survive without a host, but the Pasteur Institute researchers have found that HIV can survive outside the body, and that it can live for up to 11 days in untreated sewage.[19]

Balch says that anyone with HIV or AIDS should get involved in a treatment program which strengthens the immune system as soon as possible. A person with AIDS needs a higher amount of nutrients than normal because malabsorption is a common problem.[19]

Therapeutic Strategy

The treatment aims may be as follows:

- stress reduction and improvement to psychological health
- pain relief
- prevention of the development of opportunistic infections
- treatment for side-effects of conventional medicine
- improvement of energy levels and quality of life
- treatment to strengthen the immune system and reduce levels of virus without, or combined with, the use of allopathic medicine.[27]

Correct diet, appropriate supplements, exercise, stress reduction, a proper environment, and a healthy mental outlook all play an important role in maintaining a healthy immune system.

Aromatherapy Treatment

Aromatherapy can be used to improve the quality of life. This is achieved by offering relaxing massages, baths, mood-enhancing essential oils and emotional support.[14]

According to Davis, a possible contra-indication to the use of essential oils is chemotherapy. This may often be given to treat Kaposi's sarcoma, a rare form of cancer which affects many AIDS patients. Essential oils should not be used during chemotherapy and for some time after the treatment. She suggests that it is important that the body is detoxified before any essential oils are used by means such as special diets, gentle exercise, high dosage Vitamin C and detoxifying herbs.[14]

It is also important to stress that giving an aromatherapy treatment to a person with AIDS presents no danger to the therapist, as the virus can only be transmitted via bodily fluids such as blood and semen.

Other Treatments

Herbs

- Aloe vera contains carrisyn, which appears to inhibit the growth and spread of HIV. Balch recommends using the food grade aloe and taking 2 cups a day. Reduce the dosage if diarrhoea occurs.[19]
- Dandelion root and silymarin extract help to protect and aid in repairing of the liver and cleanse the blood stream.[19]
- Ginkgo biloba extract is good for the brain and circulation.[19]
- Liquorice and wild yam root are good for the endocrine gland function.[19]

Nutrition

- Increase the intake of fresh fruit and vegetables. Eat a diet consisting of 75% raw foods, preferably organically grown.[19]
- Eat plenty of cruciferous vegetables, such as broccoli, brussel sprouts, cabbage and cauliflower. Also consume yellow and deep-orange vegetables such as carrots, pumpkin, squash and yams.[19]
- Eat unripened paw paw (including the seeds). It is a good source of proteolytic enzymes, which is crucial for proper digestion of foods and assimilation of nutrients.[19]

- Eliminate all junk food from the diet and foods with preservatives, colourings, saturated fats, sugar and white flour.[29]

References

1. Aldridge S. *Magic bullets: How drugs work.* Cambridge University Press, United Kingdom, 1998.
2. Mills S. *The essential book of herbal medicine.* Penguin Books, England, 1991.
3. Dwyer D. *The body at war: The story of our immune system.* 2nd edn, Allen & Unwin Pty Ltd, Australia, 1993.
4. Lemonick M. *The killers all around.* Time Magazine, 1994; 37: 58–65.
5. Begley S. *The end of antibiotics.* The Bulletin, 1994 April 19: 55–60.
6. Cohen BJ, Wood DL. *Memmler's the human body in health and disease.* 9th edn, J.B. Lippincott Company, USA, 2000.
7. Tortora G, Anagnostakos N. *The principles of anatomy and physiology.* 4th edn, Harper & Row Publishers, USA, 1984.
8. Pénoël D. *Winter shield.* International Journal of Aromatherapy 1992; 4(4): 10–12.
9. Knobloch K et al. *Antibacterial and antifungal properties of essential oil components.* The Journal of Essential Oil Research 1989; 1(3): 112–128.
10. Dean C. *The safety profile of tea tree oil, and its implications for aromatherapy.* Australasian Aromatherapy Conference Proceedings, Sydney, 1998.
11. Department of Genito-urinary Medicine, *Tea tree and anaerobic (bacterial) vaginosis.* Lancet 1991; 337(8736): 300.
12. Schnaubelt K. *Potential application of essential oils in viral diseases.* The International Journal of Aromatherapy 1988/1989; 1(4): 32–35
13. Price S, Price L. *Aromatherapy for health professionals.* 2nd edn, Churchill Livingstone, UK, 1999.
14. Davis P. *Aromatherapy: An A–Z.* The C.W. Daniel Company Limited. Great Britain, 1988.
15. Schnaubelt K. *Advanced aromatherapy.* Healing Art Press, USA, 1998.
16. Tisserand R. *Aromatherapy as mind — Body medicine.* The International Journal of Aromatherapy 1994; 6(3): 14–19.
17. Moyer B. *Healing and the mind.* Doubleday, USA, 1993.
18. Bone K, Mills S. *Principles and practice of phytotherapy.* Churchill Livingstone, UK, 2000.
19. Balch J, Balch P. *Prescription for nutritional healing.* Avery Publishing Group, USA, 1997.
20. Pomeroy K, Roberts N. *Fever.* from *A textbook of natural medicine Volume 1*, edited by Pizzorno J, Murray M, Bastyr College Publications, USA, 1993.
21. Holmes P. *The energetics of western herbs Vol.1.* Artemis Press, USA, 1986.
22. Hoffman D. *The new holistic herbal.* USA, Element Books Limited, 1983.
23. Carle R, Gomaa K. *The medicinal use of matricaria flos.* British Journal of Phytotherapy 1992; 2(4): 147–157.
24. Isaac O. *Pharmacological investigations with compounds of chamomile.* Planta Medica 1979; 35: 118–124.
25. Wagner H et al. *In vitro inhibition of prostaglandin biosynthesis by essential oils and phenolic compounds.* Planta Medica 1986; 3: 184–187.
26. Osiecki H. *The physician's handbook of clinical nutrition.* Bioconcepts Publishing, Australia, 1990.
27. Murtagh J. *General practice.* The McGraw-Hill Companies Inc, Australia, 1998.
28. Davies S, Stewart A. *Nutritional medicine.* Pan Books, Great Britain, 1987.
29. Pizzorno J, Murray M. *A text book of natural medicine.* 2nd edn, Churchill Livingstone, UK, 1999.
30. Lorrondo JV et al. *Effects of essential oils on Candida albicans.* Biomed Letter 1991; 46: 269–272.
31. Hmamouchi M et al. *Illustration of antibacterial and antifungal properties of eucalyptus oils.* Plantes Med Phytother, 1990; 24(4): 278–289.
32. Soliman FM. *Analysis and biological activity of the essential oil of Rosmarinus officinalis.* Flavour & Fragrances Journal 1994; 9: 29–33.
33. Onawumni GO. *Evaluation of the antifungal activity of lemongrass.* International Journal of Crude Drugs Research 1989; 27: 121–126.
34. Garg SC et al. *Antifungal activity of some essential oil isolates.* Pharmazie, 1992; 47: 467–468.
35. Worwood V. *The fragrant pharmacy.* Macmillan, United Kingdom, 1990.
36. Wilkinson S. *ME and you.* Wellingborough, United Kingdom, 1988.
37. Duke J. *The green pharmacy.* Rodale Press, USA, 1997.
38. Tyler V. *Herbs of choice.* Pharmaceutical Products Press, USA, 1994.

Unit VI

Aesthetic Aromatherapy

Unit VI provides you with the knowledge and skills required to use aromatherapy in skin care and a day spa.

Unit VI includes the following chapters:

Aromatherapy and Skin Care

Objectives

After careful study of this chapter, you should be able to:

- define holistic aesthetic aromatherapy
- define the benefits of using natural skincare preparations
- outline the function and structure of the skin
- describe a range of skin types and skin conditions
- explain the benefits of essential oils in skin care
- outline a skin care routine
- outline the procedure for performing an aromatherapy facial treatment
- discuss the role of Chinese physiognomy in skin care.

Introduction

It was Marguerite Maury, a French biochemist and beautician, who is often given much credit for the development of holistic aromatherapy as it is practised today. While her book *The Secret of Life and Youth* does not give much practical information on the essential oils, she emphasised the importance of the essential oils not only in massage, but also as psychotherapeutic substances capable of bringing about changes in one's mood:

> *The greatest interest is the effect of fragrance on the psyche and mental state of the individual. Powers of perception become clearer and more accurate and there is a feeling of having, to a certain extent, outstripped events. They are seen more objectively, and therefore in truer perspective.*[1]

Today, aromatherapy is extensively used in beauty and aesthetic treatments for relaxation, rejuvenation, revitalisation, specific skin care and beauty treatments. Essential oils are extensively used in beauty products such as moisturisers, scrubs, masks, toners and body care products.

There is no doubt that the use of pure essential oils in skin care preparations allows the user of the products to experience the benefits of aromatherapy. However, it is disappointing to see a number of cosmetic companies promoting natural aromatherapy skin care products that contain very little, if any, essential oils or natural ingredients.

The Benefit of Essential Oils in Skin Care

Essential oils are ideally suited to skin care because they are readily absorbed through the skin and they:

- have highly antiseptic properties
- help speed up the removal of old skin cells and stimulate the growth of new cells
- improve muscle tone and blood circulation
- help eliminate waste
- reduce inflammation
- regulate sebum production
- reduce the impact of emotional stress.

Essential oils can be easily incorporated into a base cream, lotion, ointment, gel, mask, scrub, toilet water or perfume and of course most of the essential oils used in skin care have an appealing scent. When giving a facial treatment the effect of the scent is important in itself, as it is possible to achieve a considerable degree of relaxation.

Antiseptic Properties

The skin is continuously exposed to micro-organisms such as bacteria and fungi. If the skin's natural defences fail, infections, boils and other skin disorders can result. One way that the skin protects itself is its acid mantle. The acid nature of the sebum helps to neutralise bacteria.

Essential oils such as cajeput, eucalyptus, lemon, myrtle, tea tree, lavender and myrrh, that are antiseptic, bactericidal or anti-fungal, may be used to help the skin's protective functions and are excellent for treating acne and a wide variety of common skin infections.

Cytophalactics

This refers to the ability of essential oils to increase the rate at which skin cells in the germinative layer of the skin reproduce, hence promoting the rapid healing of wounds and burns and thus eliminating scarring. The ability of an essential oil to eliminate scarring is known as its cicatrisant action.

Essential oils such as carrot seed, lavender, everlasting, myrrh, frankincense, neroli, patchouli and yarrow can be used to maintain a healthy and youthful complexion, minimise stretch marks and scarring.

Circulatory Stimulants

The skin has the ability to control temperature through expansion or contraction of the superficial capillaries. It also controls the production of sweat which regulates body temperature by the evaporation of perspiration.

Rubefacient essential oils such as cinnamon bark, clove bud, ginger, black pepper and rosemary help to increase circulation and can be used to assist the skin's body temperature.

By increasing the micro-circulation in the skin, and by strengthening the capillaries, essential oils such as cypress, German chamomile, lemon, rose otto and geranium are useful for the treatment of spider veins and varicose veins.

Detoxification

Up to 25% of the body's waste products are eliminated via the skin. Problems with the elimination of wastes will place a burden on the three main organs of elimination — the kidneys, lungs and bowels. Alternatively if these organs are not functioning efficiently, the skin takes over some of their work, and this can give rise to congested skin, boils, rashes and other skin problems.

Any essential oil such as grapefruit, sweet orange, peppermint, rosemary or carrot seed, known as lymphatic stimulants or hepatics, can assist the skin, as can diuretics such as juniper berry and fennel, which stimulate the kidneys.

Reducing Inflammation

The anti-inflammatory properties of German chamomile have been thoroughly investigated and documented. Other essential oils that reduce inflammation include lavender, neroli, yarrow and everlasting. These essential oils can be used to treat eczema and dermatitis.

Regulating Sebum Production

Sebum is produced by the sebaceous glands to keep the skin supple. Essential oils such as geranium, palmarosa, rosewood and sandalwood may be used to help balance the secretions of the sebaceous glands. For example, dry skin is caused by too little sebum, while oily skin is caused by excessive sebum production.

Reducing Stress

The skin provides an interface with the world. The sensory nerves in the skin respond to the environment. The sense of touch is considered one of the most powerful and important senses, physically, emotionally and psychologically.

The skin also reflects an emotional state. Poor skin may not necessarily represent poor living habits, but may indicate the level of stress, anxiety, lost love, spiritual crisis or any other problem. The oils can be used to reduce and soothe the underlying disharmony on the emotional, psychological or spiritual level.

In Traditional Chinese Medicine the facial features and skin tissue are used as a diagnostic aid. Over the years, grief, depression, anxiety, fear and apathy, as well as joy, laughter and contentment, all leave their mark. Excessive grief and depression may affect the heart, which in turn causes redness and inflammation to appear. This does not mean that broken capillaries are always the result of grief, but it is obvious that the condition of the heart and blood vessels affects the redness and blueness of the skin.

Essential oils such as neroli and lavender can be used to soothe and calm not only the skin, but also the mind. Anger and frustration affect the liver. This may result in poorly assimilated food, often leading to dry skin. Rose, ylang ylang and rosemary will help to correct the imbalance of the mind-body relationship, while lavender, sandalwood and German chamomile will also help the skin directly.

Dehydrated skin is usually associated with fear and the kidneys. The kidneys regulate the amount of water in the body, which in turn affects the moisture content of the skin. A dehydrated skin may indicate a dehydrated body, which may be due to insufficient fluid intake or kidney dysfunction. Essential oils that can be used to assist dehydrated skin are sandalwood and geranium.

Oily skin is associated with the large intestine and worry. Worry tends to affect the diet. Worried people will often eat too much, especially the wrong foods. Constipation often results from the tension of continual thinking and worrying. Essential oils such as lemon, geranium and lavender may be of assistance.

The Benefits of Vegetable Oils

Vegetable oils are used as a base or carrier oil for aromatherapy facial treatments. They are incorporated into moisturising preparations because of their:

- emollient properties
- ability to protect the skin
- ability to prevent moisture evaporating from the skin
- ability to supply the skin with essential fatty acids and vitamins which have specific healing properties.

It is important to used cold-pressed vegetable oils because they have all the essential nutrients which are important for the health and vitality of the skin.

Natural Skin Care Preparations

The term *natural*, used in skin care, has come to imply that the product is safer, more efficacious, more environmentally friendly and its use will endow a feeling of wellbeing.

These are some of the reasons people choose to use natural skin care products:

- **Effective and empirically proven:** The effectiveness of plants has been well documented. Their complex chemical nature gives them active properties on the skin. The wise women, shamans and healers throughout history in all cultures have used plants to care for the skin and heal skin disorders.
- **Safer:** There is the perception that plants or natural ingredients are safer for the skin and general health. This is true and untrue, depending on the ingredient and the person.
- **Accessible:** Plants can be grown and harvested from our own gardens and made into skin care products in our own kitchens.

- **Part of holistic healthcare:** Often used as part of a total healthcare regime. The skin is not seen as an isolated organ to be treated separately from the rest of the body.
- **Living in harmony with nature:** From the way the plants are grown to their disposal once they have been used, harm to the environment is minimal, although this is not always the case.

While essential oils have remarkable therapeutic effects if used with proper cosmetic base materials, Schnaubelt warns us not to make unrealistic claims similar to that of the mainstream cosmetic industry.

> *Essential oils, aromatic waters and other natural substances are well suited for skin care, but a realistic outlook must be maintained toward the regeneration and rejuvenation of the skin.*
>
> *It is possible though to have a positive influence on stress-related skin problems in a relatively short period of time if genuine and authentic essential oils are used. While normal cosmetics treatment is symptom-oriented and attempts to change the skin in one way or another, the goal of essential oil treatment is always the restoration of balance. Treatment with essential oils attempts to bring the metabolic functions back into balance. It is not the purpose of holistic essential oil cosmetics to encourage the expectation of miracles as promised by the mainstream cosmetic industry.*[2]

Many people are concerned with synthetic skin care ingredients because of the possibility of:

- skin sensitisations
- allergic skin reactions
- detrimental long-term effects on the skin
- systemic effects
- toxicity
- carcinogenicity.

Reactions to cosmetics may take the form of skin irritations, allergic contact dermatitis or contact urticaria. The most common causes of irritant reactions are soaps, shampoos and deodorants, often due to detergents or preservatives. The substances that most frequently cause allergic contact dermatitis are fragrances or preservatives and dyes often used in hair colourants.[3]

Therefore, it is critical to understand the potential adverse affects of cosmetic ingredients. However, there are often many contradictions when faced with information on the adverse effects of cosmetic ingredients.

As a guide, check the reference which cites the studies conducted, whether the substance was tested on humans or animals, whether the substance was applied diluted or undiluted, the frequency with which the substance was applied, how often the substance was applied and under what conditions the substance was applied. Beware of suppositions, implications and transference of information obtained from studies. Does the information transfer directly or indirectly with your use of the substance?

When checking information on the ingredients' safe use, be aware that authors can have biases. For example, Statham says that you should avoid bicarbonate of soda because it can cause scalp, forehead and hand rash; circulation problems; it is a liver toxin; and celiac sufferers and people with a heart condition should avoid it.[4]

However, Hampton says that bicarbonate of soda relieves burns, itching, urticarial lesions and insect bites. It is often used in bath powders to help cleanse oily skin and is a common component of many homemade cosmetics and food preparations. It is an excellent tooth powder on its own, and when combined with aloe vera gel it is the best toothpaste you can use.[5]

People will often misquote information. It is hard to believe we are talking about *baking soda*, a common ingredient used in many foods and a key ingredient in many effervescent bath preparations. It is used as a gastric antacid and is considered harmless to the skin. However, if the skin is dry, it can leave an alkaline residue which may cause skin irritation.

What Makes a Skin Care Product Effective?

Whether an ingredient is plant-derived or petrochemically derived, natural or synthetic or derived from any other substance, the following factors are equally important:

- Have the most suitable ingredients been chosen to formulate a skin care product for a particular skin type or skin condition?
- Are the ingredients of high quality?
- Do the ingredients enhance or inhibit the action of each other?
- Have the most appropriate amounts (concentration) of each ingredient been employed in the formulation of a product in order to make it suitable for a particular skin type or condition?
- Has a high standard of hygiene been observed in the manufacture of the skin care product?
- Have the correct temperatures for the extraction of the raw ingredients involved been employed?
- Are the correct method of application and conditions of use for the skin care product being employed by the end user?
- Is the correct amount of product being applied to the skin by the end user?

- Is the frequency of application correct for the particular product?

The Skin

Functions

Although the skin has many functions, the most important are:

- Protection — protection of deeper tissues against the invasion of pathogenic organisms and their toxins through a mechanical barrier.[6]
- Regulation of body fluids and temperature — the skin is considered waterproof, protecting the body from dehydration. It plays a crucial role in the regulation of body temperature by dissipation of heat and secretion and the evaporation of sweat.[6]
- Sensory reception and communication — receipt of information about the environment by means of nerve endings that are profusely distributed throughout the skin.[6]
- Cutaneous absorption and synthesis — gases such as oxygen and carbon dioxide may pass through the skin and enter the bloodstream. The skin has no barrier to steroid hormones and fat-soluble vitamins (A, D, E and K). The skin plays an integral role in the synthesis of vitamin D in the presence of UV light.[6]

The outermost layer of the skin, the stratum corneum, protects the body against invasion by pathogens and against drying. These dry, dead cells, composed of keratin, are found in a tight, interlocking pattern that is impervious to penetration by organisms and by water. The outermost cells are constantly being shed, causing the mechanical removal of pathogens.

The regulation of body temperature, the loss of excess heat as well as protection from the cold, is a very important function of the skin. Indeed, most of the blood that flows through the skin is concerned with temperature regulation. The skin forms a large surface for radiating body heat into the air. When the blood vessels dilate, more blood is brought to the surface so that heat can be dissipated. The activation of the sweat glands and the evaporation of sweat from the surface of the body also help cool the body. In cold conditions, the flow of blood in the veins deep in the subcutaneous tissue serves to heat the skin and protect deeper tissues from excess heat loss.

Structure

The skin is the largest organ of the body in terms of surface area. Structurally the skin is divided into three main layers:

- epidermis — first/outer layer
- dermis — second/inner layer
- hypodermis — third/supportive layer.

Epidermis

The epidermis is the superficial protective layer of the skin and is composed of stratified squamous epithelium that varies in thickness from 0.007–0.12 mm. All but the deepest layer of the epidermis is composed of dead cells.[6]

The epidermis is composed of either four or five layers, depending on its location within the body. The names and characteristics of the epidermal layers are as follows:

- stratum basale
- stratum spinosum
- stratum granulosum
- stratum lucidum
- stratum corneum.[6]

Stratum basale: The stratum basale is composed of a single layer of cells in contact with the dermis. There are four types of cells that are found in the stratum basale: keratinocytes, melanocytes, tactile cells and nonpigmented granular dendrocytes (Langerhans cells). It usually takes between 6 and 8 weeks for the cells in the stratum basale to move to the surface of the skin.[6]

Stratum spinosum: The stratum spinosum contains several stratified layers of cells. The spiny appearance of this layer is due to the different shape of the keratinocytes. Since there is limited mitosis in the stratum spinosum, it along with the stratum basale is collectively referred to as the stratum germinativum.[6]

Melanocytes or melanin pigment cells are located in the germinative layer. These are dark coloured granules which, when triggered by UV rays, migrate to the surface giving the skin a tanned colour or freckled appearance.

Stratum granulosum: This layer consists of only three or four flattened rows of cells. The cells within this layer appear granular due to the process of keratinisation.[6]

The cells gradually begin to die in the stratum granulosum or the granular layer and by the time they reach the stratum corneum they are dead skin cells and desquamation takes place.

Stratum lucidum: This layer is quite pronounced in the thick skin of the palms and soles. It consists of several rows of clear flat, dead cells that contain droplets of a substance called eleidin. Eleidin is eventually transformed to keratin.[7]

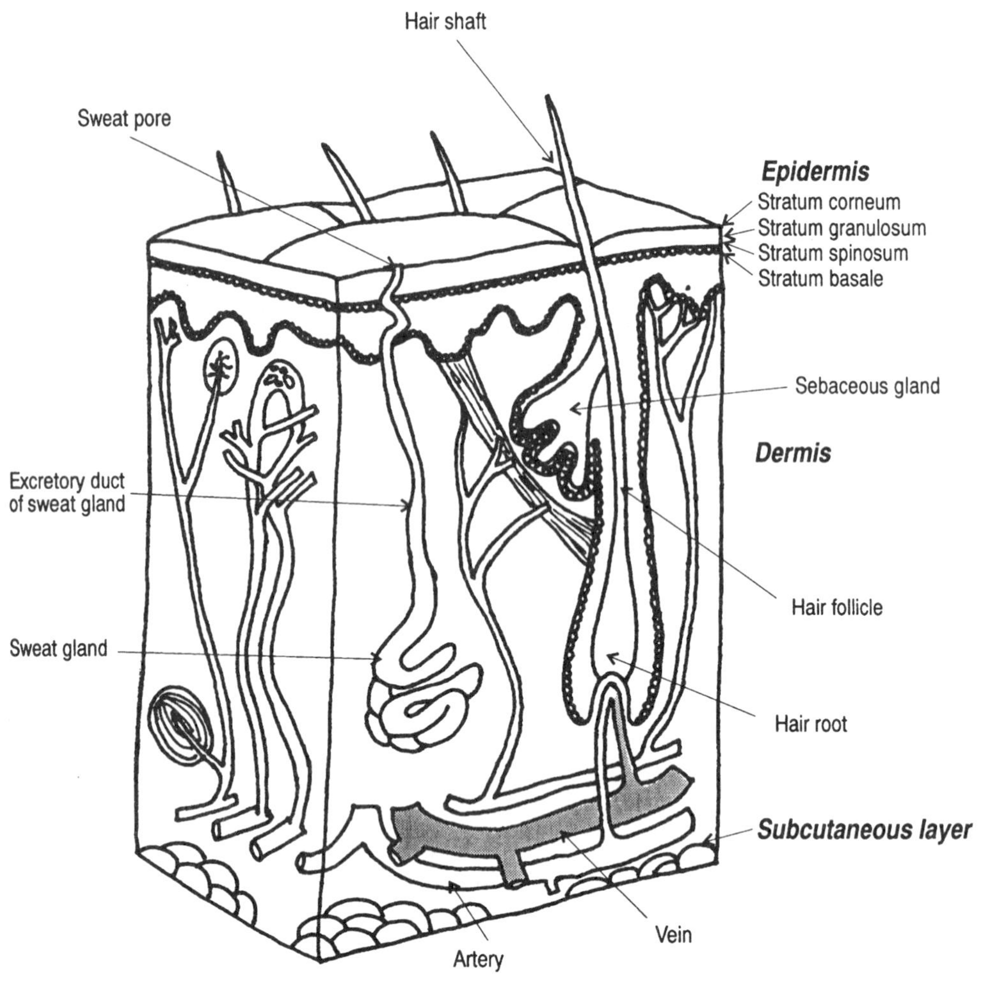

Schematic of cross section of the skin.

Stratum corneum: This layer consists of 25 to 30 rows of flat, dead cells completely filled with keratin. These cells are continuously shed and replaced. The stratum corneum serves as an effective barrier against light and heat waves, bacteria and many chemicals.

Desquamation means the natural removal of dead skin cells. It usually takes between 6 and 8 weeks for the cells to move from the stratum basale to the surface of the skin. This process slows down as we age. In an older person, it may take 50 days. In a psoriasis sufferer, it may take 3 days.

Keratinocytes are specialised cells that produce keratin, which toughens and waterproofs the skin. As keratinocytes are pushed away from the vascular nutrients and oxygen supply of the dermis, their nuclei degenerate, their cellular content is dominated by keratin and the process of keratinisation is complete.[6]

Dermis

The second principal part of the skin, the dermis, is composed of connective tissue containing collagenous and elastic fibres. The dermis is very thick in the palms and soles and very thin in the eyelids, penis and scrotum.

The dermis is well supplied with blood vessels and nerves. Most of the appendages of the skin, including the sweat glands, the sebaceous glands and the hair, are located in the dermis and may extend into the subcutaneous layer.[6]

The upper region of the dermis, about one-fifth of the thickness of the total layer, is named the papillary region or layer. Its surface area is greatly increased by small, finger-like projections called dermal papillae. These structures project into concavities between ridges in the deep surface of the epidermis and many contain loops of capillaries. Some dermal papillae contain Meissner's corpuscles, nerve endings that are sensitive to touch.[7]

The remaining part of the dermis is called the reticular region or layer. It consists of dense, irregularly arranged connective tissue containing interlacing bundles of collagenous and coarse elastic fibres. The name, reticular layer, refers to the bundles of collagenous fibres interlaced in a net-like manner. The spaces between the fibres are occupied by a small quantity of adipose tissues, hair follicles, nerves, oil glands and ducts of sweat glands.[7]

The combination of collagenous and elastic fibres in the reticular region provides the skin with strength, extensibility and elasticity. (Extensibility is the ability to stretch and elasticity is the ability to return to its original shape after extension.) Pregnancy is an example of the skin's ability to stretch.

Hypodermis or Subcutaneous Layer

The dermis rests on the hypodermis, also known as the subcutaneous layer. This layer consists of elastic and fibrous connective tissue as well as adipose tissue. The fat serves as insulation and the reserve store for energy. The major blood vessels that supply the skin run through the subcutaneous layer.[7]

Appendages of the Skin

Sweat Glands

The *sudoriferous glands* are distinguished into coiled, tube-like structures located in the dermis and the subcutaneous tissue. There are two principal types of sweat glands. *Apocrine sweat glands* are simple, branched tubular glands. Their distribution is limited primarily to the skin of the axilla, pubic region and pigmented areas (areolae) of the breasts. The secretory portion of apocrine sweat glands is located in the dermis and the excretory ducts open into hair follicles. Apocrine sweat glands begin to function at puberty and produce a more viscous secretion than the eccrine sweat gland.[7]

Eccrine sweat glands are more common than apocrine sweat glands. They are simple, coiled tubular glands. They are distributed throughout the skin except for the margins of the lips and the nail beds of the fingers and toes. The secretory portion of the eccrine sweat glands is located in the subcutaneous layer and the excretory duct projects upward through the dermis and epidermis to terminate at a pore at the surface of the epidermis. Eccrine sweat glands function throughout life and produce a secretion that is more watery than that of the apocrine sweat glands.[7]

The sweat glands function to regulate body temperature through the evaporation of sweat from the body surface.[7]

Perspiration, or sweat, consists of water with small amounts of mineral salts (mostly sodium chloride, urea, uric acid, amino acids, ammonia, sugar, lactic acid and ascorbic acid). It also helps to eliminate wastes.[7]

Hair and Nails

Hair is composed mainly of keratin and is not living. Each hair develops within a sheath called a follicle, and the new hair is formed from cells at the bottom of the follicles. Attached to most hair follicles is a thin band of involuntary muscle. When this muscle contracts, the hair is raised, forming 'goose bumps' on the skin. As it contracts, the muscle presses on the sebaceous gland associated with the hair follicle, causing a release of sebum.[7]

The primary function of hair is protection. Though the protection is limited, hair guards the scalp from injury and the sun's rays. Eyebrows and eyelashes protect the eyes from foreign particles. Hair in the nostrils and external ear canal protects these structures from dust and insects.[7]

Nails are protective structures made of hard keratin produced by the cells that originate in the outer layer of the epidermis. New cells continually form at the proximal end of the nail in the area called the nail root.[7]

Sebaceous Glands

The *sebaceous glands* or *oil glands* are sac-like structures and their oily secretion, sebum, lubricates the skin and hair and prevents drying. The ducts of the sebaceous gland open into the hair follicles.

Sebum is a mixture of fatty acids, fatty alcohols and esters, lactic acid and lactic salts, which are responsible for maintaining the acid pH of the skin at 4.5 to 6.8. This is referred to as the acid mantle of the skin. At this acid level the keratin protein of the horny layer is compact and is most effective as a barrier.[6]

Sebum helps keep hair from drying and becoming brittle, forms a protective film that prevents excessive evaporation of water from the skin and keeps the skin soft and pliable.

The activity of the sebaceous glands determines skin type. Very active sebaceous glands produce a lot of sebum resulting in greasy skin. If the skin is well balanced it produces just the right amount of sebum to prevent pimples from forming or drying the skin. The majority of people produce too much or too little sebum. Sebum production slows down in later years, so older people in general have drier skin.

Skin Types

The correct identification of skin types and conditions is important to select the most appropriate essential oils and cosmetic products to use. It is important to note that the skin type of an individual may change.

Normal Skin

Useful Oils
• German chamomile • neroli • rose absolute or otto • geranium • palmarosa • lavender • rosewood • sandalwood • ylang ylang

Normal skin has excellent hydration, muscle tone and resilience. There is strong biological activity at the basal layer, blood circulation is active and the metabolism is balanced. Normal skin looks soft, supple and has a healthy glow and colour. The surface of the skin shows a fine texture, and there are no visible wrinkles, fine lines or open pores.

The best example of normal skin is that of children, from birth usually until puberty. It is the rarest of skin types and, therefore, not really 'normal' at all. Normal skin requires proper cleansing, morning and evening. The consistent use of protective moisturisers during the day to prevent moisture loss and hydrating creams at night is essential. An occasional exfoliation is also beneficial. Sun protection is extremely important.

Essential Oils for Normal Skin

Almost any essential oil that will not irritate the skin can be used on normal skin. Essential oils such as German chamomile, geranium, lavender, rose, neroli, palmarosa, rosewood or ylang ylang can be used in a cold-pressed vegetable oil such as sweet almond, apricot kernel oil or jojoba.

Oily Skin

Useful Oils
• bay laurel • bergamot • Virginian cedarwood • clary sage • cypress • *Eucalyptus dives* • geranium • lavender • lemon • juniper berry • mandarin • myrtle • niaouli • palmarosa • spike lavender • rosemary • sandalwood • tea tree • thyme ct. linalool • ylang ylang

Oily skin can be recognised by its shiny, thick, and firm appearance. Pores look enlarged, usually due to oil entrapped in the pilosebaceous follicles. Enlarged pores become aggravated with a dehydrated condition.

An oily complexion tends to look dirty and neglected, occasionally with blemishes on the chin or the forehead area, and feels oily to the touch. Hot, humid conditions tend to exacerbate oil gland secretion, making the skin oilier.

It is a mistake to use harsh soaps and strong astringents containing lots of alcohol in an attempt to control excessive oiliness, as these tend to stimulate the skin to produce more sebum and in the long run make the situation worse.

Oily skin benefits from regular use of clay masks and steam treatments to unblock pores and prevent blackheads forming. It is most common in adolescence because sebum production is linked to the activity of the whole endocrine system, which is in a state of flux following the onset of puberty. This is a vulnerable stage of life, where appearances seem to be very important. It is little comfort to be told that a skin that is too oily in youth will age far more slowly than one which is relatively dry.[8]

Essential Oils for Oily Skin

Essential oils that can help reduce the amount of sebum produced and indirectly control the bacteria responsible for any infections are beneficial for treating oily skin. Essential oils of Virginian and Atlas cedarwood, cypress, geranium, grapefruit, lavender and sandalwood are recommended.[9,10]

Davis recommends a blend of equal amounts of lavender and geranium. This is a great synergy as geranium will regulate sebum production and is known for its balancing effect on the endocrine system, while lavender is antiseptic, healing and calming on the skin.[10]

If a carrier oil is used, oils such as apricot kernel or jojoba should be used. All traces of the carrier oil should be carefully removed using a cleanser or toner after the treatment.

Schnaubelt says that *E. dives* is traditionally used to calm hyperactive sebaceous glands. He recommends using *Inula graveolens* as it helps to dissolve hardened sebum from clogged pores. If *I. graveolens* is not available, as it is difficult to find and quite expensive, he suggests using *Myrtus communis*.[2]

Schnaubelt also recommends using camphor for its stimulating effect on skin tissue. However, as there are many risks associated with camphor he recommends using spike lavender, which contains approximately 10% camphor.[2]

Dry Skin

Useful Oils
• German and Roman chamomile • geranium • jasmine absolute • lavender • neroli • palmarosa • rose absolute or otto • rosewood • sandalwood • ylang ylang

Dry skin is the result of sebaceous gland underactivity. It is hereditary but can also result from the aging process. Dry skin also tends to be dehydrated. The lack of oil diminishes the skin's ability to retain moisture since oil in the skin acts as a barrier against moisture loss.

Dry skin tends to be very fine, overly delicate and thin. The pores are almost invisible and it tends to wrinkle easily and the skin is often filled with tiny superficial lines. Dry skin problems are aggravated by the sun, wind and heat. Improper skin care, such as insufficient lubrication and lack of protection against moisture loss especially during the day, further exacerbates this problem.

Essential Oils for Dry Skin

Floral oils such as German and Roman chamomile, jasmine absolute, neroli and rose absolute or otto are recommended. Other oils that should be considered for treating dry skin include geranium, lavender, palmarosa, rosewood and sandalwood.[9,10] Regular massage will increase circulation in the capillaries that nourish the skin, and this in turn will improve the whole health of the skin.

The best base oils to use are avocado, wheatgerm, sweet almond, apricot kernel, jojoba, evening primrose oil and infused carrot oil.

Combination Skin

Useful Oils
• geranium • lavender • neroli • palmarosa • rosewood • sandalwood

Combination skin is characterised by the existence of two or more different conditions. For example, the skin may be oily around the nose, forehead, and the chin, but dry on the rest of the face. Combination skin tends to be partly dry and partly oily and subject to blackheads and dilated pores in the T-zone area.

When treating a combination skin, each area is treated for its particular condition. For example, when applying a mask, a mask formulated for oily skin is applied to the oily areas of the face and a mask formulated for dry skin is applied to dry areas.

Essential Oils for Combination Skin

The most useful essential oils are geranium and palmarosa because of their balancing effect on the sebaceous glands. Other essential oils that can be used include sandalwood, neroli and lavender. The most suitable base oils are apricot kernel, jojoba and evening primrose cold-pressed vegetable oils.

Skin Conditions

Couperose Skin

Useful Oils
• German chamomile • lavender • neroli • rose otto • sandalwood

Couperose is temporary or chronic redness appearing on the face. It appears as small, dilated, winding, bright red blood vessels on the cheeks, around the nose and sometimes on the chin. Couperose occurs primarily as a result of poor elasticity in the capillary wall. If it is not sufficiently elastic, it will expand but may not contract again to its original shape or size. The result is a distended capillary that will hold blood cells within its structure, thus giving the appearance of diffuse or local redness.

This skin condition is aggravated by extremes of temperature either hot or cold, by the use of excessively cold or hot water, nervous disorders, digestive disorders, poor nutrition, saunas, exercise that causes the face to turn very red, drinking very hot liquids, eating spicy foods, smoking, alcohol and aggressive use of harsh products such as scrubs and alcohol-based toners.

Essential oils such as German chamomile, lavender, neroli, rose otto and sandalwood are recommended for couperose skin because they are considered gentle on the skin and will improve the microcirculation of the skin.

Dehydrated Skin

Useful Oils
• German and Roman chamomile • geranium • lavender • neroli • palmarosa • rose absolute and otto • rosewood • sandalwood

Dehydrated skin lacks sufficient moisture in the cellular system and intercellular channels. Dehydrated skin can look dull and dry, scaly and flaky. When gently pushed upward with the hand, the skin 'crinkles'. Sometimes the skin appears as if it had an additional thin layer of skin placed on top.

Dehydration may be caused and aggravated by excessive perspiration, lack of sebum to prevent evaporation of natural moisture, poor metabolism, and/or insufficient water intake, drinking tea, coffee, soft drinks or diuretics, atmospheric conditions including too much sun and wind, not using sunscreens or daytime protective moisturisers, using inappropriate skin care products and cleansing with harsh soaps and water.

Dry and oily skins can be dehydrated. When oily skin becomes dehydrated the surface layers of cells harden and block oil secretion. This is particularly detrimental in the case of someone with acne as it results in infection.

Care for dehydrated skin should include daytime protective and hydrating moisturisers. These help seal the natural moisture of the skin and reduce moisture loss and introduce moisture to the skin. Masks should be applied on a weekly or bi-weekly basis depending on the level of dehydration.

Essential oils suitable for treating dehydrated skin are geranium, lavender, German or Roman chamomile, neroli, rose absolute or otto and sandalwood.

Mature Skin

Useful Oils

• carrot seed • German and Roman chamomile
• everlasting • frankincense • lavender • neroli
• myrrh • palmarosa • patchouli
• rose absolute and otto • rosewood • sandalwood

Aging is chronological and all living things go through the process of aging from birth to death. The body's processes slow down and cells are not replaced as rapidly as they once were. Our skin has a chronological age and a physiological age. Pugliese outlines the physiological and anatomical changes seen in aging skin.[8]

Stage One (Ages 10 to 20)

At this stage, the skin should be smooth and firm with good snap and no drooping. There may be a few lines at the outer canthus in those who are avid sunbathers.[8]

Stage Two (Ages 21 to 35)

At this stage many changes have taken place. Heredity and environmental effects are more apparent. Signs include loss of skin lustre, areas of dilated veins, fine lines about the outer eyes and some under-eye puffiness. The hands may show early thinning and the neck will exhibit wrinkling, particularly under the chin. Sunbathers will exhibit a dark leathery appearance which in winter will take on a yellow hue. These physical signs occur from 28 to about 35 years of age.[8]

Stage Three (Ages 36 to 50)

The most notable change in the skin is the appearance of relaxed skin (sagging or drooping is more descriptive). The cheeks and mouth are the areas to show this change, which is due to the degeneration of the elastin fibres. The area around the nose and mouth show increased depth of the normal furrows and there is a significant increase in lines around the eyes.[8]

Stage Four (Ages 50 to 65)

Pugliese calls stage four the fixation period, because it is the time of physical and mental change that can result in a permanent 'old age attitude' and appearance. The cheekbones become more noticeable as the skin sags and the fatty tissue atrophies. The neck assumes a hatched pattern, with deep vertical folds and horizontal lines.[8]

Stage Five (Ages 66 and Older)

The wrinkles, lines and creases are more prominent due to further relaxation and deterioration of the elastin fibres. The colour of the skin varies from a sickly, yellow hue to a tawny reddish-brown. Many lesions may be visible, particularly brown, flat and raised spots; patches that represent solar type disorders and non-solar neoplastic disorders.[8]

Dermal changes are associated with elastosis in the sun-exposed areas. The weather-beaten red neck and rhomboidal lines are common in outdoor types. Deep wrinkles and creases are mainly in the direction which is transverse to the long axis of the facial muscles. The periorbital region of the eyes is yellow, thick ridges with the skin thrown into folds and afflicted with large comedones and follicular cysts. The mouth shows typical deep, furrowed lines running perpendicular to the orbicularis. The neck is also badly wrinkled.[8]

Not all individuals age uniformly. Great variations occur — many of the signs listed above are absent in individuals who have reached 90 years of age!

Treatment for Aging Skin

When treating aging skin that is at stage two, Pugliese insists that the client stops all abusive chemicals and avoids sun exposure. Carefully assess diet and lifestyle habits and evaluate levels of stress from occupation and personal relationships. Be supportive but not permissive. Design a treatment that includes diet modification, regular clinic visits and active topical products.[8]

The diet includes the elimination of high sugar containing foods. Add fruits and vegetables containing fibre and vitamins C and A. Fats should not exceed 30% of the food intake and should include unsaturated fats.

Topical treatment starts with a general facial cleansing, followed by a facial massage and a hydrating mask. This can be made using a pink clay base combined with herbal extracts such as aloe vera, seaweed, chamomile flowers, comfrey or gotu kola and essential oils of rosewood, palmarosa, lavender, neroli and sandalwood.

When treating aging skin that is at stage three and four, Pugliese says that it is important that the client has seen a doctor to ensure that there are no systemic diseases manifested by skin conditions. Start with a preventive regimen. Avoid exposure to the sun, reduce alcohol, stop smoking, improve nutrition and improve the client's concept of self with encouragement.[8]

Develop a program of monthly visits for facial cleansing and massage. A full aromatherapy massage coupled with an exercise program will greatly improve the client's feeling of wellbeing. While you should not expect any real improvement in line reduction or creases for 6 to 8 months, the general appearance of the skin, the colour and the texture, however, will improve after 30 days. Time, patience, persistence, confidence and encouragement are important to the treatment of this client.

When treating aging skin which is at stage five, Pugliese suggests that it is important to refer the client to a doctor for the evaluation of all skin lesions. While the client is primarily interested in facial appearance, do not neglect the other areas of the body. A long-term program should be developed with the client being seen on a monthly basis. As usual, attention to diet and the general wellbeing of the client should be considered.[8]

Aromatherapy Treatment for Aging Skin

Carrot seed oil has been described by Lavabre as one of the strongest revitalising essential oils for the skin.[11] Essential oils such as frankincense, patchouli, neroli and sandalwood are also recommended.[9] Davis recommends using German chamomile and rose otto if thread veins are present.[10] Carrier oils such as wheatgerm oil, avocado oil, rosehip oil and jojoba are ideal for aging skin.

Sensitive Skin

Useful Oils

• German and Roman chamomile • everlasting • lavender • neroli • rose otto • rosewood • sandalwood

Sensitive skin is described as having a very youthful appearance and is often compared to the skin of babies and young children. It is often fair, delicate and almost translucent. However, it is sensitive to heat and cold and can become dry and taut to such a degree that it is red, itchy and painful.

A sensitive skin reaction can express itself as redness, itching, burning and, in the worst of cases, as small pustules sometimes filled with a watery liquid.

Certain cosmetic ingredients aggravate skin sensitivity. Facial scrubbing and the use of astringents with high levels of alcohol will usually aggravate sensitive skin. Environmental factors such as wind, sun and heat can also aggravate sensitive skins.

People with sensitive skin should use very gentle, hypoallergenic products. Cosmetic formulations with herbs and essential oil that have anti-allergenic, soothing, healing properties are helpful, and anti-inflammatory agents are also beneficial.

Great care must be taken when selecting essential oils for sensitive skin. Essential oils such as German chamomile, everlasting, neroli, rose otto and sandalwood should be considered. Davis says that even lavender has been shown to cause irritation and redness.[10]

The essential oil dilution is much less than usual. Use a 1 to 2% for body massage and 0.5 to 1.0% for a face massage. Very light lotions and creams are more suitable bases for sensitive skin.

The most suitable base oils for sensitive skin are apricot kernel, calendula-infused oil, jojoba and evening primrose oil.

The Aromatherapy Facial

The facial usually involves a consultation, which includes an assessment of the skin to help with the choice of appropriate skin care preparations, essential and carrier oils, and finally the treatment.

A typical procedure for performing an aromatherapy facial treatment:

- client completes initial consultation form
- therapist consultation with the client
- a detailed facial skin examination
- a facial treatment
- body treatment.[12]

The Consultation and Assessment

The purpose of the consultation and a detailed skin examination is to determine:

- if there are any contra-indications to treatment, or specific essential oils.
- the type of treatment to be given.

The consultation should cover six broad areas as follows:

- basic personal history
- medical history/medication
- allergies
- emotional state
- lifestyle
- diet.[12]

Before examining the client's skin it will be necessary to remove makeup, if the client is wearing makeup.

While the role of the facial diagnosis is to determine the type of skin that the client has, you should also consider the following questions:

- What type of skin condition does your client have?
- What is the general skin tone?
- Does the skin appear slack?
- Do the muscles lack tone?
- Is there any tension being held in the muscles?
- Does the skin appear to be hydrated or dehydrated?
- Are there any nodules or swelling?
- Are there any broken capillaries?
- Are there areas of excessive oiliness?
- Are there dry or flaking patches?
- Are there any open pores?
- If there are lines, are they superficial or deep?
- Is there excessive redness?
- Does the skin have a healthy appearance, or a greyish or sallow tone?
- Is there sun damage?
- Are there signs of cosmetic surgery?
- Are there swollen lymph nodes?
- Does the sinus area feel thick and congested?

The selection of essential oils will be determined by the above factors. It is also important to consider the emotional and spiritual needs of your client.

Chinese Physiognomy

The principles of Traditional Chinese Medicine (TCM) can be incorporated into a facial examination.[13]

The face is an indicator of health or disease in the body. By studying skin conditions and changes, we can determine inner balance and stressed areas of the body. Each area of the body relates to an internal body area. Disharmony in that organ will lead to changes in complexion, moisture and texture in the corresponding facial area.

According to TCM, the skin is related to the lungs and the large intestine. The skin therefore reflects the condition of the lungs, and the ability to breathe. Eczema, psoriasis and rashes reflect an imbalance that directly relates to the lungs. Elimination is also associated with the skin, since the process of getting rid of toxins also occurs via the skin, such as acne, boils and pimples.[13]

Many skin diseases are due to stasis of blood and are related to the condition of the liver. Some skin diseases are related to stomach heat and thus are associated with the stomach — for example, eczema, hives and *Acne rosacea*. Use essential oils of bergamot, German chamomile and geranium.[13]

Breakouts, wrinkles, patches, scaliness or rashes which appear on certain areas of the face could mean that the energy of the corresponding organs is out of balance. This imbalance is reflected on the face.[13]

According to Kushi, each area of the face manifests each organ and its functions of the body. Chinese physiognomy will help to establish the connection between skin conditions and the systems of the body:[14]

- the condition of the cheeks shows the condition of the lungs and their functions
- the tip of the nose represents the heart and its functions, while the nostrils represent the bronchi connecting the lungs
- the middle part of the nose represents the stomach, and the upper part of the nose represents the condition of the pancreas
- the area between the eyebrows shows the condition of the liver, and the temples on both sides show the condition of the spleen
- the forehead as a whole represents the small intestines, and the peripheral region of the forehead represents the large intestines
- the upper part of the forehead shows the condition of the bladder
- the ears represent the kidneys
- the mouth as a whole shows the condition of the digestive system. More specifically, the upper lips show the stomach; the lower lips show the small intestines at the inner part of the lip and the large intestines at the more peripheral part of the lip. The corners of the lips show the condition of the duodenum
- the area around the mouth represents the sexual organs and their functions.

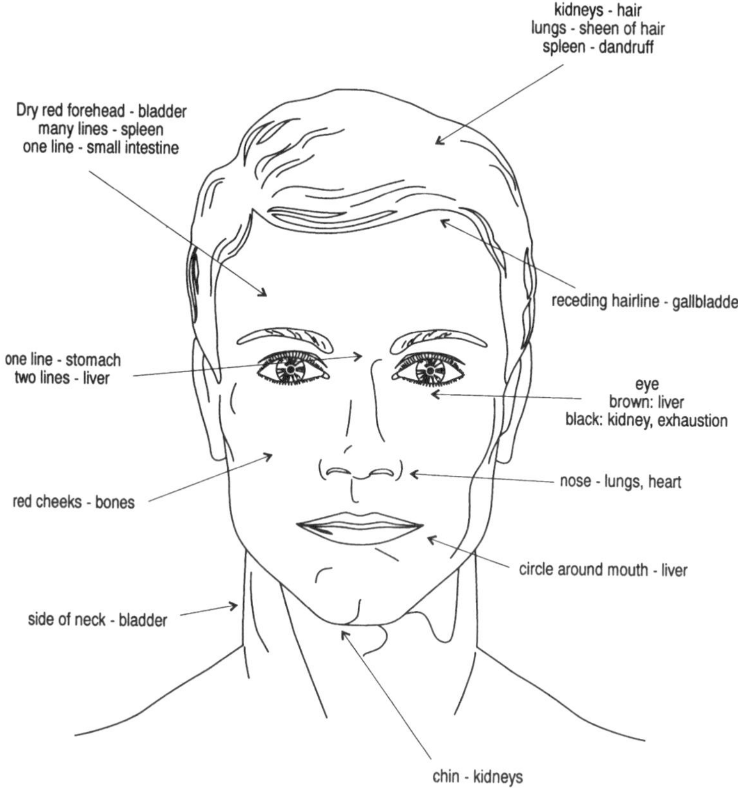

Facial diagnosis according to Traditional Chinese Medicine.

Performing an Aromatherapy Facial Treatment

It must be remembered that there are many ways to perform an aromatherapy facial treatment. They generally follow the steps outlined below:

1. cleansing
2. toning
3. compresses
4. facial massage
5. facial mask
6. application of a moisturiser
7. rest.[12]

The time for the aromatherapy facial is approximately 1 hour.

Cleansing

The most important part of caring for the skin is to cleanse it thoroughly. If the skin is not thoroughly cleansed, it can look dull and a number of skin conditions may develop or be made worse.

A cleanser should remove excess oil, perspiration, dirt, dust, pollution, make-up and naturally loosened dead skin cells from the surface of the skin and, to a certain extent, from the skin's pores.

Cleansing will help to loosen and dislodge blockages such as blackheads, and can begin to treat a skin problem. A cleanser should not disturb the acid mantle (protective layer). It should not cause the removal of too much oil or moisture or upset the skin's pH balance significantly.

A cleanser is formulated from a choice of the following basic ingredients — water (for moisture and fluidity), emollients (skin softeners), emulsifiers (hold together the water and oily components which have been mixed together), surfactants (cause foaming and help dissolve impurities), and active ingredients (chosen to heal or treat a particular skin type or condition).

Cleansers are available in the following forms: foaming cleansers for oily skins, milk cleansers for dehydrated and dry skins, creams for dry skins, gels for oily, combination and dehydrated skins, and cleansing bars for oily skins. Many commercial foaming cleansers use harsh surfactants which can be quite aggressive as they remove all traces of sebum, creating a dry and sensitive skin.

A cleanser should be applied twice; once to remove surface impurities such as pollution and make-up and again to achieve a more thorough cleansing of the pores. The cleanser should be massaged thoroughly over the entire face especially over any areas of blocked pores. It is then removed completely with damp sponges or cloths and then rinsed. The skin should feel clean, soft and hydrated. This step should be followed by skin toning.

Steaming is often used in the cleansing process as it:

- increases perspiration, which encourages the removal of wastes and cleanses the sweat pores
- softens sebum build-up and loosens dead skin cells
- improves skin hydration.[15]

If you incorporate steaming within a facial to assist with the cleansing, use only essential oils which are considered suitable for the client's skin type or condition. Some steaming machines have been specially designed for use with essential oils. While essential oils and water do not mix, the essential oils are made more volatile by the heat of the steam.

Do not steam if there are any broken veins, if the skin is hypersensitive and if there is any inflammation or sunburn.

Toning

A toner is a liquid that is used after cleansing and may be used to remove any traces of cleanser still left on the skin.

Toners help balance the skin's pH and are formulated to suit a specific skin type. A toner may contain active ingredients that help treat a skin condition. Some toners can have an astringent action and are used to treat oily skin conditions. They will also temporarily minimise pore size. The skin should feel cool, smooth and refreshed.

Avoid toners containing alcohol as they will eventually, if not immediately, cause irritation and pigmentation problems of the skin.

Floral waters, also known as hydrosols make excellent toners. Floral waters usually contain a very small amount of essential oil and water soluble extracts of the plant. The water is produced by distillation.

Commonly Used Floral Waters

Floral Water	Function
Rose water	Ideal for all skin types as a freshener or toner.
Orange flower water	Ideal for combination and sensitive skin types
Lavender water	Ideal for normal and sensitive skin types
Chamomile water	Ideal for dry, sensitive and inflamed skin
Witch hazel	Astringent, ideally suited for oily skin

A toner is the first step in adding moisture to the skin's surface and is applied to the skin just before the application of a moisturiser. Apply to damp cotton wool and wipe over the face or spray over the face.

Compresses

A compress using essential oils can be applied to the face or to the appropriate area on the body. For example, a poultice of fresh rosemary herb can be applied on the liver for detoxification.

A compress of chamomile flowers can be applied to an area of sensitive skin to decongest the skin. Alternatively, you can make a compress using essential oils. Hydrosols can also be used in a compress.

Facial Massage

Massage is one aspect of an aromatherapy facial treatment. Massage of the facial region is beneficial because:

- It stimulates the blood supply to the area, which increases the oxygen level and improves the tone of the skin.
- It relaxes facial muscle tension, softening the facial expression, especially evident if the client is under stress.
- It stimulates lymphatic circulation through the use of lymphatic drainage techniques, which can assist in the elimination of toxins.
- It can help to dispel tiredness, leaving the client feeling refreshed and relaxed.

Prepare the aromatherapy facial oil by blending the appropriate essential oils and carrier oils and apply to the face using the facial technique outlined in the Micheline Arcier aromatherapy massage.

Essential oils should always be diluted before application to the face. The percentage of essential oil in most commercially available products is likely to be between 0.1 and 1%. For products with sensitive skin the percentage is likely to be even lower.

The amount of essential oil used in a treatment will vary from client to client. This variability is dependent upon the client's skin type, tone, sensitivity, emotional state including stress and tension, any allergies or medical skin condition, whether the client is taking medication or other drugs and whether the client is pregnant.

Facial Masks

Masks are available in several forms and are used for many purposes. They can be stimulating, cleansing, drawing, pore refining, soothing and calming, toning and firming, refreshing, lightening and hydrating. There are two basic types of masks:

Setting, absorbing masks: These kinds of masks are drying, cleansing, drawing, toning and stimulating, and may contain healing ingredients. The key ingredient for all masks that draw from the skin is clay. The most commonly used is kaolin. The clays come from all over the world and in many colours. This is usually reflective of the mineral content of the clay. Although a clay mask can work by itself, the addition of essential oils which are suitable for the skin type of condition makes the clay treatment more effective.[15]

In dealing with clay-based masks it is important not to over-dry the mask on someone with oily skin.[16]

Non-setting, adsorbing masks: These kinds of masks will infuse active ingredients into the skin, hydrate, soothe and calm, heal and freshen the skin. These masks tend to remain moist on the skin and may be creamy or gel-based or made from plants, fruits, vegetables, honey, herbs or eggs.

It may be necessary to apply different masks to the face at the same time to treat different skin types and conditions. For example, you would apply a clay mask to the T-zone, which is oily and has blocked pores, while you would use a cream mask to the cheeks that may be dehydrated and sensitive.[15]

Moisturising

A moisturiser is used to protect the skin and prevent damage from the environment, including sun, wind, air-conditioning and air pollution. Moisturising creams are emulsions of water, oil and wax. The oil softens, smoothes and prevents moisture loss and protects the skin while the water adds moisture to the skin and the wax acts as an emulsifier.

A moisturiser is formulated with a selection of the following ingredients: water, emollients, emulsifiers, waxes, humectants, active ingredients, fragrances, stabilisers and preservatives.

A well-formulated moisturiser will prevent skin clogging and congestion caused by make-up, dust and air pollution. A moisturiser, as the name implies, will provide moisture to the surface layers of the skin and will prevent dehydration and dryness. It will keep the skin smooth and supple.

A moisturiser is massaged into the skin with firm upward strokes. A separate cream is generally applied to the eye area and sometimes the neck.

References

1. Maury M. *Marguerite Maury's guide to aromatherapy: The secret of life and youth.* First published in 1964, Translated and reprinted in English by The C.W. Daniel Company Limited, Great Britain, 1989.
2. Schnaubelt K. *Advanced aromatherapy.* Healing Art Press, USA, 1995.
3. Gawkrodger D. *Dermatology.* Churchill Livingstone, UK, 1997.
4. Statham B. *The chemical maze.* 2nd ed, possibility.com, Australia, 2002.
5. Hampton A. *What's in your cosmetic.* Odonian Press, USA, 1995.
6. Van De Graaff K, Fox SI, *Concepts of human anatomy and physiology.* 3rd edn, Wm.C. Brown Publishers, USA, 1992.
7. Tortora G, Anagnostakos N. *Principles of anatomy and physiology.* Harper and Row Publishers, USA, 1984.
8. Pugliese P. *Advanced professional skin care.* APSC Publishing, USA, 1991.
9. Lawless J. *The encyclopaedia of essential oils.* Element Books Limited, Great Britain, 1992.
10. Davis P. *Aromatherapy: An A–Z.* 2nd edn, The C.W. Daniel Company Limited, Great Britain, 1999.
11. Lavabre M. *Aromatherapy workbook.* Healing Art Press, USA, 1997.
12. Worwood V. *Aromatherapy for the beauty therapist.* Thomson Learning, UK, 2001.
13. Kahn L. *Aesthetic aromatherapy and oriental race diagnosis.* AROMA'95 Conference Proceedings, Aromatherapy Publications, England. 1995.
14. Kushi M. *How to see your health: Book of oriental diagnosis.* Japan Publications, USA 1980.
15. Stubbin C. *Do it yourself pure plant skincare.* The International Centre of Holistic Aromatherapy, Australia, 1999.
16. Hess S. *SalonOvations' guide to aromatherapy.* Milady Publishing Company, USA, 1996.

Aromatherapy and Day Spas

Objectives

After careful study of this chapter, you should be able to:

Define the term day spa.

- explain how aromatherapy can be incorporated into a day spa
- explain the benefits of hydrotherapy treatments
- outline the benefits and contra-indications for cold and heat in hydrotherapy treatments.
- describe a range of day spa treatments
- examine how it is possible to convert an existing clinic into a day spa.

What Is a Spa?

The word 'spa' originates from a little town of that name in Belgium, which became famous for its hot springs, reputed to be therapeutic. The use of water and bathing as a therapeutic tool has been popular since Roman times. Spas and their treatments have always been, and are still, centred on water therapies.[1]

The 'destination spa' traditionally offers overnight or longer-term stays, whereas the modern model, the 'day spa' has grown in response to the hectic pace of people today which has seen the need to create the one-day or part-day spa experience. The definition of a 'day spa' is exactly that — the destination spa experience within one day.

Technically speaking, a day spa needs water-based treatments for the title to be accurately adopted. According to Cook, every beauty salon, hairdresser, fitness facility, every hotel and resort is now converting their traditional amenities into a 'spa'.[2]

However, many of these centres do not have a drop of water in sight. Does this matter? Cook says that it is not necessary for a spa to provide every possible service, it is more important to create the atmosphere, the service, the ambiance and the emotional response that makes the spa experience unique.[2]

Daley says that it is the 'spa attitude' that is vital to the success of the spa. He says that this 'attitude' is essentially the creation and maintenance of a relaxing environment which incorporates superb customer service with a particularly nurturing and respectful quality, an atmosphere of perfect calm and peaceful ambiance offering true escape, and a focus and commitment to the holistic wellbeing of the individual.[3]

The spa concept has become an all-encompassing term for a facility that provides a wide range of personal care services. Broadly speaking, the services may include beauty, hair, nails, health and fitness. According to Daley, day spas may fall into three main categories:[3]

- professional beauty salons integrating spa services
- hairdressing salons expanding to embrace the day spa concept
- new facilities and centres being developed specifically as day spas.

The fast-paced stressful lifestyle of people today has led to a desire for a balanced and healthy lifestyle. People need a one-stop centre where they can:

- de-stress, rebalance and rejuvenate
- attend to their body's total aesthetic requirements
- take the first steps in dealing with a variety of health issues.

The Role of Aromatherapy in the Day Spa

Aromatherapy is ideally suited to the day spa. It can create a peaceful healing sanctuary for the body, mind and soul. Essential oils can be used in psychoaromatherapy, aesthetic aromatherapy, clinical aromatherapy and holistic body treatments.

Spas are seen as centres of rest, renewal, relaxation and, most importantly, centres of healing. Kahn says that clients who visit day spas do not have major diseases or illnesses. They are often seeking a holistic approach to preventative health care for imbalances in their lives. She says that the most common conditions that clients present are stress, fatigue, lethargy, headaches/migraines, insomnia, emotional imbalance, grief, hormonal imbalances, menopausal symptoms, anxiety and nervous tension, water retention, muscular tension, poor circulation, cellulite, respiratory problems and depression.[4] Aromatherapy can play a vital role in treating these conditions, alone or in combination with other modalities.

Kahn's comments are supported by a recent survey of the spa industry that indicates at least 50% of day spa operations offered aromatherapy treatments, 50% offered beauty therapy services and 33% offered hydrotherapy treatments.[5]

Spa Treatments

There are many types of treatments that can be offered in a day spa. Most of these treatments can easily incorporate the benefits of aromatherapy:

- hydrotherapy treatments
- exfoliant treatments
- body pack or masks
- massage treatments
- steam treatments
- facial treatments
- pedicures and manicures.

While the type of services and treatments offered in a day spa are many and varied, they all have one common factor — they provide clients with a unique experience which will improve their sense of wellbeing.

For information of massage treatments and facial treatments refer to the relevant chapters in this book. This chapter will examine the benefits and procedures for performing hydrotherapy treatments, exfoliation treatments, body packs and masks, steam treatments, pedicures and manicures.

Hydrotherapy

The concept of hydrotherapy is not new. It dates back to ancient Greece where hydrotherapy was the true foundation of healing and curing of disease.

Hydrotherapy is defined as the therapeutic use of water on the body at variable temperatures to induce a reaction in the body. Father Sebastian Kneipp, a Bavarian monk of West Germany (1821–1897), is regarded as the 'Father of Hydrotherapy' because he developed numerous water treatments still used today.[6]

Properties of Water

To understand the scope of hydrotherapy we need to first examine the effects of water on the body. Water has several unique properties which contribute to its effectiveness as a therapeutic agent. These include:[7]

- It has the ability to store and transmit heat, which renders it most appropriate for therapeutic purposes.
- It has excellent solvent properties, which makes it very useful in all hydrotherapy procedures. Essential oils, herbs, minerals, seaweeds and clays are added to the water to enhance its therapeutic value.
- Water is non-toxic.
- Water has the ability o change state, within a narrow, easily obtainable temperature range. As ice, it is an effective cooling agent; as a liquid it can be used in a bath, spray, compress and douche. As a vapour, it may be used in a steam bath or inhalation.
- The density of water is near that of the human body. It can therefore be used as an exercise medium for patients with paralysis, inflammations, or atrophy.
- Water is readily available — in most parts of the world.

Physiological Effects of Water

Barry classifies the physiological effects of hydrotherapy as thermal, mechanical and chemical.[7] Salvo also adds the effects of moisture and the mineral content.[6]

The thermal effect of water is produced when water is used at temperatures above or below that of the body. The greater the temperature difference between the body and the water, the greater the effect. The mechanical effects are produced by the impact of water on the surface of the body in the form of sprays, douches, frictions and spas. The chemical effects are produced when water is taken by mouth or used to irrigate a body cavity — as is the case in a colonic.

Moisture refers to the amount of humidity in the air. Steam baths help to moisten the mucous membranes of nasal passages and throat and can help keep the skin supple.[6]

The mineral content of the water also influences the therapeutic effect on the body. Many famous spas are known for the health-giving properties of the mineral waters. Three types of mineral waters have been identified — saline water which contains salts used for its purgative effects, rust-coloured water rich in iron oxide used for its restorative effects and sulphur water used for its cleansing effects.[6]

Additives may be added to duplicate these effects. Sea salt (sodium chloride), Epsom salt (magnesium sulphate) and baking soda (sodium bicarbonate) can be added to help draw out toxins as the body attempts to balance the percentage of saline content between the water and skin.[6]

Effects of Hot Applications

Heat may be applied to the body in hydrotherapy by using hot packs, fomentations, steam, baths or showers. The effects produced by hot applications will depend on the method of application, temperature and duration of the application and the condition of the client.[7]

In general, short-term application of heat has a stimulating effect on the body while prolonged application of heat has a depressing effect on the body. Some of the physiological effects of heat include:

- has an excellent anti-inflammatory and anti-infectious action
- relaxes the body
- increases blood flow
- increases metabolism
- induces perspiration and elimination of toxins
- reduces pain
- relieves stiffness and soreness
- relaxes the muscles
- stimulates the immune system and inhibits the growth of many bacteria and viruses.[6]

Contra-indications of Heat

Avoid heat applications for all of the following conditions:

- acute injury
- autoimmune diseases
- clients with an aversion to heat
- recent burns, including sunburns
- cardiac impairment
- cases of fever
- cerebrovascular accident or stroke
- oedematic conditions
- areas directly over the eyes
- hypertension or hypotension
- immediately after an injury
- inflammation
- area over prosthetic joint
- area of implants
- malignancy or chronic illness
- significant obesity
- open wounds, blisters, or abrasion burns
- phlebitis
- area over a pacemaker
- pregnancy
- rosacea
- skin infections or rashes
- areas directly over a tumour or cyst
- clients who are weak or debilitated.[6]

Effects of Cold Applications

The short application of cold has a stimulating effect on the body, while prolonged application has a depressing effect on the body. The benefits are as follows:

- reduces acute inflammation
- reduces swelling
- reduces muscle spasm
- invigorates and stimulates the body
- contracts the capillaries to assist in the reduction of swelling
- stimulates immunity
- reduces pain
- stimulates the maintenance of skin elasticity
- can help to relieve headaches.[6]

Contra-indications of Cold

Contra-indications for cold application include:

- arthritis
- aversion to cold
- cerebrovascular accident or stroke
- open wounds
- hypertension
- Raynaud's syndrome
- rheumatoid conditions
- sensory impairments
- skin infections or rashes.[6]

General Safety Guidelines for Hydrotherapy Applications

It is important to ensure that the hydrotherapy equipment is maintained in good working order and complies with public and multipurpose use standards.[6]

Ensure that all wet areas are made safe by providing non-slip mats and ensure that water that spills and collects on the floor is wiped up immediately to prevent accidents.[6]

Salvo provides us with the following guidelines for ensuring a safe and effective hydrotherapy treatment:[6]

- Ensure that the wet room is warm.
- If providing full-body treatments, consider asking the client to bring a swimming suit.
- Check and monitor the water temperature.
- Check the client's comfort level.
- Use a timer to limit treatment duration. Do not over-treat.
- Ask the client not to eat at least 1 hour before the appointment.
- Before a treatment, perform a client consultation.
- Review contra-indications.
- Explain the procedures to the client.
- Give clear instructions on where to place clothing and personal belongings, how much clothing to remove, and how to lie on the table.
- Do not wait for the client to become thirsty; offer water or juice before, after and during the treatment.
- After the treatment, allow the client to rest for at least 10 minutes, so that the body temperature can return to normal.

Hydrotherapy Treatments

Hydrotherapy treatments can be used exclusively or as part of an aromatherapy or massage treatment. Hydrotherapy treatments may involve baths, hydrotherapy tubs, Swiss showers, Vichy showers, Scotch hose, saunas or steam baths.

Baths

Baths may consist of full or partial immersions of the body into water at various temperatures. The water may contain additional substances such as salts, minerals, herbs, clays or essential oils.

Some of the commonly used bath treatments available are as follows:

The *neutral bath* which is given at the average temperature of the skin — approximately 33–35°C. The client does not have the sensation of being warm or cool. A minor variation on temperature of as little as 0.5°C may create a totally different therapeutic effect. The primary role of a neutral bath is to create a state of decreased excitation. A secondary effect is the activation of the kidneys, creating increased urinary output. Therapeutically neutral baths are used to treat insomnia, anxiety, nervous irritability, exhaustion or chronic pain.[7]

A *hot immersion bath* consists of a bath in water of 40°C for approximately 20 minutes. Generally recommended for home treatments for poor circulation, muscular stiffness and inducing perspiration. It should be followed by a cold shower. Prolonged hot tub baths are not recommended for very old or very young, weak or anaemic persons, individuals with vascular disorders or high blood pressure.[7]

The Hydrotherapy Tub

In a day spa, hydrotherapy baths play an integral role in healing and wellbeing. Generally the hydrotherapy tub has hydro jets (emits water), air jets (emits air) and a hand jet which can be used by the therapist to perform a manual massage. The jets are strategically positioned to stimulate lymphatic activity.[9]

The hydrotherapy tub can be controlled manually or it may be fully computerised with pre-set programs. Hydrotherapy tubs are designed and built for commercial use, therefore mud, seaweed and herbal additives will not clog them. They also have 'self-disinfecting' systems that ensure the health and safety of the client. Hydrotherapy tubs are considered quite expensive and require a wet room.[8]

Bath Treatments

There are three types of bath treatments available:

- plain water baths — no additives
- thalossotherapy baths — additives are seaweed or sea salts
- aromatherapy or herbal baths — additives are essential oils or herbs
- mud baths — additives are a range of clays.[8]

Seaweed baths are used to increase metabolism and blood circulation, increase the elimination of toxins and revitalise the skin.[1]

Many of the essential oils which we have discussed in this book can be used in a bath. Ensure that you use a dispersant before adding the essential oils into the bath. Do not exceed the recommended dosages that have been outlined in this book.

Showers

A shower is considered a must for a day spa. The shower is used to ensure that the client is clean and it can be used to prepare the client for treatment by warming and relaxing muscles and tension.

It is necessary to use a shower to rinse off products that have been applied during a treatment such as mud, seaweed and exfoliants.

Swiss Shower

A Swiss shower is form of water massage from a number of jets or shower heads which spray water at strategically targeted areas to a standing client to stimulate the circulation and metabolism.[8]

It is commonly used before and/or after a herbal body wrap, skin exfoliation or massage. It is recommended for the relief of tension, insomnia and stress.[9]

Vichy Shower

Vichy showers are a row of suspended shower heads, and are ideally used with wet tables. The wet room needs to be tiled to at least half way up the walls as water is splashed about with a Vichy shower.[8]

The client lies beneath the shower bar on a wet spa table (a waterproof table with a self-draining trough around its edges). The shower is turned on (not over the client as the bar will be holding cold water!) and, when the water is warm, it is directed over the client to provide a relaxing warm cascade of water.[8]

The shower heads are adjustable to provide varying pressure (light for a sedating effect and strong for a tonic effect) and are targeted to various parts of the body. They may be positioned on the chakras or over parts of the body which are in pain, onto cellulite areas or even for a soothing 'rain massage'.[8]

Vichy shower is a form of hydromassage. It is recommended for chronic fatigue, mild hypertension, lymphatic congestion and skin exfoliation.[9]

Scotch Hose

The concept of the Scotch hose is to target a strong stream of water to specific areas of the body to increase circulation and elimination. The client normally stands next to the wall holding onto handles attached to the wall while the therapist shoots water from a device similar to a fire hose from a distance of 3 metres away.[8]

The Scotch hose is indicated for arthritis in the non-inflammatory stage, chronic lumbago, muscular tension, irregular menstruation cycle and mild circulatory problems.[9]

Sauna

A sauna bath utilises hot air with temperatures ranging from 76–99°C with 10–20% humidity.[6]

Clients using saunas must be in good health and if they feel weak or dizzy, the treatment must be discontinued immediately. Saunas are often used before a body wrap, massage or other hydrotherapy treatment.[6] Salvo recommends a sauna is for general tension and insomnia, but it also increases metabolism and circulation and aids in the elimination of toxins.[6]

Because of the minerals lost during perspiration it is important that clients remain hydrated before, during and after the treatment.[6]

Steam Bath

A steam bath utilises hot vapours in a confined area to maintain temperatures between 40° and 49°C with 100% humidity. A steam bath can be used to decrease stress and assist in the removal of toxins from the body.[6]

Steam baths are often used before a body wrap, massage, or other hydrotherapy treatments. It is possible to add essential oils to the water to enhance the desired therapeutic effect.[6]

A steam canopy that fits over a wet table is an inexpensive method of offering clients the benefits of a steam bath. A steam cabinet that allows the head to be exposed is called a Russian bath.[6]

Exfoliation Treatments

Exfoliation is the process that removes dead skin cells, rancid oils, dirt and debris from the skin. This makes the skin more vibrant and allows the skin to readily accept moisturisers, nutrients and other treatments to improve the skin texture.[1]

Exfoliation is considered the first and most important treatment to be performed in a body care treatment. There are two types of exfoliants — mechanical exfoliants and enzymatic or dissolving exfoliants.[1]

Dry Brush Massage

Dry skin brushing is very stimulating to the skin. It involves using a dry natural bristle brush, a loofah sponge or mitt, or an abrasive cloth to friction massage the skin. The brushing should always be short, brisk strokes towards the heart.[6]

Dry skin brushing should be done before a body wrap or a product mask to gently exfoliate the skin and stimulate superficial glands so that the treatments work better.[6]

Body Scrub

A body scrub utilises a coarse, gritty substance to exfoliate the skin. A body scrub cleanses the skin and removes cellular debris. A wide range of scrubbing agents are available that range from gentle to abrasive. Therefore, care must be taken in choosing the most appropriate scrubbing agent. Natural scrubs include salt, ground up nuts, oatmeal or various grains. If the client complains of a burning sensation during the application, the treatment should be discontinued.[6]

Salt Glow

A salt glow involves the application of a wet salt on the skin. The salt glow is prepared by blending Epsom salt or a sea salt with a vegetable oil or liquid soap. Essential oils can also be added to a salt glow.

The purpose of salt glows is to exfoliate the skin, increase circulation to the skin and render the skin soft and supple. This invigorating treatment leaves one refreshed and centred.[6]

A salt scrub should not be done on someone with skin rashes, cuts, abrasions or someone who has just shaved. A brisk back and forth friction is used to apply the salt, while circular frictions are recommended around the joints.[6]

Kahn recommends finishing a salt glow with gentle herbal steam to assist the body in further eliminating toxins from the skin; followed by a rub down using a cloth soaked in a liniment of eucalyptus, peppermint and wintergreen.[4]

Body Packs or Mask Treatments

A body pack or mask is generally used to enhance the skin's health and appearance. Products include oil, creams, lotions, clays, herbs or seaweed.

The amount of product applied to the skin depends on the product being used and the size of the client. Heat may be used to enhance the effectiveness of the mask being used, which may add nutrients into the skin or draw out toxins from the skin. Body packs and masks are applied topically.

The procedure for applying a pack or mask is as follows:

- Before applying the mask, ensure the skin has been cleaned.
- Apply the mask according to the supplier's recommendations.
- Leave on the skin for the recommended time frame.
- Apply moisturiser to hydrate the skin.
- Remove the mask with hot towels or in a shower.

Clay

Clay has been an important part of the spa menu for hundreds of years. Clays combine extremely well with aromatherapy for body packs and may be used to soothe aches and pain, smooth the skin and aid in the elimination of toxins and the treatment of cellulite.

The properties of the clay are determined by its mineral content. Some of the commonly used clays include:

Kaolin: A fine-grained white clay used in masks for cleansing, tightening and toning the skin.[1]

Illite/Chlorite: These clays come from soils that are predominantly made of marine sediments. Illite is made when potassium is added to kaolin and chlorite is formed when magnesium is added.[1]

Smectites: These clays are predominantly found in volcanic ash. Bentonite is primarily composed of smectite clay and is commonly used in skin care. There are two kinds of bentonites — sodium bentonite and calcium bentonite. Sodium absorbs water and swells, whereas calcium bentonite (popularly known as Fuller's earth) is a non-swelling clay that is used as an absorbent clay.[1]

Clays are commonly referred to by colour, rather than by name. The colours that are commonly used are green red, yellow and white. White clay is usually kaolin and is typically used for masks.[1]

Green clay appears to be the most active, is usually a smectite/chlorite or illite combination and is used in masks for oily and congested skins.[1]

Red clays are also a smectite combination and are principally used for dry, sensitive, mature and tired skin. Yellow clay has similar characteristics to red clay.[1]

General Advice When Using Clays

- Do not mix or store clays in metal containers. It will draw out the minerals.
- It is best to heat the clay indirectly in a double boiler or inside a heating unit with water. Heat once and use. Do not reheat.
- A shower or Vichy shower is ideal for rinsing clay.

Seaweed

Seaweed is high in vitamins and minerals. The mineral salts are said to act on cell vitality and help re-energise the body, moisturise and soften the skin and the iodine in the seaweed helps to activate metabolism.[1]

Seaweed masks may be used to treat cellulite. Seaweed helps to disrupt the fat cells by breaking the chemical bonds and allows trapped waste materials to be released into the lymph for elimination.[1]

As there are so many different types of seaweed used in spas, it is important to obtain specific details and treatment procedures from your product supplier.

Other Treatments

Aromatherapy Pedicure and Manicure

Pedicures should be given in a comfortable chair. Essential oils that invigorate and stimulate circulation should be used. Essential oils such as peppermint, cypress, lemon and calendula-infused oil should be added to a lotion and massaged onto the calves and feet. A reflexology treatment may also be performed and selected oils may be used.[11]

Nails are soaked in soapy water with geranium and tea tree, used for their antiseptic and antifungal properties. Seaweeds for remineralising skin and nails may also added to the water.

Kahn recommends a blend of myrrh, frankincense, vitamin E oil and sweet almond oil should be massaged into the hands and nails. Cuticles may be conditioned with lavender essential oil in a sweet almond oil base.[10]

Scalp Treatment

Scalp treatments are designed to clean, condition and soften the scalp. Most scalp treatments involve massage with essential oils and a carrier oil.

Essential oils of rosemary, peppermint and lavender in a blend of jojoba, vitamin E and apricot kernel oil can be massaged onto the scalp and hair. A warm towel may be wrapped around the head to aid penetration.[10]

A cleansing or conditioning mask with clays or seaweed can also be applied. After the mask has been applied, the scalp may be steamed with a facial steamer, hot towels or a steam dryer.[1]

The hair is then washed with an aromatherapy shampoo that contains essential oils such as lavender or rosemary.[10]

Converting an Established Clinic to a Day Spa

The decision to expand or convert an existing salon into a day spa is a major one. Daley says that a day spa technically needs to have water-based treatments for this title to be accurately adopted.[3] However, adding a wet room can be a very costly exercise. Daley suggests that a wet room facility should increase the business by a minimum of 25% to be viable — it should not simply alter the current business mix.[3]

Before investing in a wet room you should first try dry treatments (spa treatments that can be washed away with steam towels).

If you do not have the finances to invest in a wet room, you can still provide a 'spa experience', by changing the environment of the clinic and the service you offer. Things to consider include the lighting of your clinic, the location of the reception, the waiting area and the retail selection. Withers asks:[11]

- Are they appealing, comfortable and positioned for maximum comfort and ease of use?
- Do your staff all follow a set of procedures and protocols so that the same high standard is repeated every time?
- Is your linen immaculate?
- What are your bathroom facilities like?

Even the little touches such as lighting, colours, music, aromas, carefully selected images, the choice of refreshments and how they are served, vocal tones and well placed clothes hangers all contribute to making your clients' experience one that they will be eager to return to.

When designing a day spa, Tulloh recommends dividing the spa into five categories:[12]

Dry room: for beauty therapy and massage therapy treatments.

Wet room: Vichy showers, Scotch shower, hydrotherapy bath or therapeutic spa bath, steam room.

Water experience zones: swimming pools, plunge and spa pools, baths, showers, sauna.

Common space: reception, waiting room and consultation rooms, relaxation areas, hanging rooms.

Services: plant room, storage, staff area.

Obviously the configuration of these different areas is dependent on the location, size, client base, range of treatments and services and, most importantly, the budget.

References

1. Millar E. *Day spa techniques*. Milady SalonOvations, USA, 1996.
2. Cook C. *Day Spa Developments*. Professional Beauty Magazine. Jan/Feb 1998.
3. Daley J. *Spa-Gazing in Australia*. Day Spa Magazine January 1999: 10–12.
4. Kahn L. *Holistic aromatherapy within the spa/ wellness center,* The World of Aromatherapy III Conference Proceedings, USA, 2000: 88–91.
5. Garrow J. *Asia Pacific Spa Industry Trends*. Spa Australasia, 2002; 6: 14–16.
6. Salvo S. *Massage therapy: Principles and Practice.* Elsevier Science, USA, 2003.
7. Barry R. *Hydrotherapy*. From Textbook of Natural Medicine. Vol. 1, edited by Pizzorno J, Murray M. Churchill Livingstone, UK, 1999.
8. Scior L. *Redefining H_20: Exploring the options for hydrotherapy in the Salon and Spa*. Day Spa Magazine Feb 1999: 46–49.
9. Leavy H, Bergel R. *The spa encyclopedia*: A guide to treatments and their benefits for health and healing. Thomson Learning, USA, 2003.
10. Kahn L. *Aesthetic Aromatherapy and Oriental Face Diagnosis*. AROMA'95 Conference Proceedings, Aromatherapy Publications, England. 1995.
11. Withers K. *The Spa Attraction — Raising standards in salon.* Professional Beauty Magazine Nov/Dec 99.
12. Tulloh G. *Spa architecture — The second wave*. Spa Australasia, 2002; 6: 64–70.

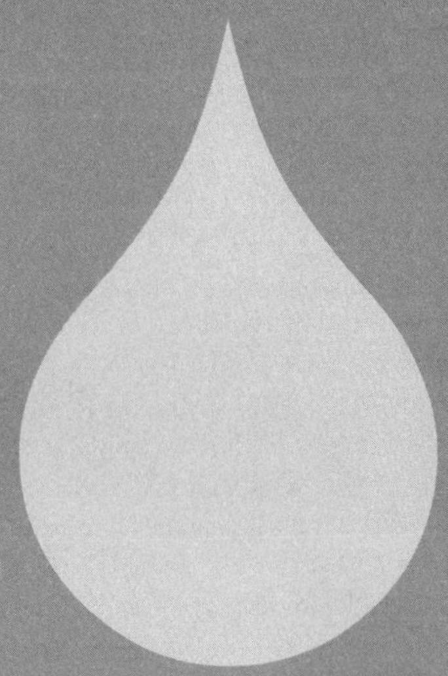

Appendices

This section includes the following appendices:

Appendix 1 ♦ **Glossary**
Appendix 2 ♦ **List of Properties**
Appendix 3 ♦ **Therapeutic Cross Reference**
Appendix 4 ♦ **List of Essential Oils**
Appendix 5 ♦ **A Typical Material Safety Data Sheet**
Appendix 6 ♦ **Summary of Cautions and Contraindications**
Appendix 7 ♦ **Accupressure**
Appendix 8 ♦ **Useful Addresses**

Appendix 1 ♦ Glossary

Absolute
Products obtained from a concrète, a pomade or a resinoid by extraction with ethanol at room temperature. The resulting ethanol solution is generally cooled and filtered to eliminate the waxes. The ethanol is then eliminated by distillation.

Adulteration
Any material added to a whole, genuine essential oil which alters its original composition or odour.

Aetiology
Study of the cause of a disease or the theory of its origin.

Albedo
The pith, or inner rind of a citrus fruit.

Alcohol
An organic compound containing one or more hydroxyl groups attached directly to carbon atoms.

Aldehyde
An organic compound containing a carbonyl group of atoms and a hydrogen atom bonded to the carbon atom of the carbonyl group.

Alkanes
A saturated hydrocarbon found in natural gas and petroleum and having the general formula $C_n H_{2n+2}$.

Alkenes
An unsaturated hydrocarbon, of which the molecules contain one or more double covalent bonds. Terpenes are alkenes with the general formula $(C_5H_8)_2$. These are important constituents of essential oils.

Alkynes
An unsaturated hydrocarbon, of which the molecules contain one or more triple covalent bonds. Alkynes and their derivatives are uncommon as constituents of essential oils.

Allelopathy
The adverse effect which one plant has on another, caused by the exudation of chemicals into the soil which suppress the growth of nearby plants.

Allergen
A substance which causes an allergic reaction.

Allergy
Tendency to react unfavourably to a certain substance that is normally harmless to most people.

Anaerobic
A type of organic respiration which does not require oxygen. Many bacteria are anaerobic.

Androgen
Masculine sex hormone produced by the testes in males and in the adrenal cortex of both sexes.

Androstenone
See Androgen.

Anosmic
Complete loss of sense of smell. May be temporary or permanent.

Antibody
Substance produced in response to a specific antigen.

Aromacology
The study of the psychological effects of odours, particularly those of essential oils used in aromatherapy.

Aromatic chemicals
Any chemical with an aroma or flavour, which is usually synthetic.

Aromatic water
Aqueous distillates, remaining from water or steam distillation after the essential oil has been separated.

Arrhythmia
Irregular or loss of rhythm of the heartbeat.

Artefact
A compound produced during distillation and other processes, or storage of an essential oil.

Arteriosclerosis
A loss of elasticity of the arteries.

Atherosclerosis
An accumulation of fatty deposits on the inner walls of the arteries.

Atom
The smallest particle of an element which can take part in a chemical change.

Atomic number
The number of protons in the nucleus of an atom, which is equal to the number of electrons that the atom contains.

ATP
Adenosine triphosphate — an energy-storing compound found in all cells.

Autoimmunity
Abnormal reactivity to one's own tissues.

Basal ganglia
Grey masses in the lower part of the forebrain that aid in muscle coordination.

Benzene ring
The molecular structure of the cyclic, unsaturated, aromatic hydrocarbon benzene C_6H_6.

Blood-brain barrier
A barrier consisting of specialised brain capillaries that prevent the passage of substances from the blood to the brain.

Bursa
Small, fluid-filled sac found in an area subject to stress around bones and joints.

Carbonyl group
The divalent group of atoms consisting of a carbon atom joined to an oxygen atom by a double bond.

Carboxylic acid
Organic compounds containing one or more carboxyl groups.

Carcinogen
A chemical substance or radiation that causes cancer.

Carcinogenesis
Refers to the inception or production and growth of cancer.

Carrier oil
A fixed oil of vegetable origin.

Cerebellum
Small section of the brain located under the cerebral hemispheres; functions in coordination, balance and muscle tone.

Cerebrum
Largest part of the brain; composed of the cerebral hemispheres.

Chassis
The arrangement of glass plates and the surrounding wooden frame used in the enfleurage process.

Chemotype
Variation in the chemical composition of an essential oil produced from two or more plants of the same species.

Chi
A term used in Traditional Chinese Medicine and holistic therapies, referring to the life force.

Chronic
Referring to a disease that develops slowly, persists over a long time, or is recurring.

Clonic
A word applied to short spasmodic movements.

Cohobation
A process of redistillation of the distillation water in order to recover dissolved essential oil.

Colonoscopy
Examination of the upper portion of the rectum with an elongated speculum.

Concrète
Extracts obtained with non-aqueous solvents from fresh, natural raw materials. A concrète consists mainly of waxy components of plant materials. Mainly prepared for the production of absolutes.

Coppiced
The regrowth of a tree in the form of thin stems after felling to leave a stump.

Coronary
Referring to the heart or the arteries supplying blood to the heart.

Corpus callosum
Thick bundle of myelinated nerve cell fibres, deep within the brain, that carries nerve impulses from one cerebral hemisphere to another.

Covalent bond
A bond between two atoms consisting of a shared pair of electrons.

Cultivar
A plant variety produced from a naturally occurring species that has been developed and maintained by cultivation.

Cutaneous
Means belonging to the skin.

Defecation
Act of eliminating undigested waste from the digestive tract.

Dermatology
The study of the histology, physiology and pathology of the skin and the treatment of skin diseases.

Diastole
Relaxation phase of the cardiac cycle.

Diencephalon
Region of the brain between the cerebral hemispheres and the midbrain; contains the thalamus, hypothalamus and the pituitary gland.

Digestion
Process of breaking down food into absorbable particles.

Distillation
The process of vaporising a substance in a distillation vessel and collecting the product by cooling the vapour in a separate vessel.

EEG
Electroencephalograph — Instrument used to study electrical activity of the brain.

Efferent
Carrying away from a given point, such as a motor neuron that carries nerve impulses away from the central nervous system.

Electron
A negatively charged particle, of a mass approximately 1/2000 of that of a proton.

Element
A substance composed of atoms. The nuclei of all the atoms contain the same number of protons.

Endometrium
Lining of the uterus.

Enfleurage
The process of extracting essential oil from flowers. The flowers are placed on trays of fat which absorbs the oil. The oil is then solvent extracted.

Essential oil
A product obtained from natural distillation or expression.

Esters
Organic compound formed by the union of an acid and an alcohol with the elimination of water.

Ether
An organic compound which is characterised by the presence of an oxygen atom bonded to two hydrocarbon chains, ring systems or other hydrocarbon molecular structures.

Evaporation
The change of a liquid or solid to a gas or vapour phase.

Expression
A mechanical method using compression and pressure for extracting essential oils from the rinds of citrus fruits.

Fixative
A material that is capable of prolonging the effects of the main fragrance theme of a perfume.

Fixed oil
Non-volatile, fatty, generally vegetable oil.

Flash point
The temperature, under standardised conditions, at which a liquid begins to evolve flammable vapours.

Flavedo
The coloured part of the rind of a citrus fruit.

Floral water
Also known as hydrosol. The water collected when plants are distilled to extract essential oils.

Fractional distillation
A distillation process in which portions of the distillate have different boiling points, or ranges of boiling points, and are collected in separate receivers.

Functional group
The smallest part of an organic molecule consisting of a single atom or group of atoms that substitutes for a hydrogen atom and has a profound effect upon the properties of the molecule as a whole.

Furanocoumarins
Derivatives of coumarins.

Gas liquid chromatography (GLC)
An analytical technique for separating the constituents of a minute sample of a mixture of volatiles and recording the results of the analysis. The results of the analysis are recorded as a series of peaks, each one corresponding with respect to its position, to a constituent of the sample.

GLA
Gamma linoleic acid — an essential fatty acid that the body requires in the diet for the manufacture of important bodily chemicals such as hormones.

GLC
See Gas liquid chromatography.

GMP
Good Manufacturing Practice.

Haemorrhage
Loss of blood.

Headspace
The space bounded by the walls of a container, the closure and the surface of its contents.

Headspace analysis
Analysis done by GLC, of the gas or vapour present in a headspace.

Heartwood
The internal, non-living art of a woody stem, branch or trunk.

Hepatotoxicity
Having a harmful or toxic effect on the liver.

Homeostasis
State of balance within the body; maintenance of body conditions within set limits.

Hormone
Secretion of an endocrine gland; chemical messenger that has specific regulatory effects on certain other cells.

Hydrocarbon
A compound composed of molecules consisting of atoms of carbon and hydrogen only.

Hydrolysis
The decomposition of a compound by water.

Hydrosol
Also known as floral water. The water that is recovered from the distillation process.

Hydroxyl group
The functional group -OH, present in water molecules and molecules of alcohols, and distinguished from the hydroxide ion by its electronic configuration and lack of negative charge.

Hypersensitivity
Exaggerated reaction of the immune system to a substance that is normally harmless to most people; allergy.

Hypothalamus
Region of the brain that controls the pituitary and maintains homeostasis.

Humectant
A substance attracting or retaining moisture.

IFRA
International Fragrance Research Association. A voluntary body based in Switzerland which advises the perfume industry on the safety of fragrance ingredients.

Immunity
Power of an individual to resist or overcome the effects of a particular disease or other harmful agent.

Inflammation
The production of redness, swelling, heat and pain in a tissue in response to chemical or physical injury, or an infection.

Infra-red spectroscopy
A spectroscopic instrumental technique measuring the absorption of infra-red radiation over a range of frequencies by molecules of a substance.

Infused oil
Produced by the immersion of plant material in a vegetable oil, often gently heated to release aromatic constituents from the plant into the oil.

ISO
The International Organization for Standardization.

Isomers
Compounds that have the same molecular formula but different structures and hence different properties.

Isoprene
The basic building unit of a group of chemicals called terpenes (2-methylbuta-1,3-diene), molecular formula C_5H_8.

Ketone
An organic compound characterised by the presence in its molecules of a carbonyl functional group bonded to two hydrocarbon radicals.

Lactone
An organic compound characterised by the presence in its molecules

of an ester functional group as part of a ring system.

LD_{50}

Lethal dose 50%. It is a traditionally accepted method of determining toxicity. The value is the dosage required to kill 50% of the group of animals used in the test (usually rats or mice). LD_{50} values are usually expressed in grams of the toxic substance per kilogram of body weight.

Lichenification

Cutaneous thickening and hardening from continued irritation.

Ligament

Band of connective tissue that connects a bone to another bone.

Limbic system

A part of the forebrain, concerned with various aspects of emotion and behaviour.

Lipophilic

Having an affinity for lipids.

Lymph node

Mass of lymphoid tissue along the path of a lymphatic vessel that filters lymph and harbours white blood cells active in immunity.

Maceration

The process of allowing a definite weight of extractable matter to soak, in a closed vessel for several days, in a definite weight of alcohol of given strength to produce a tincture.

Macrophage

Larger phagocytic cell that develops from a monocyte.

Menarche

Onset of menses.

Menopause

Time at which menstruation ceases.

Menses

Monthly flow of blood from the female reproductive system.

Molecular formula

The formula expressing the true number of atoms of the different elements present in a molecule of a compound.

Monoterpene

A terpene of molecular formula $C_{10}H_{16}$.

Myelin

A fatty material enveloping the majority of nerve cells.

Narcotic

Substance that induces stupor and eventually unconsciousness. Can be used in the relief of severe pain.

Nature identical

Designates a synthetic organic compound of the same composition and molecular structure of the same compound as it occurs in nature.

Neurotoxic

Having a harmful or toxic effect on the nervous system.

Neurotransmitter

Chemical released from the ending of an axon that enables a nerve impulse to cross a synapse.

Neutron

An electrically charged neutral article of unit mass present in the nuclei of the atoms of all elements other than hydrogen of unit atomic mass. The effect of the presence of neutrons in an atomic nucleus containing more than one proton is to bind the protons together.

Nucleus

In chemistry it refers to the positively charged central body of an atom. In biology it is the dense, organised proteinaceous body found in the protoplasm of a plant or animal cell, containing hereditary material and controlling the metabolic activities of the cell.

Occlusions

The covering of the skin with an impermeable material which prevents evaporation of a volatile substance from the skin.

Odorant

A substance having an odour.

Odour

There is no accurate description of this term. It defines what an individual perceives via the nose as the scent of any material.

Odour threshold

The least concentration, or highest dilution, at which the odour of an odorant can be detected under standardised conditions.

Oestrogen

Female sex hormone produced by the ovaries.

Olfactory

Pertaining to the sense of smell.

Olfactory tract

A bundle of axons that extend from the olfactory bulb to the olfactory regions of the cerebral cortex.

Optical isomer

See Isomers.

Optical rotation

Angle through which the plane of polarisation of light is rotated when polarised light passes through a layer of liquid. Unless otherwise specified, the measurement is by sodium light in a 1 mm layer at 20°C. Essential oils may be dextrorotatory (+) or laevorotatory (-) according to whether the plane of polarisation is rotated to the left or right.

Organic chemistry

The study of the chemical behaviour of compounds of carbon, other than carbon-containing ionic compounds such as carbonates and similar molecular compounds such as carbon dioxide.

Oxidation

The addition of oxygen to, or the removal of electrons or hydrogen from, an organic molecule.

Oxide

A compound of oxygen with another element. The most commonly occurring oxide in essential oils is 1,8-cineole.

Oxygenated constituent

A constituent of an essential oil or aromatic extract containing combined oxygen.

Pathogenic

Disease producing.

Percutaneous

By diffusion through the skin.

Periodic table
An arrangement of the chemical elements in the order of their atomic numbers showing the regular recurrence of many of their properties.

Peristalsis
Wavelike movements in the walls of an organ or duct that propel its contents forward.

pH
A measure of the acidity or alkalinity of an aqueous solution, expressed as a numerical value on a scale from 0 (extremely acidic) to 14.0 (extremely alkaline). A pH value of 7.0 expresses neutrality.

Pharmacokinetics
The way in which the body deals with a pharmacologically active substance. This includes the absorption, distribution, metabolism and excretion of the drug.

Phenols
The organic benzenoid compound C_6H_5OH or any other compound of which the molecules each have one or more hydroxy groups bonded directly to a benzene ring.

Phenyl propane derivatives
The name given to compounds of phenol that have a three-carbon-atom chain attached.

Pheromone
A chemical messenger used as a signal between individuals.

Photosynthesis
The manufacture of the sugar glucose in the leaves of a green plant from carbon dioxide and water in the presence of chlorophyll, using sunlight as a source of energy and with the evolution of oxygen.

Phototoxicity
An excessive reaction to sunlight or UV light, caused by chemicals such as furanocoumarins when applied to the skin.

Pineal
Gland in the brain that is regulated by light; involved in sleep-wake cycles.

Pituitary
Endocrine gland located under and controlled by the hypothalamus; releases hormones that control other glands.

Placebo
An inactive substance administered to a patient, usually to compare the effects with that of the real drug.

Placebo effect
The positive therapeutic effect claimed by the patient after receiving a placebo believed to be an active drug.

Polar
A term used to describe a molecule which has a partial positive and negative charge. Polar molecules are generally water-soluble.

Polarised light
Light with a specific plane of polarisation.

Polarimeter
An instrument for measuring optical rotation.

Pomade
Perfumed fat obtained as a result of enfleurage.

Progesterone
Hormone produced by the corpus luteum and placenta, maintains the lining of the uterus for pregnancy.

Prostaglandins
Group of hormones.

Proton
A positively charged particle of unit atomic mass, which occurs in the nuclei of all atoms.

Qi
See Chi.

Rectification
The process in which an essential oil is distilled a second time to remove unwanted constituents (also known as redistillation).

Refractive index
The ratio of the sine wave of the angle of incidence to the sine of the angle of refraction, when a ray of light of defined wavelength passes from a less dense to a more dense medium.

Refractometer
An instrument for measuring the refractive index.

Resinoid
An extract obtained from dried, natural, raw materials by use of non-aqueous solvents.

RIFM
Research Institute for Fragrance Materials. A voluntary organisation, based in the USA, for testing the safety of perfume ingredients.

Scarification
A process of scraping as used in the expression of citrus oils from the peel of the fruit.

Sebaceous gland
An exocrine gland in the dermis of the skin, associated with a hair follicle, that secretes sebum.

Sebum
Oil secretion that lubricates and protects the skin.

Sesquiterpene
A terpene with the molecular formula $C_{15}H_{24}$. These constituents are based on 3 terpene units.

Specific gravity
The ratio of the weight of a substance to the weight of an equal volume of water measured at a stated temperature.

Solvent
Hexane, petroleum ether, acetone or methanol are often used to extract essential oils from plant materials or their extracts.

Solvent extraction
Extraction by solvents.

Still
Any form of distillation equipment.

Still note
An unpleasant, vegetable-like note commonly found in freshly distilled essential oils, caused by the presence of organic sulphides. Still notes can be eliminated by brief aeration of the essential oils.

Structural isomer
See isomer.

Surfactant
A surface active agent such as soap or a detergent.

Synergy
The increased effect achieved by two or more substances working together. The effect of the whole is greater than the sum of its separate arts.

Systole
In the cardiac cycle, the phase of contraction of the heart muscle, especially of the ventricles.

T Cells
Lymphocyte activity in immunity that matures in the thymus gland; destroys foreign cells directly.

Tendon
Cord of fibrous connective tissue that attaches a muscle to a bone.

Teratogenic effect
Leading to the production of foetal abnormalities.

Terpeneless oil
Essential oils from which the monoterpene hydrocarbons have been removed.

Terpenes
Naturally occurring unsaturated hydrocarbon compounds.
They constitute a large number of compounds present in plants and essential oils.

Terpenoid
Essential oil constituents based on the isoprene skeleton, but containing a functional group.

Thalamus
Region of the brain located in the diencephalon; chief relay centre for the sensory impulses travelling to the cerebral cortex.

Thymus gland
Endocrine gland in the upper portion of the chest; stimulates the development of T cells.

Tincture
Solutions obtained by maceration of natural raw materials in ethanol. Such products are commonly used in herbal medicine.

Vaccine
Substance used to produce active immunity.

Volatile
A volatile substance is one capable of readily changing from a solid or liquid to a vapour or gas

Appendix 2 ♦ List of Properties

Abortifacient
An agent capable of inducing abortion.

Alterative
An agent which cleanses the blood and corrects impure blood conditions.

Analgesic
An agent that relieves or diminishes pain.

Anaphrodisiac
An agent that reduces sexual desire.

Anthelmintic
An agent that destroys or expels intestinal worms.

Antisudorific
An agent that reduces sweating.

Anti-allergenic
An agent that reduces the symptoms of allergies.

Anti-arthritic
An agent that combats arthritis.

Anticatarrhal
An agent that reduces the production of mucus.

Anticonvulsive
An agent that arrests or controls convulsions.

Anti-emetic
An agent that reduces the incidence and severity of vomiting.

Anti-inflammatory
An agent that alleviates inflammation.

Antidepressant
An agent that is uplifting and counteracts melancholy.

Antimicrobial
An agent that resists or destroys pathogens.

Antiphlogistic
An agent that reduces inflammation.

Antipruritic
An agent that relieves sensations of itching or prevents its occurrence.

Antirheumatic
An agent that helps to relieve rheumatism.

Antiseborrheic
An agent that prevents excessive secretion of sebum by the sebaceous glands.

Antiseptic
An agent that destroys or controls pathogenic bacteria.

Antispasmodic
An agent that prevents and eases spasms and relieves cramps.

Antitussive
An agent that relieves coughing.

Aphrodisiac
An agent that provokes sexual interest and excitement.

Astringent
An agent that contracts, tightens and binds tissues.

Bactericide
An agent that destroys bacteria.

Balsamic
Usually applies to a resin — which is a soothing and healing agent.

Cardiac
An agent having a stimulating effect on the heart.

Calmative
An agent that produces a sedative or tranquillising effect.

Carminative
An agent that settles the digestive system and the expulsion of gas from the intestines.

Cephalic
An agent that is stimulating and clears the mind.

Cholagogue
An agent that increases the secretion and flow of bile production into the duodenum.

Choleretic
An agent that aids the excretion of bile by the liver, so that there is a greater flow of bile.

Cicatrisant
An agent that promotes the formation of scar tissue.

Convulsant
An agent that causes convulsions.

Cordial
An agent that is invigorating and stimulating.

Cytophylactic
An agent that encourages growth of skin cells.

Decongestant
An agent that relieves or reduces congestion.

Demulcent
An agent that soothes, softens and allays irritation of mucous membranes.

Deodorant
An agent that destroys or inhibits odours.

Depurative
An agent that helps to purify the body, particularly the blood.

Diaphoretic
An agent that promotes perspiration.

Digestive
An agent that aids the digestion of food.

Disinfectant
Prevents and combats the spread of disease.

Diuretic
An agent that increases the secretion and expulsion of urine.

Emetic
An agent that induces vomiting.

Emmenagogue
An agent that promotes and regulates menstrual flow.

Emollient
An agent used externally to soothe and soften the skin.

Expectorant
An agent that expels mucus in the respiratory system.

Febrifuge
An agent that cools and reduces high body temperature.

Fungicide
An agent that destroys fungal infections.

Galactagogue
An agent that increases the secretion of milk.

Germicidal
An agent that destroys germs or micro-organisms.

Haemostatic
An agent that arrests bleeding.

Hepatic
An agent that stimulates and aids liver function.

Hypertensive
An agent that increases blood pressure.

Hypoglycaemiant
An agent that lowers blood sugar levels.

Hypnotic
An agent that produces sleep.

Hypotensive
An agent that lowers blood pressure.

Insecticide
An agent that kills insects.

Laxative
An agent that aids bowel evacuation.

Mucolytic
An agent that dissolves or breaks down mucus.

Nervine
An agent that strengthens or tonifies the nerves and nervous system.

Oestrogenic
An agent that stimulates the action of oestrogen.

Parturient
An agent that helps in the delivery in childbirth.

Prophylactic
An agent that prevents disease.

Refrigerant
An agent that lowers abnormal body heat.

Relaxant
An agent that causes relaxation of the mind and/or the body.

Rubefacient
An agent that is warming and increases blood flow.

Sedative
An agent that reduces nervousness, distress or agitation.

Soporific
An agent that induces sleep.

Spasmolytic
See antispasmodic.

Splenetic
An agent that is a tonic to the spleen.

Stimulant
An agent that stimulates the physiological functions of the body.

Stomachic
An agent that is a digestive aid and tones the stomach.

Styptic
An agent that is astringent, especially preventing external bleeding.

Sudorific
An agent that promotes or increases perspiration.

Tonic
An agent that strengthens and improves bodily performance.

Uterine
An agent that is a tonic to the uterus.

Vasoconstrictor
An agent that causes contraction of blood vessel walls.

Vasodilator
An agent that causes dilation of blood vessels.

Vermifuge
An agent that causes expulsion of worms.

Vulnerary
An agent that prevents tissue degeneration and promotes healing of wounds.

Appendix 3 ♦ Therapeutic Cross-reference

Cardiovascular System

Broken capillaries

German chamomile, cypress, geranium, rose otto.

Chilblains

Black pepper, cinnamon bark or leaf, clove bud, ginger, lavender, lemon, sweet marjoram, nutmeg, rosemary, red thyme.

Circulation, poor

Black pepper, cinnamon bark or leaf, clove bud, eucalyptus, ginger, lemon, sweet marjoram, nutmeg, pine, rosemary, red thyme.

Hypertension

Bergamot, Roman chamomile, lavender, may chang, melissa, sweet marjoram, neroli, melissa, ylang ylang.

Hypotension

Ginger, lemon, red thyme, rosemary.

Oedema

Carrot seed, cypress, sweet fennel, grapefruit, geranium, juniper berry, lemon, cold-pressed lime, mandarin, sweet orange, tangerine, sage.

Palpitations

Lavender, may chang, melissa, neroli, rose otto, ylang ylang.

Varicose veins

Lemon, cypress, calendula-infused oil, geranium, wheatgerm cold pressed oil.

Digestive System

Constipation

Black pepper, carrot seed, cinnamon bark, sweet fennel, sweet marjoram, peppermint, pine, sweet orange, rosemary.

Diarrhoea

Black pepper, cajeput, carrot seed, German and Roman chamomile, cinnamon bark, cypress, eucalyptus, sweet fennel, ginger, mandarin, neroli, peppermint.

Dyspepsia

Aniseed, black pepper, cardamom, German and Roman chamomile, cinnamon bark and leaf, sweet fennel, ginger, mandarin, sweet marjoram, neroli, nutmeg, sweet orange, peppermint, rosemary, spearmint.

Eating disorders

Bergamot, Roman chamomile, clary sage, neroli, rose otto, ylang ylang.

Flatulence

Angelica root, aniseed, black pepper, cardamom, caraway seed, German and Roman chamomile, dill seed, sweet fennel, ginger, mandarin, sweet marjoram, sweet orange, peppermint, spearmint.

Irritable Bowel Syndrome

Bergamot, German and Roman chamomile, geranium, lavender, peppermint.

Nausea and Vomiting

Black pepper, sweet fennel, ginger, peppermint, spearmint.

Periodontal disease

Sweet fennel, manuka, myrrh, peppermint, tea tree.

Reproductive and Endocrine System

Amenorrhoea

Carrot seed, clary sage, German and Roman chamomile, sweet fennel, geranium, juniper berry, sweet marjoram, myrrh, rose absolute or otto, yarrow.

Dysmenorrhoea

Clary sage, German and Roman chamomile, cypress, sweet fennel, geranium, jasmine, lavender, sweet marjoram, peppermint, rose absolute or otto, rosemary.

Endometriosis

Clary sage, Roman chamomile, cypress, sweet fennel, geranium, nutmeg, rose otto and rose absolute.

Menopause

Bergamot, German and Roman chamomile, clary sage, cypress, sweet fennel, geranium, jasmine absolute, juniper berry, lavender, neroli, rose absolute and otto, ylang ylang.

Pre-menstrual tension

Bergamot, German or Roman chamomile, carrot seed, clary sage, sweet fennel, evening primrose, geranium, juniper berry, lavender, sweet marjoram, neroli, rose absolute, rosemary, rose otto, ylang ylang.

Vaginal candidiasis

Bergamot, German chamomile, lavender, myrrh, petitgrain, tea tree.

Integumentary System

Acne

Bergamot, cajeput, German chamomile, geranium, grapefruit, lavender, lemon, lime, juniper berry, neroli, niaouli, palmarosa, petitgrain, rosemary, rosewood, *Santalum album, S. spicatum*, tea tree.

Boils and carbuncles

Bergamot, carrot seed, geranium, grapefruit, juniper berry, lavender, lemon, rosemary, tea tree.

Burns

Carrot seed, frankincense, lavender, everlasting, manuka, neroli, tea tree.

Cold sores

Bergamot, *Eucalyptus radiata*, tea tree.

Eczema and dermatitis

Bergamot, carrot seed, calendula-infused oil, Atlas and Virginian cedarwood, German and Roman chamomile, everlasting, juniper berry, lavender, myrrh, palmarosa, patchouli, *Santalum album, S. spicatum*, tea tree, yarrow, ylang ylang.

Herpes simplex

Bergamot, cajeput, geranium, lemon, melissa, niaouli, ravensara, rose otto, tea tree.

Pressure sores

Calendula-infused oil, German chamomile, geranium, frankincense, lavender.

Psoriasis

Bergamot, cajeput, calendula-infused oil, carrot seed, German or Roman chamomile, everlasting, lavender, juniper berry, *Santalum album, S. spicatum*, tea tree.

Pruritus

Calendula-infused oil, German or Roman chamomile, hypericum-infused oil, peppermint, lavender.

Scabies

Cinnamon bark, clove bud, lavender, lemon, peppermint.

Tinea

Myrrh, patchouli, tagetes, tea tree.

Wounds

Calendula-infused oil, German chamomile, hypericum-infused oil, lavender, lemon, myrrh, sage, tea tree, yarrow.

Lymphatic System

Accumulated toxins

Carrot seed, sweet fennel, geranium, grapefruit, juniper berry, lemon, cold-pressed lime, sweet orange, rosemary, tangerine.

Cellulite

Carrot seed, cypress, sweet fennel, ginger, grapefruit, geranium, lemon, cold-pressed lime, mandarin, juniper berry, sweet orange, rosemary, sage.

Lymphoedema

Carrot seed, sweet fennel, juniper berry, grapefruit, geranium.

Musculoskeletal System

Arthritis

Black pepper, cajeput, carrot seed, German chamomile, clove bud, ginger, spike lavender, lavender, juniper berry, sweet marjoram, nutmeg, pine, rosemary, thyme.

Bruises

Arnica-infused oil, black pepper, German chamomile, sweet fennel, geranium, hypericum-infused oil, hyssop, spike lavender, lemon, sweet marjoram, rosemary.

Backache

Arnica-infused oil, black pepper, cajeput, cinnamon bark, clove bud, German chamomile, eucalyptus, ginger, juniper berry, lavender, spike lavender, lemon, sweet marjoram, nutmeg, peppermint, pine, rosemary, thyme.

Bunions

German chamomile, lavender, lemon, sweet marjoram, peppermint, rosemary.

Bursitis

Cajeput, eucalyptus, ginger, juniper berry, rosemary.

Cramps

Black pepper, Roman chamomile, clary sage, cypress, geranium, lavender, sweet marjoram, thyme.

Gout

Carrot seed, juniper berry, lemon, pine, rosemary, thyme.

Muscular aches and pains

Cajeput, clove bud, eucalyptus, ginger, lavender, nutmeg, peppermint, rosemary, thyme.

Sciatica

Black pepper, cajeput, cinnamon bark, clove bud, German chamomile, eucalyptus, ginger, juniper berry, spike lavender, sweet marjoram, nutmeg, peppermint, rosemary, thyme.

Strains

Arnica-infused oil, black pepper, cajeput, cinnamon bark, clove bud, ginger, spike lavender, sweet marjoram, nutmeg, rosemary, thyme.

Sprains

Arnica-infused oil, black pepper, clove bud, German chamomile, ginger, juniper berry, spike lavender, lemongrass, sweet marjoram, nutmeg, peppermint, rosemary, thyme.

Nervous System

Anxiety

Basil, bergamot, Roman chamomile, Virginian cedarwood, cypress, frankincense, geranium, jasmine absolute, lavender, sweet marjoram, neroli, palmarosa, patchouli, rose, rosewood, vetiver, ylang ylang.

Depression

Basil, bergamot, Roman chamomile, cypress, frankincense, geranium, grapefruit, jasmine absolute, lavender, mandarin, may chang, sweet marjoram, melissa, neroli, sweet orange, rose absolute or otto, pine, peppermint, *Santalum album, S. spicatum*, tangerine, ylang ylang.

Epilepsy

Roman chamomile, lavender, sweet marjoram, neroli, melissa, ylang ylang.

Headaches and migraines

Cajeput, Roman chamomile, clary sage, eucalyptus, lavender, spike lavender, lemon, sweet marjoram, neroli, peppermint, rosemary, thyme.

Insomnia

Bergamot, Roman chamomile, lavender, lemon, sweet marjoram, neroli, petitgrain, sweet orange, *Santalum album, S. spicatum*, valerian.

Nervous exhaustion

Basil, cajeput, cardamom, cinnamon leaf or bark, clove bud, *Eucalyptus radiata, E. citriodora*, ginger, grapefruit, lemongrass, lemon, may chang, peppermint, pine, rosemary, spearmint, thyme, vetiver.

Stress

Basil, bergamot, Atlas and Virginian cedarwood, German and Roman chamomile, clary sage, frankincense, geranium, jasmine absolute, lavender, lemon, sweet marjoram, mandarin, may chang, melissa, neroli, sweet orange, patchouli, petitgrain, rose absolute and otto, rosemary, rosewood, *Santalum album, S. spicatum*, tangerine, vetiver, ylang ylang.

Respiratory System

Asthma

Aniseed, Atlas cedarwood, cajeput, clary sage, Roman chamomile, cypress, sweet fennel, frankincense, *Eucalyptus radiata, Hyssopus officinalis* var. *decumbens*, lemon, lavender, spike lavender, mandarin, sweet marjoram, myrtle, niaouli, peppermint, petitgrain, pine, rosemary, tea tree.

Bronchitis

Aniseed, basil, bay, cajeput, Atlas and Virginian cedarwood, *Eucalyptus radiata, E. dives*, everlasting, frankincense, hyssop, ginger, lavender, spike lavender, myrtle, niaouli, peppermint, pine, ravensara, rosemary, *Santalum album, S. spicatum*, tea tree, red thyme.

Catarrh

Aniseed, cajeput, Atlas and Virginian cedarwood, German chamomile, everlasting, *Eucalyptus radiata, E. dives,* sweet fennel, frankincense, ginger, *Hyssopus officinalis var. decumbens,* spike lavender, sweet marjoram, myrtle, peppermint, pine, ravensara, *Santalum album, S. spicatum*, tea tree, red thyme.

Colds and flus

Aniseed, cajeput, Atlas and Virginian cedarwood, cinnamon leaf or bark, *Eucalyptus radiata*, ginger, *Hyssopus officinalis* var. *decumbens,* lavender, spike lavender, lemon, sweet marjoram, manuka, peppermint, pine, ravensara, rosemary, tea tree, red thyme.

Coughs

Aniseed, cajeput, Atlas cedarwood, clary sage, cypress, *Eucalyptus radiata,* frankincense, ginger, hyssop, spike lavender, myrtle, pine, rosemary, thyme.

Hay fever

Cajeput, German chamomile, *Eucalyptus radiata,* lavender, spike lavender, myrtle, peppermint, petitgrain, pine, rosemary, red thyme, tea tree.

Sinusitis

Cajeput, *Eucalyptus radiata, E. dives, Hyssopus officinalis* var. *decumbens,* ginger, niaouli, myrtle, peppermint, pine, tea tree, thyme.

Skin Care

Cracked skin

Calendula-infused oil, myrrh, patchouli.

Dry skin

German and Roman chamomile, calendula-infused oil, carrot-infused oil, jasmine absolute, lavender, neroli, patchouli, palmarosa, rose absolute or otto, rosewood, *Santalum album, S. spicatum*, ylang ylang.

Insect repellent

Basil, Virginian cedarwood, citronella, clove bud, eucalyptus radiata, *Eucalyptus citriodora, E. dives,* geranium, spike lavender, lemon myrtle, peppermint, tea tree.

Mature skin

Carrot seed, fennel, frankincense, lavender, jasmine, mandarin, myrrh, neroli, palmarosa, patchouli, rose, rosewood, *Santalum album, S. spicatum.*

Nappy rash

Apricot kernel, avocado, calendula-infused oil, German chamomile, lavender, jojoba, sweet almond, wheatgerm.

Oily skin

Bay laurel, bergamot, cajeput, Virginian cedarwood, clary sage, cypress, *Eucalyptus dives,* geranium, lavender, lemon, juniper berry, mandarin, myrtle, niaouli, palmarosa, petitgrain, rosemary, *Santalum album, S. spicatum,* tea tree, ylang ylang

Perspiration, excessive

Cypress, petitgrain.

Scars and stretch marks

Frankincense, lavender, mandarin, neroli, palmarosa, rosewood, *Santalum album, S. spicatum,* tangerine.

Sensitive skin

Apricot kernel, calendula-infused oil, German and Roman chamomile, evening primrose oil, everlasting, jojoba, lavender, neroli, *Santalum album, S. spicatum.*

Sunburn

German chamomile, lavender, peppermint.

Immune System

Allergies

German and Roman chamomile, everlasting, lavender, yarrow.

Candida albicans

Bergamot, German chamomile, lavender, lemongrass, melissa, myrrh, myrtle, petitgrain, rosemary, tea tree.

Chronic fatigue syndrome

Basil, geranium, lavender, lemon, sweet orange, rosemary.

Fever

Cinnamon bark, eucalyptus, ginger, peppermint.

Inflammation

German chamomile, clove bud, cinnamon bark, everlasting, ginger, lavender, nutmeg, thyme, yarrow.

Urinary System

Cystitis

Bergamot, Atlas and Virginian cedarwood, German and Roman chamomile, juniper berry, lavender, *Santalum album, S. spicatum,* tea tree.

Appendix 4 ♦ **List of Essential Oils**

Common Name	Botanical Name	Part of Plant	Origin	Method of Extraction
Ajowan	*Trachyspermum copticum*	seeds	India	steam distillation
Ambrette seed	*Abelmoschus moschatus*	seeds	India	steam distillation
Amyris	*Amyris balsamifera*	wood & branches	Haiti	steam distillation
Angelica	*Angelica archangelica*	roots or seeds	Europe	steam distillation
Anise, Star	*Illicium verum*	seeds	China	steam distillation
Aniseed	*Pimpinella anisum*	seeds	Spain	steam distillation
Asafoetida	*Ferula asafoetida*	oleoresin from roots	Afganistan	steam distillation
Balsam, Fir	*Albies balsamea*	oleoresin	Canada	steam distillation
Balsam, Peru	*Myroxylon balsamum var. pereirae*	oleoresin	El Salvador	steam distillation
Basil (linalool)	*Ocimum basilicum*	leaves & flowering tops	France	steam distillation
Basil (methyl chavicol)	*Ocimum basilicum*	leaves & flowering tops	Comoros Island	steam distillation
Basil, Sweet	*Ocimum basilicum*	leaves & flowering tops	France	steam distillation
Bay, Laurel	*Laurus nobilis*	leaves	Morocco	steam distillation
Bay, West Indian	*Pimenta racemosa*	leaves	West Indies	steam distillation
Benzoin	*Styrax benzoin*	resin	South East Asia	solvent extraction
Bergamot	*Citrus bergamia*	fruit rind	Italy, Ivory Coast	expression
Birch	*Betula lenta*	bark	USA	steam distillation
Black pepper	*Piper nigrum*	dried peppercorns	Indonesia	steam distillation
Boldo leaf	*Peumus boldus*	leaves	Chile	steam distillation
Buchu	*Agothosma betulina*	dried leaves	South Africa	steam distillation
Cade	*Juniperus oxycedrus*	branches & heartwood	Europe	destructive distillation
Cajeput	*Melaleuca cajeputi*	leaves	Indonesia, Malaysia	steam distillation
Calamus	*Acorus calamus var. angustatus*	roots	India, Europe	steam distillation
Camphor	*Cinnamomum camphora*	wood, root stumps & branches	China	steam distillation
Cananga	*Cananga odorata*	flowers	Indonesia & Philippines	water distillation
Caraway	*Carum carvi*	seeds	Europe	steam distillation
Cardamom	*Elettaria cardamomum*	seeds	India	steam distillation
Carrot seed	*Daucus carota*	seeds	India, Europe	steam distillation
Cassia	*Cinnamomum cassia*	leaves, twigs or bark	China	steam distillation
Cassie absolute	*Acacia farnesiana*	flowers	France	solvent extraction
Cedarwood, Atlas	*Cedrus atlantica*	wood	Morocco	steam distillation
Cedarwood, Himalayan	*Cedrus deodora*	wood	Nepal	steam distillation
Cedarwood, Texas	*Juniperus ashei*	wood	USA	steam distillation
Cedarwood, Virginian	*Juniperus virginiana*	wood	USA	steam distillation
Celery seed	*Apium graveolens*	seed	Europe	steam distillation
Chamomile, German	*Matricaria chamomilla*	flowers	Europe	steam distillation
Chamomile, Maroc	*Ormenis multicaulis*	flowers	Morocco	steam distillation
Chamomile, Roman	*Anthemis nobilis*	flowers	Europe	steam distillation
Champa absolute	*Michelia champaca*	flowers	India	solvent extraction
Cinnamon	*Cinnamomum zeylanicum*	bark, leaf	Sri Lanka	steam distillation
Cistus	*Cistus ladaniferus*	resin, leaves & twigs	Mediterranean region	steam distillation
Citronella	*Cymbopogon winterianus*	leaves	Indonesia, Sri Lanka	steam distillation
Clary sage	*Salvia sclarea*	flowering tops	Europe, USA	steam distillation
Clove	*Eugenia caryophyllus*	dried flowers, leaves, stem	Indonesia, Madagascar	water distillation
Coriander	*Coriandrum sativum*	seed, leaf	Europe	steam distillation
Costus	*Saussurea costus*	dried roots	India	steam distillation
Cubeba	*Piper cubeba*	unripe berries	Indonesia	steam distillation
Cypress	*Cupressus sempervirens*	needles	Europe	steam distillation

Common Name	Botanical Name	Part of Plant	Origin	Method of Extration
Dill	*Anethum graveolens*	seed, herb	Europe	steam distillation
Elecampane	*Inula helenium*	dried roots	Europe	steam distillation
Elemi	*Canarium luzonicum*	resin	Indonesia, Philipines	steam distillation
Eucalyptus, Australiana	*Eucalyptus radiata*	leaves	Australia	steam distillation
Eucalyptus, Blue Mallee	*Eucalyptus polybractea*	leaves	Australia	steam distillation
Eucalyptus, Lemon	*Eucalyptus citriodora*	leaves	Australia	steam distillation
Eucalyptus, Peppermint	*Eucalyptus dives*	leaves	Australia	steam distillation
Everlasting	*Helichrysum angustifolium*	flowering tops	Mediterranean region	steam distillation
Fennel, Bitter	*Foeniculum vulgare var. amara*	seeds	Europe	steam distillation
Fennel, Sweet	*Foeniculum vulgare var. dulce*	seeds	Europe	steam distillation
Fir, Canadian	*Abies balsamifera*	needles & young twigs	Canada	steam distillation
Fir, Siberian	*Abies siberica*	needles & young twigs	Siberia	steam distillation
Fir, Silver	*Abies alba*	needles & young twigs	Europe	steam distillation
Frankincense	*Boswellia carteri*	resin	Somalia	steam distillation
Galangal	*Alpina officinarum*	roots	China	steam distillation
Galbanum	*Ferula galbaniflua*	resin	Middle East	steam distillation
Geranium	*Pelargonium graveolens*	leaves	Egypt, Reunion, China	steam distillation
Ginger	*Zingiber officinale*	roots	China, India	steam distillation
Grapefruit	*Citrus paradisi*	fruit rind	Australia, USA	expression
Guaiacwood	*Bulnesia sarmienti*	wood	South America	steam distillation
Hops	*Humulus lupulus*	dried cones	Europe	steam distillation
Horseradish	*Armoracia rusticana*	ground roots	Europe	steam or water distillation
Ho wood	*Cinnamomum camphora*	wood	China	steam distillation
Hyssop	*Hyssopus officinalis*	leaves & flowering tops	Europe	steam distillation
Jasmine absolute	*Jasminum officinalis*	flowers	India, Egypt	solvent extraction
Jonquil absolute	*Narcissus jonquilla*	flowers	France	solvent extraction
Juniper berry	*Juniperus communis*	berries	Serbia	steam distillation
Lavandin	*Lavandula intermedia*	flowering tops	France	steam distillation
Lavender	*Lavandula angustifolia*	flowering tops	France, Australia	steam distillation
Lavender, Spike	*Lavandula spica*	flowering tops	Europe	steam distillation
Lemon	*Citrus limon*	fruit rind	Australia, Italy	expression
Lemongrass	*Cymbopogon flexuosus*	leaves	Congo	steam distillation
Lemon myrtle	*Backhousia citriodora*	leaves	Australia	steam distillation
Lemon verbena	*Lippia citriodora*	leaves	France	steam distillation
Lime, Cold-pressed	*Citrus medica*	fruit rind	West Indies	expression
Lime, Distilled	*Citrus medica*	fruit	West Indies	steam distillation
Mandarin	*Citrus reticulata*	fruit rind	Australia, Italy, USA	expression
Manuka	*Leptospermum scoparium*	leaves	New Zealand	steam distillation
Mastic	*Pistacia lentiscus*	oleoresin	Mediterranean Region	steam distillation
Marjoram, Spanish	*Thymus mastichina*	leaves & flower tops	Spain	steam distillation
Marjoram, Sweet	*Marjorana hortensis*	leaves	Egypt, Europe	steam distillation
May chang	*Litsea cubeba*	leaves & berries	China	steam distillation
Melissa	*Melissa officinalis*	leaves	Europe	steam distillation
Mugwort	*Artemisia vulgaris*	leaves & flowering tops	Europe	steam distillation
Mustard	*Brassica nigra*	leaves & flowering tops	Europe	steam distillation
Myrrh	*Commiphora molmol*	resin	Somalia	steam distillation
Myrtle	*Myrtus communis*	leaves	Morocco, Europe	steam distillation
Neroli	*Citrus aurantium var. amara*	flowers	Morocco, France	steam distillation
Niaouli	*Melaleuca viridiflora*	leaves & twigs	Australia	steam distillation
Nutmeg	*Myristica fragrans*	seeds	Indonesia	steam distillation
Opopanax	*Commiphora erythraea*	oleogum resin	Middle East	steam or water distillation
Orange, Bitter	*Citrus aurantium var. amara*	fruit rind	West Indies, Italy	expression
Orange, Sweet	*Citrus sinensis*	fruit rind	USA, Australia, Italy	expression

Common Name	Botanical Name	Part of Plant	Origin	Method of Extraction
Oregano, Common	*Origanum vulgare*	leaves & flowering tops	Europe	steam distillation
Oregano, Spanish	*Thymus capitatus*	leaves & flowering tops	Spain	steam distillation
Palmarosa	*Cymbopogon martinii*	leaves	India, Indonesia	steam distillation
Parsley	*Petroselinum sativum*	leaf or seeds	Europe	steam distillation
Patchouli	*Pogostemon cablin*	leaves	Indonesia	steam distillation
Pennyroyal	*Mentha pulegium*	leaves	Europe, USA	steam distillation
Pepper, Black	*Piper nigrum*	seeds	Indonesia	steam distillation
Peppermint	*Mentha piperita*	leaves	USA, Australia	steam distillation
Peppermint, Japanese	*Mentha arvensis*	leaves	China	steam distillation
Petitgrain	*Citrus aurantium var. amara*	leaves	Paraguay, France	steam distillation
Pine, Dwarf	*Pinus mugo var. pumilio*	needles & twigs	Europe	steam distillation
Pine, Longleaf	*Pinus palustris*	wood chips	USA	steam distillation
Pine, Scotch	*Pinus sylvestris*	needles	Europe	steam distillation
Ravensara	*Ravensara aromatica*	leaves	Madagascar	steam distillation
Rose Cabbage	*Rosa centifolia*	flowers	Turkey, Morocco	solvent extraction or water distillation
Rose, Damask	*Rosa damascena*	flowers	Turkey, Morocco, France, Bulgaria	solvent extraction or water distillation
Rosemary (cineole)	*Rosmarinus officinalis*	leaves	Tunisia	steam distillation
Rosemary (camphor)	*Rosmarinus officinalis*	leaves	Spain	steam distillation
Rosemary (verbenone)	*Rosmarinus officinalis*	leaves	France	steam distillation
Rosewood	*Aniba rosaeodora*	wood	Brazil	steam distillation
Rue	*Ruta graveolens*	leaves	Europe	steam distillation
Sage, Common	*Salvia officinalis*	leaves	Europe	steam distillation
Sage, Spanish	*Salvia lavandulaefolia*	leaves	Spain	steam distillation
Sandalwood, Australian	*Santalum spicatum*	wood	Australia	steam distillation
Sandalwood, Indian	*Santalum album*	wood	India	steam distillation
Sandalwood, West Indian	*Amyris balsamifera*	wood	Haiti	steam distillation
Sassafras	*Sassafras albidum*	roots, bark	USA	steam distillation
Savin	*Juniperus sabina*	leaves & twigs	North America, Europe	steam distillation
Savory, Summer	*Satureja hortensis*	leaves	Europe	steam distillation
Savory, Winter	*Satureja montana*	leaves	Spain	steam distillation
Spearmint	*Mentha spicata*	leaves	USA	steam distillation
Spikenard	*Nardostachys jatamansi*	roots	India	steam distillation
Spruce	*Tsuga canadensis*	needles & twigs	USA	steam distillation
Tagetes	*Tagetes minuta*	flowers	South America	steam distillation
Tangerine	*Citrus reticulata blanco var. tangerine*	fruit rind	USA	expression
Tansy	*Tanacetum vulgare*	leaves & flowering top	Europe	steam distillation
Tarragon	*Artemisia dracunculus*	leaves	Europe	steam distillation
Tea tree	*Melaleuca alternifolia*	leaves	Australia	steam distillation
Tea tree, Lemon scented	*Leptospermum petersonii*	leaves	Australia	steam distillation
Thuja	*Thuja occidentalis*	leaves & twigs	North America	steam distillation
Thyme, Lemon	*Thymus serphyllum*	leaves	Spain	steam distillation
Thyme, Red	*Thymus vulgaris*	leaves	Europe	steam distillation
Tuberose absolute	*Polianthes tuberosa*	flowers	France	solvent extraction
Turmeric	*Curcuma longa*	roots	Indonesia	steam distillation
Turpentine	*Pinus ssp.*	oleoresin	USA	steam distillation
Valerian	*Valeriana officinalis*	roots	Europe, India	steam distillation
Verbena	*Lippia citriodora*	leaves	France	steam distillation
Vetiver	*Vetiveria zizanoides*	roots	Reunion, Indonesia	steam distillation
Violet leaf	*Viola odorata*	leaves	Europe	solvent extraction
Wintergreen	*Gaultheria procumbens*	leaves	North America	steam distillation
Wormseed	*Chenopodium ambrosioides*	whole herb	South America	steam distillation
Wormwood	*Artemisia absinthium*	leaves & flowering tops	Europe	steam distillation
Yarrow	*Achillea millefolium*	flowering top	Europe	steam distillation
Ylang ylang	*Cananga odorata*	flowers	Madagascar	steam distillation

Appendix 5 ♦ A Typical Material Safety Data Sheet

Material Safety Data Sheet According to Worksafe Australia

Date prepared: 20/11/02 Date issued: 20/05/03

STATEMENT OF HAZARDOUS NATURE: Not classified as hazardous according to criteria of Worksafe Australia

1. Company Details

[Name] ____________________

[Address] ____________________

[Telephone] ____________________

[Emergency contact] ____________________

2. Identification

Product name:	Geranium essential oil
INCI name:	Pelargonium graveolens leaf oil
CAS number:	8000-46-2
UN number:	N/A
Packing group:	N/A
Proper shipping name:	N/A
HAZCHEM code:	N/A
DG class:	N/A
Poisons schedule:	None allocated

3. Product Use

Therapeutic active in aromatherapy and perfumery raw material.

4. Physical Data

Appearance:	Pale yellow to green/olive/brown mobile liquid.
Odour:	Sweet, powerful, rosy, green-leaf odour with minty undertones.
Clarity:	Clear
Specific gravity:	0.884–0.892
Refractive index:	1.462–1.468
Flash point (closed cup):	64°C

5. Composition

The chemical composition of natural essential oils can vary. A typical chemical analysis by GC/MS for this oil is: linalool, citronellol, nerol, geraniol, citronellyl formate, geranyl formate, geranyl butyrate, geranyl tiglate, iso-menthone and guaia-6.9-diene.

6. Health Hazard Data

Acute-swallowed:	Full strength material may cause irritation to the mouth if swallowed. LD_{50} oral (rat): > 5g/Kg
Acute-eye:	Full strength material may be highly irritating to the eyes.
Acute-skin:	Full strength material in repeated or prolonged contact with skin may be irritating and cause allergic reaction in sensitive individuals. LD_{50} dermal: > 5g/Kg
Acute-inhaled:	Full strength material may cause irritation to the mucous membrane and upper airways.
Chronic:	This material is not listed as a carcinogen by NTB, IARC or OSHA.

7. First Aid

Swallowed:	Do not induce vomiting. Position to avoid aspiration should vomiting occur. Call a physician or Poisons Information Centre immediately. [In Australia] Poisons Information Centre Ph: 13 11 26
Eye contact:	Flush with copious amounts of water for 15 minutes. Seek medical attention if necessary.
Skin contact:	Remove contaminated clothing and wash affected area well with copious amounts of water and soap. If irritation occurs, seek medical advice.
Inhaled:	If discomfort is felt, remove person to a well-ventilated area with plenty of fresh air.

First aid facilities:	Eye wash and normal washroom facilities. Safety shower should be considered if large amounts are to be used.
Advice to doctor:	Treat symptomatically.

8. Precautions for Use

Exposure limits:	No exposure standards have been established for this material by Worksafe Australia. However, as a matter of course, avoid repeated or prolonged contact with the skin. Keep out of eyes. Do not ingest. Use with good ventilation.
Engineering controls:	Natural ventilation should be sufficient. However, where vapours or mists are generated, a grounded mechanical exhaust ventilation system is required.

9. Personal Protection

Respirator type:	Not usually required.
Eye protection:	Use splash-proof safety glasses and face shield where splashing is possible.
Glove type:	Use impervious rubber gloves to avoid repeated or prolonged skin contact.
Clothing:	Depending on conditions in the workplace, additional body protection should be considered.
Flammability:	N/A

10. Safe Handling and Storage

Storage:	Store in a tight container in a cool, well-ventilated place protected from light and away from sources of ignition.
Conditions to avoid:	Sparks, flame and heat.
Materials to avoid:	Strong oxidising agents and strong acids.
Safety data:	May be skin/eye irritant.
Spills and leaks:	Eliminate sources of ignition. Increase ventilation. Evacuate all unnecessary personnel. Wipe small spills with cloth. Absorb larger spills with vermiculite, sand, sawdust or similar porous material. Use clean, non-sparking tools to collect the material and place into a suitable, labelled container. If large quantities of this material enter the waterways, contact the Environmental Protection Authority, or your local waste management authority.
Disposal:	Disposal of this material should be undertaken by a licensed waste disposal contractor.

11. Fire and Explosion Hazard Information

Hazardous combustion products:	When heated to decomposition, produces acrid smoke and fumes.
Extinguishing media:	Carbon Dioxide (CO_2), Foam, Dry Chemical Powder.
Fire fighting precautions:	Wear self-contained breathing apparatus (SCBA) and full protective clothing to minimise skin exposure.

12. Other Information

Toxicology:	Found to be non-sensitising, non-irritating and non-phototoxic to human skin: see Opdyke D.L.J. *Food Cosmet. Toxicol.* (1975) 13, 451 & *FCT* (1976) 14, 781.
Biodegradability:	Data not available.
Environmental protection:	Prevent this material from entering waterways, drains or sewers.
Safety statement:	S 26 In case of contact with eyes, rinse immediately with water and seek medical advice. S 2 Keep out of reach of children. S 36 Wear suitable protective clothing.

13. Contact Point

Contact:	The Quality Assurance Manager Mon–Fri (8.00am–5.00pm) [Telephone and Fax]
Emergency contact (24 hours):	Poisons Information Centre [in Australia] Ph: 13 11 26

Disclaimer: The information contained in this Material Safety Data Sheet has been compiled from data considered to be accurate. This data is believed to be reliable, however it must be noted that due to the nature of the product, values for certain properties can vary depending upon the source of the material.

The [company] disclaims any liability for any injury or loss arising from the use of this information or the materials described. It is the responsibility of the user to determine the appropriate precautions for safe handling based on their application.

Appendix 6 ♦ Summary of Cautions and Contra-indications

Contra-indications of essential oils used in aromatherapy are likely to create debate. The following list should be used as a guide to the safe use of essential oils.

Essential oils that are not commercially available have not been listed in this appendix.

Never Use

The following essential oils are considered to be hazardous and have a very high oral and dermal toxicity. They should never be used.

Almond bitter (unrectified), basil ct methyl chavicol, birch (sweet), boldo leaf, buchu (*B. crenulata*), cade (unrectified), camphor (brown and yellow), cassia, cinnamon bark, costus, elecampane, fig leaf, horseradish, *Melaleuca bracteata*, mustard, mugwort, pennyroyal, rue, sage (Dalmatian), sassafras, tansy, tarragon, tea absolute, thuja, verbena, wintergreen, wormseed, wormwood.[1]

Never Use on Hypersensitive, Diseased or Damaged Skin

Tisserand and Balacs state that the following essential oils should not be used on hypersensitive, damaged or diseased skin such as in (normal) infants, or in eczema, dermatitis or psoriasis:

Garlic, oakmoss absolute, treemoss absolute, verbena absolute.[1]

Use with Caution on Hypersensitive, Diseased or Damaged Skin

Tisserand and Balacs state that the following essential oils should be used with caution because they can be irritating and sensitising on hypersensitive, damaged or diseased skin, such as in (normal) infants, or in eczema, dermatitis or psoriasis:

Ajowan, anise, cade (rectified), citronella, clove bud, clove leaf, clove stem, lemon scented eucalyptus, lemon myrtle, laurel, lemongrass, may chang, melissa, onion, oregano, perilla, savory, star anise, thyme.[1]

Do Not Use Orally

The following essential oils should not be taken orally:

Annual wormwood, basil, fennel, ho leaf (camphor/safrole ct), hyssop, Indian dill, lavender cotton, mace, East Indian nutmeg, parsley leaf, parsley seed.[1]

Do Not Use at all on Mucous Membrane

These essential oils may irritate the skin when used in baths or massage. Do not use at all on anyone who is known to have sensitive skin, or who is susceptible to skin reactions:

Basil (all varieties), cinnamon leaf, sweet fennel, fir needle, lemongrass, lemon, lemon verbena, melissa, bitter orange, peppermint, red and wild thyme.[1]

Use with Caution on Mucous Membrane

Tisserand and Balacs recommend that the following essential oils not be used at more than 1% on mucous membrane (inhalation, rectal or vaginal administration):

Ajowan, cade (rectified), clove leaf, clove stem, oregano, pimento leaf, savory, thyme.[1]

Tisserand and Balacs recommend that the following essential oils not be used at more than 3% on mucous membrane (inhalation, rectal or vaginal administration):

West Indian bay, betel leaf, caraway, cinnamon leaf, clove bud, cornmint, laurel, *Ocimum gratissimum*, peppermint, pimento berry, spearmint.[1]

Anticoagulants — Caution Only

Tisserand and Balacs recommend that the following essential oils should not be used internally by any individual who takes aspirin, heparin or warfarin:

West Indian bay, betel leaf, cinnamon leaf, clove bud, clove stem, clove leaf, garlic, *Ocimum gratissimum*, onion, pimento berry, pimento leaf.[1]

Epilepsy

Tisserand and Balacs say that the following essential oils should be used with caution by persons with epilepsy:

Camphor (white), lavandin, *Lavandula stoechas*, lavender cotton, peppermint, rosemary, rue, sage (Dalmatian), sage (Spanish), spike lavender, yarrow (camphor ct).[1]

These essential oils may stimulate an epileptic seizure in people who have epilepsy.

Davis recommends that the following essential oils showed not to be used by people with epilepsy:

Fennel (sweet), hyssop, rosemary, sage, wormwood.[2]

Fever

The following essential oils should never be used by anyone suffering from a fever:

Wormwood, camphor (white), ho leaf (camphor/safrole ct), hyssop, lavender cotton.[1]

Tisserand and Balacs also suggest that the following essential oils are contra-indicated orally by anyone with a fever:

Wormwood, camphor (white), hyssop, lavandin, *Lavandula stoechas*, spike lavender, rosemary, Spanish sage, yarrow (camphor ct).[1]

High Blood Pressure

Davis recommends that the following essential oils should not be used by anyone suffering from high blood pressure:

Hyssop, rosemary, sage.[2]

Liver Disease — Caution Only

Indian dill, parsley leaf, parsley seed.[1]

Kidney Disease — Caution Only

Indian dill, parsley leaf, parsley seed.[1]

Photosensitisation

If the following oils have been used topically do not expose the skin to sunlight or sunbed rays for 12 hours:

Angelica root, bergamot, cumin, grapefruit, lemon, cold-pressed lime, opopanax, bitter orange, rue, tagetes.[1]

Pregnancy

Tisserand and Balacs recommend that essential oils in the 'never use' section as well as those listed below should not be used throughout pregnancy:

Camphor (white), ho leaf, (camphor/safrole ct), hyssop, Indian dill, parsley leaf, parsley seed, Spanish sage, savin.[1]

Tisserand and Balacs recommend that the following essential oils should be used with caution throughout pregnancy:

Wormwood, *Lavandula stoechas*, lavender cotton, oakmoss absolute, rue, treemoss absolute.[1]

Davis recommends that the following essential oils should not be during pregnancy:

Basil, birch, Atlas cedarwood, clary sage, cypress, hyssop, jasmine, juniper berry, sweet marjoram, myrrh, peppermint, rosemary, tarragon, thyme.[2]

References

1. Tisserand R, Balacs T. *Essential oil safety.* Churchill Livingstone, UK, 1995.
2. Davis P. *Aromatherapy: An A–Z.* 2nd ed., The C.W. Daniel Company Limited, Great Britain, 1999.

Appendix 7 ♦ Acupressure

Introduction

Several different kinds of acupressure techniques are currently practised, although the same pressure points are used for all of them. Varying rhythms, pressure and techniques create different styles of acupressure. Shiatsu, for example, a form of acupressure originating from Japan, can be quire vigorous, with firm pressure applied at each point for only 3 to 5 seconds. Other styles of acupressure gently hold the points for a minute or more. Pressing with intermittent, fast beat is stimulating, while light pressure creates a sedating effect on the body.

How Acupressure Works

The acupressure points are junctions along special pathways called meridians, which carry the life force known as Qi. In Traditional Chinese Medicine tension and pain are caused when the Qi does not flow freely through the meridians. Acupressure will promote the free flow of Qi, thus relieving tension and pain.

Western scientists have found that when these points are stimulated by pressure or needles, endorphins — neurotransmitters that relieve pain — are released.

How to Apply Pressure

A general guideline to follow is that the pressure should be firm enough so that it 'hurts good', in other words, something between pleasant, firm pressure and outright pain. The more developed the muscles are, the more pressure can be applied. If the client is sensitive to the pressure, gradually decrease the pressure until balance is found.

Apply firm pressure on the specified point at 90° to the surface of the skin. If the skin is being pulled then the angle of the pressure is not correct.

How to Find a Point

Acupressure points are located by referring to anatomical landmarks. The correct anatomical location along with a brief description of the features and indications of each acupressure point used in this book are provided in this appendix.

A *cun* is often used as a unit of measurement. One cun is equivalent to the breadth of the client's thumb.

Acupressure Techniques

The following techniques are commonly used:

- Firm pressure is the most fundamental technique, using thumbs, fingers, palms, the side of the hand, or knuckles to apply steady, stationary pressure. To relax the area or relieve pain, apply pressure gradually and hold without any movement for several minutes.
- Slow motion kneading uses the thumbs and fingers along with the heels of the hands to squeeze large muscle groups firmly. The motion is similar to that of kneading a large mass of dough. This relieves general stiffness, shoulder and neck tension, constipation and spasms in the calf muscles.
- Brisk rubbing back and forth with the thumb, finger or palm uses friction to stimulate the blood and lymph, as well as to benefit the nerves and tone of the skin.
- Quick tapping with the finger tips stimulates muscles on unprotected, tender areas of the body such as the face. For larger areas of the body such as the back or buttocks, use a loose fist. This can improve the stimulation of energy flow and improve muscle tone.

Do not be tempted to rub or massage the entire area, unless specifically mentioned to do so. It is best to hold the point steadily with direct pressure.

The Acupressure Points

The acupressure points referred to in this book are described in detail as follows:

Bladder 2: Zan Zhu — Holding the Bamboo

Location — On the medial extremity of the eyebrow, or on the supraorbital notch.

Features — Disperses wind, calms the liver, stops pain.

Indications — Headaches, blurred vision, swelling and pain of the eyes, twitching eyelids.

Bladder 23: Shen Shu — Shu of the Kidneys

Location — 1.5 cun lateral to the inferior border of the spinous process of the 2nd lumbar vertebra.

Features — Regulates and strengthens the kidneys.

Indications — Menstrual pain, lumbar pain, weakness of the knees.

Bladder 36: Cheng Fu — Receive Support

Location — On the posterior aspect of the thigh, at the mid point of the transverse crease below the buttocks.

Features — Pain in the lower back and legs, ain in the genitals.

Indications — Lower back pain, sciatica, paralysis of lower extremities, constipation.

Bladder 40: Wei Zhong — Perfect Equilibrium

Location — At the midpoint of the popliteal crease, exactly between the tendons of the biceps femoris and semitendinosus.

Features — Earth point, clears heat from the blood.

Indications — Acute back pain and pain in the back of the legs.

Bladder 54: Zhi Bian — Order's Edge

Location — 3 cun from the median line of the back, level with the 4th posterior sacral foramen.

Indications — Pain in the lumbar sacral region, pain in the lower extremities, sciatica, diseases of the reproductive system.

Conception Vessel 6: Qi Hai — Sea of Energy

Location — On the midline of the abdomen, 1.5 cun below the umbilicus.

Features — Regulates Qi circulation and dispels damp.

Indications — Major tonification point for the whole body, abdominal pain, diarrhoea, constipation, oedema.

Gall Bladder 20: Feng Qi — Wind Pond

Location — In the depression which lies between the sternocleidomastoidus and the upper border of the trapezius, on a level with the mastoid process and just below the edge of the occipital.

Features — Soothes the liver and pacifies yang. Eliminates wind and expels heat.

Indications — Major point for wind problems of the head — internal and external, headaches, dizziness, pain and stiffness of the neck, pain in the shoulder and back, common cold.

Gall Bladder 30: Huan Tiao — Encircling Leap

Location — At the junction of the middle and lateral third of the distance between the greater trochanter and the hiatus of the sacrum.

Features — Benefits the lower back and legs, clears the channels.

Indications — Pain in the lower back and hip region, muscular atrophy, ain and weakness of the lower extremities.

Heart 7: Shen Men — Spirit Door

Location — On the wrist crease at the proximal border of the pisiform bone, in the depression at the radial side of the flexor ulnaris.

Features — Major point for the Shen.

Indications — Psychological disorders and insomnia.

Kidney 27: Shu Fu — Yu of the Palace

Location — In the depression on the border of the clavicle, 2 cun lateral to the midline.

Indications — cough, asthma, bronchitis, chest pain.

Large Intestine 4: He Gu — Joining of the Valleys

Location — On the dorsum of the hand in the middle of the 2nd metacarpal on the lateral side. At the highest point of the muscle when the thumb and index finger are held close together.

Features — Special point for wind-heat. Relieves external conditions. Major point for all problems of the head and face.

Indications — Headaches, redness and swelling of the eyes, toothache, sore throat, facial paralysis, abdominal pain, constipation.

Liver 2: Xing Jian — Active Interval

Location — Between the 1st and 2nd toe, proximal to the margin of the web.

Features — Eliminates fire and soothes the liver. Removes stagnant Qi and clears the lower heater.

Indications — Menorrhagia, headache, convulsions, insomnia.

Liver 3: Tai Chong — Supreme Assault

Location — In the depression distal to the junction of the 1st and 2nd metatarsals, just anterior to the articulation with the 1st and 2nd ciniforms.

Features — Soothes the liver and gall bladder. Calming and sedating function.

Indications — headache, insomnia.

Liver 4: Zhong Feng — Middle Sea

Location — 1 cun anterior to the medial malleolus in the depression medial to the tibialis anterior tendon.

Features — Regulates the function and eliminates congestion of the liver.

Indications — Hernia.

Liver 11: Yin Lian — Yin Passage

Location — In the inguinal groove, on the lateral border of the abductor longus.

Indications — Irregular menstruation, pain in the thigh and leg.

Lung 1: Zhong Fu — Central Palace

Location — Below the clavicle in the first intercostal space and 2 cun lateral to the nipple.

Features — First surface point of Qi circulation through the meridians.

Indications — Coughs, asthma, pain in the chest, shoulder and back.

Lung 1: Zhong Fu — Central Residence

Location — Approximately 1 cun below the lateral end of the clavicle in the lateral art of the first intercostal space.

Indications — Coughing and wheezing, throat blockage, congested nose, excessive sweating.

Lung 2: Yun Men — Cloud's Door

Location — At the inferior margin of the clavicle, between the pectoralis major and the deltoid muscles.

Indications — Cough, asthma, painful.

Pericardium 6: Nei Gaun — Inner Gate

Location — 2 cun above the transverse wrist crease of the wrist, between the tendons of the palmaris longus and flexor carpi radialis.

Features — Balances yin and yang.

Indications — Palpitations, gastric pain, vomiting, mental disorders, febrile diseases.

Spleen 4: Gong Sun — Grandfather and Grandson

Location — In the depression distal and inferior to the base of the 1st metatarsal bone, at the junction of the red and white skin.

Features — Harmonises the function of the stomach and spleen.

Indications — Eases intestinal pain, diarrhoea, dysentery.

Stomach 3: Ju Liao — Large Bone

Location — On a line with the centre of the pupil when looking straight ahead and level with the lower edge of the ala nasi, on the lateral side of the nasolabial groove.

Indications — Facial paralysis, twitching of the eyelids, toothache, rhinitis, trigeminal neuralgia.

Stomach 16: Ying Chuang — Breast Window

Location — In the 3rd intercostal space, on the mamillary line.

Indications — Cough, asthma, fullness and pain in the chest, bronchitis, neuralgia.

Stomach 36: Zu San Li — Three Mile Leg

Location — Place centre of palm over the centre of the patella, fingers slightly parted, the point is under the tip of the index finger.

Features — Harmonises the functions of the stomach and spleen. Eliminates wind and damp in the body.

Indications — Important tonic point, gastric pain, vomiting, abdominal distension, indigestion and all digestive disorders.

Tai Yang

Location — In the depression about 1 cun posterior to the midpoint between the lateral end of the eyebrow and the outer canthus.

Features — Disperses wind in the head, cools and clears the eyes.

Indications — Headache, swelling and pain of the eyes.

References

Gach M. *Acupressure's potent points.* Bantam Books, USA, 1990.

Rogers C. *Point location manual.* Acupuncture Colleges (Australia), 1981.

Foreign Languages Press. *Essentials of Chinese Acupuncture.* China, 1980.

O'Conner J, Bensky D. eds, *Acupuncture — A comprehensive text.* Shanghai College of Traditional Medicine. Eastland Press, USA, 1985.

Appendix 8 ♦ Useful Addresses

The contact details for the organisations listed below are correct at the time of publication.

Aromatherapy Courses

For a list of schools in your area offering professional practitioner training, please contact one of the associations listed below.

Associations

Australia

International Federation of Aromatherapists (Australian Branch) — IFA
PO Box 786
Templestowe Vic.
Australia 3106
Tel: +61 3 9850 9254
or 1902 240 125
Fax: +61 3 9850 5730
Email: info@ifa.org.au
Website: www.ifa.org.au

Australian Aromatic Medicine Association — AAMA
100 Dight Street
Collingwood Vic.
Australia 3066
Tel: 0500 800 579
(Int. +61 500 800 579)
Fax: 0500 800 679
(Int. +61 500 800 679)
Email: enquiries@aama-oz.org
Website: www.aama-oz.org

New Zealand

New Zealand Register of Holistic Aromatherapists — NZROHA
PO Box 18–399
Glen Innes, Auckland
New Zealand
Tel: 575 6636

USA

The National Association for Holistic Aromatherapy — NAHA
4509 Interlake Avenue N., #233
Seattle WA 98103-6773
USA
Tel: (206) 256 0741
Email: info@naha.org
Website: www.naha.org

Canada

International Aromatherapists and Tutors Association — IATA
268 Lakeshore Road East, Suite 226
Oakville ON L6J 7S4
Canada
Tel: 905 822 9603
Fax: 905 822 0856
Email: info@aroma-iata.com
Website: www.aroma-iata.com

Canadian Federation of Aromatherapists
843479 Oxford Rd. 84, R.R.#3
Lakeside, Ontario N0M 2G0
Canada
Tel: 519 475 9038
Email: officemanager@cfacanada.com
Website: www.cfacanada.com

UK

International Federation of Aromatherapists — IFA
182 Chiswick High Road
London W4 1PP
United Kingdom
Tel: +44 20 8742 2605
Email: office@ifaroma.org
Website: www.ifaroma.org

International Federation of Professional Aromatherapists — IFPA
82 Ashby Road
Hinckley
Leicestershire LE10 1SN
United Kingdom
Tel: +44 14 5563 7987
Email: admin@ifparoma.org
Website: www.ifparoma.org

Aromatherapy and Allied Practitioners' Association — AAPA
8 George Street
Croydon CRO 1PA
United Kingdom
Tel/Fax: +44 20 8653 9152
Email: aromatherapyUK@aol.com
Website: www.aromatherapyuk.net

Essential Oil Suppliers

To ensure that you are buying the best quality essential oils available choose a supplier that meets the criteria for quality control specified in this book. Refer to *Chapter 5*.

Essential Oil Research Database

An extensive essential oil research database and essential oil analysis database is available from:
Essential Oil Resource Consultants
'Au village', 83840 La Martre
Provence, France
Tel/Fax: +33 494 84 29 93
Email: mailto:essentialorc@aol.com
Website: http://www.essentialorc.com

Aromatherapy Journals

Aromatherapy Today

Aromatherapy Today is a journal for the professional aromatherapist. It is published quarterly. For more details contact:
Aromatherapy Today
PO Box 211
Kellyville NSW
Australia 2155
Tel: +61 2 9894 9933
Fax: +61 2 9894 0199
Website: www.aromatherapytoday.com

The International Journal of Aromatherapy

The International Journal of Aromatherapy is a peer reviewed journal for the professional aromatherapist. For more details contact:
Elsevier
32 Jamestown Road
London NW1 7BY
United Kingdom
Tel: +31 20 485 3757
Website: www.elsevierhealth.com/journals/ijar

Botanical Index

General Index

Notes

Notes

Notes

Notes

Notes

Notes

Notes